VIDEO CONTENTS

DIAGNOSTIC AND SURGICAL ARTHROSCOPY IN THE HORSE

DIAGNOSTIC AND SURGICAL ARTHROSCOPY IN THE HORSE

FOURTH EDITION

C. Wayne McIlwraith, BVSc, PhD, DSc, Dr med vet (h.c. Vienna), DSc (h.c. Massey), Laurea Dr (h.c. Turin), D vet med (h.c. London), FRCVS, Diplomate ACVS, ECVS & ACVSMR

University Distinguished Professor
Barbara Cox Anthony University Chair in Orthopaedics
Director, Orthopaedic Research Center
Colorado State University
Fort Collins, Colorado

Alan J. Nixon, BVSc, MS, Diplomate ACVS

Professor of Large Animal Surgery
Director, Comparative Orthopaedics Laboratory
College of Veterinary Medicine
Cornell University
Ithaca, New York
Chief Medical Officer, Cornell Ruffian Equine Specialists
Elmont, New York

Ian M. Wright, MA, VetMB, DEO, Diplomate ECVS, MRCVS

Senior Surgeon and Director of Clinical Services
Newmarket Equine Hospital
Newmarket, Suffolk, UK

DIAGNOSTIC AND SURGICAL ARTHROSCOPY IN THE HORSE   ISBN: 978-0-7234-3693-5
Copyright © 2015, 2005, 1984 by Mosby, an imprint of Elsevier Limited.
Reprinted 2014 (twice)

Copyright © 1990 by Lea & Febiger.

Notices

Knowledge and best practice in this field are constantly changing. As new research and experience broaden our understanding, changes in research methods, professional practices, or medical treatment may become necessary.

Practitioners and researchers must always rely on their own experience and knowledge in evaluating and using any information, methods, compounds, or experiments described herein. In using such information or methods they should be mindful of their own safety and the safety of others, including parties for whom they have a professional responsibility.

With respect to any drug of pharmaceutical products identified, readers are advised to check the most current information provided (i) on procedures featured or (ii) by the manufacturer of each product to be administered, to verify the recommended dose or formula, the method and duration of administration, and contraindications. It is the responsibility of the practitioner, relying on his or her own experience and knowledge of the patient, to make diagnoses, to determine dosages and the best treatment for each individual patient, and to take all appropriate safety precautions.

To the fullest extent of the law, neither the Publisher nor the authors, contributors, or editors, assume any liability for any injury and/or damage to persons or property as a matter of products liability, negligence or otherwise, or from any use or operation of any methods, products, instructions, or ideas contained in the material herein.

Library of Congress Cataloging-in-Publication Data

McIlwraith, C. Wayne, author.
   Diagnostic and surgical arthroscopy in the horse / C. Wayne McIlwraith,
Alan J. Nixon, Ian M. Wright. -- Fourth edition.
     p. ; cm.
   Preceded by Diagnostic and surgical arthroscopy in the horse / C. Wayne
McIlwraith ... [et al.] ; illustrations, Tom McCracken. 3rd ed. 2005.
   Includes bibliographical references and index.
   ISBN 978-0-7234-3693-5 (hardcover : alk. paper)
   I. Nixon, Alan J., author. II. Wright, Ian M., author. III. Title.
   [DNLM: 1. Horse Diseases--diagnosis. 2. Joint Diseases--veterinary. 3. Arthroscopy--veterinary.
4. Horses--surgery. 5. Joints--surgery. SF 959.J64]
   SF959.J64
   636.1'0897472059--dc23
                                          2014001016

Vice President and Publisher: Linda Duncan
Content Strategy Director: Penny Rudolph
Associate Content Development Specialist: Katie Starke
Publishing Services Manager: Jeffrey Patterson
Project Manager: William Drone
Designer: Jessica Williams

The publisher's policy is to use paper manufactured from sustainable forests

your source for books, journals and multimedia in the health sciences

www.elsevierhealth.com

Printed in China

Last digit is the print number: 9   8   7   6   5   4   3

Working together to grow libraries in developing countries

www.elsevier.com • www.bookaid.org

To our veterinary colleagues whose case referrals, encouragement,
and interest have continued to support advances in equine arthroscopy,
and to the horse owners whose open-mindedness, faith,
and perseverance have made this a reality.

Preface to Fourth Edition

It has been another nine years since the third edition of this text was published and it is now out of print. In that time, there has been continued evolution and development of specific arthroscopic surgery techniques, which are now included. While the more simple procedures have remained unchanged, many of these techniques have been better documented with improved levels of evidence. The latter is critical if equine veterinarians are to provide current recommendations to clients; while updating the technical aspects of arthroscopic surgery is important for surgeons, surgical residents and others in training.

In this edition, extensive descriptions of procedures, as well as updating of literature with studies supporting their value, have been made. There has been a considerable updating of the illustrations, and for the first time, we have added videos of the important procedures. We have also added a new chapter on postoperative management, adjunctive therapies, and rehabilitation procedures because of increased and improved information on options in these areas. Because we teach advanced arthroscopic surgery courses together in our three locations of work, there has been extensive exchange of information that hopefully provides a balanced consensus.

PREFACE

Preface to Third Edition

It has been 13 years since the second edition of this text was published, and it has long been out of print. In that time, arthroscopy has achieved further widespread use, and there have been many developments. The lapse of 13 years has not been due to any lack of interest on the part of clinicians interested in or actually doing arthroscopic surgery in the horse. Rather it has been an issue of publisher mergers and the economic realities of veterinary texts. The request from Elsevier Limited for me to consider having the third edition with them was gratefully received and accepted. In the third edition, we have attempted to provide information needed by all equine veterinarians giving recommendations to their clients, while at the same time preserving the technical teaching required of surgeons practicing arthroscopy, as well as surgical residents and others in training. There has been considerable progress in arthroscopic surgery in the horse since the publication of the second edition. I have been fortunate to be able to add as authors three individuals who have made significant contributions to the advancement of arthroscopic surgery: namely, Alan Nixon, Ian Wright, and Josef Boening. The format of the book is to retain the core chapters that were in the second edition, with considerable updating of all these chapters to include new information, both from the authors' personal experiences, other colleagues' advice and experience, and that available in the literature. We have then added separate chapters on diagnostic and surgical arthroscopy of the elbow joint, coxofemoral (hip) joint, proximal and distal interphalangeal joints, tenoscopic surgery, bursoscopy, arthroscopic management of synovial sepsis, arthroscopy of the temporomandibular joint, as well as separate chapters on problems and complications of diagnostic and surgical arthroscopy and arthroscopic methods for cartilage resurfacing. I am particularly grateful to Drs. Nixon and Wright for their extensive contributions to the new chapters and their review and additions to the revised chapters from the second edition, and to Dr. Boening for contributions to the interphalangeal and temporomandibular joint chapters. As in previous editions, the presentation of these techniques is augmented greatly by the excellent artwork of Tom McCracken. I am also indebted to staff at the Gail Holmes Equine Orthopaedic Research Center and Veterinary Teaching Hospital, Colorado State University, as well as Equine Medical Center, California for patience and help in acquisition of case material, and Geri Baker for her typing. The book would not have been possible without the initial efforts of Jonathon Gregory, Commissioning Editor, Elsevier Limited and the follow-up work by Zoë Youd and Joyce Rodenhuis of Elsevier.

ACKNOWLEDGMENTS

We each have individual acknowledgments to make.

C. Wayne McIlwraith is indebted to the staff at the Gail Holmes Equine Orthopaedic Research Center and Veterinary Teaching Hospital at Colorado State University, to the Equine Medical Center, California for patients and help in acquisition of case material, and to Lynsey Bosch for typing.

Alan Nixon would like to thank the Cornell University surgical operating room staff and radiology technicians, at both the Ithaca campus and the Cornell Ruffian Equine Specialists practice in New York City, and to acknowledge Amy Ingham for administrative assistance and manuscript preparation. Additionally, he would like to extend his sincere gratitude to the many surgical residents that provided diligent assistance in surgery and postoperative care, and to his surgical colleagues in consulting practices for their expert assistance.

Ian Wright would like to thank past and present members of the staff at Newmarket Equine Hospital, whose diagnostic excellence and dedicated clinical care permitted progression of the discipline and consequent improvements in patients' prognoses. In this respect, particular mention is due to Gaynor Minshall, Matt Smith, and both past and present interns. I am also indebted to Louise Harbidge and Lucy Coleman, who typed numerous drafts and coordinated communication while juggling management of the hospital office.

The book would not have been possible without the initial efforts of Penny Rudolph with Elsevier and Katie Starke with Elsevier, who took over before submission of manuscript and has been a great help in carrying this project to fruition.

C. Wayne McIlwraith, Fort Collins, Colorado

Alan J. Nixon, Ithaca, New York

Ian M. Wright, Newmarket, UK

CONTENTS

CHAPTER 1

Introduction

ARTHROSCOPIC SURGERY IN THE HORSE—ADVANCES SINCE 2005

Since 2005 magnetic resonance imaging (MRI) has become an important diagnostic technique in equine orthopedics. More specific diagnosis of conditions of soft tissues has led to further indications for diagnostic and surgical arthroscopy. There are limitations, however, and it has been demonstrated recently that the use of MRI for precise grading of the articular cartilage in human osteoarthritis (OA) is limited and that diagnostic arthroscopy remains the gold standard for grading cartilage damage, for a definitive diagnosis, and for decisions regarding therapeutic options in patients with OA (von Engelhardt et al, 2012).

Numerous publications have documented the use of electrosurgery, radiofrequency, and lasers within equine arthroscopic surgery. Clinical use of electrosurgery in the metacarpophalangeal and metatarsophalangeal joints for removal of fragments from the plantar margin of the proximal phalanx and proximal sesamoid bones (Bouré et al, 1999; Simon et al, 2004) desmotomy of the accessory ligament of the superficial digital flexor tendon (David et al, 2011) have been described. Thermal chondroplasty with radiofrequency energy (RFE) has been used frequently in humans and produces attractive visual effects, but multiple studies now suggest detrimental effects of RFE on articular cartilage (Cook et al, 2004; Lu et al, 2000, 2002) and in another study RFE was shown to exceed the damage obtained with mechanical debridement (Edwards et al, 2008). The use of radiofrequency probes for section and resection of soft tissues within joints, tendon sheaths, and bursae have also been described and may have a place in selected equine procedures (David et al, 2011; McCoy and Goodrich, 2011).

The use of intraarticular local analgesic agents to reduce the requirement for systemic anesthetic or analgesic agents, or both, has emerged. Evidence to support preoperative intraarticular administration of a combination of opiate and local anesthetic techniques have been provided in man (Hube et al, 2009), but opinions vary (Kalso et al, 2002; Rosseland, 2005). Toxicity of bupivacaine to bovine articular chondrocytes has been demonstrated (Chu et al, 2006), and in a second study bupivacaine, lidocaine or robivacaine were shown to have detrimental effects on chondrocyte viability in a dose- and duration-dependent manner (Lo et al, 2009). Using preoperative epidural morphine and detomidine has been reported to benefit horses undergoing experimental bilateral stifle arthroscopy (Goodrich et al, 2002).

In the carpus, arthroscopic approaches to the palmar aspect of the equine carpus have been detailed (Cheetham and Nixon, 2006), and comparison of magnetic resonance contrast arthrography and the arthroscopic anatomy of the equine palmar lateral outpouching of the middle carpal joint has also been described (Getman et al, 2007). Arthroscopically guided internal fixation of chip fractures of the carpal bones, which are of sufficient size and infrastructure, has been reported by Wright and Smith (2011). This technique can decrease morbidity associated with leaving large articular defects following removal.

New information in the metacarpophalangeal and metatarsophalangeal joints has included quantification of the amount of the articular surfaces of the metacarpal and metatarsal condyles that could be visualized with distal dorsal and distal palmar/plantar portals (Vanderperren et al, 2009). Declercq et al (2009) reported on fragmentation of the dorsal margin of the proximal phalanx in young Warmblood horses in which the majority underwent surgery for prophylactic reasons or to remove radiologic blemishes, or both. Osteochondral fragments within the dorsal plica have also been reported in Warmblood horses (Declercq et al, 2008). Impact fractures of the proximal phalanx in a filly have been described by Cullimore et al (2009) and the authors of this text have also seen similar lesions in the distal metacarpus.

In the palmar fetlock Byron and Goetz (2007) reported use of a 70-degree arthroscope to debride a subchondral bone defect in the distal palmar medial condyle of a third metacarpal bone; successful access to such lesions is generally limited. Schnabel et al (2006 and 2007) reported the results of arthroscopic removal of apical sesamoid fracture fragments in Thoroughbred racehorses with a higher success rate in horses that had raced previously. These authors also showed that removal when younger than 2 years of age gave comparable racing success to maternal siblings (Schnabel et al, 2007). Kamm et al (2011) evaluated the influence of size and geometry of apical sesamoid fragments following arthroscopic removal in Thoroughbreds and found no relationship to racing performance. Because 30% of the branches of insertion of the suspensory ligaments are subsynovial in the metacarpophalangeal/metatarsophalangeal joints, tears involving their dorsal surfaces can result in articular deficits and extrusion of disrupted ligament fibers into the synovial cavity; it has now been documented that such cases can be successfully treated with arthroscopic debridement (Minshall and Wright, 2006).

Further information has been recently published on fractures of the metacarpal and metatarsal condyles (Wright and Nixon, 2013; Jacklin and Wright, 2013) emphasizing the importance of articular congruity to outcome. Arthroscopically guided repair of midbody proximal sesamoid bone fractures was described, and results were reported by Busschers et al (2008), representing a substantial advance in the management of uniaxial fractures.

Recent developments in stifle arthroscopy have included publication of new and modified techniques, correlation of imaging modalities, and attempts to refine prognostic guidelines. In the femoropatellar joint, an arthroscopic approach has been described for the equine suprapatellar pouch (Vinardell et al, 2008). The use of a 10-mm diameter laproscopic cannula in the suprapatellar pouch for easier removal of debris and loose fragments has also been reported (McNally et al, 2011). Ultrasound has been noted to be a useful adjunct with femoropatellar osteochondritis dissecans (OCD) when there is high clinical suspicion but equivocal radiographic findings (Bourzac et al, 2009). A new concept of augmented healing of OCD defects has been introduced by Sparks et al (2011b), who used polydioxanone pins to reattach separated osteochondral flaps. In the femorotibial joints, arthroscopic approaches into the caudal medial and lateral compartments have been described by Watts and Nixon (2006) and a detailed comparison between ultrasonographic and arthroscopic boundaries of the normal equine femorotibial joints has been reported by Barrett et al (2012). The potential for false-positive ultrasonographic diagnoses of meniscal tears was highlighted by

Cohen et al (2009). Alternative techniques for treatment of subchondral cystic lesions (SCLs) of the medial femoral condyle (MFC) have been described since 2005, including injection of triamcinolone acetonide into the fibrous tissue of SCLs under arthroscopic guidance (Wallis et al, 2008) and chondrocytes or mesenchymal stem cells in fibrin glue implantation (Ortved et al, 2012). The classification of osteochondral lesions of the MFC initially reported by Walmsley et al (2003) using the Outerbridge human grading system has been developed further by Cohen et al (2009). A recent study of soft tissue injuries of the femorotibial joint treated with intraarticular autologous bone marrow–derived mesenchymal stem cells showed that a high percentage of horses were able to go back to work after meniscal injury (Ferris et al, 2013). Lastly, clinical symptoms, treatment, and outcome of meniscal cysts in horses were described for the first time recently (Sparks et al, 2011a).

In the tarsus four cases of SCL of the lateral trochlear ridge of the talus were treated successfully with intralesional injection of triamcinolone acetonide, simulating the protocol of Wallis et al (2008) on the MFC (Montgomery and Juzwiak, 2009). A severe SCL on the proximal medial trochlear ridge of the talus was treated with osteochondral mosaicplasty in one report (Janicek et al, 2010). Since 2005 there have been two descriptions of arthroscopic treatment of fractures of the lateral malleolus of the tibia (O'Neill and Bladon, 2010; Smith and Wright, 2011). Pure soft tissue lesions, including tears of the joint capsule and avulsions of the collateral ligaments of the tarsocrural joint, have been recently described (Barker et al, 2013).

Considerable advances have been made in tenoscopic surgery. In the digital flexor tendon sheath there have been further publications of tenoscopic identification and treatment of longitudinal tears of the digital flexor tendons and manica flexoria by Smith and Wright (2006) and Arensberg et al (2011). Although coblation has been reported as a technique for debridement and smoothing of the fibrillated edges of defects, it was found to have a negative impact on outcome (Arensberg et al, 2011). Primary desmitis of the palmar/plantar annular ligament has been more clearly defined (McGhee et al, 2005; Owen et al, 2008), and McCoy and Goodrich (2011) have described the use of a radiofrequency probe for tenoscopically guided desmotomy using the same approach as the free-handed hook knife technique.

In the carpal sheath a recent paper by Wright and Minshall (2012a) provided further morphologic information and results of treatment of osteochondromas. Tenoscopic evaluation of horses with tenosynovitis of the carpal sheath has also led to new diagnoses, including tearing of the radial head of the deep digital flexor tendon (DDFT) (Minshall and Wright, 2012b). This information, in turn, has permitted development of confident ultrasonographic diagnosis. Caldwell and Waguespack (2011) reported a tenoscopic approach for desmotomy of the accessory ligament of the DDFT in horses, illustrating use of synovial cavities for minimally invasive approaches to perithecal structures. Desmotomy of the accessory ligament of the superficial digital flexor tendon (proximal check ligament) using a monopolar electrosurgical technique has also been reported (David et al, 2011). Synoviocoeles associated with the tarsal sheath have been described by Minshall and Wright (2012a).

Finally, there have been developments with bursoscopy as well. Wright and Minshall (2012b) described intrathecal tearing of the tendinous portions of the calcaneal insertions of the SDF and disruption of its fibrocartilagenous cap, associated with lameness and tendon instability, respectively. Endoscopic surgery in the bicipital bursa was used to treat complete rupture of the lateral lobe of the biceps brachi tendon in one horse (Spadari et al, 2009) and to treat an SCL involving the bursal margins of the humerus in another (Arnold et al, 2008).

Details of a transthecal approach to the navicular bursa (reported briefly in the third edition) have been provided by Smith et al (2007) and Smith and Wright (2012). This is now considered the standard approach for the evaluation of treatment of aseptic bursae, particularly when tearing of the dorsal surface of the DDFT has been identified by MRI or as a clinical differential. Haupt and Caron (2010) compared direct and transthecal approaches to the navicular bursa.

Specific advantages of arthroscopy as a diagnostic and surgical tool are mentioned throughout this book. General advantages of the technique previously recognized include the following:

1. An individual synovial cavity can be examined through a small (stab) incision and with greater accuracy than was previously possible. With the availability of such an atraumatic technique, numerous lesions and "new" conditions that have not previously been identified by noninvasive imaging modalities can be recognized.
2. All types of surgical manipulations can be performed under arthroscopic guidance. The use of this form of surgery is less traumatic and less painful, and it provides immense cosmetic and functional advantages. Surgery is now possible in situations where previously the risks (morbidity)-benefits comparison would have precluded intervention. The decreased convalescence time with earlier return to work and improved performance is a significant advance in the management of equine joint and other synovial problems. The need for palliative therapies is decreased, as is the number of permanently compromised joints.

The initial optimism and advantages of arthroscopy suggested in the first three editions of this book have been substantiated. Arthroscopy has revolutionized equine orthopedics and continues to push forward pathobiological understanding, diagnostic accuracy and lesion-specific treatment. Problems have and will continue to be encountered, but now we know that many are avoidable. Although the technique appears uncomplicated and attractive to the inexperienced surgeon, some natural dexterity, good three-dimensional anatomic knowledge, and considerable practice are required for the technique to be performed well. Experience and good case selection are of paramount importance, and reiterating a passage from the first edition of this book remains as pertinent today:

In 1975, arthroscopy was underused and needless arthrotomies were performed. The pendulum is now swinging rapidly in the other direction. The current tendency in arthroscopy is toward overuse. Some surgeons seem to be unable to distinguish between patients who are good candidates for arthroscopy and those who are not, and the trend is toward arthroscopy in patients in whom little likelihood exists of finding any treatable disorder.

(Casscells 1984).

Three years later, another author stated:

… of those 9000 North American surgeons and the other surgeons of the world performing arthroscopy, many are ill-prepared and are therefore, not treating their patients fairly. Overuse and abuse by a few is hurting the many surgeons who are contributing to orthopedic surgery by lowering patients' morbidity, decreasing the cost of health care, shortening the necessary time of patients returning to gainful employment, and adding to the development of a skill that has made a profound change in the surgical care of the musculoskeletal system.

(McGinty 1987).

Arthroscopy remains the most sensitive and specific diagnostic modality for intrasynovial evaluation in the horse. This is somewhat in contrast to human orthopedics, where arthroscopy is predominately used for surgical interference and much of its diagnostic function has or is being replaced by MRI and computed tomography. Arthroscopy continues to be of great benefit in the horse, with increased recognition of soft tissue lesions in joints, tendons, sheaths, and bursae. However, as stated earlier, although there are many benefits, it is, and will remain, technically demanding with a continued need for training at multiple levels.

REFERENCES

Arensberg L, Wilderjans H, Simon O, Dewulf J, Boussauw B: Non-septic tenosynovitis of the digital flexor tendon sheath caused by longitudinal tears in the digital flexor tendons: a retrospective study of 135 tenoscopic procedures, *Equine Vet J* 43:660–668, 2011.

Arnold CE, Chaffin MK, Honnas CM, Walker MA, Heite WK: Diagnosis and surgical management of a subchondral bone cyst within the intermediate tubercle of the humerus in a horse, *Equine Vet Educ* 20:310–315, 2008.

Barker WJH, Smith MRW, Minshall GJ, Wright IM: Soft tissue injuries of the tarsocrural joint: a retrospective analysis of 30 cases evaluated arthroscopically, *Equine Vet J* 45:435–441, 2013.

Barrett MF, Frisbie DD, McIlwraith CW, Werpy NM: The arthroscopic and ultrasonographic boundaries of the equine femorotibial joints, *Equine Vet J* 44:57–63, 2012.

Bouré L, Marcoux M, Laverty S, et al.: Use of electrocautery probes in arthroscopic removal of apical sesamoid fracture fragments in 18 Standardbred horses, *Vet Surg* 28:226–232, 1999.

Bourzac C, Alexander K, Rossier Y, Laverty S: Comparison of radiography and ultrasonography for the diagnosis of osteochondritis dissecans in the equine femoropatellar joint, *Equine Vet J* 41:686–692, 2009.

Busschers E, Richardson DW, Hogan PM, et al.: Surgical repair of mid-body proximal sesamoid bone fractures in 25 horses, *Vet Surg* 37:771–780, 2008.

Byron CR, Goetz TE: Arthroscopic debridement of a palmar third metacarpal condyle subchondral bone injury in Standardbred, *Equine Vet Educ* 19:344–347, 2007.

Caldwell FJ, Waguespack RW: Evaluation of a tenoscopic approach for desmotomy of the accessory ligament of the deep digital flexor tendon in horses, *Vet Surg* 40:266–271, 2011.

Casscells SW: *Arthroscopy: diagnostic and surgical practice*, Philadelphia, 1984, Lea & Febiger.

Cheetham J, Nixon AJ: Arthroscopic approaches to the palmar aspect of the equine carpus, *Vet Surg* 35:227–231, 2006.

Chu CR, Izzo NJ, Papas NE, et al.: In vitro exposure to 0.5% bupivacaine is cytotoxic to bovine articular chondrocytes, *Arthroscopy* 22:693–699, 2006.

Cohen JM, Richardson DW, McKnight AL, Ross MW, Boston RC: Long-term outcome in 44 horses with stifle lameness after arthroscopic exploration and debridement, *Vet Surg* 38:543–551, 2009.

Cook JL, Marberry KM, Kuroki K, et al.: Assessment of cellular, biomechanical, and histological effects of bipolar radiofrequency treatment of canine articular cartilage, *Am J Vet Rec* 65:604–609, 2004.

Cullimore AM, Finnie JW, Marmion WJ, Booth TM: Severe lameness associated with an impact fracture of the proximal phalanx in a filly, *Equine Vet Educ* 21:247–251, 2009.

David F, Laverty S, Marcoux M, Szoke M, Celeste C: Electrosurgical tenoscopic desmotomy of the accessory ligament of the superficial digital flexor muscle (proximal check ligament) in horses, *Vet Surg* 40:46–53, 2011.

Declercq J, Martens A, Bogaert L, et al.: Osteochondral fragmentation in the synovial pad of the fetlock in Warmblood horses, *Vet Surg* 37:613–618, 2008.

Declercq J, Martens A, Maes D, et al.: Dorsoproximal phalanx osteochondral fragmentation in 117 Warmblood horses, *Vet Comp Orthop Traumatol* 22:1–6, 2009.

Edwards RB, Lu Y, Cole BJ, et al.: Comparison of radiofrequency treatment and mechanical debridement of fibrillated cartilage in an equine model, *Vet Comp Orthop Traumatol* 21:41–48, 2008.

Ferris DJ, Frisbie DD, Kisiday JD, et al.: Clinical follow-up of thirty three horses treated for stifle injury with bone marrow derived mesenchymal stem cells intra-articularly, *Vet Surg*, 2013.

Getman LM, McKnight AL, Richardson DW: Comparison of magnetic resonance contrast arthrography and arthroscopic anatomy of the equine palmar lateral outpouching of the middle carpal joint, *Vet Radiol Ultrasound* 48:493–500, 2007.

Goodrich LR, Nixon AJ, Fubini SL, et al.: Epidural morphine and detomidine decreases postoperative hindlimb lameness in horses after bilateral stifle arthroscopy, *Vet Surg* 31:232–239, 2002.

Haupt JL, Caron JP: Navicular bursoscopy in the horse: a comparative study, *Vet Surg* 39:742–747, 2010.

Hube R, Tröger M, Rickerl F, Muench EO, von Eisenhart-Rothe R, Hein W, Mayr HO: Pre-emptive intra-articular administration of local anaesthetics/opiates versus postoperative local anaesthetics/opiates or local anaesthetics in arthroscopic surgery of the knee joint: a prospective randomized trial, *Arch Orthop Trauma Surg* 129:343–348, 2009.

Jacklin B, Wright IM: Frequency distributions of 174 fractures of the distal condyles of the third metacarpal and metatarsal bones in 167 Thoroughbred racehorses (1999-2009), *Equine Vet J* 44:707–713, 2013.

Janicek JC, Cook JL, Wilson DA, Ketzner KM: Multiple osteochondral autografts for treatment of a medial trochlear ridge subchondral cystic lesion in the equine tarsus, *Vet Surg* 39:95–100, 2010.

Kalso E, Smith L, McQuay HJ, et al.: No pain, no gain: clinical excellence and scientific rigour – lessons learned from IA morphine, *Pain* 98:269–275, 2002.

Kamm JL, Bramlage LR, Schnabel LV, Ruggles AJ, Embertson RM, Hopper SA: Size and geometry of apical sesamoid fracture fragments as a determinant of prognosis in Thoroughbred racehorses, *Equine Vet J* 43:412–417, 2011.

Lo IKY, Sciore P, Chung M, et al.: Local anesthetics induce chondrocyte death in bovine articular cartilage discs in a dose- and duration-dependent manner, *Arthroscopy* 25:707–715, 2009.

Lu Y, Hayashi K, Hecht P, et al.: The effect of monopolar radiofrequency energy on partial thickness defects of articular cartilage, *Arthroscopy* 16(5):27–536, 2000.

Lu Y, Edwards RB, Nho S, et al.: Thermal chondroplasty with bipolar and monopolar radiofrequency energy: effect of treatment time on chondrocyte death and surface contouring, *Arthroscopy* 18:779–788, 2002.

McCoy AM, Goodrich LR: Use of radiofrequency probe for tenoscopic-guided annular ligament desmotomy, *Equine Vet J* 44:412–415, 2012.

McGhee JD, White NA, Goodrich LR: Primary desmitis of the palmar and plantar annular ligaments in horses: 25 cases (1990-2003), *J Am Vet Med Assoc* 226:83–86, 2005.

McGinty JB: Arthroscopy: a technique or a subspecialty? *Arthroscopy* 3:292–296, 1987.

McNally TP, Slone DE, Lynch TM, Hughs FE: Use of a suprapatellar pouch portal and laparoscopic cannula for removal of debris or loose fragments following arthroscopy of the femoropatellar joint on 168 horses (245 joints), *Vet Surg* 40:886–890, 2011.

Minshall GJ, Wright IM: Arthroscopic diagnosis and treatment of intra-articular insertional injuries of the suspensory ligament branches in 18 horses, *Equine Vet J* 38:10–14, 2006.

Montgomery LJ, Juzwiak JS: Subchondral cyst-like lesions in the talus in four horses, *Equine Vet Educ* 21:629–647, 2009.

O'Neill HD, Bladon BM: Arthroscopic removal of fractures of the lateral malleolus of the tibia in the tarsocrural joint: a retrospective study of 13 cases, *Equine Vet J* 42:558–562, 2010.

Ortved KF, Nixon AJ, Mohammed HO, Fortier LA: Treatment of subchondral cystic lesions in the medial femoral condyle of mature horses with growth factor enhanced chondrocyte grafts: a retrospective study of 49 cases, *Equine Vet J* 44:606–613, 2012.

Owen KR, Dyson SJ, Parkin TDH, Singer ER, Krisoffersen M, Mair TS: Retrospective study of palmar/plantar annular ligament injury in 71 horses: 2001-2006, *Equine Vet J* 40:237–244, 2008.

Rosseland LA: No evidence for analgesic effect of intra-articular morphine after knee arthroscopy: a qualitative systemic review, *Regional Anesthesia and Pain Medicine* 30:83–98, 2005.

Schnabel LV, Bramlage LR, Mohammed HO, et al.: Racing performance after arthroscopic removal of apical sesamoid fracture fragments in Thouroughbred horses age greater or equal than two years: 84 cases (1989-2002), *Equine Vet J* 38:446–451, 2006.

Schnabel LV, Bramlage LR, Mohammed HO, et al.: Racing performance after arthroscopic removal of apical sesamoid fracture fragments in Thoroughbred horses age less than two years: 151 cases (1989-2002), *Equine Vet J* 39:64–68, 2007.

Simon O, Laverty S, Bouré L, et al.: Arthroscopic removal of axial osteochondral fragments of the proximoplantar aspect of the proximal phalanx using electrocautery probes in 23 Standardbred racehorses, *Vet Surg* 33:422–427, 2004.

Smith MRW, Wright IM: Non-infected tenosynovitis of the digital flexor tendon sheath: a retrospective analysis of 76 cases, *Equine Vet J* 38:134–141, 2006.

Smith RMW, Wright IM: Arthroscopic treatment of fractures of the lateral malleolus of the tibia: 26 cases, *Equine Vet J* 43:280–287, 2011.

Smith MRW, Wright IM: Endoscopic evaluation of the navicular bursa; observations, treatment and outcome in 93 cases with identified pathology, *Equine Vet J* 44:339–345, 2012.

Smith MRW, Wright IM, Smith RKW: Endoscopic assessment and treatment of lesions of the deep digital flexor tendon in the navicular bursae of 20 lame horses, *Equine Vet J* 39:18–24, 2007.

Spadari A, Spinella G, Romagnoli N, Valentini S: Rupture of the lateral lobe of the biceps brachii tendon in an Arabian horse, *Vet Comp Orthop Traumatol* 22:253–255, 2009.

Sparks HD, Nixon AJ, Boening KJ, Pool RR: Arthroscopic treatment of meniscal cysts in the horse, *Equine Vet J* 43:669–675, 2011a.

Sparks HD, Nixon AJ, Fortier LA, Mohammed HO: Arthroscopic reattachment of osteochondritis dissecans cartilage flaps of the femoropatellar joint: long-term results, *Equine Vet J* 43:650–659, 2011b.

Vanderperren K, Martens A, Haers H, et al.: Arthroscopic visualization of the third metacarpal and metatarsal condyles in the horse, *Equine Vet J* 41:526–533, 2009.

Vinardell T, Florent D, Morisset S: Arthroscopic surgical approach in intra-articular anatomy of the equine suprapatellar pouch, *Vet Surg* 37:350–356, 2008.

von Engelhardt LV, Lahner M, Klussmann A, Bouillon B, David A, Haage P, Lichtinger TK: Arthroscopy vs. MRI for a detailed assessment of cartilage disease in osteoarthritis: diagnostic value of MRI in clinical practice, *BMC Musculoskeletal Disorders* 11:75–83, 2012.

Wallis TW, Goodrich LR, McIlwraith CW, Frisbie DD, Hendrickson DA, Trotter GW, Baxter GM, Kawcak CE: Arthroscopic injection of corticosteroids into the fibrous tissue of subchondral cystic lesions of the medial femoral condyle in horses: a retrospective study of 52 cases (2001-2006), *Equine Vet J* 40:461–467, 2008.

Walmsley JP, Philips TJ, Townsend HGG: Meniscal tears in horses: an evaluation of clinical signs and arthroscopic treatment of 80 cases, *Equine Vet J* 35:402–406, 2003.

Watts AE, Nixon AJ: Comparison of arthroscopic approaches and accessible anatomic structures during arthroscopy of the caudal pouches of equine femorotibial joints, *Vet Surg* 35:219–226, 2006.

Wright IM, Minshall GJ: Clinical, radiological and ultrasonographic features, treatment and outcome in 22 horses with caudal distal radial osteochondromata, *Equine Vet J* 44:319–324, 2012a.

Wright IM, Minshall GJ: Injuries of the calcaneal insertions of the superficial digital flexor tendon in 19 horses, *Equine Vet J* 44:136–142, 2012b.

Wright IM, Nixon AJ: Fractures of the condyles of the third metacarpal and metatarsal bones. In Nixon AJ, editor: *Equine Fracture Repair*, ed 2, Blackwell, 2013, Hoboken, NJ.

Wright IM, Smith MRW: The use of small (2.7 mm) screws for arthroscopically guided repair of carpal chip fractures, *Equine Vet J* 43:270–279, 2011.

CHAPTER 2

Instrumentation

A large selection of instrumentation is available for human arthroscopic surgery, but much of it is unsuitable and unnecessary for routine equine arthroscopy. Many of the operating instruments are expensive, fragile, and manufactured for a specific task in a specific joint. For equine use a limited amount of equipment is generally essential and appropriate. From a practical standpoint, numerous versions of hand instruments that perform similar tasks add to the clutter on the surgery table and to the expense of cleaning and resterilizing. The descriptions and recommendations in this text are based on the authors' experiences and personal choices, and numerous substitutions can be made. Obviously, the potential for variation is extreme, and it is necessary to continue to evaluate new instrumentation as it becomes available or as new arthroscopic procedures are developed. This chapter represents the authors' current views on instrumentation.

ARTHROSCOPES

The available arthroscopes vary in outer diameter, working length, and in lens angle, which may be straight (0 degrees) or angled from 5 to 110 degrees. Many manufacturers market 4-mm diameter arthroscopes with 0-, 30-, or 70-degree lens angles and working lengths of 160 to 175 mm. The field of view is often 115 degrees or more, leading to their classification as "wide-field-of-view" arthroscopes. Most manufacturers produce small arthroscopes, usually 2.7-mm diameter arthroscopes with 30- or 70-degree lens angles; a short 2.7-mm diameter arthroscope with 30- or 70-degree lens angles; and a 1.9-mm diameter arthroscope with a 30-degree lens angle. Generally, surgeons should choose the largest-diameter arthroscope that can safely be inserted and maneuvered without causing damage. Small-diameter arthroscopes with appropriate operating instrumentation have been developed for use in human carpal, metatarsophalangeal, and temporomandibular joints (Poehling, 1988). However, these are fragile, allow less illumination, and provide a much smaller field of view (90 degrees for a 2.7-mm scope and 75 degrees for a 1.9-mm scope). Small-diameter arthroscopes usually also have a shorter working length (50 to 60 mm) because the excessive flexibility of a longer instrument increases the risk of breakage (Poehling, 1988). More recently, a complete range of sizes has also become available in video arthroscopes, which are coupled directly to the video camera. This obviates the need for a coupler and eliminates the potential for fogging between the arthroscope eyepiece and camera (Jackson & Ovadia, 1985). Flexible arthroscopes have also had a period of limited use but generally failed to provide true flexibility and optical clarity (Takahashi & Yamamoto, 1997). Combined approaches, using a rigid arthroscope for most of the procedure and a flexible arthroscope to access difficult areas of the hip, ankle, or knee in people, have added to the more thorough evaluation of these joints (Takahashi & Yamamoto, 1997). Similarly, a small-diameter flexible arthroscope inserted through an 18-gauge needle (see Chapter 7) has been successfully used in standing stifle diagnostic arthroscopy for several years (Frisbie et al, 2013).

A 4-mm diameter arthroscope with a 25- or 30-degree lens angle fulfills most needs of the equine surgeon (Fig. 2-1). A 4-mm, 70-degree arthroscope can occasionally provide improved visualization of specific areas of some joints such as the tarsocrural, shoulder, and palmar/plantar aspect of the metacarpo/tarsophalangeal joints. However, none of the authors now use a 70-degree arthroscope routinely and believe additional portals generally replace the need for a 70-degree scope. Figure 2-2 illustrates the different fields of view of a 25-degree arthroscope and a 70-degree arthroscope in the same position in a tarsocrural joint. Popular choices in an arthroscope for routine equine arthroscopy include the 30-degree videoarthroscope and direct-view arthroscopes from Smith & Nephew—Dyonics[a] (Fig. 2-3), the 30-degree Hopkins® II rod lens telescope made by Karl Storz,[b] and the 30-degree direct view and videoarthroscopes made by Stryker.[c] Comparable-sized arthroscopes are also available from Linvatec,[d] Richard Wolf,[e] Zimmer,[f] Olympus[g] (True-View II), Arthrex,[h] and other companies. The advantages of the 25- to 30-degree angled lens are that (1) it provides an increased field of vision; (2) rotating the arthroscope increases the visual field without moving the arthroscope; and (3) the end of the arthroscope can be placed at some distance from the lesions, allowing easier access to the area with instruments and minimizing the risk of damaging the arthroscope.

All arthroscopes are used within a protective stainless steel cannula, which is also commonly referred to as a *sleeve* or *sheath* (Fig. 2-4). For a 4-mm arthroscope the cannula has a 5- or 6-mm diameter and is connected to the arthroscope through a self-locking system that varies among manufacturers. The cannula has one or two stopcocks for ingress or egress fluid systems, or both. The second stopcock is useful if the surgeon uses gas and fluid distention interchangeably during arthroscopy; otherwise, a cannula with one stopcock offers greater freedom of movement. A rotating stopcock is critical to allow the ingress fluid line to be positioned away from the limb or instruments, or both, as required. The space between the cannula and arthroscope allows flow of ingress fluid. Some cannulas have a wider diameter (5.8 to 6.0 mm compared with 4.5 to 5.0 mm) and have several holes adjacent to the open end. These so-called "high-flow" sheaths are useful in some large-joint applications in the horse.

A conical obturator is used for insertion of the cannula in almost all situations. In joints with a thick fibrous capsule this necessitates puncture of the joint using a stab incision with a No. 11 or 15 scalpel blade. In joints with a thin fibrous capsule, the conical obturator can be used to penetrate the capsule. Separate sharp trocars for insertion and blunt obturators for intrasynovial positioning before placement of the

---

[a]Smith & Nephew—Dyonics, 150 Minuteman Road, Andover, MA 01810. Tel: (978) 749-1000. www.smith-nephew.com

[b]Karl Storz Veterinary Endoscopy, 175 Cremona Drive, Goleta, CA 93117. Tel: (800) 955-7832. www.ksvea.com

[c]Stryker, 5900 Optical Court, San Jose, CA 95138. Tel: (800) 624-4422. www.stryker.com/en-us/

[d]Linvatec-Conmed Co, 11355 Concept Blvd., Largo, FL 33773. Tel: (800) 237-0169. www.conmed.com

[e]Richard Wolf, 353 Corporate Woods Parkway, Vernon Hills, IL 60061. Tel: (800) 323-1488. www.richardwolfusa.com

[f]Zimmer, PO Box 708, 1800 West Center St., Warsaw, IN 46581. Tel: (800) 348-2759. www.zimmer.com

[g]Olympus America Inc., 3500 Corporate Parkwaycenter Valley, PA 18034. Tel: (800) 848-9024. www.olympusamerica.com

[h]Arthrex, Inc. 1370 Creekside Blvd, Naples, FL 34108. Tel: (800) 933-7001. www.arthrex.com

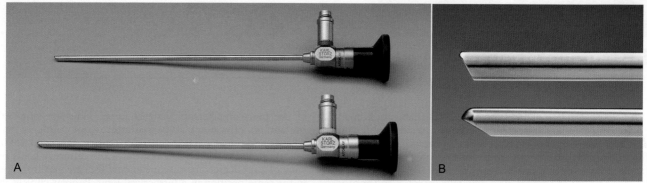

Figure 2-1 Standard arthroscope types. **A,** Panoview arthroscopes (Karl Storz Veterinary Endoscopy): 4-mm outside diameter 30 degrees (above) and 70 degrees (below). **B,** Close-up view of angled lens.

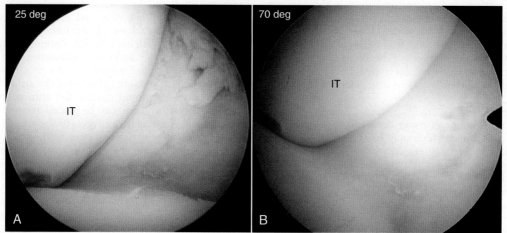

Figure 2-2 Effect of 70-degree arthroscope. Views with **A,** a 25-degree arthroscope and **B,** a 70-degree arthroscope of the same area of the tarsocrural joint with the tip of the arthroscopes in the same position. *IT,* Intermediate ridge of tibia.

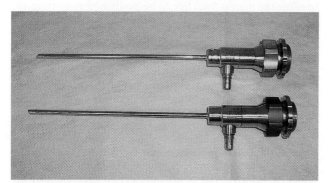

Figure 2-3 Videoarthroscopes (4 mm, 30 degrees Smith & Nephew—Dyonics), which couple directly to the video camera, eliminate fogging, and maintain optical clarity. The regular forward oblique viewing arthroscopes (top) is also available in a tenoscopy version (bottom), with the field of view angled toward the light post to facilitate annular ligament transection and other procedures where the light cable tends to interfere with the limb.

arthroscope in the cannula are now largely redundant. Illumination to the arthroscope is provided by a fiberoptic light cable from a light source. The cable should be a minimum of 10 and preferably 12 feet (3 to 3.5 meters) long to provide adequate working length across the horse. Connections between light sources and cables are unique to each manufacturer, but adapters are available so that cables can be fitted to different light sources.

Light Sources

With the increasing use of extremely light-sensitive video cameras, most small fiberoptic light generators will suffice for routine arthroscopy. Figure 2-5 depicts a small, portable 175-W LED light projector made by Karl Storz that is inexpensive, has a long bulb life, and is satisfactory for most arthroscopic examinations. Photographs can be taken with these light sources using video printers; however, careful control of the white balance of the arthroscope control system is necessary to avoid yellow and brown tint. A high-intensity light source (usually with xenon bulbs) is useful to produce high-quality photographs or video for publication. A light source with a flash unit is largely obsolete due to the advent of photographic and video capture systems that have replaced still photography.

Continuous high-intensity light is useful for videotape and digital video capture. The sources may be high-intensity tungsten illumination, xenon arc lamps (100 to 500 W), or mercury vapor lamps (McGinty, 1984). The xenon light source is still considered premier; however, the replacement bulbs are expensive ($400 to $500). The authors use a Karl Storz Xenon Nova cold light fountain with 175- or 300-W lamp (Fig. 2-6), Stryker X8000 300W xenon source, Stryker L9000 LED light source (Fig. 2-7), and an Arthrex Synergy combination LED light source/camera control. The xenon bulbs last from 350 to 500 hours, which represents a recurring cost for busy practices. Recently introduced LED sources have bulb life of up to 17,000 hours, which is a major improvement.

Light sources that automatically adjust the light intensity are useful to minimize the need for manual adjustment

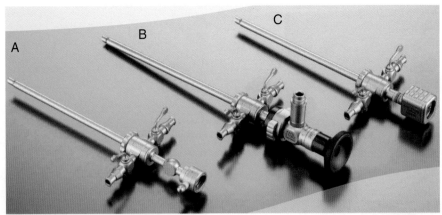

Figure 2-4 Arthroscope cannulae vary in locking mechanisms. A variety of 5.8-mm outside diameter (OD) self-locking cannulae made by the same manufacturer for use with a 4-mm OD arthroscope and varying in locking mechanism from standard rotation **(A),** bimanual snap-in release **(B),** or automatic lock-in coupling mechanism **(C).** All are inserted with a 4-mm conical obturator. The sharp trocar is rarely used. *(Image adapted from Karl Storz.)*

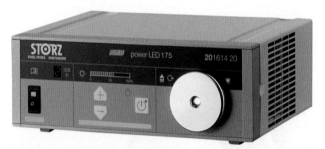

Figure 2-5 Storz 175W LED light source provides a versatile illuminator with adjustable outlet to suit most light cables in use today. *(Image courtesy Karl Storz.)*

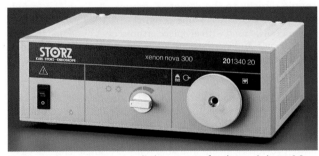

Figure 2-6 Intense xenon light source for large joints. More intense xenon light sources such as the Karl Storz Nova 300 W provide ample illumination for most joints. *(Image courtesy Karl Storz.)*

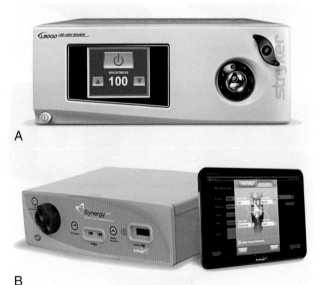

Figure 2-7 LED light sources. Cool and powerful LED light sources such as **(A)** the Stryker L9000 (500 W) and **(B)** the Arthrex Synergy HD3 combined LED light source/camera control/storage system provide state-of-the-art illumination with extremely long bulb life. *(Images courtesy Stryker Endoscopy and Arthrex Inc.)*

of light intensity. Most have a feedback electrical signal from the camera control to light source for intensity adjustment. The Stryker L9000™ light source and the Karl Storz light sources employ useful intensity feedback control. Most have the option to use this in an automatic mode or to switch to manual to override the iris control. Additionally, many new digital video camera control systems now also compensate for variation in light intensity, which reduces the need for light source intensity changes.

Video Cameras

Diagnostic and surgical arthroscopy should not be performed by direct visualization through the arthroscope. The improved comfort of erect body posture, lack of eyepiece contamination by the surgeon's eye, and better depth perception make the

direct viewing approach obsolete. The risks of contaminating the surgical field and instruments are obvious. In addition, depth perception and ability to perform fine movements are severely compromised with the monocular vision of a small image. Projection of images through a video screen corrects these deficiencies and allows simultaneous observation of the procedure by several participants (Jackson & Ovadia, 1985). Additionally, video documentation through still image capture, video recorders, and digital video capture systems (described later) provide sound surgical training, client satisfaction, and legal sense. Lightweight video cameras are attached directly to the eyepiece of the arthroscope (Fig. 2-8), eliminating the need for the eye to go to the arthroscope. This also provides a more comfortable operating position because the surgeon can stand up straight and the hands can be placed at any level. It is also possible for an assistant to hold the camera, which allows the surgeon use of both hands to manipulate instruments for fine control or access to difficult sites.

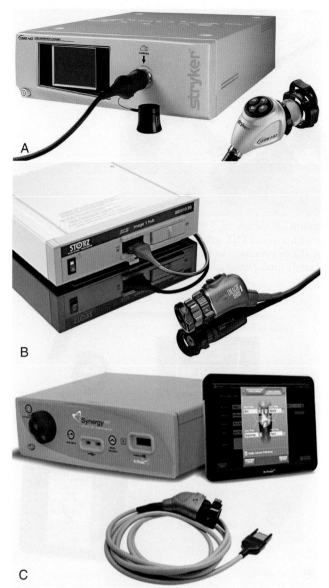

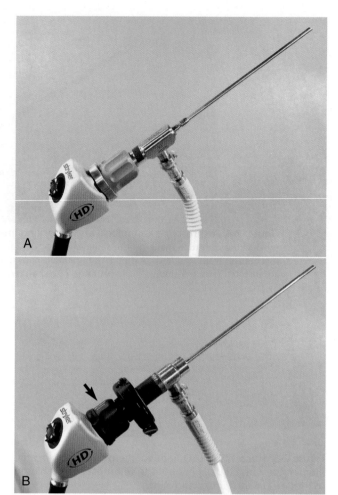

Figure 2-9 Videoarthroscopes do not have an eyepiece and couple directly to the camera C-mount. **A,** Examples include the Stryker videoarthroscope coupled to a 1088 camera. **B,** The camera can be used with eyepiece arthroscopes by adding the coupler *(arrow)*. Videoarthroscopes cannot be viewed by the naked eye, which is an important drawback if the video camera fails.

Figure 2-8 High-definition video cameras. Examples of high-definition single-chip or three-chip video camera models include the **A,** Stryker 1288; **B,** Storz SCB Image 1 hub; and **C,** Arthrex Synergy HD3. *(Images courtesy Stryker Endoscopy, Karl Storz, and Arthrex Inc.)*

Solid-state video cameras are now conveniently small and light and can be attached directly to videoarthroscopes, eliminating the coupler and any chance of fogging (Fig. 2-9). The united arthroscope and camera can be cold soaked or gas sterilized, or both. The solid-state cameras currently available produce an image from either one or three chips or, more accurately, closed coupled device (CCD) chips (Whelan & Jackson, 1992; Johnson, 2002). These chips produce excellent image quality. Most modern cameras use digital enhancement of the image, including motion correction algorithms, but still output as an analog signal (Johnson, 2002). Fully digital cameras such as the Stryker 1288™ video camera can write directly to a CD or DVD without capture devices and provide a dense 1920 × 1080p image that requires an upgraded monitor to derive the most benefit from its circuitry. Durable and high image-quality video cameras used by the authors are available from Karl Storz (Image 1 Hub camera), Smith & Nephew—Dyonics (ED-3 and D3 three-chip cameras; HD900 single-chip camera), Stryker Endoscopy (1288 and 1488 three-chip cameras), and Arthrex (Synergy system). Several manufacturers produce autoclavable

cameras (e.g., the Stryker 1188 HD three-chip camera, which can be sterilized using the flash autoclave cycle, in addition to more routine methods). These cameras are well sealed with a laser-welded titanium seal design, making them durable, but have previously been available only as single-chip devices, reducing the image quality. Availability and the need for auto-clavable cameras have declined in recent years. The authors' preferred method of sterilization is with ethylene oxide gas (see Sterilization of Equipment later). This requires a minimal exposure/ventilation time of 12 hours and, therefore, is usually suitable only for the first surgery each day. Cameras for subsequent surgeries can then be sterilized by immersion techniques or covered by a sterile sleeve. In countries where ethylene oxide is not permitted, immersion techniques are employed routinely.

Fluid or moisture between the arthroscope and camera lens can produce frustrating fogging and loss of image detail. This is reduced with cameras that have large, open vents on the camera coupler. If a "closed" camera coupler with narrow or no vents is employed, the problem can be limited by careful drying before attaching the camera to the arthroscope and also by using warm irrigating fluid. Antifogging solutions such as Fred™ (US Surgicalⁱ) tend to be ineffective.

ⁱUS Surgical, North Haven, CT 06473. Tel: (203) 492-5000.

Fluid Irrigation System

Sterile polyionic fluid is used for joint distention and irrigation during surgical arthroscopic procedures. The original systems consisted of an intravenous set connected to the ingress stopcock on the arthroscopic sheath and supplied by a bottle with attached bulb pump to apply pressure. This method is now rarely used because many facilities purchase sterile irrigating fluids in 1-, 3-, or 5-L bags (Travenol Laboratories)[j], rather than mix and sterilize polyionic solutions in reuseable bottles. Most equine arthroscopy procedures require fluid pressures greater than those derived from gravity feed developed by suspending the fluids above the surgical field, as commonly practiced in human arthroscopy. Flow rates using gravity flow through narrower arthroscope cannulas used in human small joint surgery are also frequently inadequate (Oretorp & Elmersson, 1986). Pressurized cuffs to surround 1- to 5-L bags of fluids have been developed for high rates of intravenous fluid delivery (Travenol). These have been used for joint distention and arthroscopy and allow the surgeon to broadly control the degree of distention, as well as the irrigation flow rate. Because these often deliver through intravenous drip sets, they tend to be slow and unresponsive to demands for rapid redistension for most equine arthroscopic applications. Additionally, a relationship between fluid pressure and fluid extravasation into the soft tissues has been recognized in man (Morgan, 1987); extravasation occurs at approximately 50 mm Hg, and pressure limiting is not a feature of pressurized cuff bags (Noyes et al, 1987). Control of fluid pressure is better provided by mechanical pumps.

The most popular system for fluid delivery is now a motorized pump. Such pumps can provide both high flow rates and high intraarticular pressures. The simplest and favored pump for two of the authors (C.W.M. and I.M.W.) is an infusion pump[k] such as the one illustrated in Figure 2-10. Such pumps are relatively inexpensive (Table 2-1) and provide high flow rates on demand, which is particularly useful for distention of large synovial spaces (see also Chapter 3), but automatic control of the pressure is lacking (Bergstrom & Gillquist, 1986; Dolk & Augustini, 1989). If an outflow portal is not open, excessive intraarticular pressures may cause joint capsule rupture (Morgan, 1987). Extravasation of fluid is also a complication whenever excessive pressures are generated, and compartment syndrome has occurred using mechanical pressure delivery systems in man.

The ideal pressure and flow automated pump should be capable of delivering necessary flow rates on demand, keep pressure at adequate yet safe levels, and include safety features such as intraarticular pressure-sensitive shutdowns and alarms (Ogilvie-Harris & Weisleder, 1995). Many new pumps meet these criteria, including pumps made by Arthrex, Stryker Endoscopy, Smith & Nephew—Dyonics, Karl Storz, and Linvatec (see Table 2-1; Figs. 2-11 to 2-13). Most provide pressures from 0 to 150 mm Hg and fluid flows as high as 2 L/min. All modern pumps sense joint pressures through the single-delivery fluid line. These features facilitate visualization when large joints or motorized equipment results in a demand for high fluid flows. From a reliability perspective, the roller pump design of the Arthrex, Stryker, and Karl Storz pumps provide advantages over the centrifugal and piston pump design of other manufacturers. The significant cost of these sophisticated fluid delivery systems can be reduced by tubing lines that do not require complete replacement of the entire pump assembly during multiple case schedules. An example

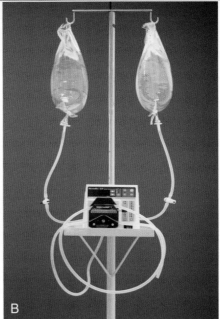

Figure 2-10 Simple roller pumps are affordable and reliable but provide no pressure sensing. A simple and inexpensive pump consists of a flow-regulated roller pump (Cole-Parmer Masterflex) **(A)**, which provides manual control of flow rates via a simple tubing system **(B)**. Flow rates up to 2.3 L/min can be achieved.

is the Arthrex pump assembly (see Fig. 2-11), which replaces only the sterile line to the patient between cases, providing new fluid delivery for less than one-third the cost of a complete roller pump and patient line setup. Pressure and flow automated pumps are more expensive (see Table 2-1) and involve a more complex setup procedure during preparation for surgery. However, equipment prices are often reduced or rolled into a minimum purchase of tubing, so the actual equipment cost can be passed on to each case. Setup and calibration are simpler on some pumps than others (see Table 2-1). A nitrogen-driven flutter valve pump with no electrical parts (Davol[l]) is a cost-effective intermediate-style pump that bridges between gravity feed and pressure-driven pumps (Fig. 2-14). This system has been occasionally used by one author

[j]Travenol Laboratories, Inc., Baxter Health Care Corp, One Baxter Parkway, Deerfield, IL 60015. Tel: (847) 948-2000. www.baxter.com
[k]Cole-Parmer Instrument Company, 625 East Bunker Court, Vernon Hills, IL 60061. Tel: (800) 323-4340. www.coleparmer.com

[l]Davol Inc., 100 Sockanossett Crossroad, PO Box 8500, Cranston, RI 02920. Tel: (800) 556-6275. www.davol.com

Table • 2-1

Summary and Comparison of Fluid Pumps Commonly Used for Equine Arthroscopy

PUMP MANUFACTURER	PUMP	PUMP TYPE	TUBING STYLE	INTEGRATED SUCTION	PRESSURE SENSING	MAX PRESSURE (mm Hg)	MAX FLOW (L/MIN)	REUSABLE TUBING	EQUIPMENT COST (U.S.$)	COST PER PATIENT (U.S.$)	SIMPLICITY OF SET-UP	RELIABILITY
Cole-Parmer	Masterflex L/S	Roller	Single line	No	No	31	2.3	Yes	1,205	68*	Simple	Excellent
Conmed Linvatec	24k Fluid System	Roller	Single line or dual line	Yes	Yes	10–150	500 mL/min	No	9,430†	24K100 $73 10K100 $90	Moderate	Excellent
Smith & Nephew—Dyonics	InteliJET	Centrifugal	Single line	No	Yes	150	N/A	No	10,084†	90	Moderate	Fair
Karl Storz	Endomat	Roller	Single line	Yes	Yes	200	1.0	No	7,000	69	Moderate	Good
Stryker	Arthroscopy pump	Roller	Single line	No	Yes	150	2.0	No‡	9,167†	89	Simple	Good
Arthrex	Continuous Wave III	Roller	Single line	No	Yes	100	1.6	Yes	3,920†	58 20	Simple	Good
Davol	Arthro-Flo Irrigator	Flutter	Single line	No	Yes	313 (14 feet§)	1.5	No‡	1,170	61*	Simple	Fair

*Cost of tubing can be significantly reduced by ethylene oxide (EtO) sterilization and reuse.
†Pump is provided without charge if pump agreement to purchase minimum number of tubing sets is established.
‡Not recommended by manufacturer but can be rinsed and EtO sterilized.
§Gravity equivalent.
N/A, Not available.

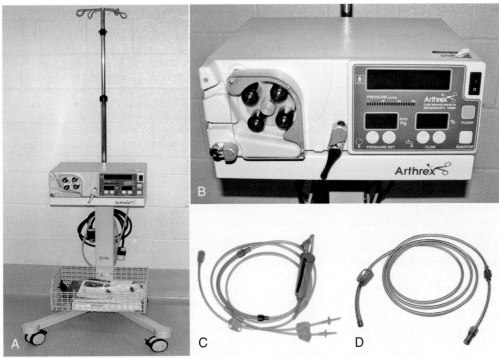

Figure 2-11 Arthrex roller pump is reliable and fully flow and pressure regulated. **A,** Arthrex Continuous wave III pump, which provides flow and pressure regulation and is easy to set up. **B,** The roller pump is simple to set up and prime and is highly reliable. **C,** The primary tube line provides dual bag spikes, silastic roller pump segment, filter, connection to the transducer, and a sealable line to the horse. **D,** An additional benefit is the reusable portion of the pump tubing, which lowers patient costs by 65% by eliminating the need to replace the entire pump and reservoir bag line for additional cases each day.

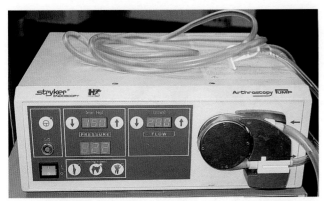

Figure 2-12 The Stryker roller pump is reliable and provides multiple adjustments and various joint presets and over-pressure warning. The Stryker arthroscopy pump provides flow- and pressure-regulated fluid, is easy to set up, and delivers up to 2 L/min.

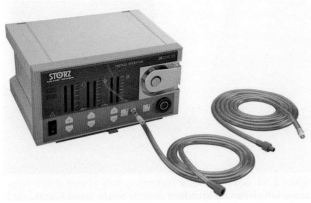

Figure 2-13 Storz Endomat pump provides pressure and flow regulated fluid delivery. Some pumps also provide built-in suction. *(Image courtesy Storz.)*

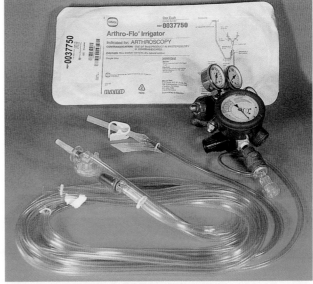

Figure 2-14 Nitrogen gas–driven flutter valve assembly (Davol) provides inexpensive pressure-sensing high fluid flows, with maximum pressures of 313 mm Hg. The system has no moving mechanical parts, and the tubing can be rinsed, gas sterilized, and reused.

(A.J.N.) for many years and is economical, simple to set up, and pressure sensing. It can also deliver high flow rates (Smith & Trauner, 1999). The disadvantages are the relatively slow recognition of pressure drops in the joint, the noise of the flutter valve pump assembly, and the need for a compressed nitrogen tank to drive the system.

The use of a balanced electrolyte solution such as lactated Ringer solution rather than saline for joint distention has been recommended on the basis of studies that show saline is not physiologic and inhibits normal synthesis of proteoglycans by the chondrocytes of the articular cartilage (Reagan et al, 1983). Any matrix depletion of the cartilage during normal arthroscopic procedures would be minor and certainly not permanent (Johnson et al, 1983), but when the cost of each fluid is similar, the use of the most physiologic solution is logical. The results of another study evaluating the acute effects of saline and lactated Ringer solution on cellular metabolism demonstrated an acute stress to both chondrocytes and synoviocytes immediately after irrigation with both fluids, although this was greater with saline. These stress patterns (monitored by evaluating relative ATP regeneration) are apparent after 24 hours, appear to be returning toward normal by 48 hours, and are not significantly different from control values 1 week later. On the basis of these results, protection from full activity during this time period was considered advisable (Straehley, 1985).

Gas insufflation has been used occasionally in equine arthroscopy by two of the authors (C.W.M and A.J.N.). Several types of gas insufflators are available. Most have a small internal reservoir gas tank, including the Karl Storz and Stryker units (Fig. 2-15). Others such as those from Linvatec, Stryker, and Directed Energy[m] use a direct step-down valve system from a commercial tank (Fig. 2-16). Arguments have been advanced for the use of gas insufflation of the joint rather than fluid distention during arthroscopy (Eriksson & Sebik, 1982); the gaseous medium (carbon dioxide, helium, or nitrous oxide) results in a sharper image with higher contrast. As well as being useful for photographs, some evidence exists that it may offer an increased degree

of accuracy in assessing cartilage damage in some situations (Eriksson & Sebik, 1982). In addition, it can prevent synovial villi from interfering with the visual field. However, a pressure-regulating device and a special system are necessary for gas insufflation. In addition, gas escapes easily after removal of any appreciable fragment through an instrument portal. Gas emphysema, pneumoperitoneum, pneumoscrotum, and gas emboli have been identified as complications in human arthroscopy (Jager, 1980). Subcutaneous emphysema is common in horses after gas insufflation, and can extend up the limb. Reports of air embolus, cardiac insufficiency, and death have been attributed to gas insufflation of body cavities and, to a lesser extent, joints (Menes et al, 2000). Both carbon dioxide and helium have been used for gas insufflation. Helium has been increasingly favored because it is inert, does not induce acidosis in the joint or peritoneal cavity, and dissipates rapidly from the subcutaneous tissues if any leakage develops. However, inadvertent gas embolus of helium has serious consequences due to poor solubility of helium in the blood, compared with carbon dioxide, and the persisting bubbles can lead to cardiac insufficiency, coronary emboli, and cerebral infarction (Neuhaus et al, 2001). Carbon dioxide should be used in equine arthroscopy for these safety reasons. Currently, there remain few reports of more widespread use of gas in human arthroscopy. In the experience of the authors, gas does have several advantages. It is relatively inexpensive, is simple to use, provides better visualization when synovial proliferation or hemorrhage obscures the field, and provides a medium in which cancellous bone graft and fibrin- or platelet-rich plasma (PRP) based cartilage repair vehicles can be used in subchondral bone and

---

[m]Directed Energy Inc, 11661 San Vicente Blvd, Suite 203, Los Angeles, CA 90049.

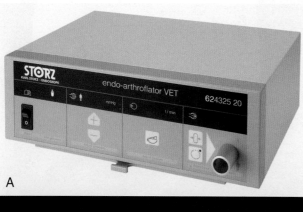

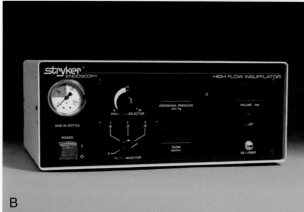

Figure 2-15 Gas insufflators. Gas insufflation systems include **(A)** Karl Storz arthroflator VET and **(B)** Stryker insufflator, both of which require refilling of the smaller internal gas tank.

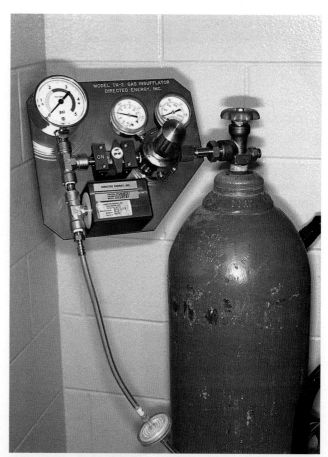

Figure 2-16 Gas insufflator consisting only of step-down regulators, which can be attached directly to the large K and J tank sizes. High gas flows are available, but pressure is limited to 2 psi.

cartilage procedures. Gas also prevents large mobile fragments from floating away when grasped for extraction. This can be especially useful in the hock and stifle. Gas leakage does form local emphysema, which may take several days to dissipate, but many procedures start with liquid distention and only use gas for short periods of defined activity, which limits emphysema. Removal of small particles by suction obviously requires a fluid medium, and fluid irrigation will also be necessary at the end of any procedure for lavage and removal of debris.

At this stage, the authors consider the use of fluid irrigation more convenient and experience with the use of fluid can eliminate many of the problems associated with synovial villi obstructing visualization. No additional equipment is necessary, and although the images obtained have somewhat less contrast compared with images from gas-filled joints, superficial damage to the articular cartilage and other lesions are seen more readily in the form of floating strands. Nonetheless,

the addition of gas may be a necessary and convenient step in the future if bone grafting, laser surgery, or clottable biologics as vehicles for cell grafting become an important feature of arthroscopic surgery.

Egress Cannula

An egress cannula (Fig. 2-17) is a necessary item for most arthroscopic procedures. It has an accompanying locking trocar with either a sharp stylet or conical obturator. The cannula is used to flush fluid through the joint in order to clear blood and debris and optimize visibility. The outer end has a Luer attachment through which fluid can be aspirated or to which a long, flexible egress tube can be attached to transmit fluid to a bucket on the floor rather than having it spill over the surgical site or equipment. The authors use a 2- or 3-mm egress cannula (see Fig. 2-17A) routinely at the beginning of the arthroscopic procedure to flush the joint and to probe and manipulate lesions. A larger-diameter (4.5-mm) cannula (see Fig. 2-17C) can be used at the end of the procedure for clearing debris. The 3-mm cannula is usually inserted without the use of the stylet because a portal has been made with a blade. A stylet or conical obturator (see Fig. 2-17D), however, is useful to facilitate placement of the larger 4.5-mm cannula at the end of the procedure.

Hand Instruments for Arthroscopic Surgery

As mentioned previously, a myriad of instruments are available from arthroscopic equipment manufacturers (Caspari, 1987; Gross, 1993; Ekman & Poehling, 1994), most of which are neither suitable nor necessary for equine arthroscopic surgery. The instruments presented in this section are those used by the authors to perform the procedures described in this book. It is accepted that there are alternative, and possibly better, ways to perform any given task and techniques certainly will change. The current list is written with the philosophy of keeping arthroscopy simple and practical without compromising standards. A combination of specialized arthroscopic instruments and instruments not designed specifically for arthroscopic surgery is used.

Blunt Probe

This standard arthroscopic instrument (Fig. 2-18) is necessary for diagnostic and surgical arthroscopy. Suitable probes are available from all arthroscopic instrument manufacturers.

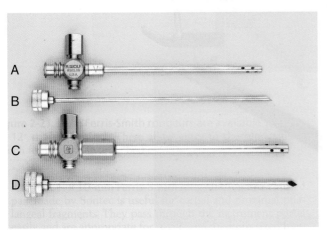

Figure 2-17 Egress cannulae. A 3-mm egress cannula **(A)** with stylet **(B)** and a 4.5-mm egress cannula **(C)** with sharp obturator **(D).** Both egress cannula sizes have a role in equine arthroscopy, but the smaller cannula is more suitable for routine flushing on entry to the joint, "probing" lesions, and postprocedure flushing. The 4.5-mm cannula can be used to evacuate debris, place drains into the joint for antibiotic delivery, and for debridement using the open end as a combination elevator and automatic flush.

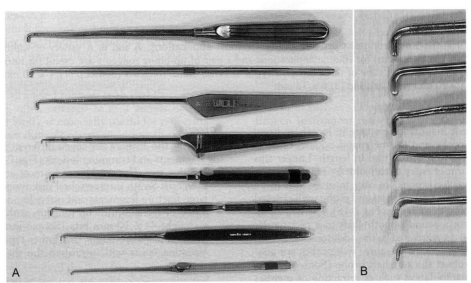

Figure 2-18 Arthroscopic probes. A, Variety of arthroscopic probes, from large to small format, and with round, rectangular, and thumb plate handles. **B,** Probe ends vary in shape and size.

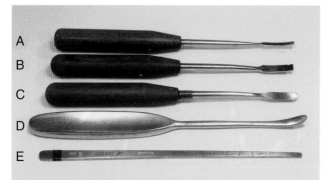

Figure 2-24 Various elevators and osteotomes are essential. **A,** Small (3 mm) Synthes periosteal elevator, used for fine cartilage debridement; **B,** medium Synthes elevator (6 mm) for sharp separation of tissues such as apical sesamoid fracture dissection; **C,** round-nose Synthes elevator, used for further separation of chip fractures and debriding OCD flaps; **D,** Freer elevator for nontraumatic separation or endoscopic reduction of intraarticular slab fractures; **E,** a 4-mm osteotome (Sontec) for separating bony exostoses or partially reattached chip fractures.

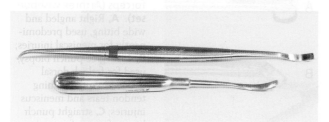

Figure 2-25 Two types of Foerner elevator (Sontec Inst) for dissecting apical sesamoid fractures from the intersesamoidean ligament. The double-ended Foerner elevator (top) with large and small ends for apical sesamoid fracture dissection and the original single-ended elevator. The versatility of exchanging from large to smaller ends, depending on the need for concentrated force, makes the double-ended elevator useful.

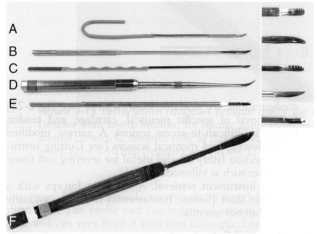

Figure 2-26 A selection of arthroscopic cutting instruments. **A,** Smith & Nephew—Dyonics curved banana blade. The handle has been bent back on itself to improve grip and dexterity; **B,** Sontec curved serrated knife; **C,** Smith & Nephew—Acufex straight serrated banana knife; **D,** Richard Wolf curved knife (detachable knife system); **E,** Beaver Arthro-Lok™ blade[p] (curved left); **F,** Sontec flat sesamoid knife.

[p]Beaver Surgical Products, Becton-Dickinson, BD Medical Systems, 1 Becton Drive, Franklin Lakes, NJ 07417. Tel: (800) 237-2762. www.bd.com

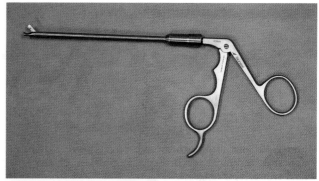

Figure 2-27 Sontec arthroscopic scissors are useful cutting instruments for dense tissue.

elevator is also occasionally useful (see Fig. 2-24). A markedly curved sharp-end periosteal elevator (Fig. 2-25) is useful for removing apical sesamoid fragments (Foerner elevator; Sontec Instruments; see Chapter 5).

Cutting Instruments

Numerous cutting instruments are available. Their use is limited to specific situations. If sharp severance of structures is required, special arthroscopic cutting instruments should be used. The authors have used both reusable blades and disposable blade systems (Fig. 2-26, made by Karl Storz,[b] Wolf,[e] Beaver,[p] Dyonics, Acufex-Smith & Nephew,[q] Concept-Linvatec-Zimmer, and Bard-Parker. Sheathed blades are also available and eliminate the risk of inadvertent damage to other structures when introducing the blade.

Use of straight and curved arthroscopic scissors (Fig. 2-27) has several advantages in tight situations such as carpal canal release, villonodular mass resection, and opening of the T ligament during digital sheath approaches to the navicular bursa (Fig. 2-28). Serrated or plain curved and straight scissors are available from Karl Storz, Sontec Instruments, and Arthrex Instruments. Another scissor-type cutting instrument is the narrow basket forceps (Arthrex or Scanlan-McIlwraith scissor action rongeur) (see Fig. 2-23).

The authors have found few indications for the retrograde or hook knives, other than those available for arthroscopic annular ligament transection (see Chapter 12). A meniscotome can be useful for breaking down fibrous capsule attachments when freeing a chip because it makes a cleaner cut than a periosteal elevator.

Curettes

Curettes are used for debridement of most osteochondral defects, including those remaining following removal of traumatic or developmental fragmentation, evacuation of subchondral bone cysts, and debridement of foci of infection. Closed spoon curettes are suitable for most purposes, but open ring curettes may be preferable for the center of lesions (Fig. 2-29). Straight and angled spoon curettes, either 0 or 00 in size, are generally preferred for routine applications (see Fig. 2-29). Smaller and more angled curettes are also useful for fine cartilage debridement and cyst curettage, respectively. A rasp is rarely necessary for smoothing debrided bone regions in joints but may be useful for smoothing larger areas such

[b]Karl Storz Veterinary Endoscopy, 175 Cremona Drive, Goleta, CA 93117. Tel: (800) 955-7832. www.ksvea.com

[e]Richard Wolf, 353 Corporate Woods Parkway, Vernon Hills, IL 60061. Tel: (847) 913-1113. www.richardwolfusa.com

[q]Acufex Microsurgical Inc., Smith & Nephew, 150 Minuteman Road, Andover, MA 01810. Tel: (978) 749-1000. www.smith-nephew.com

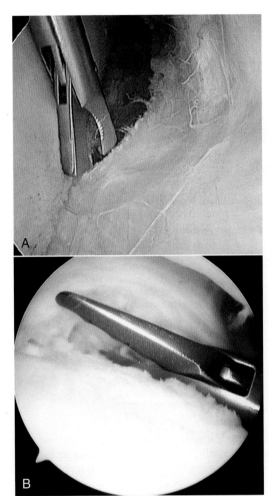

Figure 2-28 Arthroscopic scissors being used in confined spaces. **A,** Carpal canal showing retinaculum release with Sontec arthroscopic scissor. **B,** Digital sheath approach to navicular bursa with Arthrex scissor being used to divide the T ligament.

as after radial osteochondroma and physeal exostosis removal. These instruments are available in straight, offset convex and concave, and push-cut and pull-cut designs from various manufacturers, including Sontec Instruments and Stainless Manufacturing Inc.[r]

Microfracture Awls

Microfracture has become an established technique in man and horses to improve the bulk of repair tissue in confined cartilage erosions (see Chapter 16). Various manufacturers market awls, which have angled tips varying from 30 degrees to 90 degrees (Fig. 2-30). Use of the 30- and 45-degree awls is common in select applications in the authors' practices. Quality of the steel and handle construction varies, but more expensive instruments such as those from Linvatec (Conmed-Linvatec[d]) are robust and remain sharp.

Self-Sealing Cannulae

The use of self-sealing sleeves or cannulae (Fig. 2-31) is a logical answer to the loss of fluid through instrument portals. These devices have application in large joints, particularly the shoulder and femoropatellar joints, but they are not useful in the carpus and fetlock because of the close proximity of

---

[r]Stainless Manufacturing Inc., 225 West Allen Avenue, San Dimas, CO 91773. www.stainlessmd.com

joint capsule and lesion. Disposable self-sealing 4.5- to 10-mm operating cannulae are available through several manufacturers (Arthrex, Smith & Nephew—Dyonics). They are useful for repeatedly introducing small forceps, hand tools, and shavers, but in the horse, removal of osteochondral fragments is the most common procedure, and this can only rarely be done through such cannulae. A 10-mm (I.D.) threaded self-sealing disposable cannula with insertion obturator (Arthrex) has been useful in shoulder arthroscopy (see Fig. 2-31); otherwise, operating cannulae are still rarely used in equine arthroscopic surgery. The limitation is often associated with reduced protruding working length of the hand instrument (Fig. 2-32), which depends on long slender instrument shafts and relatively short cannulae. Flexible silicone self-sealing cannulae (see Fig. 2-31) (Passport; Arthrex Instruments) overcome some of these issues but are more difficult to place.

Suction Punch Rongeurs and Vacuum Attachments

Various instruments, including forceps and curettes, are available with attachments so that suction can be applied as they are used. The 5.2-mm DyoVac (Smith & Nephew—Dyonics) or larger 8.0-mm Sontec biopsy rongeur (Fig. 2-33) are used by two of the authors (A.J.N. and C.W.M.) for minor synovial resection, cartilage and soft bone removal, or larger soft tissue pad or meniscus trimming. As such, the Dyonics 5.2-mm suction punch rongeur provides a versatile debriding instrument that gets more use than most instruments in routine arthroscopy. Further, it often prevents having to set up motorized equipment. The larger-diameter suction punch rongeurs (Sontec Instruments) are useful for resection of substantial soft tissue masses such as meniscal flaps, villonodular masses, and tenosynovial growths but can be difficult to establish primary entry due to the large external shaft diameter. Use of suction enables instant removal of debris as it forms during debridement within the joint. However, with the high fluid pressures used in equine arthroscopy, suction is often unnecessary because free material is spontaneously flushed out through the suction channel. The use of suction during any procedure requires an increased rate of ingress fluid delivery. In general, the authors prefer to perform hand debridement without suction, reserving it for use with motorized instruments or to remove debris at the end of surgical procedures.

Motorized Instrumentation

A large assortment of motorized arthroscopic instruments is available from most of the equipment manufacturers. Although motorized equipment should be used only with due consideration to the synovial environment and tissues, these instruments are extremely efficient and some surgical procedures can only be done effectively with such equipment. Synovial resection, whether performed locally to improve visualization of lesions or therapeutically on a subtotal basis, can only be performed effectively with motorized apparatus. Similarly, some large areas of osseous debridement such as in shoulder or stifle osteochondrosis become impossible to complete reasonably without such equipment. The basic concept of motorized instruments is a rotating blade within a sheath to which suction can be applied. This pulls soft tissue into the mouth of the blade and removes debris (Graf and Clancy, 1987). Most currently available systems are powered electrically and consist of a control unit attached by an electrical cord to a motorized handpiece. The latter may be operated by buttons on the handpiece or via a foot pedal to the control unit (Fig. 2-34). Given the intense concentration required for careful motorized resection, assigning the shaver control to a foot pedal is generally advisable. This leaves the fine control of arthroscope and shaver tip to the hands of the surgeon. Voice command, cordless foot control, and combination radiofrequency shaver units (Crossfire; Stryker) also improve the focus of the surgeon.

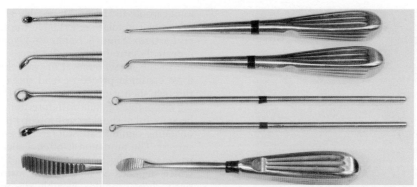

Figure 2-29 Curettes and rasps. Spoon curettes include, from top to bottom, a small (2/0) straight curette, a small 2/0 curved spoon curette, straight and curved ring curettes (Wolf or Sontec), and a rasp (Stainless Manufacturing, Inc. or Sontec Instruments).

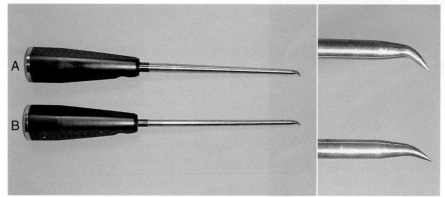

Figure 2-30 A and B, Microfracture awls (ConMed Linvatec) for perforating the subchondral bone in focal cartilage erosions. Tip angles vary from 30 degrees (bottom) to 70 degrees, but the 45-degree angle (top) is preferred in most equine joints.

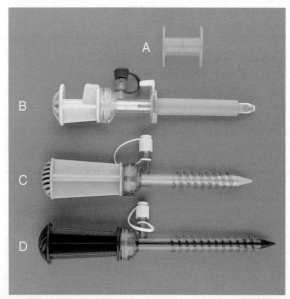

Figure 2-31 Self-sealing cannulae are useful but have limited application. Cannulae are used occasionally in equine joints and include **A,** the self-sealing push-insertion flexible silastic cannula (Passport, Arthrex); **B,** pop-out wing self-retaining cannula (Arthrex); **C** and **D,** screw-in cannula of differing lengths for instrument portals. The length should be determined by depth of the joint capsule from the skin but in general needs to be minimized to maintain effective working instrument length within the joint.

Cutting heads or blades for the motorized units can be divided into three broad groups: (1) blades designed to remove soft tissues such as synovium, plicae, and ligament remnants; (2) blades to trim denser soft tissues such as menisci; and (3) burrs for debriding bone. These blades are mostly available in disposable forms, although renewed interest in reusable blades has resulted from the economic downturn in medical practice and the more aggressive design of some of these blades. However, even disposable blades can be cleaned, sterilized, and reused for a limited number of procedures (not recommended by manufacturer). In the authors' experience, this has been a safe practice. Generally, "fatigue" damage to the blades occurs at the plastic attachment to the handpiece or in the drive shaft of curved synovial resectors.

The authors have experience with the Smith & Nephew—Dyonics Arthroplasty System™, the Stryker Core Formula 180 system, and the Karl Storz Unidrive III Arthro system. Dyonics developed the original shaver, and the current Dyonics systems (Power Shave) and Stryker Formula are still popular. Current shavers have integrated suction with hand control of suction intensity. Some manufacturers such as Smith & Nephew—Dyonics, Storz, and Stryker also have speed and rotation direction controls on the handpiece. Rotation speeds up to 12,000 rpm and bidirectional capabilities are useful. The hand units of the Dyonics and Stryker shavers are relatively heavy compared with Storz Unidrive shavers, but the heavier units are generally more powerful. All modern shaver motors can be autoclaved, and most can be flash-autoclaved or cold-sterilized as needed. Most shaver motors recognize the blade type that the user has inserted and control the motor speed range accordingly. Foot control of shaver speed and direction, including oscillation mode, is standard. Fully enclosed totally waterproof foot

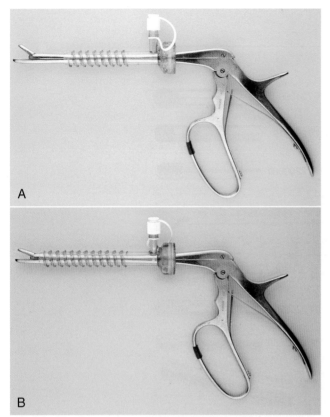

Figure 2-32 Effect of cannula length on working distance of rongeurs in a large joint such as the shoulder. **A,** A short cannula accommodates a Ferris-Smith rongeur while leaving adequate protruding length to work in the joint. **B,** A longer cannula is rarely required in horses and leaves too little protruding rongeur to manipulate in the joint.

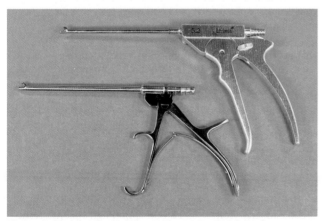

Figure 2-33 Dyonics DyoVac 5.2-mm suction punch rongeurs (top) are useful for soft tissue removal and cartilage debris cleanup. The use of suction is generally unnecessary as debris ejects out the suction port each time the jaws are opened. The cutting jaw action is protected by an aluminum shear pin. More robust tissue can be safely removed with Sontec 8-mm (O.D.) suction punch rongeurs. These are stronger but can be difficult to insert in some joints.

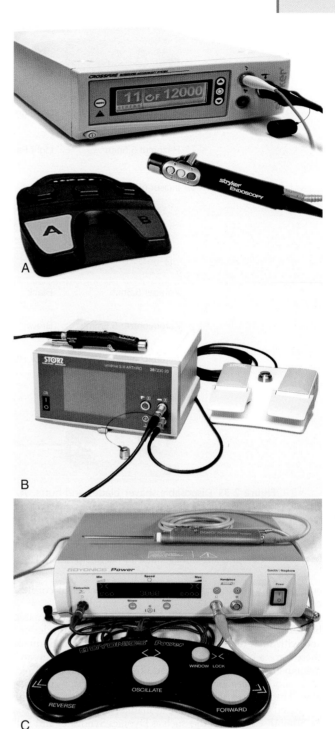

Figure 2-34 Shaver systems include variable speed control with oscillate mode, foot switch, and hand-piece with suction attachment. Common units include **A,** the Stryker Crossfire with cordless foot pedal and deactivateable handpiece controls; **B,** the Storz Unidrive SIII ARTHRO, and **C,** the Dyonics Power Shaver. All have essentially similar components, including the power control unit, waterproof foot pedal, and shaver motor drive with optional hand controls for forward, backward, and oscillate. Suction can be varied by the valve on the drive handpiece.

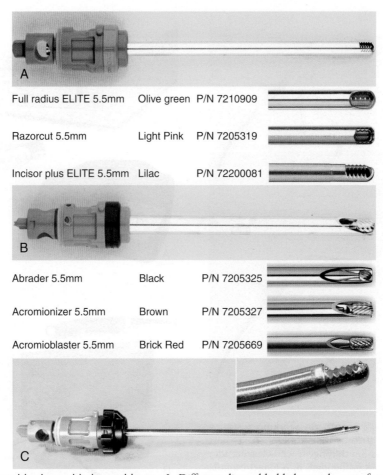

Full radius ELITE 5.5mm	Olive green	P/N 7210909
Razorcut 5.5mm	Light Pink	P/N 7205319
Incisor plus ELITE 5.5mm	Lilac	P/N 72200081
Abrader 5.5mm	Black	P/N 7205325
Acromionizer 5.5mm	Brown	P/N 7205327
Acromioblaster 5.5mm	Brick Red	P/N 7205669

Figure 2-35 Disposable shaver blades and burrs. **A,** Different disposable blade attachments for the Dyonics Power shaver line include the full radius Elite resector in 4.5-mm or 5.5-mm diameter, the razorcut in similar sizes, and the aggressive incisor plus Elite in 4.5- and 5.5-mm diameters. **B,** Bone burrs include the Abrader, Acromionizer, and Acromioblaster blades, varying from less aggressive to more aggressive burr styles, and available in sizes from 3.5-mm to 5.5-mm diameter. **C,** A useful disposable blade style is the curved 4.5-mm Orbit rotatable incisor plus, which can be adjusted to expose the cutting aperture throughout a 360-degree position. The flexible drive shaft can break during lengthy demanding cases.

control units such as the Stryker iSwitch Universal cordless control (see Fig. 2-34A) provide durable portability.

Each manufacturer provides a broad range of disposable blades, which often come with six to eight cutting tip designs and with shaft diameter sizes of 5.5, 4.5, or 3.5 mm. Some of these have a curved shaft 2 cm from the tip to allow greater maneuverability around joints. Additionally, a miniblade range of 2- and 2.9-mm cutters with a variety of tip ends are available. Three broad types of disposable blades (which can be subjected to multiple uses) are available (Fig. 2-35):

1. Smooth-edged resectors such as Dyonics Synovator and Full Radius blades (in 3.5-, 4.5-, and 5.5-mm diameter sizes)
2. Toothed-edged resectors such as Dyonics Orbit Incisor, Incisor Plus ELITE, RazorCut, full radius ELITE, and Turbowhisker blades (in 3.5-, 4.5-, and 5.5-mm diameter sizes)
3. Burrs such as Dyonics Abrader and Notch-Blaster in round burrs and Dyonics Acromionizer, Acromioblaster, and StoneCutter in oval, elongated burrs (in 2.5-, 3.5-, 4-, and 5.5-mm sizes).

The smooth-edged resector blades are appropriate for synovectomy. The toothed-edged resector (for trimming denser soft tissue) can be used for more extensive synovectomy, articular cartilage debridement, villonodular pad removal, and meniscus and soft bone debridement. The round or oval burrs are used for bone exostosis and osteophyte debridement in chronic degenerate joints, although other toothed resector blades have some value in similar situations. Large oval burrs

are particularly useful for removal of large extensor process and lateral malleolus fractures and smoothing of radius exostoses.

Modern synovial resector units are much more useful than previous types. Design changes, including larger apertures, higher speeds, narrower-diameter drive shafts (easier debris clearance), spiral flutes down the length of the drive shaft, and application of suction, have all contributed to better soft tissue resection and less clogging. The oscillating mode capability of the motor (the unit switches automatically between forward and reverse) facilitates cutting of fibrous tissues and decreases clogging between the blade and housing. The speed control is computerized, with a variable speed capacity from 0 to 12,000 rpm. High speeds are necessary when using the burr, whereas slower speeds are used with the soft tissue blades.

Stocking of all the blade types is unnecessary; most surgeons develop a preference for 1 or 2 soft tissue blades and a burr. In the Dyonics Power range, the authors prefer the 5.5-mm full radius blade (#7205307) or the 5.5-mm Incisor Plus Elite (#72200081) for villonodular pads and menisci, the 4.5-mm rotatable curved orbit incisor (#7205320) or Incisor Plus (#7205687) for most other soft tissue resection, and the 4-mm Acromionizer (oval burr; #7205326) or 4-mm Abrader (round burr; #7205324) for bone debridement (see Fig. 2-35). For large bone resection purposes, the larger 5.5-mm Acromionizer (#7205327) is effective but often requires both hands to control the cutting head, so a surgical assistant is necessary to control the arthroscope. Recently, a range of dual-use combination tips (Dyonics BoneCutter) that resect both soft tissue and bone have been introduced. These are available in synovator and full-radius styles, and they minimize both inventory and the need to switch blades in surgery.

Use of suction on shavers generally improves cutting performance. However, attention to the degree of filling of the suction bottle is required to prevent the automatic suction shut-off engaging, which can then allow fluid to flow back from nonsterile tubing and couplers at the bottle through the sterile patient line and out the shaver into the joint or onto the sterile field. It has been recognized as a potential risk in the use of shavers for some time (Bacarese-Hamilton et al, 1991), and it is particularly likely to happen when the fluid ingress runs out at that same moment, removing the positive pressure forcing joint fluid into the suction line. Prevention requires suction to be maintained on the tubing at all times, or at least ensuring the joint is pressurized during suction bottle exchange.

Electrosurgical and Radiofrequency Devices

Considerable interest and concurrent concern surrounds the use of radiofrequency (RF) electrosurgical devices for cartilage and synovial soft tissue procedures (Polousky et al, 2000; Medvecky et al, 2001; Lu et al, 2001; Lee et al, 2002; Sherk et al, 2002). RF devices use extremely high-frequency alternating current (e.g., 330 kHz compared with the 60 Hz of regular alternating current), which passes to the tissue at the applicator tip and then through the body to exit at a wide grounding plate, essentially as for all electrosurgical units. The cutting and vaporizing capability depends on the power and waveform settings. High-power settings and low voltage tends to cut, whereas low-power settings at relatively high voltage denatures and coagulates tissues (Sherk et al, 2002). Used in the liquid environment of the joint, both of these modes have found a place for excision of tissue (plica, adhesions, villonodular masses) or denaturation of cartilage (cartilage sculpting or chondroplasty). RF devices used in a cutting mode, at the lowest settings that will still cut plica, ligament, menisci, or masses, seem to be safe if the probe is directed away from cartilage and does not dwell on bone (Polousky et al, 2000; Lee et al, 2002). Similarly, thermal capsular shrinkage using low-power settings has many proponents and seems relatively low risk (Medvecky et al, 2001). However, RF devices used for thermal chondroplasty at recommended settings penetrate to the subchondral bone and cause chondrocyte death (Lu et al, 2000, 2001). Despite the apparent smoothness of cartilage after RF chondroplasty, the later necrosis can be devastating and is the subject of ongoing debate, investigation, and litigation (Lee et al, 2002). A recent review of RF chondroplasty was less critical, although still cautious, and presented three units as potentially preferable to others (Kosy et al, 2011). Second-look arthroscopy after RF chondroplasty in the human knee showed that more than 50% of patients had improved appearance with smooth cartilage and no progression or recurrence of fibrillation (Voloshin et al, 2007). More recent double-blind, controlled studies in the human knee also suggest that RF chondroplasty may result in improved outcome compared with mechanical debridement (Spahn et al, 2010). A study in the horse also suggested improved cartilage appearance and reduced permeability, without the previous thermal necrosis attributable to RF penetration (Uthamanthil et al, 2006). Given the current information, RF for chondroplasty should be used with caution until further studies define safe equipment and settings for the horse. The use of RF probes in cutting modes for capsule, check ligament, apical sesamoid fracture dissection, or annular ligament transection should use the minimal power settings that still achieve the desired effect and should absolutely avoid cartilage and underlying

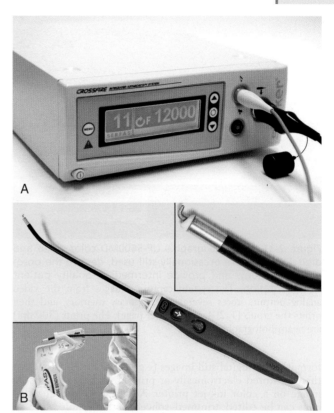

Figure 2-36 Radiofrequency generator and probe. **A,** Stryker radiofrequency probe and Crossfire control system. **B,** The probe tip is angled 90 degrees (inset), and the shaft of the wand can additionally be contoured (lower inset) to optimize entry to tight regions.

bone. Numerous manufacturers market RF systems, including Stryker, Arthrex, and ArthroCare. One of the authors (A.J.N.) has used probes from all three manufacturers for noncartilaginous procedures, including check desmotomy, navicular bursal adhesion resection, and apical sesamoid fracture removal, and has used the 90-degree probe for most of these applications (Fig. 2-36).

Still Photography

Historically, still photographic images were recorded on 35-mm film using a camera with a quick mount adaptor to the arthroscope. However, film photography has rapidly become obsolete, and even adapters to fit a digital camera to the arthroscope are cumbersome and risk contaminating the field. The current standard is digital image capture, either to a dedicated capture device (described next) or a computer with capture software. The best-quality images and the capability to capture still and video simultaneously only come from the dedicated capture units.

Video Documentation

Capture of video clips as analog video on a ½-inch video camera recorder (VCR) is now almost as obsolete as film photography. Despite its simplicity for capture, it is largely useless as case documentation because it is analog and nonsearchable. Moreover, it is difficult to find VCR equipment to play back clips in most practices. However, video and s-video formatted VCRs have become cheap and are better than no documentation. Further, simple video digitizing programs such as Windows Moviemaker™ (Microsoft), iMovie™ (Apple), VideoStudio 6™ (ULead Systems), or Pinnacle Studio Version 7™ (Pinnacle Systems, Inc.) provide a means to capture video from ½-inch tapes as digital video (e.g., MPEG

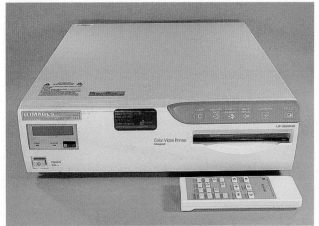

Figure 2-37 Sony Mavigraph® UP-5600MD color video and digital printers are occasionally still used, despite the obsolete technology, and provide intermediate-quality patient documentation. The system captures images from the video analog output, stores several to temporary memory, and then prints the group (1, 2, 4, 8, or 16 per page). The prints (300 dpi) are near-photographic quality.

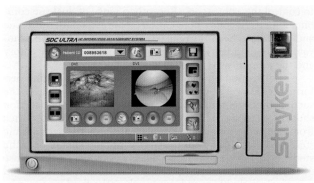

Figure 2-38 Stryker SDC Ultra HD™ high-definition digital video and still image storage and printing system. The system saves direct digital still images (jpg or bmp) and video clips (mpg-1 or -4) in separate patient folders, allowing image adjustment, annotation, and labeling. Then it outputs to a printer, digital files on CD or DVD, or a direct wired or wireless Internet connection. *(Image courtesy Stryker.)*

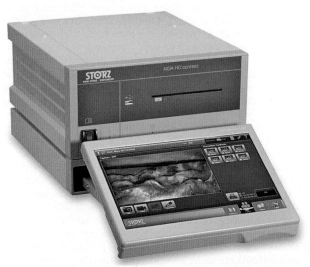

Figure 2-39 The Storz AIDA HD Connect high-definition digital image capture and storage device gathers still image and video clips for output via CD, DVD, or Blu-ray DVD. The touch screen is user friendly and rotates upward for different viewing angles. *(Image courtesy Storz.)*

format) or as digital still images (e.g., JPEG format) that can then be stored electronically or printed for several cents an image on a color ink-jet printer. Additionally, digital video clips can be edited, trimmed, spliced, and assembled into an annotated presentation using these programs. Other capture systems using Hi8 video capture have been described, and for a complete review of arthroscopic image documentation, the reader is directed to a recent review that provides an in-depth comparison of systems, cabling, connectors, and output devices (Frisbie, 2002).

Digital Image Capture and Storage Devices

Arthroscopic image capture and storage have undergone significant improvement along with the electronic revolution of the previous decade. The simplest technique for image documentation is electronic capture and printing on good-quality print paper in an ink-jet printer. These have replaced dye sublimation printers such as the Sony Mavigraph, which were previously state of the art (Fig. 2-37) (Brown, 1989; Johnson, 2002). Capture of short digital video recorder clips, or the entire arthroscopic procedure, on a digital video device (DVD) recorder/player allows full documentation. Copies can be made for distribution to owner and trainer as needed, but capture of digital video recorder (DVR) video files to still digital images requires conversion software packages such as MPEG Video Wizard. It is preferable to capture direct still images as JPEG (.jpg) or BITMAP (.bmp) images. If a dedicated capture device is not available, this can be done on a laptop computer running simple software programs that capture still and video imagery via USB connection (Arthrex Instruments).

Complete digital capture and storage devices for arthroscopic use are now in widespread use and considered the most versatile method to document digital still and video images of surgical cases. Leaders in this field include Karl Storz, Stryker, Arthrex, and Dyonics. All four units are expensive but store both digital still images (BMP or TIFF format for high detail or JPEG formats for routine use) and digital video clips (MPEG-1, -2, or -4), with the touch of a button on the camera head. The Stryker SDC HD and Ultra devices, Arthrex Synergy system, and Storz AIDA HD Connect are the more sophisticated units in the field of digital storage devices (Figs. 2-38 to 2-40). The units have touch screen patient input and image editing for still image output. Image printing can be done during surgery by attaching an inexpensive HP inkjet printer, and still

and video images can be saved on the system's hard drive. At the completion of each case, the files are saved on a CD, DVD, Blu-ray HD DVD, or USB device. The software in the unit provides versatile settings that allow extensive customization of image capture and compression, image editing, output styles, text addition, and Internet access. Retail prices range from $18,000 to $26,000.

Sterilization of Equipment

Repeated steam autoclaving shortens the useful life of an arthroscope by causing deterioration of the adhesives between the major lenses. Seals and bonding between materials may deteriorate from thermal shock; various materials expand and contract at different rates in response to the rapid temperature changes in a steam autoclave. Some manufacturers sell autoclavable arthroscopes and even autoclavable video camera systems (1188 High Definition Autoclavable 3-Chip camera; Stryker Endoscopy), which provide a more durable arthroscope and camera for steam sterilization. Gas sterilization with ethylene oxide is effective and safe, but it is not always available, is time consuming, and does not allow

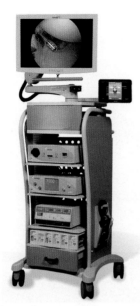

Figure 2-40 Arthrex Synergy systems provide integrated camera control, an intense LED light source, and ultra high-definition video and image capture and storage. A wireless detachable tablet can be included in the sterile field for scrubbed personnel to control camera and storage functions, as well as wireless connectivity for image sharing, consultation, teaching, or archiving. *(Image courtesy Arthrex Inc.)*

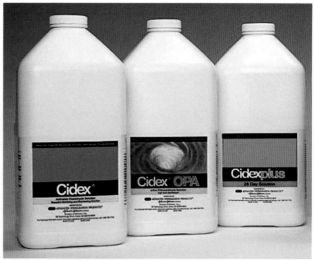

Figure 2-41 Cidex, Cidex Plus, and Cidex OPA. Cold soaking of instruments in Cidex or Cidex Plus has been popular among equine surgeons, although Cidex fumes are toxic. Cidex Plus extends the useful life after reconstitution to 4 weeks, compared with 2 weeks for Cidex. Cidex OPA provides similar sterilizing capabilities with reduced toxicity issues and 75-day shelf life after initial use.

multiple procedures in a day using a single set of instruments. Many units require certified ventilation for ethylene oxide, and growing concerns over atmospheric contamination may eventually force a ban on ethylene oxide sterilizers.

Consequently, the use of a 2% solution of activated dialdehyde (Cidex®, ASP; division of Ethicon[t]) was developed as an agent for cold sterilization procedures. Cidex® Plus has a 30-day shelf life after reconstitution, compared with the 14-day span of Cidex®, which provides cost savings for frequent users. The safety and effectiveness of Cidex® have been documented in 12,505 human arthroscopic procedures (Johnson et al, 1982). A 0.4% infection rate was noted in this series. The arthroscope and surgical instruments are soaked for a minimum of 10 minutes. It has been stated that more than 30 minutes of soaking can be damaging to the lens system of the arthroscope (Minkoff, 1977). Glutaraldehyde polymerizes on standing. When this occurs, crystals can form and cause clouding of arthroscope lenses.

The surgeon or assistant should be double gloved. He or she removes the instruments from the Cidex and places them in a sterile tray. The instruments are washed with sterile water or saline (Figs. 2-41 and 2-42) and transferred to the surgery table, where they are dried after the surgeon's outer gloves are removed. Ancillary instruments (towel clamps, scalpel handle, needle holder, and thumb forceps) can be previously autoclaved within the tray, which is then used for washing the soaked instruments. Rinsing of the equipment must be done with care to avoid damage to the camera and arthroscope from sharp-edged hand tools.

The 2% dialdehyde solution is properly classified as a disinfectant. The chemical is considered bactericidal in 10 minutes, destroying all bacteria, including *Myobacterium, tuberculosis, Pseudomonas aeruginosa,* and viruses. It is sporicidal in 10 hours and, therefore, considered a sterilizing agent after use for 10 hours (Johnson et al, 1982).

A number of glutaraldehyde-based disinfecting solutions are available. Use of a solution that does not contain a surfactant is recommended (Cidex-activated dialdehyde solution does not contain a surfactant). Surfactants may leave a residue, causing stiffening of moving parts and potential electrosurgical malfunction. Because surfactants lower the surface tension of the disinfection solution, the disinfectant can penetrate small cracks and crevices. This penetration creates a rinsing problem because high surface tension prevents water from entering the cracks and crevices and removing the disinfectant. As this disinfectant residue accumulates, stopcocks and other moving parts cease to function smoothly. Surfactant-containing solutions can also erode epoxy and other thermal plastics. Another recommendation is that plastic basins be used to soak instruments (McDonald, 1984). These basins reduce electrolytic corrosion, which can occur when metal instruments are soaked in metal pans.

The question of the potential for Cidex® to cause a chemical reaction in joints was addressed in the literature (Harner, 1988). Results of studies in rabbits showed that Cidex® induced a diffuse synovial inflammation when present intraarticularly at concentrations of 10 ppm or greater. The degree of synovial inflammation is proportional to the concentration of Cidex®. At 1000 ppm, chondrolysis occurs. When using a single-rinse basin, the concentration of Cidex® in the rinse basin is 100 to 300 ppm; if the same rinse solution is used, the concentration can be 1000 ppm by the fifth procedure. Clearly, fresh-rinse solutions should be used for each procedure. A double rinse reduces the Cidex® concentration in the second rinse to the order of 1 ppm. After irrigation of the joint with 1 L of saline, however, the intraarticular concentration of Cidex® is less than 1 ppm, regardless of the rinse technique (Harner, 1988).

Shelf life and toxicity issues of Cidex® and Cidex® Plus are partially overcome by a more recently introduced *ortho*-phthalaldehyde (0.55%) solution known as Cidex® OPA ASP; division of Ethicon Cidex. OPA has efficacy against bacteria, fungi, and viruses; works with a 12-minute soak time at room temperature; and requires no mixing or activation. Additionally, the product is less volatile (reduced vapor pressure) and less corrosive to endoscopes than Cidex®. It has a 75-day shelf life at room temperature after opening.

---

[t]ASP, Advanced Sterilization Products, division of Ethicon, a Johnson & Johnson Company, 33 Technology Drive, Irvine, CA 92618. Tel: (800) 595-0200. www.aspjj.com/us/

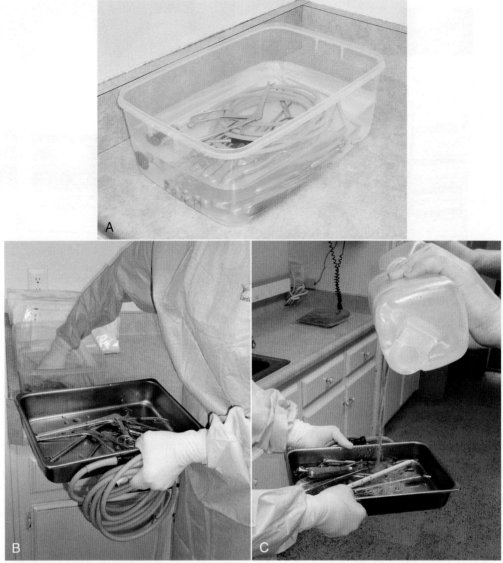

Figure 2-42 Cidex (dialdehyde) cold soak sterilization and rinsing of instruments. **A,** Instruments are immersed in Cidex for 10 to 12 minutes. Stopcocks and cannulated instruments need to be in the open position. **B** and **C,** Rinsing instruments with sterile water or saline after removal from Cidex reduces glutaraldehyde residue to safe levels.

Toxicity and safety issues have reduced the use of Cidex in many practices. An effective and less toxic alternative is the peracetic acid Steris™ system,[u] which uses a liquid peracetic acid (35%), acetic acid (40%), hydrogen peroxide (6.5%), and sulfuric acid (1%) soak, followed by a water rinse, for a total of four cycles in a closed system, to provide sterile and virtually dry equipment for arthroscopy (Fig. 2-43). Each sterilizing run has a chemical indicator strip (minimum 1500 ppm) included to verify the sterility of the instruments. The disadvantages are the cost of the unit, and the process requires 30 minutes rather than 10 minutes to complete, so emergency sterilization for a dropped instrument still requires Cidex.

Larger clinics have been moving away from ethylene oxide sterilization for arthroscopes and other heat and moisture sensitive instruments by using low-temperature hydrogen peroxide gas plasma sterilizers (Sterrad®; Advanced Sterilization Products, Ethicon Inc.). Systems vary in size from portable units suitable for operating room support areas (Fig. 2-44) to larger units designed for central sterilizing facilities. Sterrad units can sterilize a wide range of instruments, including multiple single-channel flexible endoscopes, cameras, rigid arthroscopes, light cords, batteries, and power drills. Cycle times can be as little as 28 minutes for nonlumen endoscopes and arthroscopes. Instruments are exposed to vapor phase concentrated hydrogen peroxide and come out dry. Instrument cases and trays need to be perforated but can be wrapped in paper or linen drapes, similar to ethylene oxide and autoclave systems. With the growing concern over ethylene oxide toxicity, Sterrad® sterilizers are an increasingly popular solution. Availability of Sterrad systems to the veterinary market is still limited.

In many parts of Europe, the use of Cidex® is no longer permitted. A safe alternative for soaking sterilization is MedDis™ instrument disinfectant,[v] which relies on halogenated tertiary

[u] Steris 20, Steris Corp, 5960 Heisley Road, Mentor, OH 44060. Tel: (800) 548-4873. www.steris.com

[v] Medichem International, PO Box 237, Seven Oaks, Kent TN15 O2J, UK. http://www.medi-mark.co.uk/

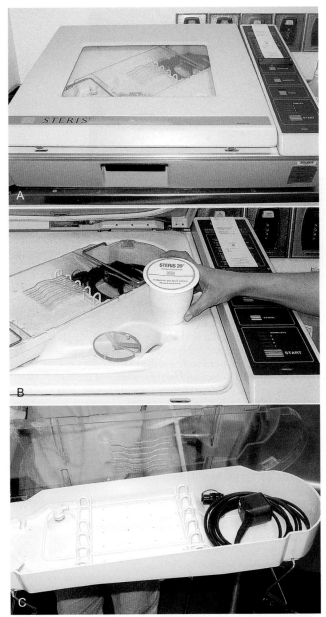

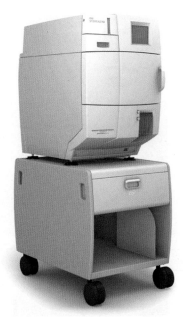

Figure 2-44 Sterrad NX gas plasma sterilizer. Temperature- and moisture-sensitive equipment that once had to be gas sterilized in ethylene oxide can now be sterilized in hydrogen peroxide gas plasma sterilizers (Sterrad®; Advanced Sterilization Products, Ethicon Inc.). Cycle times can be as short as 28 minutes. Availability to veterinary market is limited.

Figure 2-43 Steris™ cold sterilization system. **A,** The Steris™ sterilization system uses peracetic acid, acetic acid, hydrogen peroxide, and sulfuric acid to sterilize instruments, followed by extensive water rinses. **B,** The items to be sterilized are placed in the tray, and the sterilizing agents are added in a closed draw-off cup each time. The cycle takes 30 minutes. **C,** The sterile items are relatively dry after completion of the cycle.

amines, hexamethylene biquanide hydrochloride, ethyl alcohol, dodecyclamine, and sulfonic acid to sterilize instruments. This solution is diluted to 5% and is then bactericidal, fungicidal, and virucidal after a 10-minute exposure. It is tuberculocidal and sporicidal within 30 minutes. Shelf life after activation is 14 days. It also has safety advantages in that it is nonirritant, nonfuming, and noncorrosive, and there have been no reported effects on metal or glass endoscope components.

Surgical Assistants

Because of the unique instrument requirements and the need to have a smooth sequential system during the operation, scrub nurses or technicians participating in operative arthroscopy must be especially trained. It cannot be overemphasized

that an assistant totally familiar with the instruments and technique is as essential as a competent surgeon.

Drapes

Drapes and draping systems tend to be determined by the surgeon's preference, cost of drapes, and safety and comfort zone required for minimal or extensive draping by the surgeon. Drapes can vary from simple reusable cloth drapes to complete disposable packages that contain a drape large enough to cover the horse, several small drapes for preliminary draping, several tape strips to bind the drape to the limb, and a table cover to prepare the instrument table. The use of adhesive sticky drapes (Ioban, 3M[w]) is an effective method to provide a wide, sterile, impervious field for arthroscopy. Cloth drapes are generally unsatisfactory due to the lack of resistance to strike-through by the large volumes of liquid used in arthroscopy. Application of an adhesive drape followed by one or two surrounding impervious drapes, and finally a large disposable drape, is standard (Fig. 2-45). For simplicity, a large sticky drape provides a good sterile field to which an experienced user can then apply a large disposable drape directly, to complete the sterile setup. It is critical that the surgeon and assistants not drag the disposable drape across the prepared joint (double shuffling) or the inner surface of the disposable drape that has contacted the unprepared surfaces of the limb will then rest over the joint to be operated. Inexperienced users should add a quadrant of additional draping between the adhesive drape and the large arthroscopy drape to increase the margin of safety. Large drape systems are manufactured by Gepco[x] and Veterinary Surgical Resources.[y] Purpose-designated

[w]3M Orthopedics Products Division, 3M Center, St. Paul, MN 55144-1000. Tel: (888) 364-3577. www.mmm.com
[x]Gepco, General Econopak Inc., 1725 North 6th Street, Philadelphia, PA 19122. Tel: (888) 871-8568. www.generaleconopak.com
[y]Veterinary Surgical Resources, Inc., PO Box 71, Darlington, MD 21034. Tel: (800) 354-8501. www.vetsurgicalresources.com

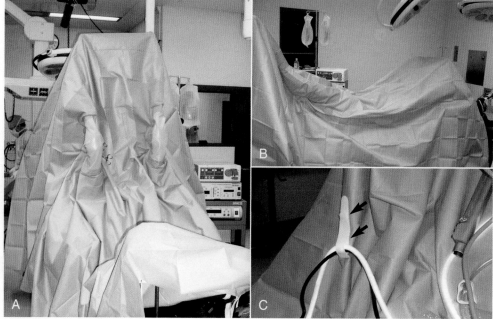

Figure 2-45 Arthroscopic drapes with self-contained rubber dam and velcro cable and line tie-downs. **A,** Application of large drapes with separate rubber dams for each joint provides an expansive integrated sterile field (Surgical Resources). Both carpi have been draped with a sheet that includes coverage of the head and caudally to cover the torso. **B,** Bilateral arthroscopy drape on the hocks showing selective draping of the hock region and broad coverage of the rest of the horse. **C,** Unilateral and bilateral drapes from Surgical Resources include a Velcro closure *(arrows)* for securing lines without the need for clamps. Many packs include smaller drapes and initial table cover.

arthroscopy drapes from Surgical Resources now have Velcro tie-downs to accommodate the light cable, video cord, and fluid line (see Fig. 2-45). Some arthroscopy packs also contain disposable gowns. In general, most manufacturers offer a range of pack contents, so individual preferences can be accommodated. Clearly, the complete systems lack nothing but can be expensive (up to $102). The arthroscopy drape pack can be ordered for unilateral or bilateral arthroscopy, the latter providing two rubber-dammed areas, one per joint, with 30 to 38 inches between them. These can be cumbersome to apply but provide exceptional large sterile fields without the need for other body sheets. The authors also vary the type of draping to the situation; numerous drapes around the foot will limit access for coffin joint arthroscopy or digital sheath tenoscopy, whereas full draping systems are easy to apply around the stifle or hock, and provide ready access to all the joints comprising these articulations.

Care and Maintenance of Equipment

Most care and maintenance issues should be covered by instructions with individual equipment items. However, repair of arthroscopes is a costly and all too frequent concern in equine arthroscopy. All arthroscope vendors repair their own telescopes. However, the cost can vary (depending on the extent of damage) from $1,000 to $2,200 (almost the cost of a new arthroscope). Third-party vendors repair arthroscopes from most manufacturers. One of the larger repair companies is Instrument Makar.[z] The cost of repair generally ranges from $350 to $600. However, the repair vendor should always provide a free assessment of damage and a quote for repair. A more informed decision for repair or replacement can then be made. Sharpening of instruments can be done by instrument vendors or independent companies.

[z]Instrument Makar, Division of Smith & Nephew Inc, Endoscopy Division, 150 Minuteman Road, Andover, MA 01810. Tel: (800) 343-5717. www.endoscopy1.com

REFERENCES

Bacarese-Hamilton IA, Bhamra M, Jackson AM: Arthroscopic meniscal shavers: a potential hazard of sepsis, *Ann R Coll Surg Engl* 73:70–71, 1991.

Bergstrom R, Gillquist J: The use of an infusion pump in arthroscopy, *Arthroscopy* 2:41–45, 1986.

Brown Jr CH: Producing still images in arthroscopy, *Arthroscopy* 5: 87–92, 1989.

Caspari RB: Current development of instrumentation for arthroscopy, *Clin Sports Med* 6:619–636, 1987.

Dolk T, Augustini B-G: Three irrigation systems for motorized arthroscopic surgery: a comparative experimental and clinical study, *Arthroscopy* 5:307–314, 1989.

Ekman EF, Poehling GG: Principles of arthroscopy and wrist arthroscopy equipment, *Hand Clin* 10:557–566, 1994.

Eriksson E, Sebik A: Arthroscopy and arthroscopic surgery in a gas versus a fluid medium, *Orthop Clin North Am* 13:293–298, 1982.

Frisbie DD: Arthroscopic documentation, *Clin Tech Equine Pract* 1:270–275, 2002.

Frisbie DD, Barrett MF, McIlwraith CW, Ullmer J: Diagnostic arthroscopy of the stifle joint using a needle arthroscope in standing horses: a novel procedure, *Vet Surg*, 2013 In Press.

Graf BK, Clancy Jr WG: Motorized arthroscopic instruments: a review, *Arthroscopy* 3:199–204, 1987.

Gross RM: Arthroscopy. Basic setup and equipment, *Orthop Clin North Am* 24:5–18, 1993.

Harner CD: Cidex induced synovitis, *Proc 34th Ann Mtg Orthopaedic Research Society* 18:332, 1988.

Jackson DW, Ovadia DN: Videoarthroscopy: present and future developments, *Arthroscopy* 1:108–115, 1985.

Jager R: Technical and instrumental requirements of arthroscopy of the knee joint, *Endoscopy* 12:261–264, 1980.

Johnson DH: Basic science in digital imaging: storage and retrieval, *Arthroscopy* 18:648–653, 2002.

Johnson LL, Shneider DA, Austin MD, et al.: Two percent glutaraldehyde: a disinfectant in arthroscopy and arthroscopic surgery, *J Bone Joint Surg Am* 64:237–239, 1982.

Johnson RG, Herbert MA, Wright S, et al.: The response of articular cartilage to the in vivo replacement of synovial fluid with saline, *Clin Orthop* 285–292, 1983.

Kosy JD, Schranz PJ, Toms AD, Eyres KS, Mandalia VI: The use of radiofrequency energy for arthroscopic chondroplasty in the knee, *Arthroscopy* 27:695–703, 2011.

Lee EW, Paulos LE, Warren RF: Complications of thermal energy in knee surgery – Part II, *Clin Sports Med* 21:753–763, 2002.

Lu Y, Edwards III RB, Cole BJ, Markel MD: Thermal chondroplasty with radiofrequency energy. An in vitro comparison of bipolar and monopolar radiofrequency devices, *Am J Sports Med* 29:42–49, 2001.

Lu Y, Hayashi K, Hecht P: The effect of monopolar radiofrequency energy on partial-thickness defects of articular cartilage, *Arthroscopy* 16:527–536, 2000.

McDonald R: Rigid endoscopes. Proper care and maintenance, *AORN J* 39:1236–1242, 1984.

McGinty JB: Photography and arthroscopy. In Casscells SW, editor: *Arthroscopy: diagnostic and surgical practice*, Philadelphia, 1984, Lea & Febiger.

Medvecky MJ, Ong BC, Rokito AS, Sherman OH: Thermal capsular shrinkage: basic science and clinical applications, *Arthroscopy* 17:624–635, 2001.

Menes T, Spivak H: Laparoscopy: searching for the proper insufflation gas, *Surg Endosc* 14:1050–1056, 2000.

Minkoff J: Arthroscopy – its value and problems, *Orthop Clin North Am* 8:683–706, 1977.

Morgan CD: Fluid delivery systems for arthroscopy, *Arthroscopy* 3:288–291, 1987.

Neuhaus SJ, Gupta A, Watson DI: Helium and other alternative insufflation gases for laparoscopy, *Surg Endosc* 15:553–560, 2001.

Noyes FR, Good ES, Hoffman SD: The effect of flexion angle on pressure–volume relationships in the human knee. *Proc Ann Mtg AANA*, 1987.

Ogilvie-Harris DJ, Weisleder L: Fluid pump systems for arthroscopy: a comparison of pressure control versus pressure and flow control, *Arthroscopy* 11:591–595, 1995.

Oretorp N, Elmersson S: Arthroscopy and irrigation control, *Arthroscopy* 2:46–50, 1986.

Poehling GG: Instrumentation for small joints: the arthroscope, *Arthroscopy* 4:45–46, 1988.

Polousky JD, Hedman TP, Vangsness Jr CT: Electrosurgical methods for arthroscopic meniscectomy: a review of the literature, *Arthroscopy* 16:813–821, 2000.

Reagan BF, McInerny VK, Treadwell BV, Zarins B, Mankin HJ: Irrigating solutions for arthroscopy. A metabolic study, *J Bone Joint Surg Am* 65:629–631, 1983.

Sherk HH, Vangsness CT, Thabit III G, Jackson RW: Electromagnetic surgical devices in orthopaedics. Lasers and radiofrequency, *J Bone Joint Surg Am* 84–A: 675–681, 2002.

Smith CF, Trauner KB: Arthroscopic laser surgery: a revisitation, *Am J Knee Surg* 12:192–195, 1999.

Spahn G, Klinger HM, Muckley T, Hofmann GO: Four-year results from a randomized controlled study of knee chondroplasty with concomitant medial meniscectomy: mechanical debridement versus radiofrequency chondroplasty, *Arthroscopy* 24:410–415, 2008.

Straehley D: The effect of arthroscopic irrigating solutions on cartilage and synovium, *Trans 31st Ann Mtg ORS* 15:260, 1985.

Takahashi T, Yamamoto H: Development and clinical application of a flexible arthroscopy system, *Arthroscopy* 13:42–50, 1997.

Uthamanthil RK, Edwards RB, Lu Y, Manley PA, Athanasiou KA, Markel MD: In vivo study on the short-term effect of radiofrequency energy on chondromalacic patellar cartilage and its correlation with calcified cartilage pathology in an equine model, *J Orthop Res* 24:716–724, 2006.

Voloshin I, Morse KR, Allred CD, Bissell SA, Maloney MD, Dehaven KE: Arthroscopic evaluation of radiofrequency chondroplasty of the knee, *Am J Sports Med* 35:1702–1707, 2007.

Whelan JM, Jackson DW: Videoarthroscopy: review and state of the art, *Arthroscopy* 8:311–319, 1992.

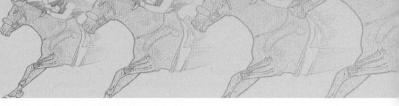

CHAPTER 3

General Technique and Diagnostic Arthroscopy

GENERAL TECHNIQUE FOR ARTHROSCOPY

The general principles of arthroscopic technique are presented with the middle carpal (intercarpal) joint used as an example. These principles are applicable to all diarthrodial joints, as well as arthroscopic evaluation of tendon sheaths and bursae. The specific portals for both the arthroscope and the instruments, along with the specific maneuvers in the different joints, are discussed in the individual chapters. Throughout this chapter the term *arthroscopic* is used to designate procedures in all synovial cavities and, in the interest of brevity, *articular* may also refer to tendon sheaths and bursae.

Preoperative Evaluation of the Patient

Every patient undergoing an arthroscopic procedure for a known or suspected intraarticular problem must first be evaluated by history, physical examination, and radiographic examination. Ultrasonographic evaluation of tendon sheaths and bursae are equally important and may be contributory to the preoperative evaluation of joints. Increasingly, other imaging modalities such as magnetic resonance imaging (MRI) and computed tomography (CT) may provide further useful information. However, it should be noted that direct visualization and palpation remain the best techniques for assessing the surfaces of structures bordering or within synovial cavities. To date, correlative studies between imaging modalities are lacking. In humans arthroscopic evaluation of abnormalities identified by MRI and CT is common, but incidental findings of no clinical relevance are commonplace and such evaluations should not be considered a substitute for conventional clinical evaluation of the patient (Dandy, 2010).

Preoperative Preparation

The patient is prepared for arthroscopy in the same fashion as for any other aseptic orthopedic procedure, and these principles are well recognized. Although the vast majority of arthroscopy is performed under general anesthesia, a few procedures have been performed under standing sedation and local analgesia (Elce & Richardson, 2002). Short skin incisions, multiple entries of instruments, and frequent use of percutaneous needles raise the potential for introducing hair. The authors' practices range from close clipping (e.g., No. 40 blades) to shaving. On the basis of a small study in horses evaluating skin bacterial flora before and after aseptic preparation of clipped and non-clipped arthrocentesis sites, it has been concluded that aseptic preparation of the skin over the midcarpal and distal interphalangeal joints can be accomplished without hair removal in horses (Hague et al, 1997). However, shaving of the arthroscopy sites precludes the likelihood of hair going into the joint at arthroscopy. Aseptic preparation of the skin and surgical scrub for the surgeon is routinely done with either povidine iodine or chlorhexidine gluconate. The iodophors have several disadvantages, including diminished effectiveness in the presence of organic matter, a high incidence of dermal irritation, unreliable residual activity, and toxicity (Phillips et al, 1991; Rosenberg et al, 1976). Chlorhexidine has a broad spectrum of antimicrobial activity, has good residual activity (even in the presence of organic material), and causes minimal skin irritation (Stubbs et al, 1996). However, it should be noted that in a study comparing the efficacy of povidone iodine with chlorhexidine as surgical scrub solutions, both povidone iodine and

chlorhexidine were equally effective in decreasing bacterial numbers on the skin, given a variety of contamination levels present before the scrub procedure (Wan et al, 1997).

The authors perform all arthroscopic surgical procedures in the carpus, dorsal fetlock, tarsus, and stifle joints, with the horse in dorsal recumbency, except in isolated instances when the facilities do not allow this positioning.

Although there are numerous individual draping products and techniques, because of the fluid involved, an impervious draping system is mandatory (Fig. 3-1). There is also merit in the use of adhesive barrier drapes, although surgeons should be cognizant of the potential to push such material through skin portals. Adhesion is variable, but Ioban[a] is currently considered to be the best available.

Arthroscope Insertion and Positioning

When draping is complete, light and camera cables and the fluid ingress line can be connected and secured to the drapes. Fluid is run through the latter to eliminate air and can be used to provide fluid for inflation. If a sterile sleeve is used over the camera, this should be applied with a watertight seal created around the eyepiece of the arthroscope.

Dependent on the individual cavity under investigation, a skin portal for insertion of the arthroscope may be made before or following distension. In some situations such as the fetlock joint, distension aids appropriate location of the arthroscopic portal, aids insertion of the cannula, and reduces the potential for iatrogenic damage to internal tissues during this process. In the carpal joints, the skin incisions for the arthroscopic and instrument portals are made before distension, one between the extensor carpi radialis and common digital extensor tendons for a lateral portal and the second medial to the extensor carpi radialis tendon for a medial portal, to avoid penetration of those tendon sheaths. The incision should be 6 to 10 mm in length and should always penetrate the periarticular tissues and joint capsule (Fig. 3-2). A No. 11 or No. 15 scalpel blade is used for both incisions. The joint is then distended (Fig. 3-3). The incision through the joint capsule is then made as a straight perpendicular stab. A triangular incision, with its apex being the joint penetration and base the skin incision, should minimize accumulation of extravasated fluids in periarticular soft tissues.

A conical obturator is placed within the arthroscopic cannula, and this combination is used to insert the cannula through the fibrous joint capsule. The cannula should follow the perpendicular trajectory of the portal created. It is inserted through the fibrous joint capsule with hand pressure and a gentle twisting motion (Fig. 3-4). Directional and insertion control, avoiding sudden entry and potential for intraarticular excoriation, is given by using the thumb of the noninserting hand as a friction bridge. Only when the cannula is within the joint should the trajectory be changed from perpendicular, to locate the cannula at a more distant position to the portal before the obturator is replaced with the arthroscope. The light cable and ingress fluid system are then attached and the cavity is distended (Fig. 3-5). The authors no longer use the sharp trocar for insertion of the

[a]3M, St. Paul, MN, USA

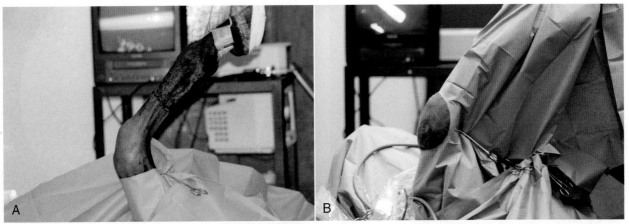

Figure 3-1 Limb suspended for arthroscopic surgery **(A)** and draped with impervious drapes before bilateral carpal arthroscopic surgery. **(B)** The horse is positioned in dorsal recumbency.

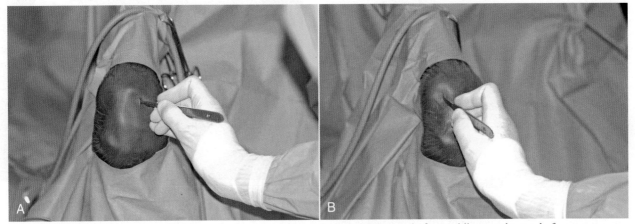

Figure 3-2 Skin incisions being made for lateral **(A)** and medial **(B)** portals for middle carpal joint before joint distention.

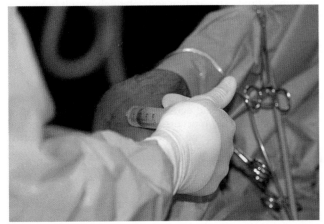

Figure 3-3 Distention of middle carpal joint with sterile fluid before entry of arthroscope.

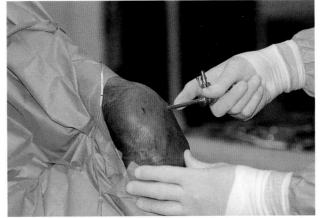

Figure 3-4 Insertion of arthroscopic sheath with conical obturator through fibrous capsule.

arthroscopic sleeve in any joint. Figure 3-6 illustrates creation of the medial instrument portal into the joint under arthroscopic visualization.

Frequently, some degree of lavage is necessary to optimize visibility and systematic assessment of the cavity. In some locations (e.g., the carpal joints) this is readily achieved by insertion of the small egress cannula through a previously created instrument portal (Fig. 3-7). In others, this may be achieved by insertion of percutaneous needles allowing later creation of instrument portals at sites relevant to subsequently identified lesions. This process will require ingress fluid levels to be adjusted in line with the bore of the egress. It is important to note that all holes in the egress cannula must be within the joint cavity; if holes are outside the joint in the subcutaneous tissues this will promote rapid extracapsular extravasation of fluid.

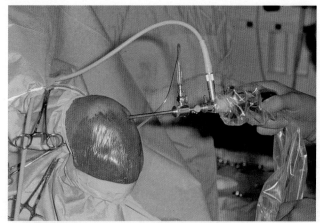

Figure 3-5 Arthroscope inserted and light cable and fluid ingress line are attached.

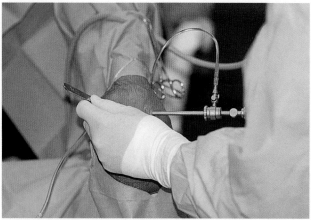

Figure 3-6 Completion of positioning of arthroscope within the middle carpal joint and medial instrument portal into joint being completed.

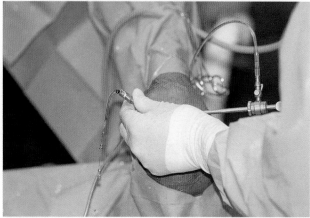

Figure 3-7 Placement of egress cannula in the joint to allow flushing.

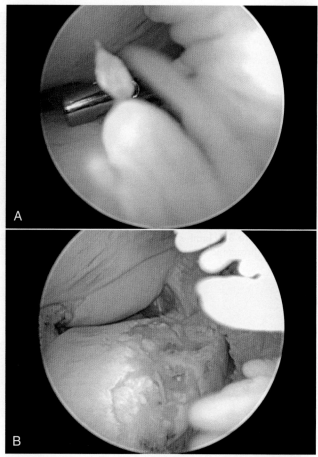

Figure 3-8 Arthroscopic view of same area of a middle carpal joint with egress cannula open **(A)** and closed **(B)**. Note the difference in degree of interposition of synovial villi in the visual field.

Once the view is clear, the stopcock on the egress cannula is closed and/or the egress cannula is withdrawn. Operation with an open cannula causes villi to obstruct the visual field (Fig. 3-8). Once an egress cannula is closed or removed it is important that the flow rate (when using a flow regulated system of fluid administration) is lowered to a minimal level. The requirement for joint distention in equine arthroscopy is

quite high, but it is important to be aware that pressure can exacerbate fluid extravasation and potentially result in rupture of the joint capsule. This has been recognized in the human knee at about 200 mm Hg pressure (Noyes & Spievack, 1982). For these reasons the authors do not recommend the use of constant pressure fluid administration systems. The choices of fluid systems were discussed in Chapter 2.

During arthroscopic surgery, once a large instrument or fragment passes through a portal in the joint capsule, some degree of constant fluid egress is unavoidable. Consequently, some villi interposition occurs. For this reason, the diagnostic examination must be completed before surgical removal of large fragments from the joint. For the same reason, a small (2.7 to 3 mm) egress cannula is used for an initial flush. This avoids a large instrument portal and the continuous fluid flow during the initial examination.

The arthroscopist should be continually reminded that visualization is enhanced by rotating the arthroscope. Simply by rotating the arthroscope (without changing its position), the visual field of view is greatly increased. This generally obviates the need for a 70-degree arthroscope.

Arthroscopic Surgery and the Principle of Triangulation

Although the details of arthroscopic surgery for each joint are presented in later chapters, the principle of arthroscopic surgery needs introduction here because the use of both the egress cannula and the arthroscopic probe are important to the diagnostic examination, and they are used according to the principle of triangulation.

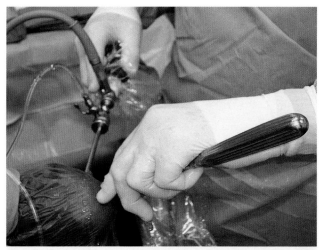

Figure 3-9 Use of probe to palpate under arthroscopic visualization.

Two basic techniques have been developed for arthroscopic surgery. The first involves an operating arthroscope (Carson, 1984; O'Connor, 1977), which has a channel through which instruments are passed down the optical line of the instrument; the technique has not been used in equine surgery and therefore is not discussed in this text.

The second technique is triangulation, which involves bringing one or more operating instruments through separate portals and into the visual field of the arthroscope with the tips of the instrument and the arthroscope forming the apex of a triangle. It is the common technique used in human arthroscopic surgery (Jackson, 1983). The principle is illustrated in Figures 3-9 and 4-20 and is used to handle all of the various surgical requirements in equine joints. It is the basic technique to master for effective diagnostic and surgical arthroscopy. To be able to use this technique effectively, the surgeon must develop the bimanual psychomotor skills of manipulating two objects in a confined space while using monocular vision, which eliminates the convergence that provides depth perception.

For arthroscopic surgery, instrument portals are made in various positions, depending on the joint and the site of the lesions. Cannulas or sleeves are rarely used at instrument portals for reasons mentioned in Chapter 2. To create an instrument portal, a skin incision is made followed by a stab through the joint capsule with the use of a No. 11 or 15 scalpel blade. These techniques have been noted previously (see Fig. 3-6).

Use of the Probe in Diagnostic Arthroscopy

For effective diagnostic arthroscopy, the use of a probe through an instrument portal is important, both to evaluate defects that cannot be discerned with vision alone and to provide an index of size by comparison of the lesions with the probe (see Fig. 3-9). In the carpus, the egress cannula is often used as a probe to palpate lesions. This technique is a shortcut, often eliminating the need for another instrument insertion. On the other hand, the blunt, hooked probe is important in assessing suspect articular cartilage in cases of osteochondritis dissecans, and its use is a routine part of the procedure. Elsworth et al (1986) noted, "arthroscopy without the use of the probe is an incomplete investigation," and that routine use of the probe is essential in training for arthroscopic surgery.

Postarthroscopic Irrigation and Closure

When the arthroscopic procedure is completed, using an open egress cannula and pumping fluid through the joints effectively flushes debris from the joint. Typically, the larger, 4.5-mm cannula is used so that all debris is removed (in the femoropatellar joint a larger 6-mm cannula is used).

No sutures are required to close the joint capsule portals. One or two sutures are placed in the skin incisions. One suture is usually sufficient. The authors prefer a simple interrupted pattern to a cruciate pattern, to avoid inverting the skin edge. In human arthroscopy, some authors have made a case for not suturing skin incisions (Williamson & Copeland, 1988). Cosmetic advantages have been proposed, and some individuals believe hematoma or stitch abscesses are less likely to occur. Suturing is considered the safer alternative in the horse, although adherent Steri-Strips are gaining popularity. Specific postoperative management is discussed in the individual joint chapters.

DIAGNOSTIC ARTHROSCOPY

In the 28 years that have elapsed since the first edition of this book (McIlwraith, 1984), arthroscopic surgery has become the norm. Techniques have developed for almost all synovial surgery to the point that there are now no practicing surgeons who would consider an arthrotomy for any surgical interference other than in exceptional circumstances. Of equal, but often overlooked, importance has been the contribution of arthroscopic evaluation to the diagnosis and pathogenesis of synovial-based lameness in horses. This in turn has led to the development of more rational treatment protocols. Examples are found in each successive edition of the book highlighted, particularly in the last two editions, by identification of lesions involving synovial soft tissues. Nonetheless, it should always be remembered that arthroscopy is an adjunctive diagnostic technique; it does not replace traditional methods including palpation, radiography, ultrasonography, etc. The hazards of not evaluating a joint radiographically before arthroscopy have long been understood in man (Joyce & Mankin, 1983) and strict adherence to such principles cannot be overemphasized. It has also been demonstrated recently that the use of MRI for precise grading of the articular cartilage in osteoarthritis (OA) is limited and that diagnostic arthroscopy is of outstanding value when a grading of the cartilage is crucial for a definitive decision regarding the therapeutic options in patients with OA (von Engelhardt et al, 2012).

Arthroscopy is invaluable in assessing synovial membrane, articular cartilage, intraarticular ligaments, and menisci (in the stifle). The ability to perform diagnostic arthroscopy of parts of the equine femorotibial joints has furnished considerable amounts of new information, and much progress has been made in this area since the last edition of this text.

Knowledge of Normal Anatomy

Before valid interpretations of changes in the joint can be made, the surgeon must have a good knowledge of arthroscopic anatomy. This prerequisite, in turn, means relearning joint anatomy, which constitutes the first learning step in arthroscopy, be it diagnostic or surgical. It introduces concepts not reported in anatomic texts including variations of the morphology of intraarticular ligaments and plicae and in the distribution of synovium (Fig. 3-10). There is also a dynamic component to arthroscopic anatomy. The appearance and consistency of some tissues vary according to joint position. Additionally, evaluation of the latter involves palpation, generally with an arthroscopic probe. This demands a working knowledge of variables including the thickness of articular cartilage, which varies between joints but also in location within an individual joint. Failure to recognize normal variations in morphology is a common pitfall for the inexperienced surgeon. Another pitfall is overinterpretation because of magnification.

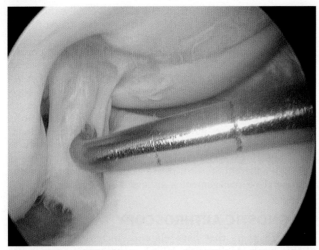

Figure 3-10 Use of probe to palpate the medial palmar intercarpal ligament and distinguish between the lateral and medial portions.

Observation of Synovial Fluid

Frequently the appearance of synovial fluid will be a useful guide to intrasynovial pathologic change. The information is subjective and crude because observations are generally made on drops of fluid at the time of initial joint distension or after inflation and usually during preevaluation lavage of the cavity. Sanguineous fluid suggests acute or recurrent tissue disruption, or both, while xanthochromia of reducing degrees follows as blood pigment is removed. Intrasynovial debris can vary between large osteochondral or chondral fragments to fine sandlike particles suspended in the irrigating fluid. As the joint is distended, loose bodies will usually gravitate to dependent parts of the cavity determined in large part by the positions of the horse and the limb; this is frequently consistent in individual joints (e.g., the suprapatellar cul-de-sac of the femoropatellar joint). Close inspection of these sites is important whenever free floating material is present or has been created during surgery, particularly at the end of procedures in order to ensure its removal. Microscopic evaluation of suspended debris has been reported in human knee arthroscopy (Mori, 1979) but has not recently been pursued.

Evaluation of Synovial Membrane (Synovium)

The distribution of villus or non-villus synovium is consistent for each cavity. Synovium can act as a sentinel of synovial insult, but it has a relatively narrow range of visible change. Depending on the insult, synovium will respond throughout the cavity but this is usually the greatest adjacent to primary lesions, particularly when these involve areas of villus synovium. These features can be visualized better with arthroscopy performed with fluid distention. Under gas distention, use of arthrotomy incisions, or at postmortem, villi are not suspended and their features are less distinct (Bass, 1984). Transillumination and magnification of the arthroscopy image enhance assessment of villi, including information regarding villous vascularity. The magnification of the arthroscope also facilitates definition. The degree of magnification varies, however, depending on the distance of the object from the end of arthroscope. If the end of the arthroscope is 1 mm from the object, the magnification is 10 times; at a 1 cm distance, no magnification is noted (Crane, 1984). Use of a magnifying arthroscope (microarthroscopy) has been reported in humans (Fizziero, 1986) and horses (Serena et al, 2005), both with and without use of vital stains. Excellent images have been obtained, but clinical application is pending. Recognition and knowledge of normal anatomy is critical, and the presence and morphology of normal synovial plicae and the normal intraarticular ligaments need to be known (see Fig. 3-10).

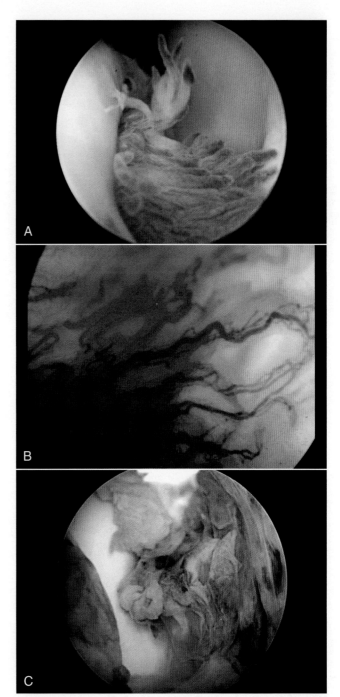

Figure 3-11 A, Hyperemic synovial villi in a case of acute synovitis of the carpus. **B,** View of acute synovitis using magnifying arthroscope. **C,** Severe fibrinous synovitis associated with penetrating injury and focal fracture of lateral trochlear ridge of talus.

Recording the morphologic features of synovial villi in the horse was one of the first publications on equine arthroscopy (McIlwraith & Fessler, 1978). The surgeon needs to recognize the many variations of normal synovium that exist and the degree of change that can occur with minimal clinical compromise. Synovitis manifests in a number of forms that have yet to be completely characterized:
1. Hyperemia, which is typical of peracute synovitis (Fig. 3-11A and B). It may be accompanied by some degree of edema and fibrin deposition (see Fig. 3-11C)
2. Petechiation, which usually occurs at the tips of villi in acute synovitis

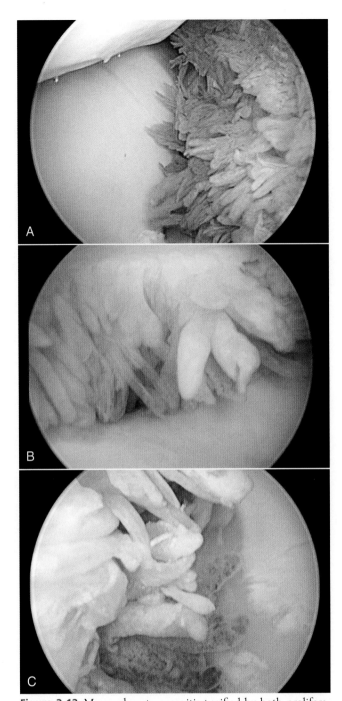

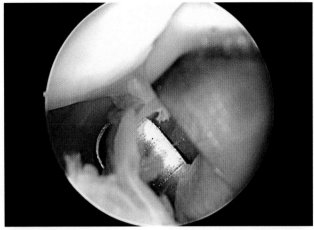

Figure 3-13 The use of a motorized resector to remove proliferated synovial membrane. This is most commonly done for enhancement of visualization.

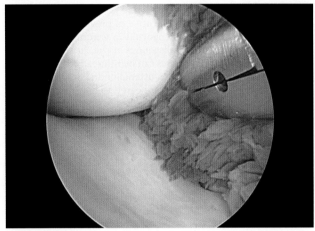

Figure 3-14 Brown discoloration (believed to be hemosiderosis) in antebrachiocarpal joint with recurrent hemarthrosis and with a synovial biopsy being obtained.

Figure 3-12 More subacute synovitis typified by both proliferation and thickening of synovial villi, which are still hyperemic **(A)** to more chronic synovitis in the dorsal aspect of the metacarpophalangeal joint (where villi are typically narrow and relatively translucent) **(B)** and medial aspect of the middle carpal joint **(C).**

3. Thickening of villi apparently by fluid accumulation (frequently described as edematous swelling) (Fig. 3-12)
4. Apparent coalescence and increase in density of villi
5. Changes in villi morphology (e.g., cauliflower-like villi)
6. Formation of plump polypoid villi with detachment of these masses to form "rice bodies"
7. Atrophy of villi and total flattening of villous areas with fibrin deposition and adhesion formation
8. Deposits of brown pigment within villi, presumed to be hemosiderin and described as hemosiderosis (Fig. 3-13), and are thought to indicate recurrent intrasynovial hemorrhage

(not found following single hemorrhagic insults such as intraarticular fracture)
9. In the proximal aspect of the dorsal compartment of the metacarpophalangeal joint there is a synovial pad that can be thickened or enlarged, and it manifests as chronic, fibrotic proliferation (Fig. 3-14)

Reliable synovial biopsy requires arthroscopy in order for samples to be obtained from appropriate/affected areas. It has been demonstrated in humans that macroscopic signs of inflammatory activity in the synovium vary considerably within a single joint (Lindblad & Hedfors, 1985). A limited range of responses possible in synovium mean that there are limitations to the conclusions that can be drawn from its histologic evaluation (McIlwraith, 1983). Nonetheless, it is useful in the diagnosis and antimicrobial management of synovial infections.

Clots and proteinaceous material overlying, and with varying degrees of adherence to, the synovium represent marked breakdown of the synovial barrier such that high-molecular-weight (clotting) proteins access the synovial cavity. This occurs most commonly with infective processes. Occasionally there will be a synovial disruption while the underlying fibrous capsule remains intact producing a synovial hernia (Fig. 3-15). Adhesions can form between any disrupted intrasynovial surfaces, but in the horse synoviosynovial adhesions are most common. Dependent

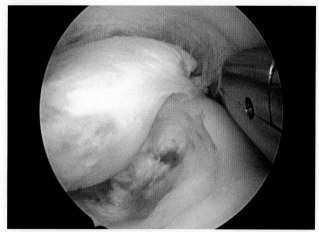

Figure 3-15 Fibrous thickening of the dorsal synovial pad (villo-nodular pad) above the medial condyle of the metacarpus.

on their stage of pathogenesis these may be fibrinoid and friable or well organized and fibrous. They are of questionable significance in themselves but are indicative of previous insult. Intrasynovial masses have been recognized in a number of cavities and result from disrupted collagenous tissue. In some, usually osteoarthritic joints, such masses can be mineralized; some have the appearance of chondral or osteochondral fragments that were first adherent to and then appeared to have been covered by synovium, whereas others, devoid of visible infrastructure, are consistent with foci of dystrophic mineralization.

The changes observed in experimentally induced synovitis illustrate the sequential nature of villous change (McIlwraith & Fessler, 1978). They also highlight that repeated examinations provide a good dynamic understanding of the synovium. In this study, in which synovitis of the middle carpal joint was induced by using filipin, there was an initial marked hyperemia. Petechiation of the villi and abnormal development of small hyperemic villi were frequent findings. Abnormal membranous fanlike and cauliflower-like villi were also seen. In more severely inflamed joints, there was fusion of villi, the presence of fibrinoid strands, and adhesion formation. Chronic fibrotic changes were noted in the later stages, with the villi becoming thicker and denser as the disease progressed.

Localized synovectomy is commonly performed to enhance visualization, particularly in the palmar compartment of the metacarpophalangeal and metatarsophalangeal joints and in the femoropatellar joint (Fig. 3-16). It is rare to do widespread synovectomy as a therapeutic procedure because of potential complications.

Disruption of the Fibrous Joint Capsule

Under normal circumstances the fibrous capsule of joints and tendon sheaths is covered by synovium, although where this is non-villus, the fibrous capsule may be visible. Varying degrees of tearing and avulsion of fibrous joint capsules may be seen as sole injuries or in combination with other lesions. Complete tears will result in abnormal outpouchings of the synovial cavity. In the acute phase, disrupted tissue is visible while chronic cases are covered by varying degrees of fibrous tissue, sometimes with a smooth, presumed non-villus synovial covering. Avulsions of the fibrous joint capsule can expose areas of bones that would normally not be visible, and again the appearance of the disrupted tissue is dependent on the chronicity of the injury (Fig. 3-17).

Plicae

Articular plicae are remnants of embryonic mesenchyme that produce folds of fibrous joint capsule. They have a

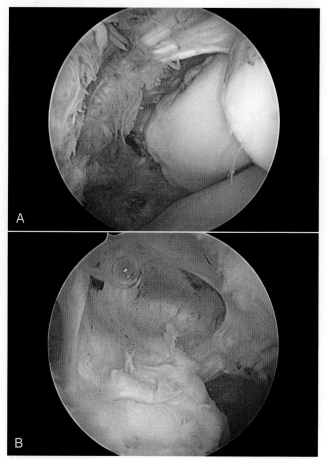

Figure 3-16 Long-standing tear of antebrachiocarpal joint capsule adjacent to intermediate carpal bone **(A)** viewed from a dorsomedial instrument portal **(B)** viewed from a dorsolateral instrument portal.

complex and controversial contribution to joint pain in man, particularly in the knee. Abnormalities are frequently seen with concomitant lesions and sometimes are the only identifiable explanation of symptoms; in these cases it is reported that resection can resolve clinical signs (Diduch et al, 2004). They have consistent locations within individual synovial cavities, but their degree of development varies among individuals. They are subject to pathologic changes consistent with other synovial tissues such as tearing and avulsion but additionally exhibit the potential for proliferation (e.g., in the dorsal compartment of the metacarpophalangeal joint in response to recurrent irritation). The visual appearance is usually the best guide to abnormality, but palpation is also contributory and use of the probe is frequently necessary to look beneath the plicae, where there may be additional lesions.

Articular Ligaments

Ligaments associated with joints may be extraarticular, periarticular or intraarticular (Getty, 1975). Extraarticular ligaments can be distinct but are frequently blended with or form part of the fibrous capsule. Periarticular ligaments lie within the fibrous capsule, and both these and intraarticular ligaments are covered by a thin layer of synovium. Intraarticular ligaments are increasingly recognized as important contributors to articular pathophysiology in many (and perhaps most) joints. They are consistent in location but exhibit morphologic variability among individuals, and appreciation of this is important in making arthroscopic assessments. Tearing and avulsion

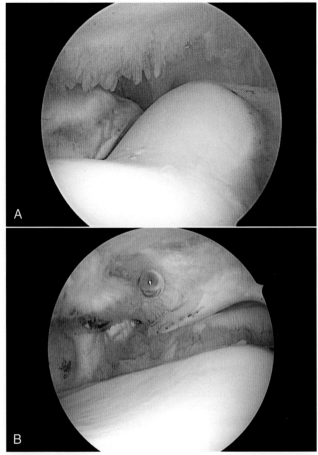

Figure 3-17 Long-standing tearing/avulsion of metacarpophalangeal joint capsule. **A,** Dorsal compartment creating an abnormally large space. **B,** Palmar compartment demonstrating avulsion from the palmar surface of the third metacarpal bone.

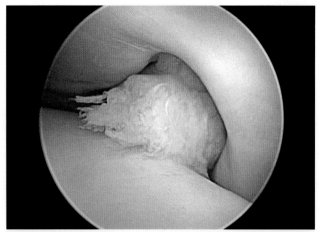

Figure 3-18 Mild tearing of the lateral portion of the medial palmar intercarpal ligament.

Evaluation of Articular Contours

The shape, congruity, and margins of articular contours in individual joints are consistent among individuals. They may be altered as a result of periarticular osteophytes or marginal modeling/remodeling or by entheseals new bone. Radiologists consider periarticular osteophytes to be pathognomonic for the presence of osteoarthritis (OA); however, equine arthroscopic experience has demonstrated the presence of periarticular osteophytes in many high-motion joints in the absence of other morphologic evidence of OA. Osteophytes by definition are found at the articular margins. Entheseal new bone is laid down at or within sites of insertion of joint capsules or articular ligaments. Because most are intracapsular, it is not usually arthroscopically visible. The transverse dorsal intercarpal ligament between the intermediate and ulnar carpal bones viewed from the middle carpal joint is an exception.

Evaluation of Articular Cartilage

Assessment of articular cartilage is central and critical to the evaluation and management of any joint disorder, and arthroscopy is the modality of choice for a direct assessment (McIlwraith & Fessler, 1978; McIlwraith, 1984 and 1990; Brommer et al, 2004 and 2006; Casscells, 1984). The principal parameters used are color, translucency, surface integrity, thickness, stiffness, resilience, and attachment to subchondral bone. Several of these features often occur together and to varying degrees in individual cases. Changes in articular cartilage are also rarely uniform throughout the joint, and it is important therefore that the surgeon comments also on location and extent of change. Reference will be made to these characteristics in discussing individual lesions, but it is frequently the composite assessment that ultimately leads to a conclusion regarding the status of the joint and hence the prognosis. Evidence of pathologic changes in the cartilage can be recognized radiographically only when lesions extend into the subchondral bone or over sufficient area to cause loss of joint space. Many situations of cartilage compromise are less severe than this, but they may still represent significant clinical problems. In man a number of classification systems have been employed in attempts to provide some objectivity to assessments (Dougadous et al, 1994; Hjelle et al, 2002). These are not readily applicable to the range of lesions found in equine arthroscopy. The authors prefer and recommend descriptions and assessments of individual parameters within each joint (Figs. 3-20 to 3-28) except for the femorotibial articulation, where systems that are modifications of the Outerbridge classification have been proposed by others (Walmsley et al, 2003; Cohen et al, 2009).

of intraarticular ligaments have been documented as the sole identifiable lesion in joints to which lameness has been localized and have been seen as parts of more complex injuries. Some (e.g., suspensory ligament branch lesions) are readily identifiable preoperatively (Minshall & Wright, 2006). Others such as the medial palmar intercarpal ligament (McIlwraith, 1992; Phillips & Wright, 1994) are only found at arthroscopy (Fig. 3-18). Tearing and avulsion usually result in extrusion of disrupted ligament fibrils into the synovial environment. The appearance of such lesions is determined by both severity and longevity of the injury.

Menisci

The importance of lesions of the fibrocartilagenous menisci and their associated ligaments to lameness in horses was first appreciated following diagnostic arthroscopy (Walmsley, 2002; Walmsley et al, 2003). To date no imaging modality provides a comprehensive evaluation of mensci, but arthroscopic evaluation of both cranial and caudal compartments of the femorotibial joints permits evaluation of the margins that (currently) are most implicated in clinical disease. Palpation and manipulation with an arthroscopic probe are critical parts of these evaluation processes. Lesions can vary from surface fibrillation, through clefts running parallel to the meniscal margins, to defects that are axially complete, resulting in hinged protuberances (Fig. 3-19). Meniscal lesions occur most commonly in the cranial compartments.

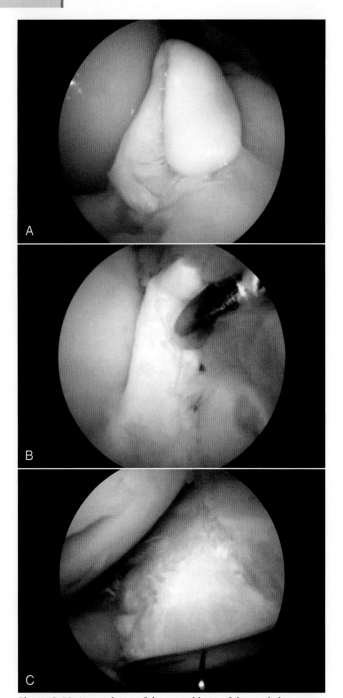

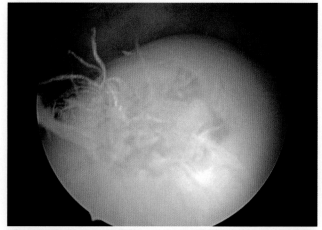

Figure 3-20 Focal fibrillation of articular cartilage on sagittal ridge of third metacarpus.

Figure 3-19 An axial tear of the cranial horn of the medial meniscus resulting in a hinged flap (**A** and **B**) and following removal of flap (**C**).

Normal articular cartilage is white and translucent. Its surfaces should be smooth and continuous over areas of articular contact. However, there are a number of sites where normal ridges or defects occur such as in the intertrochlear groove of the femur (consistent in location but varying in size and morphology). Additionally, "synovial fossae," which are areas devoid of articular cartilage and are normal, are found in various locations, but the best example is the intertrochlear groove of the talus.

There is a spectrum of pathologic change in cartilage, from fibrillation, when its surface layers disintegrate and discontinuous collagen fibrils become suspended in irrigating fluid (see Fig. 3-20), to punctate erosions and linear erosions (most commonly seen in the middle carpal joint). Focal articular defects may be caused by impingement of an adjacent incongruent

articular surface, whereas more widespread lesions can be caused by loose osseous, osteochondral, or chondral debris within the joint. Although sometimes the causative fragments can be found, these frequently become milled by the articular surfaces before arthroscopy, which precludes identification of discrete pieces. Wear lines are linear defects in articular cartilage that are aligned in the plane of motion of an individual joint (see Fig. 3-21). These are typically found in the distal dorsal metacarpus or metatarsus in the dorsal pouch of the fetlock or on the articular surfaces of the sesamoid bones in the palmar or plantar pouches. Over the years there has been much speculation regarding their etiology. Theories such as turbulent flow in synovial fluid, a minor subchondral incongruity, slight joint instability, and microscopic articular debris have been implicated. Although their etiology is unproven, they are generally considered to have a negative prognostic influence on joint function and a reduction in racing success has been associated with their presence (Kawcak & McIlwraith, 1994). Focal areas of cartilage erosion are also seen regularly in the carpus (see Fig. 3-22) and on the dorsal aspect of the medial condyle in the metacarpophalangeal joint (see Fig. 3-23).

Focal articular cartilage lesions of the medial femoral condyle have been reported as a cause of lameness in 11 horses (Schneider et al, 1997). Cartilage change was revealed at diagnostic arthroscopy despite normal radiographs. All the horses had lameness, which was improved by intraarticular analgesia. Diagnostic arthroscopy in 12 affected joints in 11 horses revealed dimpled, wrinkled, and folded cartilage, and a blunt arthroscopic probe could be inserted into the subchondral bone. In addition to focal lesions, 4 of the 11 horses had generalized damage to cartilage on the medial femoral condyle. These focal lesions on the femoral condyle were debrided. Six of seven horses with focal cartilage lesions treated by debridement recovered completely and resumed previous activity. Arthroscopic visualization of such lesions is common in horses with lameness localizing to this joint (see Fig. 3-24).

An important part of the examination of articular cartilage is subjective evaluation of the stiffness by use of an arthroscopic probe. Recognition of normal is critical. Whereas a degree of indentation is normal in the femoropatellar joint, it is not so in the thinner cartilage of the carpus or metacarpophalangeal joint. Instruments have been developed to measure stiffness objectively, but in one study in metacarpophalangeal joints (Brommer et al, 2006) the instrumentation lacked sensitivity and it was suggested it may be related to thinness and stiffness of equine cartilage compared with other species. The first author (C.W.M.) has tested the ARTSCAN® device in femoropatellar joints, where the cartilage is indeed thicker, but consistent

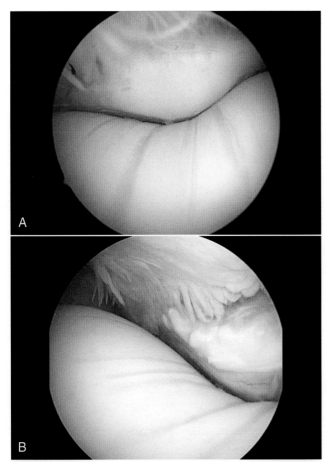

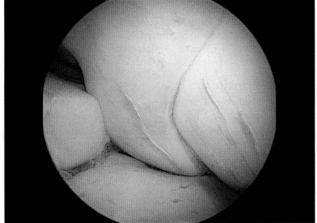

Figure 3-21 A, Multiple wear lines on the medial condyle and sagittal ridge of the third metacarpal bone found at diagnostic arthroscopy but with no primary cause identified. **B,** Partial-thickness wear lines on medial condyle and sagittal ridge of the third metacarpal bone adjacent to long-standing fragmentation of the proximal phalanx.

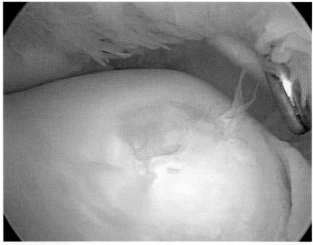

Figure 3-23 Articular cartilage defect on medial condyle of distal metacarpus in association with osteochondritis dissecans of sagittal ridge of McIII.

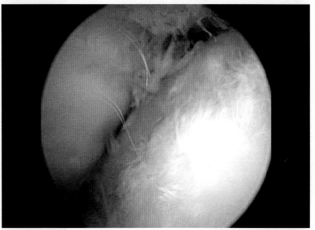

Figure 3-24 Full-thickness erosion on the medial femoral condyle in association with osteoarthritis of the femorotibial joint.

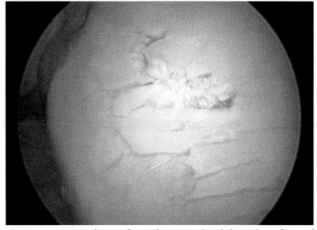

Figure 3-22 Multiple full- and partial-thickness cartilage defects in the middle carpal joint associated with loose fragments and milled debris.

Figure 3-25 Cracking of cartilage on distal lateral surface of radius.

readings could still not be obtained. Another study has revealed similar results testing femoropatellar, tarsocrural, and metacarpophalangeal joints ex vivo (Garcia-Seco et al, 2005). Variations in cartilage thickness also affect the outcome of indentation measurements (Töyräs et al, 2001). In the meantime it is

believed that experience makes indentation with the probe a fairly consistent technique for evaluating cartilage properties.

Other manifestations of articular cartilage disease are illustrated in Figures 3-25 to 3-28 and include cracking of articular cartilage, varying degrees of partial-thickness articular cartilage

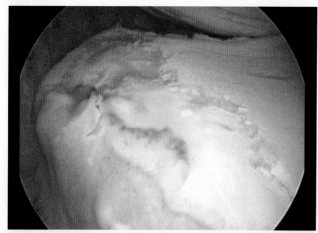

Figure 3-26 More diffuse articular cartilage erosion on the distal aspect of the radial carpal bone.

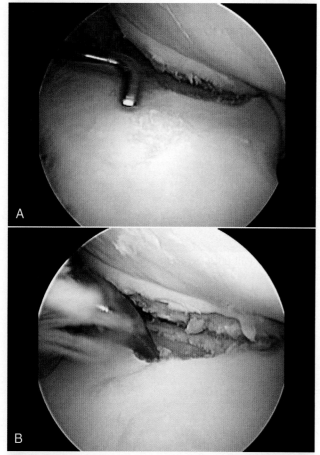

Figure 3-27 Osteochondral erosion in the palmar aspect of the visible articulation in the middle carpal joint **(A)** and micropicking of debrided defect in radial carpal bones **(B).**

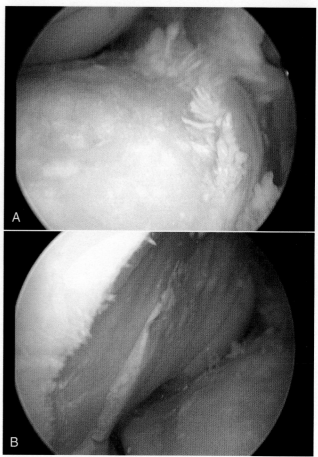

Figure 3-28 Severe full-thickness articular cartilage erosion on the surfaces of the distal radial carpal bone **(A)** and proximal third carpal bone **(B).**

erosion, and extensive osteochondral erosion. Figure 3-27 demonstrates a case of osteochondral erosion in the palmar aspect of the middle carpal joint found at diagnostic arthroscopy in the absence of radiographic change but increased technetium uptake on scintigraphy.

With the use of arthroscopy, osteochondral fractures or flaps that were not evident on radiographs are found regularly (see Chapters 4 to 8). The integrity of attachment between articular cartilage and subchondral bone is critical to joint function. Clinically, separation can occur through the junction of mineralized cartilage and subchondral bone or at the tide mark of mineralized and nonmineralized cartilage. All loose flaps or fragments need to be removed. Subchondral bone disease is a common lesion found at diagnostic arthroscopy. In some instances it may be predicted by a radiograph (Fig. 3-29), but, as detailed in Chapter 4, there are multiple sites where lesions can only be identified at arthroscopy.

Surgical Principles

General principles of arthroscopic treatments are based on the pathobiology and healing of articular and other synovial tissues. Current concepts could be summarized as (1) viable, mechanically stable tissues are required for primary healing; (2) healing of unstable fragments is slow and incomplete (because these fragments are initially the product of pathologic bone processes); (3) loose fragments and articular debris produce mechanical trauma; and (4) inflammatory mediators are produced by and in response to disrupted tissues.

Cartilage healing and repair is reviewed along with management to enhance cartilage repair in Chapter 16. The principal goals of the arthroscopic surgeon are (1) reconstruction of articular surfaces or congruity, or both; (2) removal of osteochondral fragments and other separated cartilage and bone; (3) debridement of lesions to viable tissue margins with the capacity to heal; and (4) synovial lavage. These techniques are discussed in individual chapters as they pertain to specific locations and lesions. In skeletally mature animals, the subchondral margins of lesions are generally considerably clearer than in juveniles. Joints that are operated on at an age before

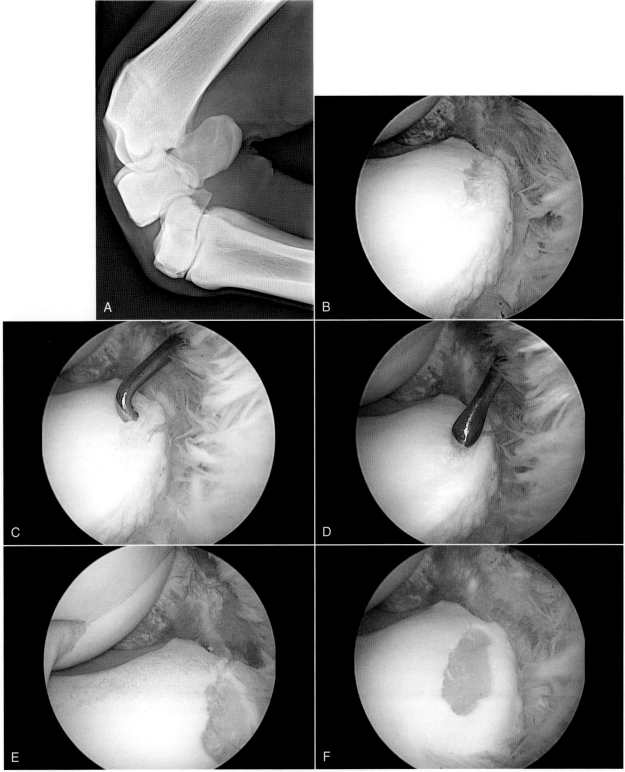

Figure 3-29 Chondral bone disease on the distal aspect of the radial carpal bone **(A)** manifesting as an irregular concavity in the distal articular surface of the radial carpal bone. **B,** Defect found at arthroscopy. **C,** Evaluation of the defect with a probe. **D,** Commencement of debridement with a 2-mm closed cup curette. **E,** Debris produced by debridement before lavage. **F,** Lesion at the end of debridement leaving stable attached osteochondral margins and viable subchondral bone within.

subchondral bone plates have formed, when there is little differentiation between mineralized layers of the articular epiphyseal complex and the underlying epiphyseal spongiosa, pose challenges. Differentiation of normal and abnormal is often not clear. The bone is soft on palpation and has an open granular appearance. Historically, this is likely to have led to excessive debridement of lesion margins.

"Second look arthroscopy" has much to commend it as a means of assessing healing or disease progression, or both. In the absence of persistent or recurrent clinical compromise it is infrequently performed in horses. In humans it is considered a useful guide to patient management and recommendations regarding return to athletic activity, whereas in small animal orthopedics it is useful (Fitzpatrick et al, 2009a, b; Hulse et al, 2010) but has attracted controversy (Houlton, 2009).

Arthroscopic Synovectomy

The remainder of this book deals in large part with arthroscopic surgery to correct various conditions of the joint. One procedure that has been performed relatively infrequently in any equine joint, and is not addressed elsewhere in this text, is that of synovectomy. It is frequently used in a local manner in the horse to facilitate the diagnostic process by allowing examination of an otherwise obscure region. Synovectomy is greatly facilitated by improved soft tissue blades for motorized units (see Chapter 2).

Arthroscopic synovectomy has been performed in man to reduce joint pain and improve function in severe inflammatory conditions such as recurrent hemarthrosis associated with haemophilia (Limbrid & Denis, 1987; Tamurian et al, 2002); proliferative synovitis of the knee (Chow et al, 2002); and rheumatoid arthritis (Rosenburg et al, 1996; Kampen et al, 2001). Synovectomy can be performed arthroscopically, chemically, or with radiation (Kampen et al, 2001; Mäkelä et al, 2003). Equivalent indications may be found in the horse; Figure 3-16 illustrates hemarthrosis and the biopsy of a piece of synovial membrane. Early experimental studies predominantly in rabbits suggested regeneration of synovium between 35 and 110 days after synovectomy (Mitchell & Blackwell, 1968; Bentley et al, 1975). However, later studies in the horse reported limitations. There was no evidence of synovial regeneration at 30 days (Jones et al, 1994) and incomplete regeneration at 120 days (Theoret et al, 1994) after arthroscopic synovectomy with a motorized resector in the normal equine carpal joint. Neither of these studies nor that from Doyle-Jones (2002) identified any villous regeneration at periods of up to 6 months following synovectomy. Palmer et al (1998) also reported deterioration in both biochemical (reduced proteoglycan synthesis) and mechanical (stiffness) properties of cartilage from middle carpal joints that had undergone experimental synovectomy 2 or 6 weeks earlier. It was also suggested that synovectomy in inflamed joints could be more deleterious to articular cartilage integrity than inflammation alone. In a comparative study, there were no detectable benefits between use of monopolar radiofrequency energy and a motorized synovial resector by arthrotomy at 2 weeks and 3 months in rabbit femoropatellar joints (Davis et al, 2004).

The authors of this textbook are also concerned about capsular defects and fibrosis following synovectomy. They recommend localized synovial resection to improve visualization but caution against using more generalized synovial resection as a therapeutic measure, at least in traumatic joint disease. It is clear that synovectomy is irreversible in the horse, and there are potentially deleterious sequelae. Motorized instruments cut indiscriminately, and resultant damage to fibrous capsules can readily produce restrictive fibrosis. The use of the resector for eliminating fibrin in infected joints is another issue and is discussed in Chapter 14.

Assessment of Fractures

In addition to the diagnosis and treatment of intraarticular osteochondral fragmentation, larger intraarticular fractures requiring internal fixation are repaired under arthroscopic visualization. The articular manifestations of these fractures are discussed in their respective chapters.

Osteochondritis Dissecans

Osteochondritis dissecans (OCD) occurs in a number of joints and is dealt with in detail in the chapters on these joints.

However, a unique part of the management of OCD is delineation of the lesion margins using the probe because in many instances there are areas of undermined or loose cartilage. Arthroscopic evaluation is critical to the accurate assessment of which regions of separated articular cartilage and bone need to be removed and what can be retained.

USE OF ELECTROSURGERY, RADIOFREQUENCY, AND LASERS

Electrosurgery

Monopolar electrosurgical equipment can be used to cut, cauterize, or coagulate intrasynovial soft tissue. The cutting effect results from a constant low voltage current that produces heat rapidly and vaporizes tissue (David et al, 2011). Clinical use has been reported in the metacarpophalangeal and metatarsophalangeal joints and the carpal sheath for removal of fragments from the plantar margin of the proximal phalanx and proximal sesamoid bones and desmotomy of the accessory ligament of the superficial digital flexor tendon, respectively (Bouré et al, 1999; Simon et al, 2004; David et al, 2011). It has been used for meniscal surgery in man (Kramer et al, 1992), but sharp dissection and mechanical debridement remain the most popular techniques for meniscectomy (Soto & Safran, 2004).

The principal advantage of electrosurgery is hemostasis. However, with judicious limb positioning (principally dorsal recumbency) and the use of tourniquets this is rarely a limiting factor during surgery. In addition, the edges of devitalized tissue that result from and remain following electrosurgical procedures challenge current concepts of intrasynovial healing.

Electrocoagulation of intrathecal bleeding points can occasionally be useful (Nixon, 2002; David et al, 2011). When electrosurgical electrodes are used for coagulation, they deliver a high-voltage current intermittently. This results in less tissue heat than when these are used in cutting mode and results in a coagulum (David et al, 2011).

Thermal Chondroplasty with Radiofrequency Energy

Both monopolar and bipolar radiofrequency energy (RFE) can be used to thermally modify intraarticular soft tissues. This causes shrinkage of collagenous tissues, including articular cartilage. In humans it has been used frequently for chondroplasty; the visual effect is said to be enticing because at the end of surgery smoother margins are obtained than those achieved with mechanical debridement (Edwards et al, 2008). At that time these authors suggested that 18% of articular cartilage debridement procedures in humans were performed with RFE. However, there are now multiple studies suggesting detrimental effects of RFE on articular cartilage. In a study using canine cartilage explants, bipolar radiofrequency chondroplasty produced marked degenerative changes, including cell death and reduced type II collagen content with increased degradative matrix metalloproteinase content (MMP-13) (Cook et al, 2004), which supports similar work in other species (Turner et al, 1998; Horstman et al, 2009; Lu et al, 2000 & 2002). Edwards et al (2008) reported comparison of RFE monopolar and bipolar probes with mechanical debridement for chondroplasty of an experimentally created partial-thickness cartilage defect in equine patellae. A prototype, power-controlled monopolar RFE probe resulted in less chondrocyte death than the bipolar unit while maintaining the advantage of controlled cartilage debridement and contouring. Nonetheless, damaging effects still exceeded that obtained with mechanical debridement.

The visual benefits of RFE has attracted use in other situations such as the digital flexor tendon sheath. Experimental work to evaluate the advantages and disadvantages of this has yet to be published. The authors are therefore currently cautious regarding its adoption.

Noncartilaginous Application of Radiofrequency Probes

Radiofrequency probes for section and resection of soft tissues within joints, tendon sheaths, and bursae have been described and may have a place in selected equine procedures. Manufacturers provide a range of probe tips for division of tissues, including 90-degree probes, which are described for annular ligament transection and desmotomy of the accessory ligament of the SDFT (David et al, 2011; McCoy and Goodrich, 2012) and diffuse multielectrode tips for soft tissue ablation of synovial masses and adhesions. Resection of large dorsal synovial (villonodular) masses and plantar osteochondral fragments in the fetlock have also been expedited by RF probe use for one of the authors (A.J.N.), but RF probes are by no means essential.

Lasers in Arthroscopy

The case for the use of lasers has also been made in joints (Palmer, 1996). Similar to the drawbacks with RF probes, use of laser for debridement of cartilage and drilling of subchondral bone in the carpus resulted in bone necrosis alongside the entry points (Nixon et al, 1991). Evaluation in clinical cases also revealed unwanted subchondral bone necrosis when an articular cartilage lesion is debrided. Where the cartilage can be avoided, such as with resection of the metacarpophalangeal dorsal synovial pad, the results are satisfactory (Murphy et al, 2001). However, the use of laser is now overshadowed by RF probe use, which is safer and more versatile for noncartilage applications.

ARTHROSCOPIC LAVAGE AND DEBRIDEMENT

The usefulness of lavage in traumatic arthritis had been claimed before arthroscopic surgery became routine (Norrie, 1975). The adjunctive lavage that goes with arthroscopic surgery has always been considered beneficial, although there is little documentation of this effect (Kalunian et al, 2000). However, the benefit of partial-thickness chondrectomy where there is cartilage fibrillation or minor exfoliation is more controversial (Fig. 3-30). The use of such debridement along with joint lavage has been commonly touted, but controlled work is necessary. In one study, articular cartilage was shaved on the underside of rabbit patellae with no evidence of repair in either the superficially or deeply shaved areas (Mitchell & Shephard, 1987).

Ultrastructural studies after arthroscopic cartilage shaving question regeneration and suggest deleterious effects (Schmid & Schmid, 1987). An article describing what the authors considered to be a controlled trial of arthroscopic surgery for osteoarthritis of the knee in humans caused considerable controversy (Moseley et al, 2002). The authors concluded that the outcomes after arthroscopic lavage or arthroscopic debridement were no better than those after a placebo procedure. However, there has been considerable debate regarding bias and defective experimental design (Johnson, 2002; Poehling, 2002). Results of arthroscopic lavage and debridement of osteoarthritic knees, based on the severity of degeneration, continue to need critical documentation (Jackson & Dietreichs, 2003).

In the horse, the authors feel that lavage is an important beneficial part of arthroscopic procedures by reducing inflammatory mediators. Debridement of articular cartilage should only be done when there are separated pieces or flaps, or undermined cartilage. A useful rule is that if articular cartilage is attached to subchondral bone, it should be left alone. Second-look arthroscopies provide an opportunity to examine the amount of healing that has occurred in previously debrided defects (Fig. 3-31).

LEARNING ARTHROSCOPIC TECHNIQUE

Clinicians may learn and widen their experience by observing arthroscopic procedures in clinical cases, reading papers and books, attending seminars, and viewing video recordings. However, "hands-on" training and practice are essential. Instruction and practice on cadavers is the most common way veterinary clinicians have improved their skills before embarking on clinical cases. Animal cadavers have also been used in the training of arthroscopy in humans (Voto et al, 1988). Artificial models have also been used successfully. More recently, there has been some development of equine artificial bones with joint capsules, but at present, cadaver material is inexpensive and readily available.

An interesting prospect for the future is the development of computer-based simulations of arthroscopic surgery for training and testing of arthroscopic skills (Medical Simulations, Inc., Williamstown, MA). Use of simulators will increase, particularly in learning human arthroscopic techniques.

ANALGESIA FOR ARTHROSCOPIC SURGERY

Since the development and adaptation of techniques in horses, analgesia for the majority of arthroscopic surgery has been provided by anesthetic agents and perioperative nonsteroidal

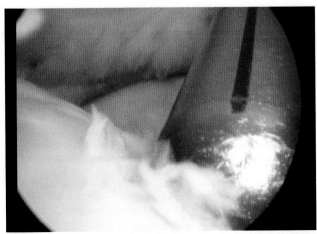

Figure 3-30 Debridement of fibrillated cartilage on the sagittal ridge of the third metacarpus bone.

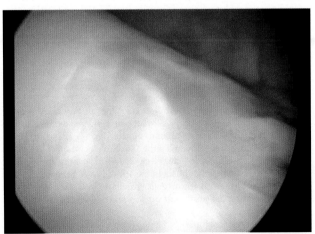

Figure 3-31 Follow-up examination of a defect previously debrided for osteochondritis dissecans. Fibrocartilage fills this defect.

antiinflammatory drugs. In recent years, this has been reviewed. It has been suggested, although not substantiated, that use of intraarticular local analgesic agents might reduce the requirement for systemic anesthetic or analgesic agents, or both. When performing arthroscopy in conscious patients, of whatever species, there is clear necessity. Evidence to support preoperative intraarticular administration of a combination of opiate (fentanyl) and local anesthetic (bupivacaine) has been provided in humans (Hube et al, 2009). Kalso et al (2002) concluded that intraarticular opioids (morphine) injected at the end of surgery reduce postoperative knee pain for up to 24 hours in human patients, but this has been subsequently challenged (Rosseland, 2005). However, more recently it has been demonstrated in vitro that bupivacaine is cytotoxic to bovine articular chondrocytes (Chu et al, 2006), and in another study with bovine articular cartilage discs, bupivacaine, lidocaine, and ropivacaine were all shown to have detrimental effects on chondrocyte viability in a dose- and duration-dependent manner (Lo et al, 2009). The conclusion was that high-dose, long-term intraarticular administration of local anesthetic should be performed with caution. Given the toxicity associated with long-term exposure to bupivacaine, one of the authors (A.J.N.) uses bupivacaine during distension before all arthroscopic and tenoscopic procedures, but complete lavage of the synovial structure is performed during initial arthroscopic examination within minutes of infusion, which may limit chondrocyte toxicity. Conversely, administration of bupivacaine at closure after arthroscopy is avoided.

Perineural analgesia can be a useful adjunct for highly invasive distal limb surgery in horses. However, the authors have concerns regarding the risks-versus-benefits ratio when considering proprioceptive loss in horses recovering from arthroscopy under general anesthesia. Central analgesia effected by preoperative epidural morphine (0.2 mg/kg) and detomidine (30 μg/kg) has been reported to benefit horses undergoing experimental bilateral stifle arthroscopy (Goodrich et al, 2002). Potential benefits in clinical cases have yet to be published. The pharmacologic properties and clinical use of nonsteroidal antiinflammatory drugs are well recognized and documented (Kallings, 1993; MacAllister et al, 1993), and there is a large corporate body of experience in their use in horses.

REFERENCES

Bass AL: Lesions of the synovium. In Casscells SW, editor: *Arthroscopy, diagnostic and surgical practice*, Philadelphia, 1984, Lea & Febiger.

Bentley G, Dreutner A, Ferguson AB: Synovial regeneration and articular cartilage changes after synovectomy in normal and steroid-treated rabbits, *J Bone Joint Surg (Br)* 57:454–462, 1975.

Bouré L, Marcoux M, Laverty S, et al.: Use of electrocautery probes in arthroscopic removal of apical sesamoid fracture fragments in 18 Standardbred horses, *Vet Surg* 28:226–232, 1999.

Brommer H, Laasasen MS, Brama PAJ, et al.: In situ and ex vivo evaluation of an arthroscopic indentation instrument to estimate the health status of articular cartilage in the equine metacarpophalangeal joint, *Vet Surg* 35:259–266, 2006.

Brommer H, Rijkenhuizen ABM, Brama PAJ, et al.: Accuracy of diagnostic arthroscopy for the assessment of cartilage damage in the equine metacarpophalangeal joint, *Equine Vet J* 36:331–335, 2004.

Carson RW: Meniscectomy and other surgical techniques using the operating arthroscope. In Casscells SW, editor: *Arthroscopy, diagnostic and surgical practice*, Philadelphia, 1984, Lea & Febiger.

Casscells SW: Lesions of the articular cartilage. In Casscells SW, editor: *Arthroscopy, diagnostic and surgical practice*, Philadelphia, 1984, Lea & Febiger.

Chow JC, Hantes M, Houle JB: Hypertrophy of the synovium in the anteromedial aspect of the knee joint following trauma: an unusual cause of knee pain, *Arthroscopy* 18:735–740, 2002.

Chu CR, Izzo NJ, Papas NE, et al.: In vitro exposure to 0.5% bupivacaine is cytotoxic to bovine articular chondrocytes, *Arthroscopy* 22:693–699, 2006.

Cohen JM, Richardson DW, McKnight AL, Ross MW, Boston RC: Long-term outcome in 44 horses with stifle lameness after arthroscopic exploration and debridement, *Vet Surg* 38:543–551, 2009.

Cook JL, Marberry KM, Kuroki K, et al.: Assessment of cellular, biomechanical, and histological effects of bipolar radiofrequency treatment of canine articular cartilage, *Am J Vet Res* 65:604–609, 2004.

Crane J: Technique of diagnostic arthroscopy. In Casscells SW, editor: *Arthroscopy, diagnostic and surgical practice*, Philadelphia, 1984, Lea & Febiger.

Dandy D: Imaging and clinical judgement, *Equine Vet J* 42:287, 2010.

David F, Laverty S, Marcoux M, Szoke M, Celeste C: Electrosurgical tenoscopic desmotomy of the accessory ligament of the superficial digital flexor muscle (proximal check ligament) in horses, *Vet Surg* 40:46–53, 2011.

Davis KM, King DS, Philips L, et al.: Comparison of surgical techniques for synovectomy in New Zealand white rabbits with induced inflammatory arthritis, *Am J Vet Res* 65:573–577, 2004.

Diduch DR, Shen FH, Ong BC, et al.: Knee: Diagnostic arthroscopy. In Miller MD, Cole BJ, editors: *Textbook of Arthroscopy*, Philadelphia, 2004, Saunders, pp 471–487.

Dougadous M, Ayral X, Listrat V, et al.: The SFA system for assessing articular cartilage lesions at arthroscopy of the knee, *Arthroscopy* 10:69–77, 1994.

Doyle-Jones PS, Sullins KE, Saunders GK: Synovial regeneration in the equine carpus after arthroscopic mechanical or carbon dioxide laser synovectomy, *Vet Surg* 31:331–343, 2002.

Edwards RB, Lu Y, Cole BJ, et al.: Comparison of radiofrequency treatment and mechanical debridement of fibrillated cartilage in an equine model, *Vet Comp Orthop Traumatol* 21:41–48, 2008.

Elce YA, Richardson DW: Arthroscopic removal of dorsoproximal chip fractures of the proximal phalanx in standing horses, *Vet Surg* 31:195–200, 2002.

Elsworth CF, Drabu K, Hodson J, Noble J: To probe or not to probe. In: Proceedings and Reports of Universities, Colleges, Councils, Associations and Societies, *J Bone Joint Surg (Br)* 68:842, 1986.

Fitzpatrick N, Yeadon R, Smith T, et al.: Techniques of application and initial clinical experience with sliding humeral osteotomy for treatment of medical compartment disease of the canine elbow, *Vet Surg* 38:261–278, 2009a.

Fitzpatrick N, Yeadon R, Smith TJ: Early clinical experience with osteochondral autograft transfer for treatment of osteochondritis dissecans of the medial humeral condyle in dogs, *Vet Surg* 38:246–260, 2009b.

Fizziero L, Zizzi F, Leyhissa R, Ferruzzi A: New methods in arthroscopy. Preliminary investigation, *Ann Rheum Dis* 45:529–533, 1986.

Garcia-Seco E, Wilson DA, Cook JL, et al.: Measurement of articular cartilage stiffness of the femoropatellar, tarsocrural, and metatarsophalangeal joints in horses and comparison with biomechanical data, *Vet Surg* 34:571–578, 2005.

Getty R: General syndesmology. In Getty R, editor: *The Anatomy of the Domestic Animals*, Philadelphia, 1975, WB Saunders, pp 34–38.

Goodrich LR, Nixon AJ, Fubini SL, et al.: Epidural morphine and detomidine decreases postoperative hindlimb lameness in horses after bilateral stifle arthroscopy, *Vet Surg* 31:232–239, 2002.

Hague BA, Honnas CM, Simpson RB, Peloso JG: Evaluation of skin bacterial flora before and after aseptic preparation of clipped and non-clipped arthrocentesis sites in horses, *Vet. Surg* 26:121–125, 1997.

Hjelle K, Solheime Strand T, Muri R, Brittberg M: Articular cartilage defects in 1000 knee arthroscopies, *Arthroscopy* 18:730–734, 2002.

Horstman CL, McLaughlin RM, Elder SH, et al.: Changes to articular cartilage following remote radiofrequency energy and with or without Cosequin therapy, *Vet Comp Orthop Traumatol* 22:103–112, 2009.

Houlton J: Advances in canine elbow disease, *Vet Surg* 38:133–134, 2009.

Hube R, Tröger M, Rickerl F, Muench EO, von Eisenhart-Rothe R, Hein W, Mayr HO: Pre-emptive intra-articular administration of local anaesthetics/opiates versus postoperative local anaesthetics/opiates or local anaesthetics in arthroscopic surgery of the knee joint: a prospective randomized trial, *Arch Orthop Trauma Surg* 129:343–348, 2009.

Hulse D, Beale B, Kerwin S: Second look arthroscopic findings after tibial plateau leveling osteotomy, *Vet Surg* 39:350–354, 2010.

Jackson RW: Arthroscopic surgery (current concepts review), *J Bone Joint Surg (Am)* 65:416–420, 1983.

Jackson RW, Dietreichs C: The results of arthroscopic lavage and debridement of osteoarthritic knees based on the severity of degeneration: a 4 to 6 year symptomatic follow-up, *Arthroscopy* 19:13–20, 2003.

Johnson LL: Letter to the editor, *Arthroscopy* 18:683–687, 2002.

Jones D, Barber S, Jack S, et al.: Morphological effects of arthroscopic partial synovectomy in horses, *Vet Surg* 23:231–240, 1994.

Joyce KJ, Mankin HJ: Caveat arthroscopes. Extra-articular lesions of bone simulating intra-articular pathology in the knee, *J. Bone Joint Surg. (Am.)* 65:289–292, 1983.

Kallings P: Nonsteroidal anti-inflammatory drugs, *Vet Clin North Am Eq Pract* 9:523–541, 1993.

Kalso E, Smith L, McQuay HJ, et al.: No pain, no gain: clinical excellence and scientific rigour – lessons learned from IA morphine, *Pain* 98:269–275, 2002.

Kalunian KC, Moreland LW, Klashman DJ, Brion PH, Concoff AL, Myers S, Singh R, Ike RW, Seeger LL, Rich E, Skovron ML: Visually-guided irrigation in patients with early knee osteoarthritis: a multicenter randomized controlled trial, *Osteoarthritis and Cartilage* 8:412–418, 2000.

Kampen WU, Brenner W, Kroeger A, Sawula JA, Bohuslavizki KH, Henze E: Long-term results of radiation synovectomy: a clinical follow-up study, *Nucl Med Commun* 22:239–246, 2001.

Kawcak CE, McIlwraith CW: Proximal dorsal first phalanx osteochondral chip fragmentation in 336 horses, *Equine Vet J* 26:392–396, 1994.

Kramer J, Rosenthal A, Moraldo M, Mueller KM: Electrosurgery in arthroscopy, *Arthroscopy* 8:125–129, 1992.

Lindblad S, Hedfors E: Intra-articular variation in synovitis. Local macroscopic and microscopic signs of inflammatory activity are significantly correlated, *Arthritis Rheum* 2:977–986, 1985.

Lo IKY, Sciore P, Chung M, et al.: Local anesthetics induce chondrocyte death in bovine articular cartilage discs in a dose- and duration-dependent manner, *Arthroscopy* 25:707–715, 2009.

Lu Y, Edwards RB, Nho S, et al.: Thermal chondroplasty with bipolar and monopolar radiofrequency energy: effect of treatment time on chondrocyte death and surface contouring, *Arthroscopy* 18:779–788, 2002.

Lu Y, Hayashi K, Hecht P, et al.: The effect of monopolar radiofrequency energy on partial thickness defects of articular cartilage, *Arthroscopy* 16:527–536, 2000.

MacAllister CG, Morgan SJ, Borne AT, et al.: Comparison of adverse effects of phenylbutazone, flunixin meglumine, and ketoprofen in horses, *J Am Vet Med Assoc* 202:71–77, 1993.

Mäkelä O, Sukura A, Penttilää P, et al.: Radiation synovectomy with holmium-166 ferric hydroxide macro aggregate in equine metacarpophalangeal and metatarsophalangeal joints, *Vet Surg* 32:402–409, 2003.

McCoy AM, Goodrich LR: Use of radiofrequency probe for tenoscopic-guided annular ligament desmotomy, *Equine Vet J* 44:412–415, 2012.

McIlwraith CW: *The use of arthroscopy, synovial fluid analysis and synovial membrane biopsy in the diagnosis of equine joint disease. In: Equine medicine and surgery*, 3rd edn, Santa Barbara, 1983, American Veterinary Publications.

McIlwraith CW: Diagnostic and Surgical Arthroscopy in the Horse. Veterinary Publishing Company, *Kansas*, 1984.

McIlwraith CW: *Diagnostic and Surgical Arthroscopy in the Horse*, 2nd edition, Lea & Febiger, 1990.

McIlwraith CW: Tearing of the medial palmar intercarpal ligament in the equine midcarpal joint, *Equine Vet J* 24:547–550, 1992.

McIlwraith CW, Fessler JF: Arthroscopy in the diagnosis of equine joint disease, *J Am Vet Med Assoc* 172:263–268, 1978.

Minshall GJ, Wright IM: Arthroscopic diagnosis and treatment of intra-articular insertional injuries of the suspensory ligament branch in 18 horses, *Equine Vet J* 38:10–14, 2006.

Mitchell N, Blackwell P: The electron microscopy of regenerating synovium after subtotal synovectomy in rabbits, *J Bone Joint Surg (Am)* 50:675–686, 1968.

Mitchell N, Shephard N: Effective patellar sharing in the rabbit, *J Orthop Res* 5:388–392, 1987.

Mori Y: Debris observed by arthroscopy of the knee, *Orthop Clin North Am* 16:579–593, 1979.

Moseley JB, O'Malley K, Petersen NJ, et al.: A controlled trial of arthroscopic surgery for osteoarthritis of the knee, *N Engl J Med* 347:81–88, 2002.

Murphy DJ, Nixon AJ: Arthroscopic laser extirpation of metacarpophalangeal synovial pad proliferation in eleven horses, *Equine Vet J* 33:296–301, 2001.

Nixon AJ: Arthroscopic surgery of the carpal and digital tendon sheaths. Clin Tech, *Equine Pract* 4:245–256, 2002.

Nixon AJ, Krook LP, Roth JE, King JM: Pulsed carbon dioxide laser for cartilage vaporization and subchondral bone perforation in horses. Part II: Morphologic and histochemical reactions, *Vet Surg* 20:200–208, 1991.

Norrie RD: The treatment of joint disease by saline lavage. Proceedings 21st Annual Meeting of the American Association of Equine Practitioners, Boston, MA, 1975, 91–94.

Noyes FR, Spievack ES. Extra-articular fluid dissection in tissues during arthroscopy. A report of clinical cases and a study of intra-articular and thigh pressures in cadavers, *Am J Sports Med* 10:346–351, 1982.

O'Connor RL: *Arthroscopy*, Philadelphia, 1977, JB Lippincott.

Palmer JL, Bertone AL, Malemud CJ, Mansour J: Changes in third carpal bone articular cartilage after synovectomy in normal and inflamed joints, *Vet Surg* 27:321–330, 1998.

Palmer SE: Instrumentation and techniques for carbon dioxide lasers in equine general surgery, *Vet Clin North Am Equine Pract* 12:397–414, 1996.

Phillips MF, Vasseur PB, Gregory CR: Chlorhexidine diacetate versus povidone-iodine for pre-operative preparation of the skin: a prospective randomized comparison in dogs and cats, *J Am Anim Hosp Assoc* 27:105–108, 1991.

Phillips TJ, Wright IM: Observations on the anatomy and pathology of the palmar intercarpal ligaments in the middle carpal joints of Thoroughbred racehorses, *Equine Vet J* 26:486–491, 1994.

Poehling GG: Degenerative arthritis. Arthroscopy and research (editorial), *Arthroscopy* 18:683–687, 2002.

Rosenberg A, Alatatry SD, Peterson AF: Safety and efficacy of the antiseptic chlorhexidine gluconate, *Surg. Gynecol. Obstet* 143:789–792, 1976.

Rosseland LA: No evidence for analgesic effect of intra-articular morphine after knee arthroscopy: a qualitative systemic review, *Regional Anesthesia and Pain Medicine* 30:83–98, 2005.

Schmid A, Schmid F: Ultrastructural studies after arthroscopical cartilage shaving (abstract), *J Arthroscopy* 3:137, 1987.

Schneider RK, Jenson P, Moore RM: Evaluation of cartilage lesions on the medial femoral condyle as a cause of lameness in horses: 11 cases (1988–1994), *JAVMA* 210:1649–1652, 1997.

Serena A, Hanson RR, Kincaid SA: Synovial membrane microarthroscopy of the equine midcarpal joint, *Vet Surg* 34:310–317, 2005.

Simon O, Laverty S, Bouré L, et al.: Arthroscopic removal of axial osteochondral fragments of the proximoplantar aspect of the proximal phalanx using electrocautery probes in 23 Standardbred racehorses, *Vet Surg* 33:422–427, 2004.

Soto G, Safran MR: Arthroscopic meniscectomy. In Miller MD, Cole BJ, editors: *Textbook of arthroscopy*, Philadelphia, 2004, Saunders, pp 507–516.

Stubbs WP, Bellah JR, Vermaas-Hekman D, Purich B, Kuplis PS: Chlorhexidine gluconate versus chloroxylenol for pre-operative skin preparation in dogs, *Vet Surg* 25:487–494, 1996.

Tamurian RM, Spencer EE, Wojtys EM: The role of arthroscopic synovectomy in the management of hemarthrosis and hemophilia patients: Financial prospective, *Arthroscopy* 18:789–794, 2002.

Theoret C, Barber S, Moyana T, et al.: Repair and function of synovium after total arthroscopic synovectomy of the equine antebrachiocarpal joint, *Vet Surg* 23:418, 1994.

Töyräs J, Lyyra-Laitinen T, Niinimäki M, et al.: Estimation of the Young's modulus of articular cartilage using an arthroscopic indentation instrument and ultrasonic measurement of tissue thickness, *J Biomech* 34:251–256, 2001.

Turner AS, Tippett JW, Pavers BE, et al.: Radiofrequency (electrosurgical) ablation of articular cartilage: a study in sheep, *Arthroscopy* 14:585–591, 1998.

von Engelhardt LV, Lahner M, Klussmann A, Bouillon B, David A, Haage P, Lichtinger TK: Arthroscopy vs. MRI for a detailed assessment of cartilage disease in osteoarthritis: diagnostic value of MRI in clinical practice, *BMC Musculoskeletal Disorders* 11:75–83, 2012.

Voto SJ, Clark RN, Zuelzer WA: Arthroscopic training using pig knee joints, *Clin. Orthop* 226:134–137, 1988.

Walmsley JP: Arthroscopic surgery of the femorotibial joint, *Clin Tech Equine Pract* 1:226–233, 2002.

Walmsley JP, Phillips TJ, Townsend HCG: Meniscal tears in horses; an evaluation of clinical signs and arthroscope treatment of 80 cases, *Equine Vet J* 35:402–406, 2003.

Wan PY, Blackford JT, Bemis DA, et al.: Evaluation of surgical scrub methods for large animal surgeons, *Vet Surg* 26:382–385, 1997.

Williamson DM, Copeland SA: Suturing arthroscopy wounds: brief report, *J Bone Joint Surg (Br)* 70:146, 1988.

CHAPTER 4

Diagnostic and Surgical Arthroscopy of the Carpal Joints

The earliest applications of arthroscopy in horses were centered on the carpus. The development of techniques appropriate for clinical use and reports of successful treatment served as a springboard for the discipline (McIlwraith, 1983, 1984; McIlwraith et al, 1987). Carpal injuries have long been recognized as major limiting factors in the training and racing of horses. The morbidity, convalescence, and results associated with arthrotomy promoted conservative/medical management frequently to the long-term detriment of joints and horses. This chapter reviews arthroscopic techniques in the carpal joint and, while remaining comprehensive, will attempt to highlight developments that have occurred since the last edition of the book (McIlwraith et al, 2005), including further experiences in fracture repair and in the palmar compartments of both antebrachiocarpal and middle carpal joints.

The carpal joints illustrate perfectly the concept that arthroscopic examination permits a more detailed and comprehensive evaluation of a joint than any or even multiple open (arthrotomy) approaches whether antimortem or postmortem. In most circumstances, dorsal compartments of antebrachiocarpal and middle carpal joints can be evaluated from a single arthroscopic portal. Complete lateromedial passage of the arthroscope is not possible in the palmar compartments, which require separate lateral and medial portals.

DIAGNOSTIC ARTHROSCOPY OF THE CARPAL JOINTS

Comprehensive arthroscopic evaluation of a synovial cavity is the necessary prelude to all surgical procedures (Fig. 4-1).

This can be performed in a timely manner and forms an essential part of good surgical practice. In the carpal joints it permits identification of radiologically silent lesions, including articular cartilage defects, nonmarginal (and therefore not seen in radiographic profile) osteochondral fragmentation, and lesions of intraarticular ligaments that currently are only reliably identified by arthroscopic examination. Arthroscopy of the carpal joints can be performed with the animal in lateral or dorsal recumbency. The latter has greater versatility and has been almost universally adopted. The surgical techniques can also be adapted readily to most other locations. For these reasons, all descriptions are presented in this manner (i.e., proximal is below and distal is above). Learning arthroscopic anatomy in this manner is an important prerequisite to performing surgery. Initially, the most important aspect is to learn the specific landmarks that allow orientation. These are described later and in the accompanying video recordings.

The carpal joints are evaluated in varying degrees of flexion to permit insinuation of the arthroscope and instruments between the composite joint surfaces (see Fig. 4-1). The middle carpal joint opens primarily as a hinge, whereas movement in the antebrachiocarpal joint is principally rotational with some glide. Differential movement of the proximal row of carpal bones is evident in both. Due to the anatomic differences, examination and surgery of the middle carpal joint is easier than the antebrachiocarpal joint. The gliding movement of the latter tends to tuck the dorsal edge of the radius beneath the joint capsule, and the joint capsule attaches closely to the proximal marginal edge of the intermediate and radial carpal

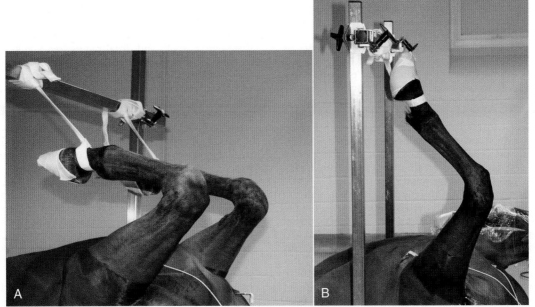

Figure 4-1 A, Limbs positioned for bilateral arthroscopy of the dorsal aspect of the middle carpal joint. **B,** Limb position for arthroscopy of the dorsal antebrachiocarpal joint.

bones. In addition, the convex curvature of the distal medial and lateral aspects of the radius make access to the medial and lateral joint angles slightly more difficult. The narrow angle between the radius and the proximal radial carpal bone in the medial aspect of the joint can also make instrument manipulation more difficult in this area.

In most circumstances, adequate examination of the dorsal compartments of both middle and antebrachiocarpal joints are possible through a single dorsal arthroscopic portal for each joint. Use of two separate dorsal portals improves visualization and reduces the tendency to slip out of the joint when examining areas close to the arthroscopic portal (Martin and McIlwraith, 1985). Two portals are also used for surgery to be performed on both sides of the joint. In addition, villi in the area of arthroscopic entry will sometimes compromise visualization of that area. Two standard arthroscopic portals are described for the middle carpal and antebrachiocarpal joints: dorsal lateral and dorsal medial. The former is better for visualizing the medial aspect of the joint and vice versa. In either or both circumstances a contralateral portal is used for instrument entry, and interchange of portal use is frequently useful.

Initially, the most important aspect is to learn the specific landmarks that allow orientation within the carpal joints. These are described in the following examination techniques.

▶ Arthroscopic Examination of the Middle Carpal (Intercarpal) Joint

For the majority of procedures, the dorsal compartment of the middle carpal joint is most readily accessed with the carpus flexed to an angle of approximately 70 degrees (see Fig. 4-1). The choice of arthroscopic portal depends on the principal area the surgeon wants to examine. However, if there is no primary focus of attention, the lateral portal is the most convenient and most comprehensive alternative. The technique of insertion of the arthroscope through a lateral portal in the middle carpal joint has been previously demonstrated in Chapter 3. The lateral portal is halfway between the extensor carpi radialis tendon and the common digital extensor tendon and midway between the two rows of carpal bones. The medial arthroscopic portal is made approximately 10 mm medial to the extensor carpi radialis tendon, to avoid its tendon sheath, and creates an opening dorsal and lateral to the medial dorsal intercarpal ligament. In contrast to other joints, the skin incision for these portals is made before distention of the joint to avoid damage to the tendon sheaths. The joint can then be distended, and the arthroscope can be inserted as described in Chapter 3.

Systematic examination of the joint can be performed in a number of ways (e.g., commencing medially and moving the arthroscope in a circular motion with the lens moving from medial to lateral to inspect the distal row of carpal bones and then from lateral to medial to examine the proximal row). Alternatively, a single sweep can be made from medial to lateral, inspecting proximal and distal rows of carpal bones by rotating the arthroscope lens to alternately view proximally and distally while traversing the joint.

Examination with the arthroscope inserted through the lateral portal commences with the visual field in the medial aspect of the middle carpal joint (Fig. 4-2). The dorsal medial intercarpal ligament extends between the radial and second carpal bones. It is predominantly intracapsular, but frequently a portion of radial insertion is intrasynovial (previously described as a synovial plica by McIlwraith, 1990). Withdrawing the arthroscope and angling the lens proximad allows inspection of the articular surface and dorsal margin of the radial carpal bone. Continued withdrawal of the arthroscope allows visualization of the junction between

the radial and intermediate carpal bones and, moving laterally, the intermediate carpal bone and ulnar carpal bone. The articular surface of the intermediate carpal bone is divided by a dorsopalmar ridge into two facets. Rotation of the arthroscope allows inspection of the palmar aspect of the joint and the articulation between the radial, intermediate, and third carpal bones (see Fig. 4-2). Also in this view is the synovial fossa in the medial palmar aspect of the third carpal bone and the medial palmar intercarpal ligament (MPICL). This fossa is normal; it is a site of communication with the palmar pouch of the middle carpal joint and may be a site for lodgment of small particles that break free during arthroscopic surgery. During examination of the articular margins of the radial and intermediate carpal bones, the joint capsule attachment is some distance from the articular rim, allowing excellent visualization of the dorsal margins of these bones. Moving the arthroscope back laterally allows visualization of the lateral palmar intercarpal ligament (see Fig. 4-2).

The arthroscope is advanced back to the medial side of the joint, and the arthroscopic lens is angled distad to visualize the second carpal bone and the medial portion of the third carpal bone. Slight withdrawal allows additional visualization of the remaining dorsal margin and body of the radial facets of the third carpal bone. If the arthroscope is then moved so that the tip sweeps laterad and the eyepiece mediad, the intermediate facet of the third carpal bone and the more central aspects of the joint can be visualized. By continuing this motion, the lateral aspect of the joint can be visualized. A palmar view at this point reveals the four-way junction of ulnar, intermediate, fourth, and third carpal bones. Between them is the lateral palmar intercarpal ligament, the fibers of which are frequently seen to twist in their course. Rotation back distad allows examination of the fourth carpal bone and the lateral half of the third carpal bone. A transverse dorsal intercarpal ligament is usually visible between the dorsal surface of intermediate and ulnar carpal bones. The remaining dorsal joint capsule is covered by villous synovium (see Fig. 4-2).

▶ Arthroscopic Examination of the Antebrachiocarpal (Radiocarpal) Joint

Arthroscopic examination of the antebrachiocarpal joint is conducted in the same fashion as the middle carpal joint, except that the flexion angle in the carpus is decreased (i.e., leg is extended) to 120 to 130 degrees to facilitate maximal visualization of the dorsal aspects of the radial and intermediate carpal bones and distal radius (see Fig. 4-1). As in the middle carpal joint, the dorsolateral arthroscopic portal is halfway between the common digital extensor and the extensor carpi radialis tendons, and the dorsomedial portal is medial to the extensor carpi radialis tendon. The site of the medial portal is at the center of a triangle formed by the extensor carpi radialis, the distal rim of the radius, and the dorsal rim of the radial carpal bone. The joint narrows markedly at this point, so the surgeon must be careful when inserting the arthroscope to minimize the risk of iatrogenic cartilage damage.

The arthroscope is inserted through the lateral portal, and evaluation of the joint begins medially. The rotating nature of the joint necessitates proximal and distal movement of the arthroscopic tip, in addition to lens rotation, in order to evaluate the dorsal margins of the articular surfaces. The dorsal distal radius is separated by dorsopalmarly oriented ridges into two medial concave and one lateral convex facets corresponding with the proximal row of carpal bones. The articular surface is more convex in the palmar region. Differential movement between radial and intermediate carpal bones is again evident, and this reveals capsular plicae but there are no visible intraarticular ligaments in this joint. The distal radius

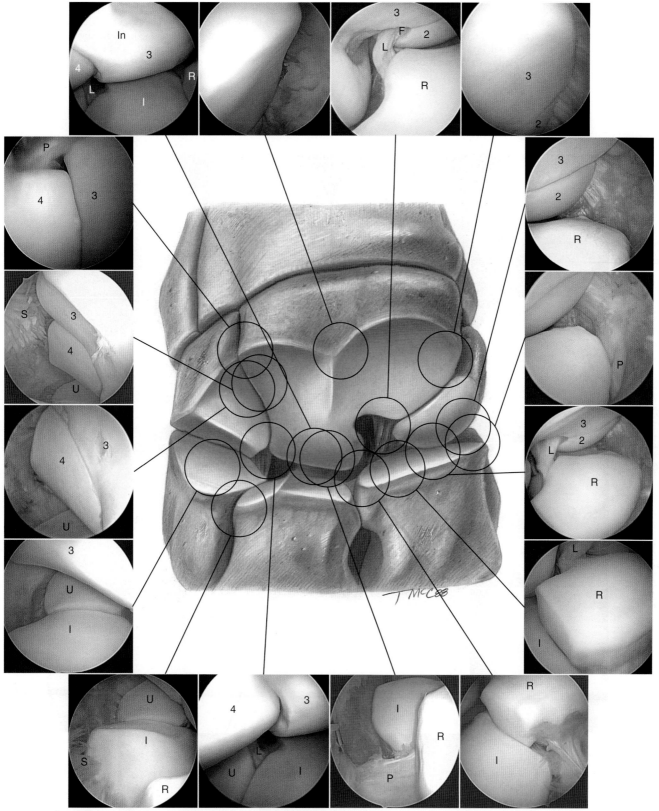

Figure 4-2 Composite of arthroscopic images obtained from middle carpal joint using dorsolateral arthroscopic approach. Distal radial carpal bone *(R)*; *2*, Second carpal bone; *3*, Third carpal bone; *L*, medial palmar intercarpal ligament; *4*, fourth carpal bone. *CD*, Common digital extensor tendon; *ECR*, extensor carpi radialis tendon; *I*, intermediate carpal bone *P*, dorsal to medial intercarpal ligament; *S*, synovial membrane; *U*, ulnar carpal bone.

and the proximal radial carpal bone form the medial joint angle. Rotation of the lens distad allows close inspection of the medial portion of the proximal articular surface of the articular surface of the radial carpal bone (Fig. 4-3). Withdrawing the arthroscopic slightly allows examination of the entire proximal radial carpal bone to the level of its junction with the intermediate carpal bone (see Fig. 4-3).

The arthroscope is then rotated so that the lens is angled proximad to examine the medial aspect of the distal articular surface of the radius (see Fig. 4-3). As in the middle carpal joint, the lateral aspect of the joint can be examined through the same lateral arthroscopic portal by moving the eyepiece mediad and the tip laterad and then rotating the scope appropriately. For purposes of palpation and surgery, however,

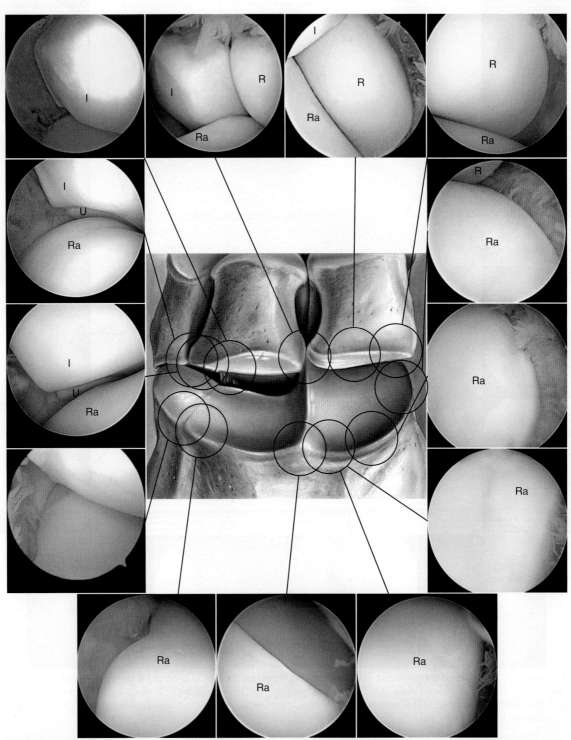

Figure 4-3 The same composite images obtained from antebrachiocarpal joint using dorsomedial arthroscopic approach. *I,* Proximal surface of the intermediate carpal bone; *R,* proximal articular surface of the radial carpal bone; *Ra,* distal radius; *U,* proximal surface of the ulnar carpal bone.

examination of the lateral aspect of the joint is best performed through a medial arthroscope portal.

By switching to a medial portal, the most lateral aspect of the antebrachiocarpal joint is examined. The arthroscope is rotated with the lens pointed distad to visualize the proximal articular surface of the ulnar carpal bone and the lateral aspect of the proximal articular surface of the intermediate carpal bone. Withdrawing the arthroscope allows examination of the entire proximal surface of the intermediate carpal bone, and tilting of the arthroscopic tip distad allows inspection of the junction of the intermediate and radial carpal bones (see Fig. 4-3).

By returning the tip of the arthroscope to the lateral aspect of the joint and rotating the arthroscope so that the lens is directed proximad, the lateral aspect of the distal radius can be examined. On a close lateral view, the articular groove between the lateral styloid process and the distal epiphysis of the radius (fused in the adult) can be seen; in a young horse, it can appear as a completely separated fissure. With withdrawal and rotation, the entire lateral half of the joint can be scanned including the midsagittal ridge of the distal radius (see Fig. 4-3). Grooves in the central portion of the radius are commonly observed and are considered normal.

Arthroscopic Examination of the Palmar Pouches of the Middle Carpal and Antebrachiocarpal Joints

Cheetham and Nixon (2006) described the synovial anatomy and reported techniques suitable for evaluation of the palmar compartments of the middle and antebrachiocarpal joints, although surgical procedures in these areas had previously been recorded (Dabareiner et al, 1993; McIlwraith, 1990 & 1996; Wilke et al, 2001). Prominent lateral and medial palmar outpouchings are evident in both the middle carpal and antebrachiocarpal joints (Figs. 4-4 and 4-5). Firm attachment of the capsule and palmar carpal ligament to the intermediate and lateral portion of the third carpal bones makes movement across the palmar surfaces from medial to lateral palmar pouches impossible. Hence surgical triangulation used routinely in the dorsal aspects of the carpal joints has to be modified to allow arthroscope and instrument entry in the one palmar outpouching. This places the arthroscope and instruments in close proximity and makes surgery in the palmar region more challenging. Additionally, the thin palmar joint capsule allows leakage of distending fluid, which rapidly accumulates in the subcutaneous region, obscuring palpable landmarks.

Arthroscopic Examination of the Palmar Compartment of the Antebrachiocarpal Joint

These compartments are evaluated with the carpus slightly (20 to 30 degrees) flexed. In most circumstances, if both dorsal and palmar compartments are to be examined, the dorsal compartment is examined initially and the entry for the palmar compartment is then made with the joint fully distended to make identification of the palmar outpouching easier. The palmaromedial pouch of the antebrachiocarpal joint is more voluminous than the corresponding pouch of the middle carpal joint. It is approached palmar to the medial collateral ligament at the level of the distal radius, dorsal to the tendon of insertion of flexor carpi radialis and medial palmar vein (Cheetham & Nixon, 2006). The arthroscope cannula is inserted in a 45-degree palmaromedial to dorsolateral trajectory to avoid entry to the carpal sheath (Fig. 4-6). The palmar surface of the radial carpal bone and corresponding facet of the distal radius

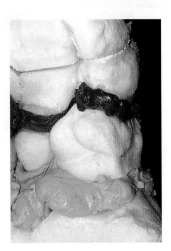
Figure 4-5 Latex model of middle (red) and antebrachiocarpal (yellow) joints with limb positioned in dorsal recumbency, showing palmaromedial pouches in both joints.

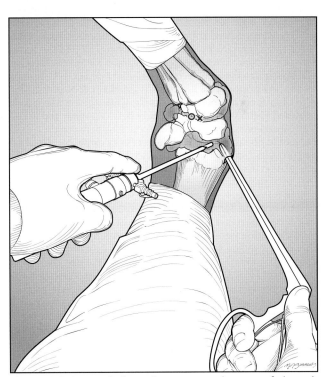
Figure 4-6 Approach for arthroscopic exploration of the palmaromedial pouch of the antebrachiocarpal joint. Positions for arthroscope (O) and instrument (**X**) entry for access to the palmaromedial aspect of the middle carpal joint are shown.

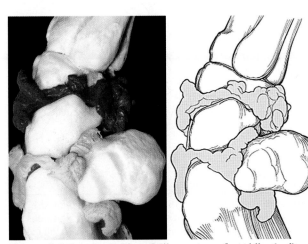
Figure 4-4 Latex model and illustration of middle (red) and antebrachiocarpal (yellow) joints with limb positioned in dorsal recumbency, showing palmarolateral pouches in both joints.

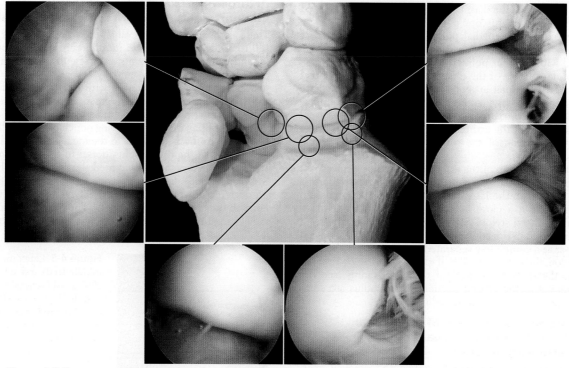

Figure 4-7 Structures visualized in the palmaromedial aspect of the antebrachiocarpal joint, including the caudomedial surface of the radius and palmar surface of the radial carpal bone.

are readily visualized from this portal (Fig. 4-7). Leaving adequate space for the anticipated instrument portal is vital in the planning of portal position. The most frequent target is a fracture of the palmaromedial corner of the radial carpal bone, for which the instrument portal is made closer to the medial collateral ligament (see Fig. 4-6), using a needle to verify appropriate instrument angle for fragment removal and bone debridement.

The palmarolateral approach to the antebrachiocarpal joint is made more complex by several outpouchings around the accessory carpal bone. Latex injection techniques identified three lateral pouches to the antebrachiocarpal joint (see Fig. 4-4), formed by the accessorio carpal ligaments (Cheetham & Nixon, 2006). The distal pouch proved inaccessible while the middle pouch provided visibility of the articulation between ulnar and accessory carpal bones. The proximal outpouching between the caudal radius and proximal margin of the accessory carpal bone is larger and provides clinically useful access to the accessoriocarpal radial articulation. Creation of an arthroscopic portal at the proximal margin of this outpouching leaves room for the distal instrument portals immediately adjacent to the articular surfaces.

The position for placing the arthroscope in the lateral palmar aspect of either carpal joint is most easily ascertained by joint distention (see Fig. 4-4). With distention of the joint from the front, swelling will be revealed. In the case of the antebrachiocarpal joint, the swelling is proximal to the perceived joint line. A No. 11 or 15 blade is then used to create a portal in the most proximal region of the palmarolateral cul-de-sac, and the arthroscope can be inserted in a palmarolateral to dorsomedial direction, angling distally to enter near the accessorio-radial articulation (Fig. 4-8). Figure 4-9 shows arthroscopic views of the lateral aspect of the palmar pouch of the antebrachiocarpal joint. The proximal articular surface of the accessory carpal bone and articulation with the caudal radius are easily visible. A proximal acessorio-radial ligament makes a useful proximal landmark. With more carpal flexion the arthroscope can be manipulated down the lateral aspect of the accessory to view the middle palmarolateral pouch of the antebrachiocarpal

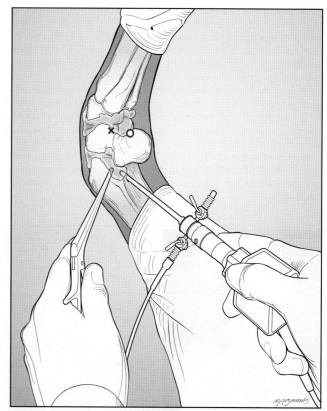

Figure 4-8 Approach for arthroscopic exploration of the palmarolateral pouch of the antebrachiocarpal joint. Positions for arthroscope (O) and instrument (X) entry for access to the palmaromedial aspect of the middle carpal joint are shown.

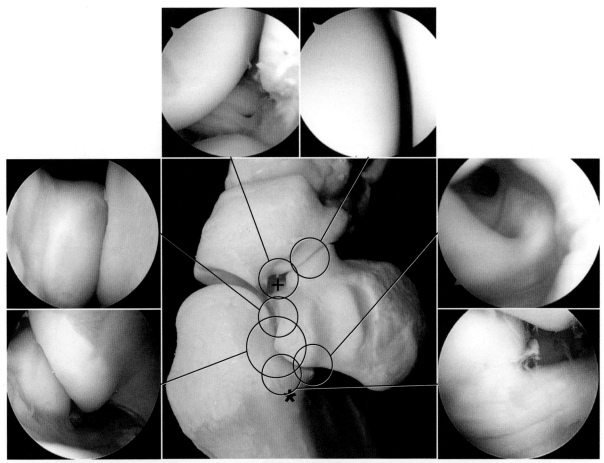

Figure 4-9 Structures visualized in the palmarolateral aspect of the antebrachiocarpal joint, with the arthroscope inserted into the proximal cul-de-sac *(asterisk)*. The caudolateral surface of the radius and articular surfaces of the accessory carpal bone are accessible. With the arthroscope in the midaccessory entry (+), the distal aspect of the accessory carpal and proximal perimeter of the palmar surface of the ulnar carpal bone can be viewed.

joint and part of the palmar surface of the ulnar carpal bone (see Fig. 4-9). However, it is usually necessary to selectively enter the midaccessory palmar pouch to view this region.

Arthroscopic Examination of the Palmar Compartment of the Middle Carpal Joint

The palmar compartments of the middle carpal joints are also evaluated with the carpus slightly (20 to 30 degrees) flexed. Examination of the palmar regions of the middle carpal joint is not as frequently indicated as the antebrachiocarpal joint. Most fractures of the palmar surfaces of the ulnar, fourth, and radial carpal bones are solitary and without concurrent cartilage injury to the central weight-bearing surfaces. The exception is severe joint trauma with multiple small comminuted fragments that have migrated into the palmar pouches of the middle carpal joint. When only the palmar approach will be used, inflation should be performed through the dorsal compartment until a clearly defined outpouching is evident palmarly. An arthroscopic portal is created in a conventional manner in the center of the appropriate medial or lateral outpouching. If fragments are being removed from both medial and lateral palmar pouches, skin incisions should be made medially and laterally while the distended outpouchings are readily identifiable. Medially this is located between radial and second carpal bones palmar to the medial collateral ligament (see Fig. 4-5). The outpouching and synovial spaces are small, and both carpal fascia and joint capsule are thicker medially than laterally. The portal is created and cannula inserted in a medial 45-degree palmar to dorsolateral oblique trajectory angling slightly (20 degrees)

proximal to distal (see Fig. 4-6) (Cheetham and Nixon, 2006). The arthroscopic cannula and conical obturator are inserted cautiously using the thumb of the opposite hand as a friction bridge to minimize the potential for iatrogenic damage to articular surfaces as the space available for the cannula in the joint is limited. Similarly, once the arthroscope is in place, fluid flow should be kept to the minimum necessary for visualization in order to reduce periarticular extravasation.

This approach permits evaluation of the palmar margins of radial and second carpal bones, part of the third carpal bone, and the palmar surface of the medial palmar intercarpal ligament (Fig. 4-10). Axially (laterally) the latter is the most useful landmark for orientation. Lateromedial movement of the arthroscope is limited, and visualization of the various surfaces is done more by rotation of the arthroscope tip than medial to lateral movement. Instrument portals are made with the aid of percutaneous needles. The size of the outpouching dictates that these are close to the arthroscopic portal, which allows only a minimal triangulation angle for surgical procedures.

The lateral palmar pouch portal is made in the location used for synoviocentesis and analgesia of the middle carpal joint when the limb is loaded (see Fig. 4-4). This is between the ulnar and fourth carpal bones palmar to the lateral collateral ligament and between the accessoriocarpal ulnar and accessoriocarpal quartal ligaments. The carpal fascia is thinner laterally, and this is a more voluminous cavity than its medial counterpart. The technique for insertion of the arthroscope is similar to that described for the medial approach with a slightly distally inclined palmarolateral to dorsomedial trajectory. As with the medial technique, mediolateral movement of the arthroscope is limited. It permits evaluation of the palmar margins of the ulnar and fourth carpal bones (Fig. 4-11).

The palmar lateral aspect of the third carpal bone, lateral palmar intercarpal ligament, and palmarodistal aspect of the intermediate carpal bone are not visible from either palmar approach. Capsular resection is required to expose any of these structures, and the consequences are unknown.

Maintenance of Joint Distention

The arthroscopist must direct the operation to ensure the maintenance of joint distention. This is not usually a problem at the time of initial examination when the only patent portal is that for the arthroscope. If an egress cannula is placed in the other side, varying the closure of the cannula still easily controls distention. However, once there is a patent instrument portal and manipulations have been performed, some flow of fluid from the joint is inevitable. This requires an increased rate of fluid input to maintain distention sufficient to continue the arthroscopic procedure and several key points help avoid the development of subcutaneous fluid. One of the most important of these is the shape of a portal; incisions should always be linearly triangular, diverging from the joint in order to minimize resistance to fluid outflow. External pressure, such as placing a finger, over the skin incision to stop or reduce fluid flow is usually counterproductive and promotes filling in the subcutaneous and periarticular tissue. If the high fluid input rate on a skin portal is obstructed by instruments, this similarly promotes extravasation to periarticular tissues. Fluid ingress rates should therefore be modulated during instrument manipulations.

Commonly, switching of arthroscope and instrument portals is necessary during surgical procedures (e.g., in the presence

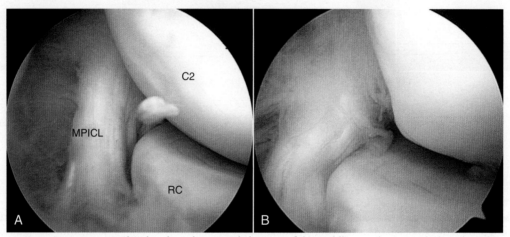

Figure 4-10 A, Structures visualized in the palmaromedial aspect of the middle carpal joint, including the palmaromedial surface of the radial carpal bone *(RC)* and second carpal bone *(C2)*, and the medial palmar intercarpal ligament *(MPICL)*. **B,** Flexion of the joint relaxes the MPICL.

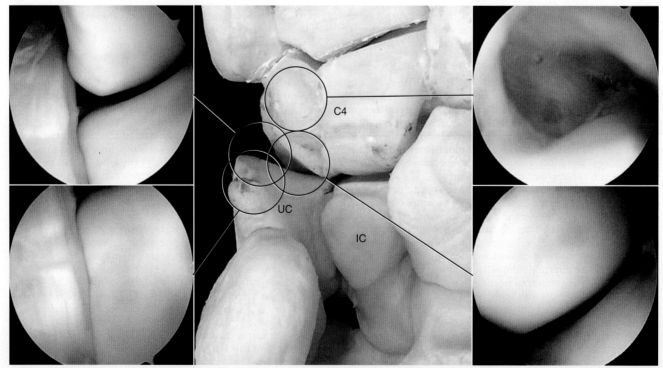

Figure 4-11 Structures visualized in the palmarolateral aspect of the middle carpal joint. The palmarolateral surface of the ulnar *(UC)* and fourth carpal *(C4)* bone are easily viewed. The intermediate carpal bone *(IC)* is not accessible without synovial and capsular resection.

of multiple, commonly biaxial lesions). Reinsertion of the arthroscope into a nondistended joint must be done with care to avoid iatrogenic damage. This can be obviated by use of a second arthroscopic cannula placed through the instrument portal before withdrawing the arthroscope from its initial location. "Switching sticks" have been described (Johnson, 1986); these are simple long obturators without a flanged end that can be placed into the joint under arthroscopic guidance and then serve as a guide to reposition the cannula from its current position. They obviate the need to use two arthroscope cannulae during a procedure. Whenever the arthroscope is removed from one portal and placed in another, there will be transient loss of joint distension. This is usually associated with hemorrhage, which is readily cleared by the insertion of an egress cannula and transient high fluid flow.

ARTHROSCOPIC SURGERY FOR REMOVAL OF OSTEOCHONDRAL CHIP FRAGMENTS

Current Status and Advantages of Arthroscopic Surgery

The potential to return horses to training and racing more quickly following arthroscopic surgery was initially perceived as its principal advantage over both conservative management and removal by arthrotomy. However, it is now widely understood that minimally traumatic removal of unstable osteochondral fragments also has major pathophysiological advantages for the joint and its continued function. Poor results can often be related to inadequate surgical ability, experience, or practice. Many problems can be avoided by good surgical techniques, and one of the main purposes of this textbook is to steer the beginning arthroscopist past some of the predictable pitfalls. Good technique requires skill and practice and demands a disciplined systematic approach. The techniques presented in this chapter are not the sole means of performing surgery but have worked for the authors and veterinarians who have undertaken the arthroscopic training courses that the authors have conducted worldwide. Modification and refinement of techniques continue, and it is the authors' philosophy to disseminate this information through training courses and publications.

Presurgical Information

As with any surgical candidate, as complete a history as possible is obtained. Particular emphasis should be placed on previous intraarticular corticosteroid medication, although the authors are not aware of any associated complications. There is wide variation in the clinical features associated with carpal fragmentation, but severity generally reflects the amount of articular damage. As with other work-related injuries, bilateral radiographic examination is mandatory. Bilateral or clinically silent lesions, or both, are common.

There is also a lack of correlation between radiographic and arthroscopic findings, with the latter frequently more severe than predicted (McIlwraith et al, 1987). Arthroscopy will also reveal osteochondral lesions that are not predicted by radiographs frequently at sites which cannot be imaged in profile by any radiographic projections. Other imaging modalities such as magnetic resonance imaging (MRI) may be able to predict such lesions, but this remains unknown.

Relevant Pathobiology

Carpal fragmentation frequently presents with acute clinical signs, and in some instances the radiologic features and subsequent arthroscopic examination are consistent with acute injury. However, in most cases fragmentation appears to have occurred at the end of a pathologic process. Some fragments come from articular margins previously altered by subchondral bone disease (Pool & Meagher, 1990). It is also now increasingly recognized that many intraarticular fractures result from cumulative micro damage in subchondral bone (Kawcak et al, 2000 & 2001).

Osteochondral fragmentation has direct physical effects on the joint because of the loss of the smooth articular surface and indirect effects due to the release of articular cartilage and bone debris, which leads in turn to synovitis. Severe compromise of the articular surfaces leads to instability, as does tearing of fibrous joint capsule and ligaments. The synovial membrane responds directly to mechanical trauma and indirectly to injury elsewhere in the joint. Increased intraarticular pressures generated by synovial effusion compromises the microstability. Damage to synoviocytes also liberates matrix metalloproteinases, aggrecanase, prostaglandins, free radicals, and cytokines (principally interleukin-1 [IL-1]), which can lead to articular cartilage degeneration and osteoarthritis (OA) (McIlwraith, 2005). Chronic articular insult results in fibrosis of the joint capsule and consequent loss of motion. Arthrofibrosis is recognized as an important problem in humans. The cause is still unknown, but the use of skilled arthroscopic techniques is considered critical in the minimization of arthrofibrosis in man (Finerman & Noyce, 1992).

Thus, from the joint's perspective, the primary indication for surgical treatment of osteochondral fragments in the carpus is to minimize the articular insult and prevent development of osteoarthritis (McIlwraith & Bramlage, 1996). It is recognized that following loss of articular surface, the joint is not returned to normal. All articular defects produce incongruity, mal-loading of adjacent surfaces and microinstability. These features, in turn, are limited by a conservative approach to lesion debridement following fragment removal such that as much viable osteochondral tissue as possible is retained. Following these principles and the techniques that follow, horses that sustain osteochondral chip fractures can be returned to full athletic function (McIlwraith et al, 1987).

Location of Intraarticular Fragments

McIlwraith et al (1987) reported the incidence and location of osteochondral fragments in the dorsal compartments of 1000 carpal joints in 591 horses (Box 4-1). All but 11 were racehorses comprising 220 Thoroughbreds, 349 Quarter Horses, 5 Appaloosas, and 6 Standardbreds. The others included 2 barrel-racing Quarter Horses, 3 roping Quarter Horses, and 6 other riding horses.

Of the 591 horses, 278 horses were 2 years old, 196 were 3 years old, 52 (55%) were 4 years old, 47 were 5 years or older, and 18 did not have their age documented. In 326 horses, osteochondral fragments were noted in one carpus, whereas 265 (45%) horses had bilateral lesions. Multiple joint involvement was more common in Quarter Horses in which 1 joint was operated in 144, 2 joints in 130, 3 joints in 46, and 4 joints in 30 horses. In Thoroughbreds, a single joint was involved in

Box • 4-1

Distribution of Carpal Chip Fragments

540 Intercarpal (Midcarpal) Joints

Distal radial carpal bone	475
Distal intermediate carpal bone	106
Proximal third carpal bone	60
Total	641

460 Radiocarpal (Antebrachiocarpal) Joints

Distal lateral radius	167
Distal medial radius	96
Proximal radial carpal bone	168
Proximal intermediate carpal bone	273
Proximal ulnar carpal bone	1
Total	705

From McIlwraith CW, Yovich JV, Martin GS. Arthroscopic surgery for the treatment of osteochondral chip fractures in the equine carpus, *J Am Vet Med Assoc* 191:531–540, 1987.

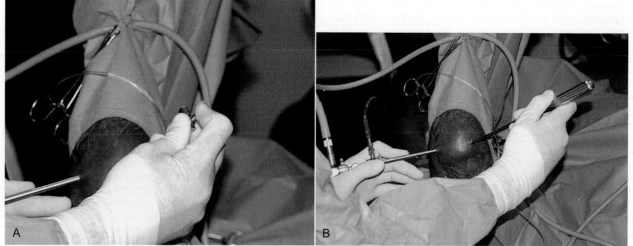

Figure 4-12 Manipulation of carpal fragment with a closed egress needle **(A)** and a probe **(B)** to evaluate the mobility of a carpal chip fragment in the intercarpal joint.

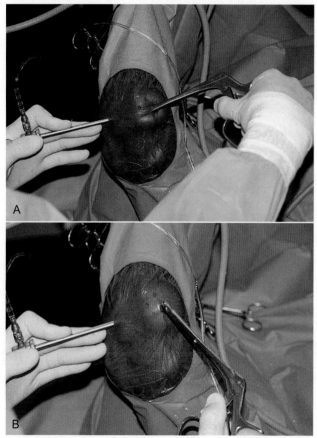

Figure 4-13 Removal of a carpal chip fragment from the intercarpal joint using Ferris-Smith cup rongeurs: **A,** grasping of the fragment; **B,** removal of fragment through the skin.

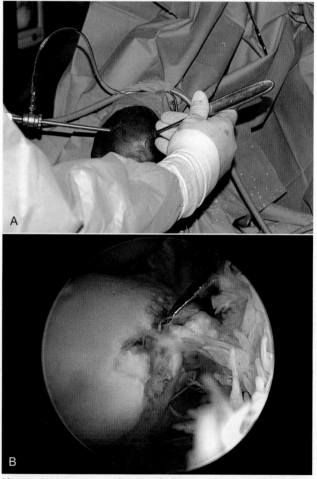

Figure 4-14 A, External view of elevating fragment. **B,** Internal arthroscopic view of elevating fragment.

142 horses, 2 joints in 70, 3 joints in 14, and 4 joints in 1 horse (McIlwraith et al, 1987).

There is geographic and breed/use variability. In the middle carpal joint of European Thoroughbreds, the relative frequency of fragments from the proximal third and distal intermediate carpal bones is reversed, and in the antebrachiocarpal joint fragmentation of the intermediate facet of the distal radius is the commonest focus (IMW, unpublished data). Fragmentation in the antebrachiocarpal joint of Standardbreds is uncommon, and lesions of the proximal third and distal radial carpal bones are by far the most common sites. The combined date of the two principal papers (Palmer, 1986; Lucas et al, 1999) gives a total of 251 Standardbreds with fragmentation of the proximal third carpal bone in 177, distal radial carpal bone in 150, distal intermediate carpal bone in 3, proximal radial carpal bone in 2, distal radius in 2, and proximal intermediate carpal bone in 1 horse.

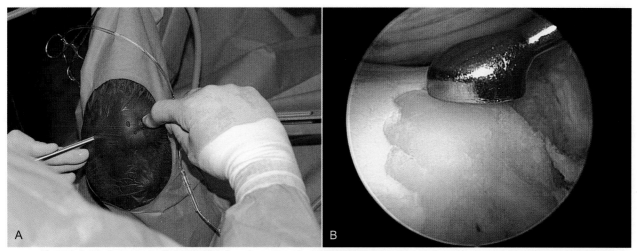

Figure 4-15 Curettage of undermined and separated cartilage at edge of lesion using a curette. **A,** External view. **B,** Arthroscopic view.

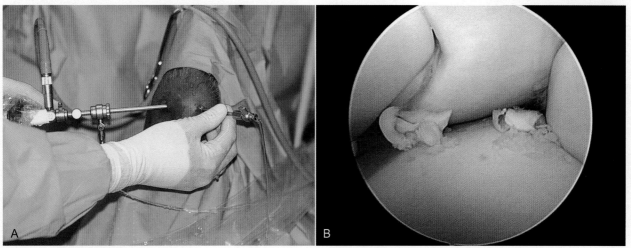

Figure 4-16 Flushing debris from central area of middle carpal joint. **A,** External view. **B,** Arthroscopic view.

General Technique

Removal of carpal fragmentation uses the technique of triangulation as described in Chapter 3 (Figs. 4-12 to 4-14). Specific details on the arthroscopic and instrument approaches for individual fragment locations follow, but generally for fragments on the medial side of the joint, the arthroscope passes through the lateral portal and the instruments enter through a medial portal and vice versa.

The basic protocol for surgery of all carpal fragmentation is similar. A diagnostic arthroscopic examination is always performed first. If there is hemorrhage or other discoloration of the synovial fluid, the egress is used to flush the joint. When the view is clear, the egress is closed and the joint evaluated. This should include palpation of lesions with a probe (see Fig. 4-12), including assessment of size and degree of attachment of fragments. If multiple lesions are present, the surgeon should decide an appropriate order of surgery. As a general principle, smaller and less accessible lesions should be treated first.

If the fragment is fresh and mobile on palpation, immediate insertion of appropriately sized Ferris-Smith arthroscopic rongeurs is done. The fragment is grasped, and the forceps are rotated to free the chip of soft tissue attachments (if these are significant), before it is removed (see Fig. 4-13). A Ferris-Smith jaw size is chosen to enclose the fragment as completely as possible to minimize loss, as this is brought through the joint capsule, subcutis, or skin (see Fig. 4-13). Rongeurs

with a jaw size of 4 × 10 mm are suitable for most carpal fragments and locations. Tearing a fragment loose from its soft tissue attachment by twisting the forceps may not seem as aesthetically pleasing or relate as well to basic surgical principles as sharp severance of the attachments, but it minimizes the risk of creating a free-floating fragment.

If attachments at the fracture line are strong and the fragment cannot be displaced with initial probing, a small elevator is used to separate the chip from the parent bone (see Fig. 4-14). Also, when the chip has considerable fibrous capsular insertions, as typically occurs with fragmentation of the distal lateral radius, then an elevator or a fixed blade arthroscopy knife can also be used to separate these attachments before removal of the fragment with forceps. It is important in either of these situations that the rongeurs are not used to twist or lever the fragment because these maneuvers frequently break the instrument jaws.

Following fragment removal, debridement is performed according to the principles described in Chapter 3 (Fig. 4-15). Other osseous defects may also be debrided at this time. Kissing lesions are evaluated, but when they are of partial thickness and cartilage is attached to bone, they are not debrided.

At the end of the procedures, thorough, directed, high-pressure lavage of the joint is important to remove all particulate debris and the larger 4.5-mm egress cannula is used (Fig. 4-16). The egress can also be used to rub off small tags of cartilage and bone (see Fig. 4-16). Lavage should continue

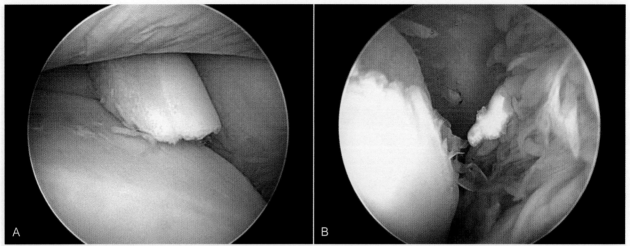

Figure 4-17 Free fragment in the joint **(A)** and adhered to synovial membrane **(B).**

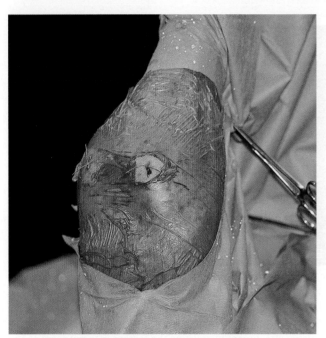

Figure 4-18 Skin sutures in portals.

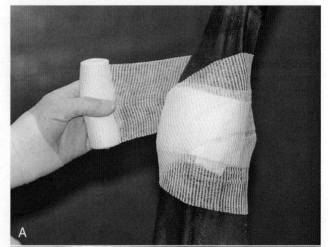

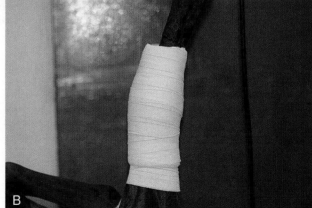

Figure 4-19 Bandage on carpal joint for recovery of anesthesia. **A,** Telfa pad and Kling are initially placed. **B,** A firm cotton wrap is then placed over the Kling bandage and Elasticon® taped over this.

until the joint is macroscopically cleared of debris. Occasionally, a fragment migrates away from the fracture site and is either free floating or attached to synovial membrane (Fig. 4-17). In such cases, it is removed with forceps.

At the completion of irrigation of the joint, the portals are closed by using skin sutures only (Fig. 4-18). Single or double simple interrupted sutures are recommended. Cruciate or other mattress patterns can be used but have no advantage and increase the amount of material pulled through the subcutis on removal. The incisions are covered with a sterile nonadhesive dressing and adhesive gauze, before an elastic or padded bandage is applied (Fig. 4-19).

The size of fragments that can be removed arthroscopically is limited only by the size of the secure grasping instrument that can be safely inserted in the joint. The skin incision has to be extended in some instances, but additional incising of the joint capsule is not usually required. Failure to lengthen the skin incision can result in the fragment being lost or trapped in the subcutis. Closure of large portals usually involves only additional skin sutures; repair of the joint capsule is rarely necessary (see Fig. 4-19).

Postoperative or intraoperative radiographs to ensure removal of all fragments are recommended. Although it is important that no loose fragments remain in the joint, some osseous densities in the radiographs may not be candidates for removal. In addition, osteophytes away from the articular margin and within the joint capsule (or enthesophytes) are of less concern. For any fragment or spur completely buried within the joint capsule, dissection out of the capsule is unnecessary and is excessively traumatic. The surgeon should be certain

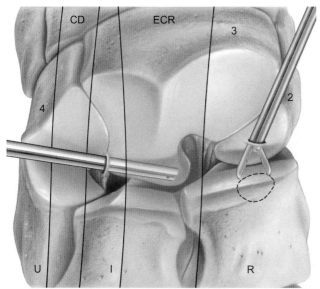

Figure 4-20 Diagram of positioning of arthroscope and instrument used during operations involving fragmentation of the distal radial carpal bone. *R*, Radial carpal bone; *I*, intermediate carpal bone; *U*, ulnar carpal bone; *3*, third carpal bone; *ECR*, extensor carpi radialis tendon; *CD*, digital extensor tendon.

that such fragments are indeed outside the joint cavity, and it is important to recognize that one should treat the patient rather than the radiograph. Veterinarians involved in obtaining follow-up radiographs of arthroscopic surgery patients should also be aware of this principle before proclaiming to the client or the trainer that "a chip has been left in the joint."

If radiographs reveal evidence of a fragment remaining in the joint, further arthroscopic examination is performed. When a fragment has lodged subcutaneously, the area is palpated and swept with a pair of hemostats. When the fragment is located, it is brought to the skin incision and grasped. Any soft tissue attachments to the fragment are severed while the fragment is held with forceps or a towel clamp. Occasionally, insertion of the arthroscope into subcutaneous pockets, with either no or little fluid flow, can assist in location of fragments.

Specific Sites of Carpal Chip Fragmentation

▶ *Dorsodistal Radial Carpal Bone*

The dorsodistal aspect of the radial carpal bone is both the most common and the most readily accessed site for carpal fragmentation but has the greatest range of pathologic change. The arthroscope is placed through the lateral portal with the lens angled proximad, and the instruments are brought through the medial portal (Fig. 4-20). Fragmentation can occur anywhere along the distal dorsal margin of the bone.

The fragmentation is imaged in profile in lateromedial (LM) and dorsolateral-palmaromedial oblique (DL-PaMO) radiographic projections (Figs. 4-21 to 4-25). Although traditionally the flexed lateromedial radiographic view has been used to assess the size of fragments and the amount of bone loss, it is important to recognize that (1) the chip is not always seen in this view and is detected only in the DL-PaMO oblique view and (2) that the correlation between radiographic and arthroscopic findings at this site is particularly poor. In addition, chip fractures have been found on the distal radial carpal bones that were not visualized on any of the radiographic views. Generally, these fragments are on the dorsolateral corner of the radial carpal bone (see Fig. 4-37), which is never projected in profile.

As with any chip fractures, the size of distal radial carpal bone lesion varies widely. The smallest lesions manifest radiographically as a small, mineralized density or as a small lucency in the

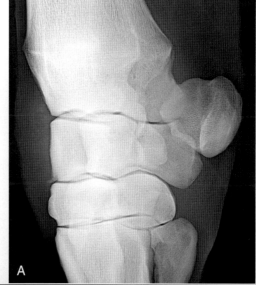

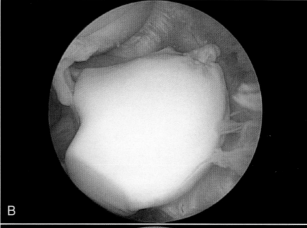

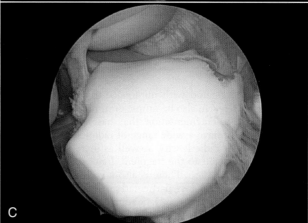

Figure 4-21 Small acute chip fracture of the dorsal distal radial carpal bone. **A,** Dorsolateral-palmaromedial oblique radiograph. **B,** Arthroscopic appearance of the fragment. **C,** Arthroscopic appearance following fragment removal and debridement.

distal dorsal margin (see Figs. 4-21 and 4-22). When examined arthroscopically, such lesions usually manifest as a small osteochondral fragment (see Figs. 4-21B and C) or a focus of fragmentation. Occasionally, an erosive defect is all that is found.

Larger osteochondral fragments are easily identified radiographically (see Figs. 4-22 to 4-24). At arthroscopy, the size and degree of displacement vary (see Fig. 4-24). Acute fragments

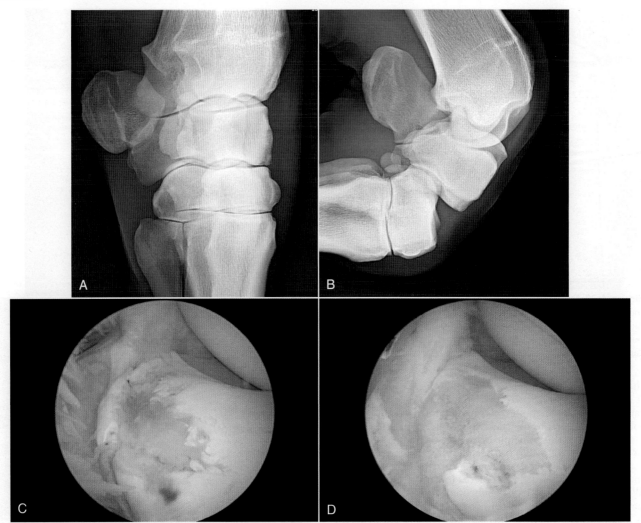

Figure 4-22 Dorsolateral-palmaromedial oblique **(A)** and flexed lateromedial **(B)** radiographic projections of a large chip fracture of the dorsodistal radial carpal bone. Demineralization of the fracture fragment and adjacent bone are consistent with chronicity. **C,** Arthroscopic appearance of the fragmentation. **D,** Arthroscopic appearance following fragment removal and debridement.

are sharply marginated with minimal disruption of adjacent parent bone. They can also be simple or multiple and displaced or nondisplaced. Fragmentation that has followed previous bone disease can have a wide range of radiologic appearances, including loss of radiodensity, as well as increased density in parent bone adjacent to the fragment, frank fragmentation, or crumbling degeneration. There is also a wide range of associated articular cartilage loss, particularly palmar to the fragmentation (see Figs. 4-23 and 4-24). Grading the degree of articular cartilage damage is discussed more fully in a subsequent section.

Radiographs also do not often predict accurately the extent of bone fragmentation found at arthroscopy. Both the amount of cartilage degeneration that extends back from the edge of the defect and the amount of subchondral bone loss vary considerably. Loss of bone is typically related to finding soft defective bone at surgery, which requires debridement. Such changes in the distal radial carpal bone can be severe when the radiographic changes appear rather mild. Often the degree of clinical compromise (lameness and synovial effusion) is a better indicator of the state of the joint than the radiographs. The presence of bloody or brown synovial fluid on initial entry is also usually a strong indicator of severe damage within the joint. In some instances, radiographs provide an indication of marked bone loss in association with chip fractures (Figs. 4-25

and 4-26), but usually the bone loss is more than is anticipated (see Figs. 4-25 and 4-26). In either case, when loss of bone is marked, there is loss of joint congruity and, potentially, instability. In instances where bone remains but there is Grade 3 articular cartilage loss, radiographs do not predict the amount of damage at all (Fig. 4-27). After removal of fragmentation, detached cartilage is removed and exposed subchondral bone debrided to healthy margins (see Fig. 4-27).

The prognosis is related to the amount of cartilage or bone loss, or both, and decreases with loss of bone along the entire dorsal margin of the bone. The relationship between prognosis and articular cartilage loss is more difficult to predict, particularly in racing Quarter Horses where the first author (C.W.M.) has had horses with complete loss of articular cartilage from the distal radial carpal bone that have come back and won at stakes level (see Fig. 4-27). Actual figures based on follow-up with these cases are presented in a subsequent section.

Fragmentation will frequently be found adjacent to the medial dorsal intercarpal ligament (MDIC) (Wright, 1995). On arthroscopic examination, its degree of confluence with the joint capsule is quite varied and the ligament cannot always be identified. The MDIC ligament may function as part of the medial collateral ligament, resist carpal bone displacement during weight bearing, or assist in production of "closed-pact" position in preparation for loading

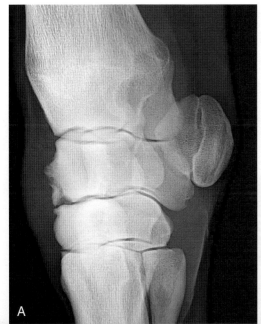

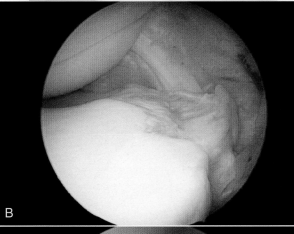

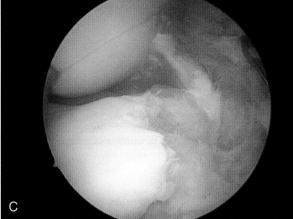

Figure 4-23 A, Large, long-standing chip fracture of the dorso-distal radial carpal bone. The fragment is displaced, and there is a degree of malunion. A large area of subchondral bone loss is evident at and adjacent to the articular margin of the fracture. The fragment is devoid of infrastructure. Densification is evident in the adjacent parent bone, which has a convex dorsal surface including substantial entheseous/capsular new bone. The adjacent dorsal margin of the third carpal bone is also remodeled and protuberant. **B,** Arthroscopic appearance of the fracture depicted in **A.** The fragment protrudes dorsally beyond the dorsomedial intercarpal ligament, and fibrous tissue bridges the fracture plane. **C,** Arthroscopic appearance following fragment removal and debridement.

(Wright, 1995). There is no doubt that the origin of the ligament is commonly involved in degeneration and fragmentation of the dorsodistal medial aspect of the radial carpal bone, but all evidence suggests that this is not causative. Removal of fragments attached to the DMIC ligament will result in tearing and frayed tissue (Fig. 4-28) that can be debrided with basket forceps or a motorized synovial resector.

▶ Dorsodistal Intermediate Carpal Bone

Fragmentation of the dorsodistal aspect of the intermediate carpal bone is usually recognized on the flexed LM and the dorsomedial-palmarolateral oblique (DM-PaLO) projections (Fig. 4-29). Differentiation from periarticular remodeling and osteophytosis can sometimes be difficult. Most fragments are from the medial facet; some from the lateral facet can be radiographically silent. Fragmentation can be seen in young animals that have not yet commenced training and may be a manifestation of the osteochondrosis syndrome.

The approach for operating on the distal intermediate carpal bone lesions is illustrated in Figure 4-30. The arthroscope is placed through the medial portal, and the instrument enters through the lateral portal. Visualization is usually good (Fig. 4-31), but the instrument angle is not as convenient for these lesions as for those on the distal radial carpal bone. Because the distance from the instrument portal to the lesion is often small, opening forceps inside the joint is sometimes difficult. This can be aided (if fragmentation at this site is predicted preoperatively) by making the lateral portal closer to the distal row of carpal bones. Lesions on the most medial portion of the intermediate carpal bone can be more difficult to visualize completely because differential movement between radial and intermediate carpal bones when the carpus is flexed produces a "step" in the middle carpal joint.

Lesions of the distal intermediate carpal bone vary in size, but most are small and discrete. In these cases, the prognosis is good. Fragmentation at this site can also be found in horses with other lesions within the middle carpal joint (Fig. 4-32). As always, complete evaluation of the joint at the beginning of surgery is mandatory when lesions can be logged and a logical order of approach made. Radiographically silent lesions on the lateral aspect of the radial carpal bone are commonly encountered when operating on distal intermediate carpal bone fragmentation (and can usually be treated using the same lateral instrument portal).

▶ Dorsoproximal Third Carpal Bone

Fragmentation of the dorsoproximal third carpal bone most commonly involves its radial facet but can occur at any point along its distal margin. Schneider et al (1988) in a series of 371 third carpal bone fractures in 313 horses recorded fragmentation of the dorsal margin of the radial facet in 171 and from the intermediate facet in 4 horses. The former comprised large chip fractures in 140 cases, smaller fragments in 18 cases, and medial corner fractures in 13 cases. Fractures of the third carpal bone are commonly associated with fragmentation at other sites. Twenty-four percent of the cases reported by Schneider et al (1988) had fragmentation of ipsilateral radial or intermediate carpal bones, or both, and 21% of horses with large chip fractures of the radial facet of the third carpal bone had fragmentation of the contralateral third carpal bone.

Fragmentation of the radial facet of the third carpal bone may be visualized in lateromedial, dorsolateral-palmaromedial oblique (DL-PaMO) and flexed dorsoproximal-dorsodistal (DPr-DDi) oblique (Fig. 4-33A and B) projections. In 10% of the cases reported by Schneider et al (1988), fractures were visible only in the latter projection. The less commonly encountered fragmentation of the dorsal margin of the intermediate facet of the third carpal bone can be identified in dorsomedial-palmarolateral (DM-PaLO)

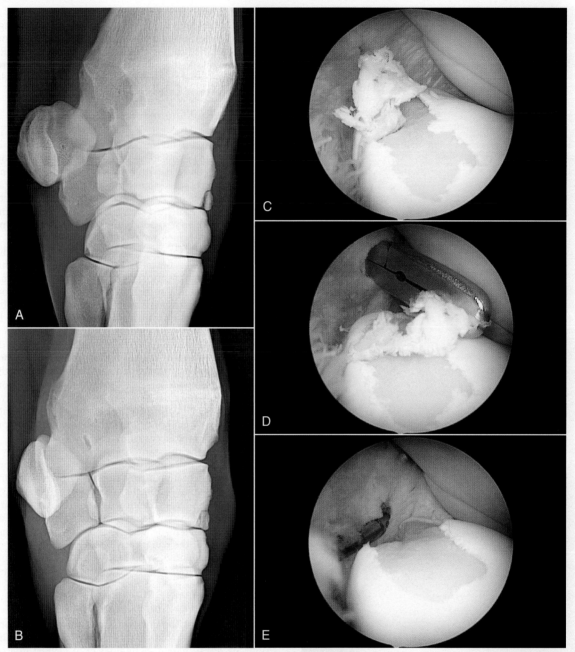

Figure 4-24 A and **B,** Two dorsolateral-palmaromedial oblique projections of a large chip fracture of the dorso-distal radial carpal bone illustrating how fracture assessment can be altered by small changes in projection angle. **C,** Arthroscopic appearance of the fracture depicted in **A** and **B** demonstrating also palmar comminution and a full-thickness cartilage defect extending laterally from the principle fracture fragment. **D,** Arthroscopic ronguers removing palmar comminution. **E,** Arthroscopic appearance following fragment removal and debridement.

projections. The radiologic features associated with acute fragmentation of the third carpal bone are similar to other sites. When this has occurred at the end of the degenerative process, there is commonly densification of the parent bone. This involves a generalized increase in radiodensity, most commonly of the radial facet, and loss of regular dorsopal-marally oriented trabecular infrastructure in the flexed dor-soproximal-dorsodistal oblique (DPr-DDiO) projections. Irregular lucencies in the proximal subchondral bone plate may also be recognized and are commonly found at arthros-copy to be associated with nonmarginal fragmentation.

Figure 4-34 illustrates the surgical technique for operat-ing on fragments of the third carpal bone. The arthroscope

is placed laterally, and the instruments are placed medially. Because of the central location of the chip, the reversed posi-tion could be used, but the triangulation technique described and illustrated here is preferable because the distal radial car-pal bone surface is further away from the third carpal bone than is the intermediate. Therefore, manipulation of instru-ments onto the third carpal bone is more convenient with a medial approach. Third carpal bone fractures may be typi-cal chip-type fragments, which are separated from the bone and simple to remove (Fig. 4-35A). Partial slab fractures that extend halfway down the bone distad and exit dorsad within the joint capsule attachment (Fig. 4-36) or complete slab fractures are also amenable to arthroscopic surgery. Thin slab

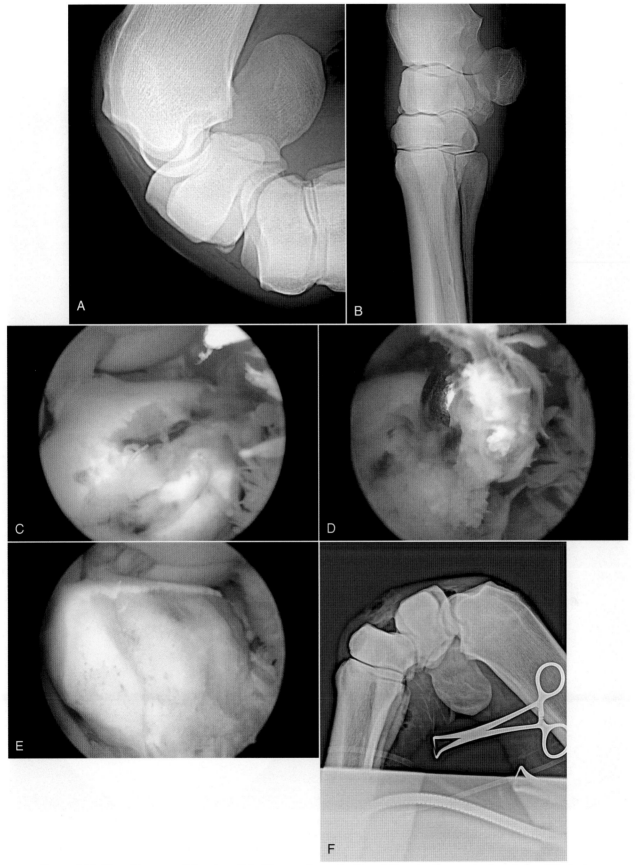

Figure 4-25 Flexed lateromedial and medial oblique radiographs (**A** and **B**) and arthroscopic views before (**C**), during fragmentation removal (**D**) and after removal and debridement (**E**) of grade IV fragmentation of distal radial carpal bone. **F,** Postoperative radiographs showing beveling on radiographs, but there is more dramatic demonstration of the bone loss in arthroscopic views.

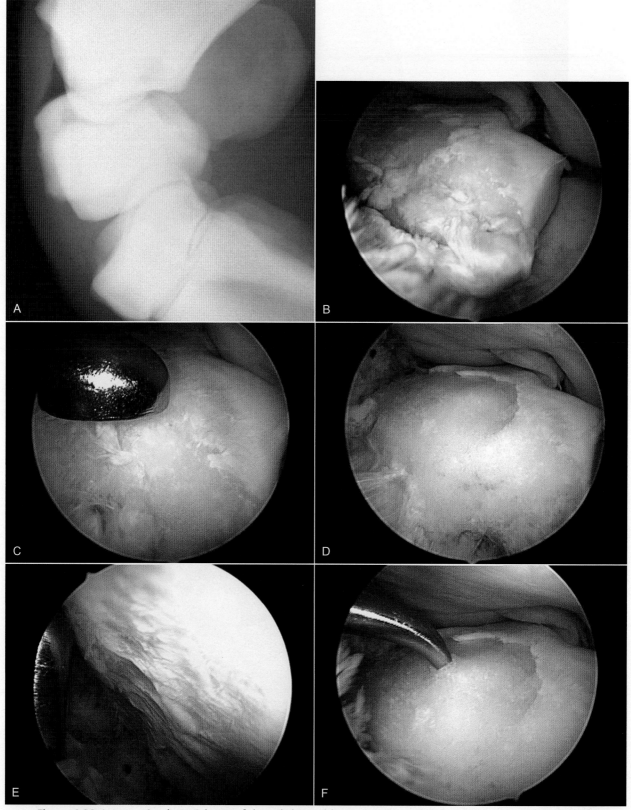

Figure 4-26 A severe (grade 3–4) lesion of the radial carpal bone on radiograph **(A)** and arthroscopic views before **(B)**, during **(C)**, and after debridement **(D).** Note the fragment off the lateral corner not visible on radiographs. Kissing lesion on the opposite third carpal bone **(E)** and microfracturing of palmar aspect of the radial carpal bone defect **(F).**

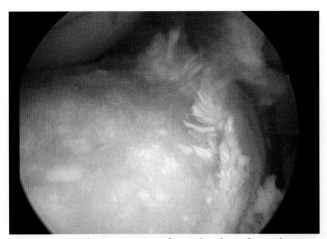

Figure 4-27 Arthroscopic view of complete loss of articular cartilage from visible area of distal radial carpal bone. Radiographs did not show significant change in the distal radial carpal bone. This horse came back and won at Grade I level after this surgery and was champion racing Quarter Horse in U.S. that year.

fractures through entire thickness of the third carpal bone can also be removed by using arthroscopic technique, although cutting the carpometacarpal joint capsule attachments with these is difficult. The less common fragmentation of the dorsal margin of the intermediate facet can be managed using either dorsomedial or dorsolateral instrument approaches. The most common single site of fragments from the radial facet lies beneath the tendon of insertion of the extensor carpi radialis and its sheath, and with the joint flexed there is closer contact between the joint capsule and dorsal surface of the bone. Joint distention is therefore more critical at this site than for lesions of the radial and intermediate carpal bone, so when these are present concomitantly, lesions of the third carpal bone should be managed first.

The general technique for fragment removal is as described previously. Larger fragments frequently extend into the dorsal capsular reflection (so-called partial slab fragments) and may require dissection before removal. Sometimes this will involve portions of the transverse dorsal intercarpal ligaments. Visualization and removal can be facilitated by extending the joint more than is usual for most middle carpal joint procedures.

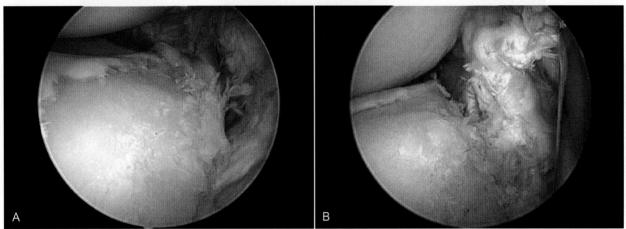

Figure 4-28 Fraying of the medial plica (medial dorsal intercarpal ligament) in association with fragmentation off the distal radial carpal bone. **A,** Mild case. **B,** More severe case. This injury commonly accompanies such fragmentation.

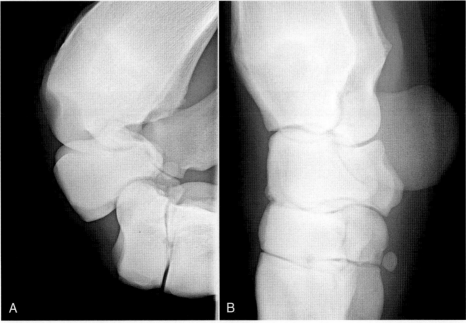

Figure 4-29 Flexed lateromedial and dorsomedial-palmarolateral oblique (DM-PaLO) views demonstrating small (**A** and **B**) fragments off the distal intermediate carpal bone.

Continued

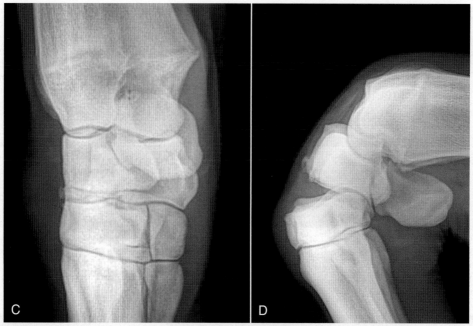

Figure 4-29, cont'd Flexed lateromedial and dorsomedial-palmarolateral oblique (DM-PaLO) views demonstrating large (**C** and **D**) fragments off the distal intermediate carpal bone.

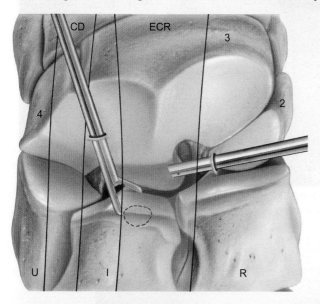

Figure 4-30 Diagram of positioning of arthroscope and instrument during operations involving a distal intermediate carpal bone chip fragment. *R,* Radial carpal bone; *I,* intermediate carpal bone; *U,* ulnar carpal bone; *2,* second carpal bone; *3,* third carpal bone; *4,* fourth carpal bone; *ECR,* extensor carpi radialis tendon; *CD,* common digital extensor tendon.

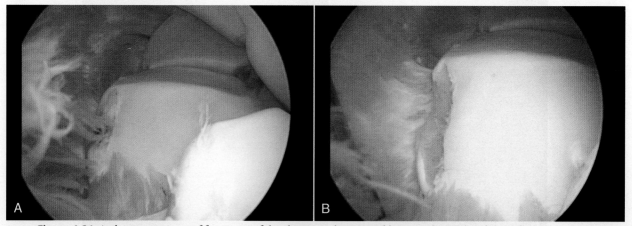

Figure 4-31 Arthroscopic views of fragments of distal intermediate carpal bone (radiographs of these fragments are in Fig. 4-29A and B). **A,** Fragment before removal. **B,** After removal.

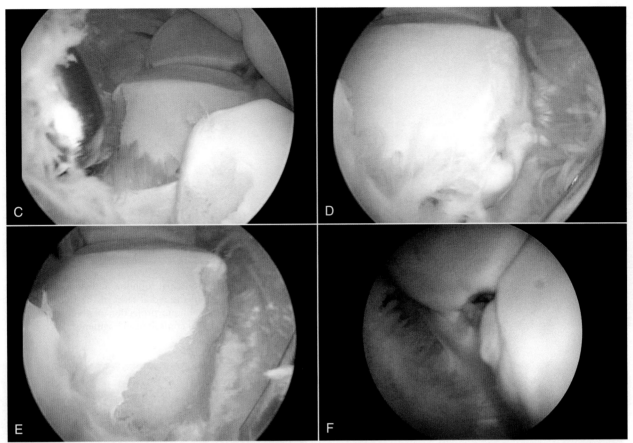

Figure 4-31, cont'd C, View after removal of additional fragment off distal radial carpal bone using same lateral instrument portal. **D** and **E,** Larger fragment off distal intermediate carpal bone. **F,** Fragment on lateral margin adjacent to ulnar carpal bone.

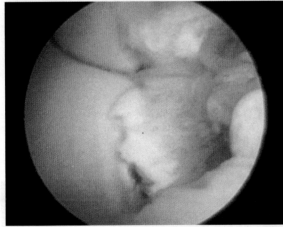

Figure 4-32 Fragment on distal intermediate carpal bone found during diagnostic arthroscopy for removal of a fragment on distal radial carpal bone. The fragment is on the most-medial margin of the distal intermediate carpal bone and in this case was removed using a medial instrument portal.

Dorsoproximal Radial Carpal Bone

The technique for operating on fragmentation at this site is illustrated in Figure 4-37. These fractures are usually identified preoperatively with flexed lateromedial, but may also be identified with dorsolateral-palmaromedial (DL-PaM) oblique and standing LM radiographs. As with other sites, the size of lesions can vary widely (Figs. 4-38 and 4-39). The arthroscope is placed through a dorsolateral portal, and instruments enter through a dorsomedial portal. The narrow dorsomedial portal and underlying joint space limit instrument maneuverability. Rongeurs usually have to be introduced into the joint, passed slightly lateral to the fragmentation, opened, and then withdrawn to enclose the fragment(s). This maneuver blocks free fluid flow from the instrument portal. Flow rates therefore should be reduced appropriately in order to limit periarticular extravasation.

Occasionally, a lateral arthroscopic portal can be used (Fig. 4-40). Generally fragments of the proximal margin of the radial carpal bone are accompanied by less subchondral compromise and palmar cartilage loss than their distal counterparts.

▶ Dorsoproximal Intermediate Carpal Bone

The technique for operating on fragmentation at this site is illustrated in Figure 4-41 using dorsomedial arthroscopic and dorsolateral instrument portals. Fragments are most frequently seen in profile in flexed lateromedial (LM) projections but may also be identified on dorsomedial-palmarolateral (DM-PaL) oblique (Fig. 4-42) projections. These fragments can be small, distinct, and easily removed (see Fig. 4-42), but often they are large and extend a considerable distance into the joint capsule attachments (Fig. 4-43). In such cases, prior separation of capsular attachments in addition to separation at the fracture line is recommended. Dissection from the capsular attachments, in line with general principles, should be performed with minimal soft tissue trauma. Similarly, surgeons should debride only cautiously beyond the capsular reflection.

Proximal Ulnar Carpal Bone

Fragments at this site are rare. To perform arthroscopic surgery for this lesion, the arthroscope is placed dorsomedially and instruments are placed dorsolaterally.

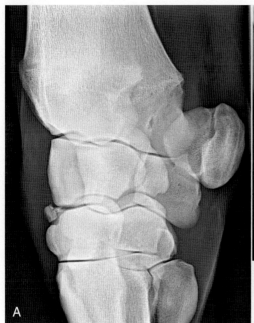

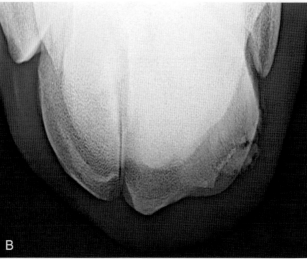

Figure 4-33 A, Dorsolateral-palmaromedial oblique radiograph depicting a comminuted displaced chip fracture of the radial facet of the third carpal bone. **B,** Flexed dorsoproximal-dorsodistal oblique projection of fracture depicted in **A** demonstrating additional small, dorsal comminuted fragments.

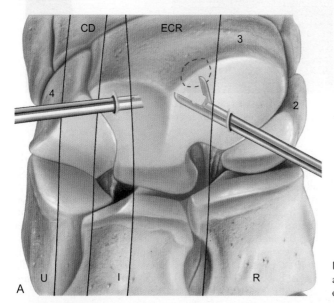

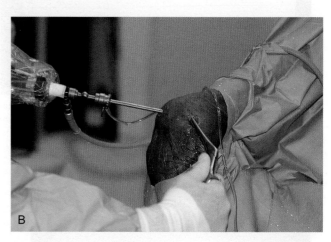

Figure 4-34 Diagram of arthroscope and instrument during operations involving chip fragments off the third carpal bone **(A)** and external view **(B).**

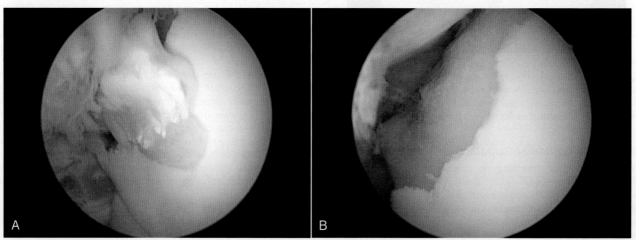

Figure 4-35 Arthroscopic views (**A** and **B**) of removal of fracture fragments from the third carpal bone (case in Fig. 4-33).

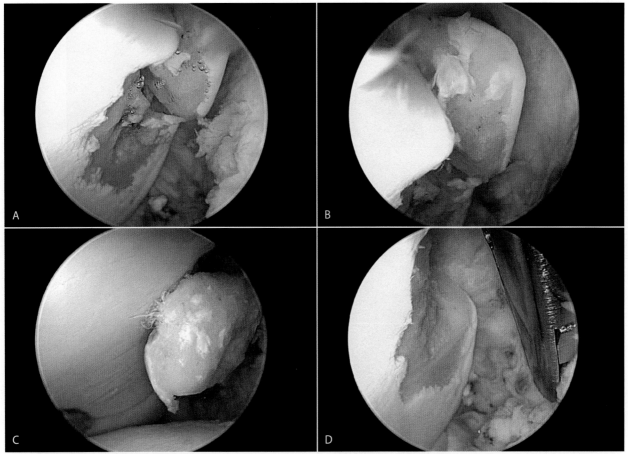

Figure 4-36 Arthroscopic views of a partial slab fragment of the third carpal bone. **A** and **B,** Surface defect at proximal-distal length of the fragment, respectively. **C,** At removal of the fragment. **D,** At debridement.

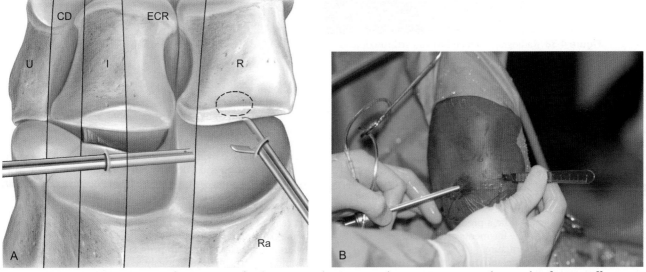

Figure 4-37 A, Diagram of positioning of arthroscope and instrument during operations involving a chip fracture off the proximal aspect of the radial carpal bone. **B,** Making instrument portal. *R,* Radial carpal bone; *I,* intermediate carpal bone; *U,* ulnar carpal bone; *ECR,* extensor carpi radialis tendon; *CD,* common digital extensor tendon; *Ra,* distal radius.

▶ *Distal Lateral Radius*

Fragmentation of the distal lateral radius almost invariably involves the dorsal margin of its intermediate facet and specifically the convexity at the distal margin of the ridge that forms the groove in the dorsodistal radius between extensor carpi radialis and the common digital extensor tendons and their sheaths.

Fragments at this site are usually profiled in dorsomedial-palmarolateral (DM-PaL) oblique radiographs (Fig. 4-44). This projection will usually delineate the proximal limit of the fracture, which frequently is long and extends beyond the joint capsule reflection from the distal radius. As a result of this feature, horses with fractures at this site will commonly, in addition to distension

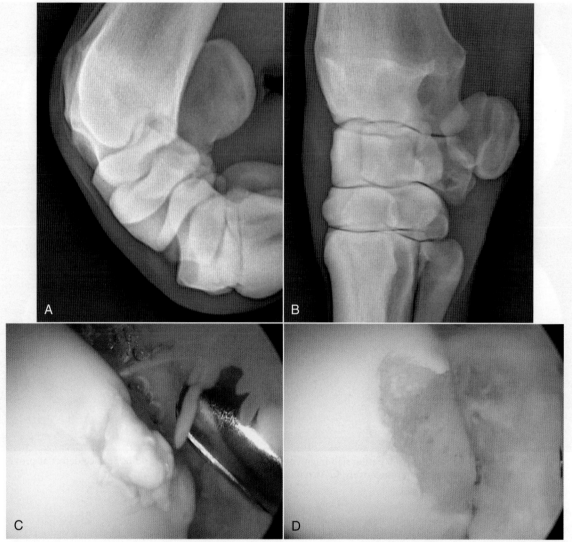

Figure 4-38 Radiographs (**A** and **B**) and arthroscopic views before (**C**) and after (**D**) removal of a small fragment from the proximal aspect of the radial carpal bone.

of the antebrachiocarpal joint, exhibit soft tissue swelling dorso-laterally over the distal radial epiphysis and metaphysis. Fractures that are long-standing or that have occurred following long-standing osseous failure will frequently exhibit periosteal and capsular new bone at this site. This swelling is usually seen between the extensor carpi radialis and common digital extensor tendons and their sheaths (see Fig. 4-44). Occasionally, the DM-PaL oblique radiograph will not demonstrate clearly a fracture. In this event, a flexed dorsoproximal-dorsodistal (DPr-DDi) oblique projection of the distal radius will be a predictor of fragmentation at this site (see Fig. 4-44E). The fragments often have reduced radiodensity and loss of infrastructure.

Dorsomedial arthroscope and dorsolateral instrument portals are employed as illustrated in Figure 4-45. The position of the fragments necessitates that instruments are directed distad so that their shafts lie at an angle close to the dorsal aspect of the carpus. The fragments are usually large (≥1 cm wide), with the most proximal portion attached to the fibrous joint capsule. These fractures are also commonly comminuted with a wedge-shaped osteochondral fragment palmar to the largest dorsal fragment. Damage is usually limited to the defect created by the fragments only, and cartilage loss does not usually extend peripheral to the defect (Figs. 4-46 and 4-47). The arthroscopic appearance depends on the age of the fragments.

In many such cases the dorsal fragment appears to be acute and the palmar wedge-shaped fragment appears to be longer standing (see Fig. 4-47). In acute fragmentation there is usually hemorrhage within the fracture. When there are multiple fragments, the larger fragment is usually beneath smaller superficial comminution and a deep search is important in these cases. With long-standing fractures, these fragments may coalesce, are associated with less debris, and often can be removed en masse.

Before retrieval, large fragments are elevated. Varying degrees of dissection from the joint capsule are necessary. Some fragments can simply be grasped and twisted free, whereas others benefit from prior sharp dissection. Dissection should be performed judiciously in order to minimize disruption of the joint capsule and specifically to avoid creation of a defect into the common digital extensor (or less commonly the extensor carpi radialis) tendon sheath because this can result in a permanent synovial communication (fistula) and distension of the sheath. Most fragments can be removed with 4- × 10-mm Ferris-Smith arthroscopic rongeurs, but occasionally 6- × 10-mm rongeurs are necessary and may require a concomitantly increased skin incision. Figure 4-47 depicts a chronic distal lateral radius fragment that was associated with osteochondral disease peripheral to the fracture. Damage is rarely more extensive than that noted here, unless the lesion is

Text continued on p.74

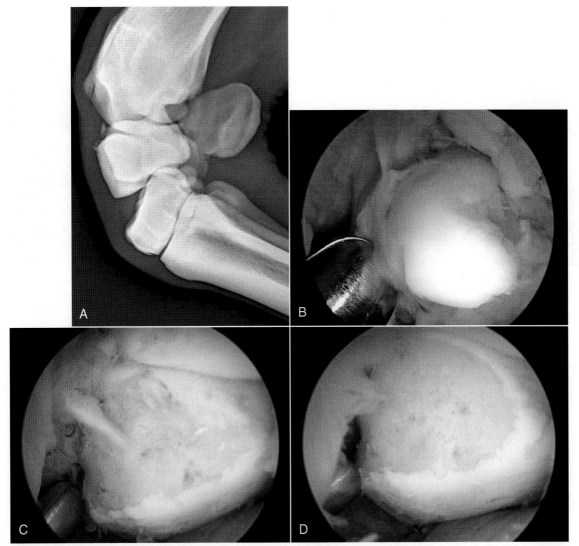

Figure 4-39 Flexed lateral to medial radiograph **(A)** and arthroscopic views **(B)** before removal. **C,** After removal. **D,** After debridement of larger displaced chronic fragment from the dorsoproximal margin of the radial carpal bone. (Note there was also fragmentation of the distal lateral radius and proximal intermediate carpal bone.)

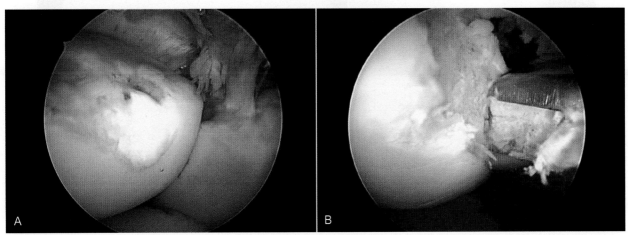

Figure 4-40 A and **B,** Fragmentation of the proximal radial carpal bone encountered during removal of a proximal intermediate carpal bone fragment and being removed using a lateral instrument portal.

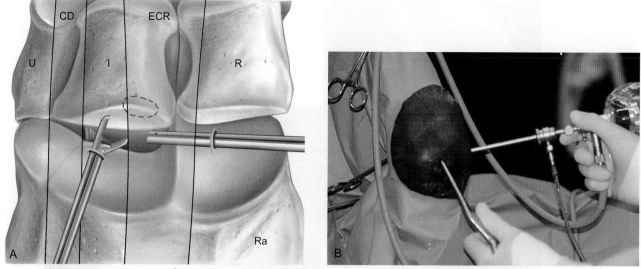

Figure 4-41 A, Diagram of positioning of arthroscope and instrument during operations involving fragmentation of the proximal aspect of the intermediate carpal bone. **B,** External view. *R,* Radial carpal bone; *I,* intermediate carpal bone; *U,* ulnar carpal bone; *ECR,* extensor carpi radialis tendon; *CD,* common digital extensor tendon; *Ra,* distal radius.

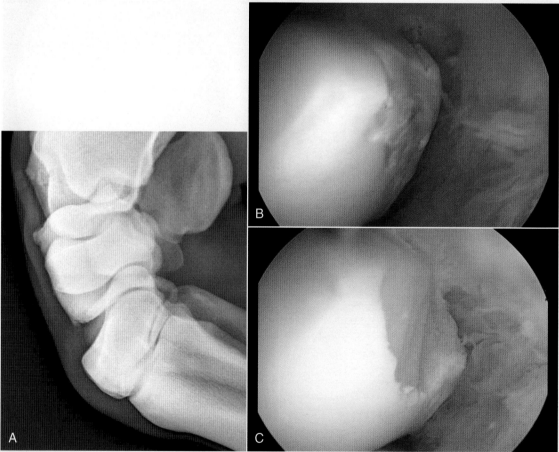

Figure 4-42 A, Flexed lateromedial radiograph demonstrating a fragment off the proximal intermediate carpal bone. **B,** Arthroscopic view of the fragment prior to removal. **C,** After fragment removal and debridement.

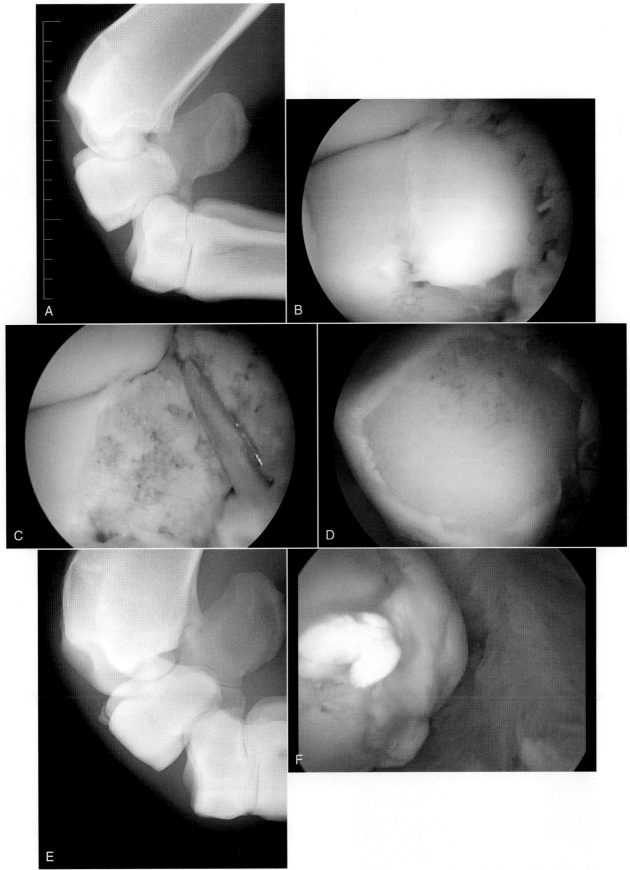

Figure 4-43 Radiographic view of carpus **(A)** with fragmentation of proximal intermediate carpal bone before removal **(B)**, after removal but before debridement **(C)**, and after debridement of defect **(D)**. Note absence of evidence of a fragment on preoperative radiograph (there is a small fragment on the proximal radial carpal bone). **E,** Flexed lateral to medial radiograph of larger fragment of proximal intermediate carpal bone. **F,** Prior to removal.

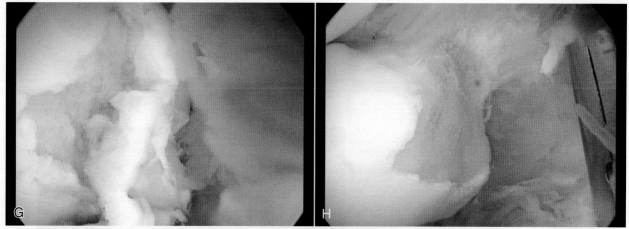

Figure 4-43, cont'd G, During elevation, and **H,** after debridement.

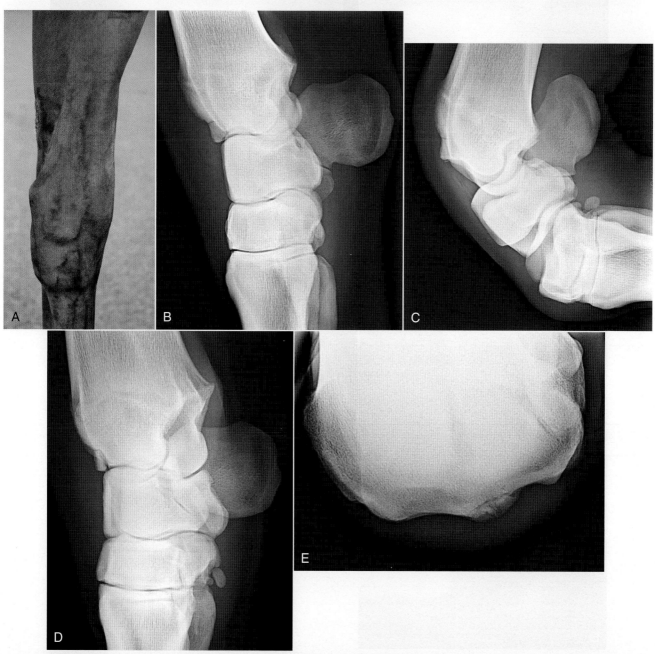

Figure 4-44 Osteochondral fragmentation of the dorsolateral radius **(A).** Clinical appearance demonstrating distention of the antebrachiocarpal joint and soft tissue swelling extending proximally between extensor carpi radialis and common digital extensor tendons and their sheaths. **B,** Lateromedial radiograph. **C,** Flexed lateromedial radiograph. **D,** Dorsomedial-palmarolateral oblique radiograph. **E,** Flexed dorsoproximal-dorsodistal oblique radiograph.

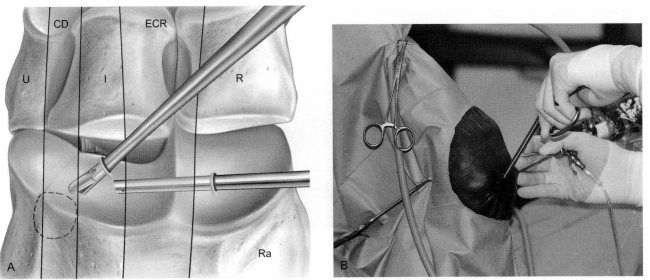

Figure 4-45 Diagram **(A)** and external view **(B)** of arthroscope and instrument during operations involving a chip fracture off the distal lateral radius.

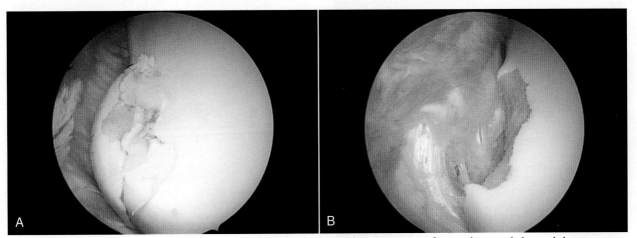

Figure 4-46 A, Arthroscopic appearance of the fracture depicted in Figure 4-44 from a dorsomedial portal demonstrating palmar comminution and dorsal displacement of the principle fracture fragment. **B,** Arthroscopic appearance following fragment removal and debridement demonstrating extension of the fragmentation into the dorsal capsular reflection.

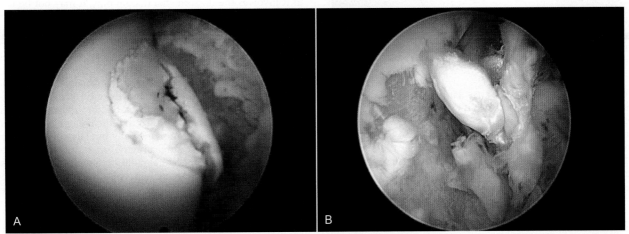

Figure 4-47 A, Arthroscopic view of large fresh fragment of distal lateral radius of right carpus. A fresh fragment associated with clear visualization of palmar osteochondral wedge.

Continued

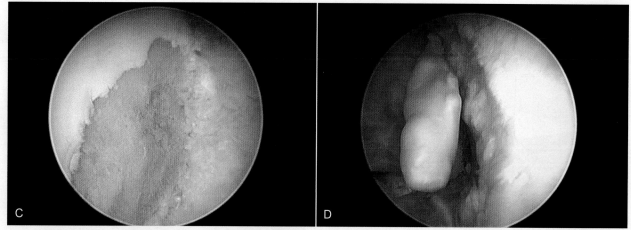

Figure 4-47, cont'd Arthroscopic views (**B** and **C**) of chronic distal lateral radius fragmentation in which the pieces were removed with Ferris-Smith rongeurs and deeper tissue debrided using a curette. **D,** Single, chronic fragment in opposite antebrachiocarpal joint.

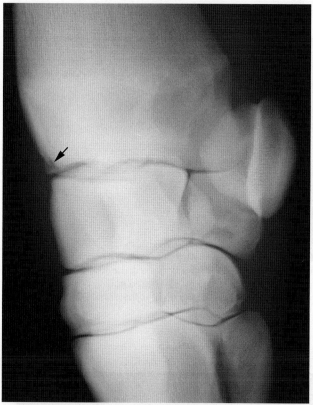

Figure 4-48 Dorsopalmar lateral to medial oblique radiograph demonstrating fragment off distal medial radius.

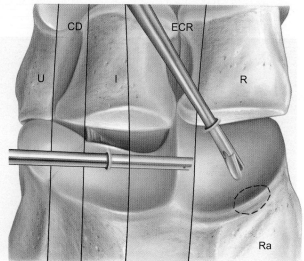

Figure 4-49 Diagram of positioning of arthroscope and instruments during operations involving a chip fracture off the distal medial radius. *R,* Radial carpal bone; *I,* intermediate carpal bone; *U,* ulnar carpal bone; *ECR,* extensor carpi radialis tendon; *CD,* common digital extensor tendon; *Ra,* distal radius.

chronic and mobile. Although articular defects associated with these fractures can be quite large, it does not appear to have a negative prognostic influence. Commonly, fractures at this site can be accompanied by defects or fragments on the adjacent intermediate carpal bone, and in many instances these are not radiographically obvious before surgery. When these fractures are of long duration, the fracture line may be obscured and the fragment is usually recognized by the presence of articular erosions and irregularities.

Distal Medial Radius

Fragmentation at this site is best demonstrated in dorsolateral-palmaromedial (DL-PaM) oblique radiographs (Fig. 4-48).

If it involves the dorsomedial margin only, it may not be identifiable in any other projection including flexed, dorsoproximal-dorsodistal (DPr-DDi) oblique projections. The technique for removing fracture fragments from the medial aspect of the distal radius is illustrated in Figure 4-49. Dorsolateral arthroscopic and dorsomedial instrument portals are used; as with distal lateral radius fragments, the instruments are angled rather flatly against the knee and directed proximad. These fragments are similar to their lateral counterparts in that the surface damage is usually localized to the area of the fragment. Small fragments are common medially, but large ones can occur (Fig. 4-50). Methods of surgical removal are the same as those described previously for lateral radius fragments, but the dorsomedial portal and underlying joint space are limited. Fragment size can vary, but the fractures are usually discrete and rarely extend into the joint capsule. Most do not require elevation or other dissection. Rongeurs usually have to be passed lateral to the fragment before the jaws are opened, and the instrument is withdrawn to grasp and remove the fragmentation. Fluid levels should be restricted to minimize extravasation at this time.

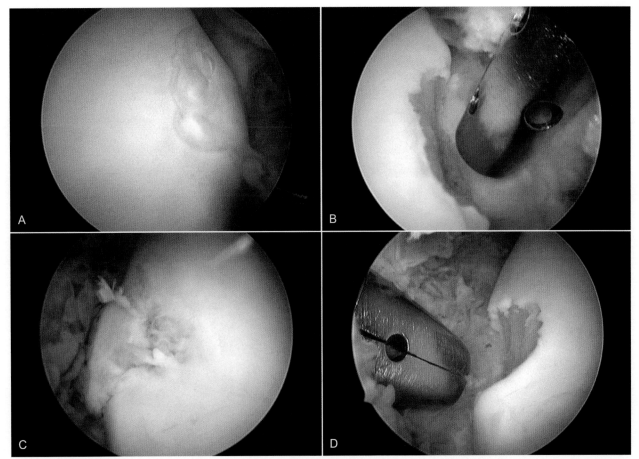

Figure 4-50 Arthroscopic views of small (**A** and **B**) and larger (**C** and **D**) fragments from the distal medial radius.

Debridement follows in line with previously described principles. The surface manifestation of these fragments varies like distal lateral chips, and the use of the curette may be necessary for chronic lesions (Fig. 4-51). Although uncommon, large fragments can extend sufficiently laterad to underlie the extensor carpi radialis tendon and its sheath. In such circumstances, the surgeon should minimize soft tissue dissection or debridement in order to reduce the risk of trauma to the same and consequential fistula formation and tenosynovitis (Fig. 4-52).

Fragmentation at Multiple Sites

Arthroscopic surgery is particularly suited to the removal of fragments from multiple sites. Particularly in the Quarter Horse, surgical procedures often involve both middle carpal and both antebrachiocarpal joints. In this situation it is recommended that the middle carpal joint(s) is/are operated on first because subcutaneous fluid extravasation is more likely to occur in the antebrachiocarpal joint. The loss of irrigating fluid after creation of a large instrument portal means that the surgeon will need to switch to the opposite side of the joint to operate on a chip on the other side and insert the arthroscope into a relatively nondistended joint. If time has passed between the two entries, some blood may be in the joint, which can be cleared by irrigation. The bleeding is usually from a previously debrided subchondral bone defect and occurs after loss of joint distention. With joint distention and irrigation, subchondral bleeding is usually not observed.

Removal of Osteophytes or Spurs

The removal of spurs or osteophytes is appropriate if these have fractured off or if their interposition into the joint makes them likely candidates for later fracture. Figure 4-53 demonstrates spurs that were removed. These spurs may be removed with Ferris-Smith rongeurs, curettage, an osteotome, or a burr.

Most spurs that are visible radiographically are not candidates for removal. In many instances the experienced surgeon can predict whether an attempt at removing a spur is appropriate by examining the radiographs. As a general rule, however, the surgeon should maintain an open mind and examine the spur at the time of arthroscopic surgery. This statement is not to say that every carpus with a spur is a candidate for arthroscopic surgery. As experienced clinicians know, many small spurs noted in 2-year-old horses are purely evidence of previous synovitis and capsulitis and are of no current clinical importance.

Classification of Articular Defects Associated with Carpal Fragmentation

McIlwraith et al (1987) reported four grades of articular defect resulting from fragmentation of carpal bones:
1. Minimal fibrillation or fragmentation at the edge of the defect left by the fragment, extending no more than 5 mm from the fracture line (Fig. 4-54A and B).
2. Articular cartilage degeneration extending more than 5 mm back from the defect and including up to 30% of the articular surface of that bone (see Fig. 4-54C and D).
3. Loss of 50% or more of the articular cartilage from the affected carpal bone (see Fig. 4-54E).
4. Significant loss of subchondral bone (usually distal radial carpal bone lesions) (see Fig. 4-54F and G).

These grades are illustrated in Figure 4-54. Significant bone loss causes loss of cuboidal congruency (see Fig. 4-54F and G).

This suffers from limitations common to all clinical grading systems but logically groups cases in order to assess the influence of the articular deficit itself on case outcome. This in turn

Text continued on p. 79

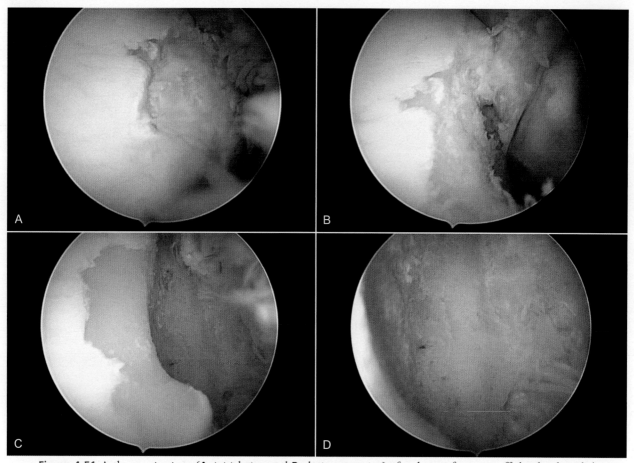

Figure 4-51 Arthroscopic views (**A,** initial view and **B,** during curetting) of a chronic fragment off the distal medial radius requiring progressive removal. After removal and debridement (**C** and **D**). **D,** Note fibrous joint capsule exposed.

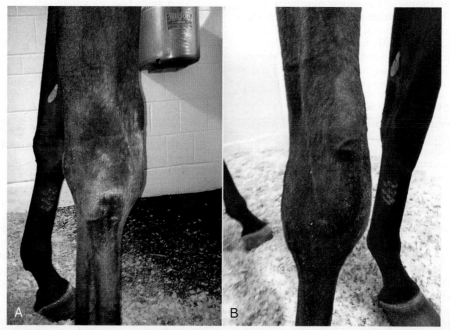

Figure 4-52 A and **B,** Tenosynovitis following removal of large fragment from distal medial radius.

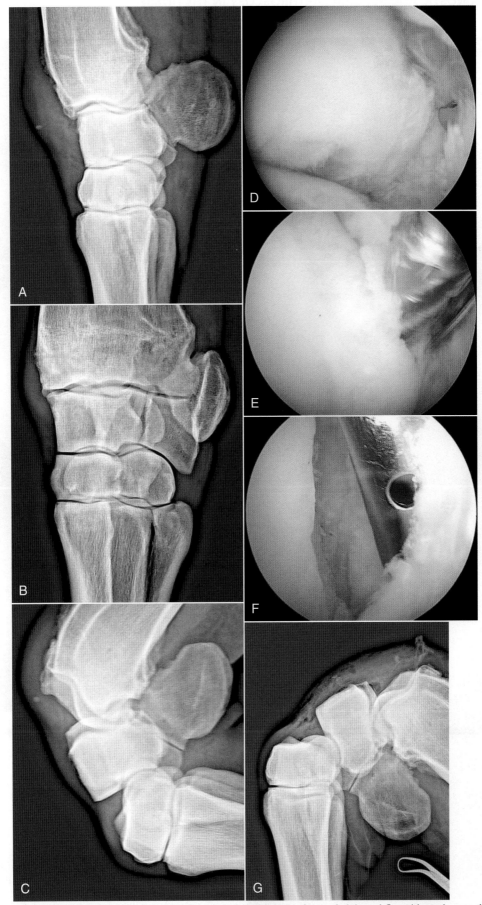

Figure 4-53 Lateromedial **(A)**, dorsolateral-palmaromedial oblique radiograph **(B)**, and flexed lateral to medial radiograph **(C)** of osteophytosis of the distal medial radius and proximal radial carpal bone. Arthroscopic views **(D)** of spur on proximal radial carpal bone prior to removal. **E,** Osteophyte on distal medial radius at commencement of removal and **F,** after removal of osteophytosis with the motorized burr. **G,** Intraoperative lateral to medial radiograph showing removal of osteophytosis.

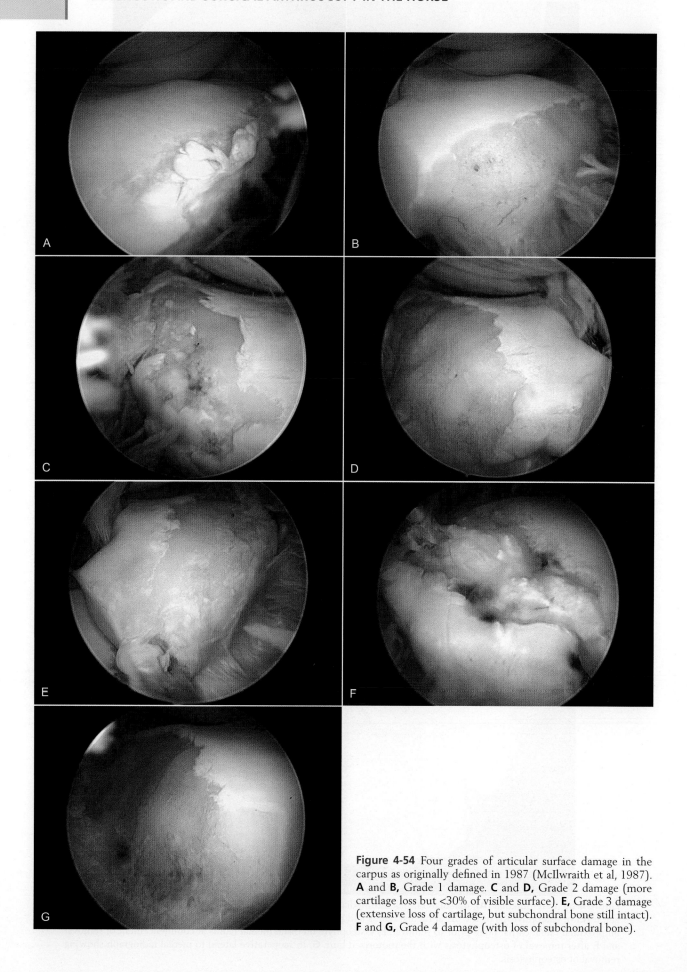

Figure 4-54 Four grades of articular surface damage in the carpus as originally defined in 1987 (McIlwraith et al, 1987). **A** and **B,** Grade 1 damage. **C** and **D,** Grade 2 damage (more cartilage loss but <30% of visible surface). **E,** Grade 3 damage (extensive loss of cartilage, but subchondral bone still intact). **F** and **G,** Grade 4 damage (with loss of subchondral bone).

has led to improved understanding and both development and refinement of techniques to limit the defects resultant from fragmentation. These have required better understanding of osteochondral healing; a summary of this and techniques of enhancement are provided in Chapter 16.

Debridement of Defects after Chip Fracture Removal

Details on debridement and techniques to limit the defects, as well as improve osteochondral healing, are detailed in Chapter 16. However, in summary the authors advocate a relatively conservative approach to debridement. Rough edges or adjacent undermined or fragmented cartilage are removed. This protocol is based on the belief that loose cartilage is irritating and may detach while its prospects of healing onto bone are virtually nil. Partial-thickness erosion adjacent to a full-thickness defect is not subjected to curettage if the cartilage that remains is attached solidly to the bone. Full-thickness defects are debrided to the level of subchondral bone. Any soft defective bone is also removed.

Postoperative Management

The principles of perioperative medication including antimicrobial and analgesic drugs are discussed in Chapters 3 and 17. It is generally recommended that sterile wraps or bandages are applied postoperatively and maintained for 7 to 10 days with changes as needed. Sutures are usually removed approximately 10 days postoperatively. The use of antiinflammatory and chondroprotective agents together with potential regenerative therapies are discussed in Chapter 17.

Injured and healing tissues can be modulated by physical activity. There are no appropriate scientific studies, and recommendations are necessarily empiric in nature. Nonetheless, on the basis of current understanding, it is recommended that exercise is avoided for the first week after surgery in order to enable a stable blood clot to form in osseous defects. Physiotherapy in the form of carpal flexion exercises and hand walking can begin 7 days postoperatively. The level of exercise is then progressively increased in line with the severity of articular compromise. Horses with simple, fresh fragments creating grade 1 lesions may begin training 6 weeks after surgery. As the damage in the joint increases, the convalescent time should be appropriately increased such that horses with grade 3 and 4 lesions are usually recommended to have 4 to 6 months' rest. Other forms of exercise such as swimming, saltwater walking, and water treadmill use may also assist in rehabilitation. Recent evaluation of water treadmilling has shown significant amelioration of post–chip fragment osteoarthritis in the horse and is the first demonstration in a controlled, scientific study of rehabilitation benefit.[a]

Case Selection, Prognosis, and Results

Although fragments of all ages and size are amenable to arthroscopic surgery, not all horses are good surgical candidates. Cases should be assessed on an individual basis taking into account causation, predisposing factors, size and location of fragments, pathologic changes in the parent and other carpal bones, and the presence of other lesions within the joint. Following assessment, accurate communication with owners and trainers is important, particularly before embarking on complex cases with less certain prognoses. In general terms, a better result can be expected with a horse that has proven racing ability and an owner that understands the prognosis.

In general terms, the prognosis is related to the amount of cartilage or bone loss, or both, and decreases when there is loss of subchondral bone along the entire dorsal rim of a bone. Subchondral incongruity appears particularly unforgiving with respect to athletic function. The relationship between prognosis

and articular cartilage loss is more difficult to predict, particularly in racing Quarter Horses that have raced at stakes level despite complete loss of articular cartilage on the dorsodistal radial carpal bone. A similar situation may exist when comparing the outcomes of Thoroughbred sprinters and Thoroughbreds that run over middle and staying distances; subjectively, the athletic potential of the former appears less compromised with large articular deficits compared with the latter. Postoperative performance may also be influenced by differences in medication regulations between racing authorities.

McIlwraith et al (1987) reported on the postoperative performance of 445 racehorses. After surgery, 303 (68.1%) raced at a level equal to or better than the preinjury level, 49 (11%) had decreased performance or still had problems referable to the carpus, and 23 (5.2%) were retired without returning to training. Of those that returned to training, 28 (6.3%) sustained another chip fracture, 32 (7.2%) developed other problems, and 10 (2.2%) sustained collapsing slab fractures while racing. When grouped by size of articular defect, the performance of the two most severely affected groups was significantly inferior. One hundred thirty-three of 187 horses with grade 1 damage (71.1%), 108 of 144 with grade 2 damage (75%), 41 of 77 with grade 3 damage (53.2%), and 20 of 37 horses with grade 4 damage (54.1%) returned to racing at a level equal to or better than the preinjury level. These comprised 277 Quarter Horses, of which 81 of 112 (72.3%) with grade 1, 72 of 96 (75%) with grade 2 lesions, 26 of 46 (56.5%) with grade 3 lesions, and 13 of 23 (56.5%) with grade 4 lesions returned successfully to racing. Of 164 Thoroughbreds, 51 of 73 (69.9%) with grade 1, 36 of 47 (76.6%) with grade 2, 14 of 30 (46.7%) with grade 3, and 7 of 14 (50%) with grade 4 lesions performed successfully postoperatively.

The influence of site of fragmentation was assessed by comparing results of horses with single foci (Table 4-1). In racing Quarter Horses, the prognosis associated with the third carpal bone was significantly worse than with lesions at other sites, whereas in Thoroughbreds, third and radial carpal bone lesions had the poorest prognoses. Postoperative performance in racing Thoroughbreds appeared unaffected by affliction of middle or antebrachiocarpal joints when 66.2% and 65.5%, respectively, successfully returned to racing. In Quarter Horses 83.3% of horses with fragmentation in the middle carpal and 82.7% fragmentation in the antebrachiocarpal joint successfully returned to racing. There was no evidence of diminution in performance if both middle and antebrachiocarpal joints were involved (see Table 4-1).

Since the publication of these data 15 years ago, there have been a number of changes in clinical practices that may influence future results, including the following:

1. Earlier intervention and therefore a higher percentage of grades 1 and 2 lesions being presented for surgery
2. New techniques to enhance osteochondral healing (see Chapter 16)
3. More aggressive postoperative protocols, including medication and physiotherapy

Variable healing follows debridement of defects after osteochondral fragment removal in the carpus (Fig. 4-55).

Lucas et al (1999) reported results following arthroscopic surgery in 176 Standardbreds comprising 117 pacers and 59 trotters. Overall 130 (73.8%) made at least one start postsurgery, but pacers (96; 82.1%) had a greater frequency of return to racing than trotters (34; 57.6%). The majority (52; 69.3%) of horses of both gaits that had raced before surgery decreased their median race mark (i.e., ran faster postsurgery). However, using median earnings per start as an indicator of performance, both trotters and pacers had reduced earnings postsurgery. There was no information relating outcome and site of fragmentation.

Table • 4-1

Results of Surgery for Carpal Chip Fracture Relative to Location

LOCATION	QUARTER HORSE N = 187 (%)*	THOROUGHBRED N = 133 (%)
Distal radial carpal bone	70.6	55.4
Distal intermediate carpal bone	80.0	100
Proximal third carpal bone	29.4	58.8
Distal radius	80.0	74.2
Proximal intermediate carpal bone	89.7	61.5
Proximal radial carpal bone	100	75.0

*Percentage of horses racing at a level equal to or better than preinjury level, relative to the location of the carpal chip fracture.
From McIlwraith CW, Yovich JV, Martin GS. Arthroscopic surgery for the treatment of osteochondral chip fractures in the equine carpus. *J Am Vet Med Assoc* 1987;191:531–540.

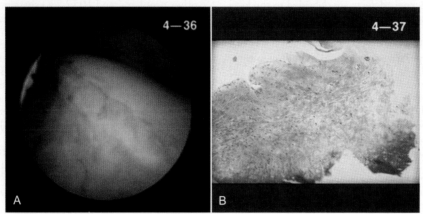

Figure 4-55 A and **B,** Follow-up arthroscopic views and histologic analysis of defect in the radial carpal bone 1 year after fragment removal and debridement.

ARTHROSCOPIC SURGERY FOR OSTEOCHONDRAL FRAGMENTS IN THE PALMAR ASPECT OF THE CARPAL JOINTS

Palmar Fractures in the Antebrachiocarpal Joint

Fractures originating from the proximal palmar articular margin of the radial carpal bone are more frequent than any other palmar surface (Wilke et al, 2001) and can occur alone or in combination with other lesions. These include comminuted fractures of the palmar radial carpal bone and/or concurrent fractures of intermediate and ulnar carpal bones and palmar distal radius. Despite this, these are still considered uncommon fractures compared with those developing on the dorsal margins of the radial carpal bone and are not generally athletic injuries. They can follow falls or in recovery from general anesthesia, where the horse may be seen to collapse onto one or both knees with the carpus fully flexed. In one study, most of the recognized fractures resulted during recovery from anesthesia, with only one horse falling onto its knees during race training (Wilke et al, 2001).

Fragments from the proximal palmar articular margin of the radial carpal bone are most readily identified in LM or DM-PaLO projections (Fig. 4-56), but a full radiographic examination is mandatory in all cases to evaluate other carpal bones. Nonetheless, particularly in the acute phase, some fractures remain radiologically undetectable and radiographs frequently underestimate the complexity of the lesions. Alternative imaging modalities such as computed tomography (CT) and MRI have the potential to establish a diagnosis in questionable circumstances and provide therapeutic and prognostic information (Fig. 4-57). Time to acquire MRI series

limits its use to preoperative assessment, whereas CT can be performed under the same anesthetic episode on the way to surgery.

When removable fragments are identified, the palmaromedial portion of the antebrachiocarpal joint is arthroscopically assessed as described in the diagnostic arthroscopy portion of this chapter. Ideally the arthroscopic portal is made at the palmar margin of the joint in order to optimize lesion identification and instrument manipulation. Generally the arthroscope is positioned more palmar and proximal in the palmaromedial pouch, leaving the distended pouch closer to the medial collateral available for an instrument portal directly over the palmaromedial corner of the radial carpal bone (the predisposed site for fracture). The exact position of the instrument portal is identified by placement of a percutaneous needle. Synovial proliferation rapidly follows fracture fragmentation at this site, and insertion of a motorized resector to clear access to the fragment is a vital initial step. The proximity of the shaver to the tip of the arthroscope must always be recognized during this phase. Once exposed, most fragments from the proximal palmar radial carpal bone are unstable and readily removed with arthroscopic rongeurs. The bone often feels soft and crumbly, and judicious debridement is necessary (see Fig. 4-56). Comminuted fractures that extend distally involve extensive palmar carpal ligament attachments, which, if removal is elected, require dissection. The prognosis for (apparently) simple fractures is guarded and for complex fractures is poor. Wilke et al (2001) reported a series of 10 cases. Six underwent surgery, of which 3 returned to ridden work. Experience with additional cases suggests early intervention can improve outcome for proximopalmar radial carpal bone fractures.

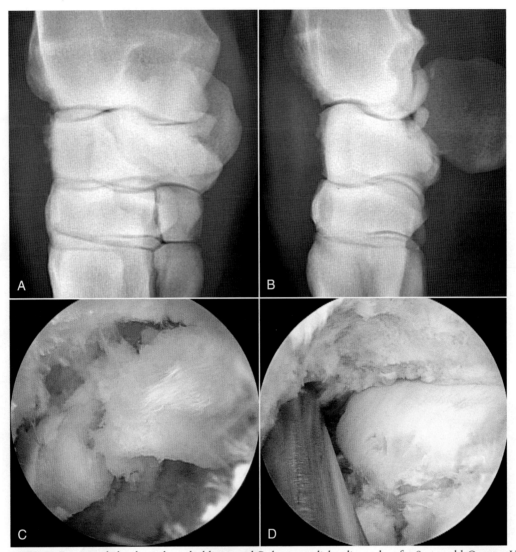

Figure 4-56 A, Dorsomedial-palmarolateral oblique and **B,** lateromedial radiographs of a 9-year-old Quarter Horse that had undergone colic surgery 4 weeks before re-presentation. The palmaromedial corner of the radial carpal bone has a substantial fracture, and the soft tissue swelling is extensive. **C,** Arthroscopic view during removal showing the wide fracture fragment, which has been cracked in two for easier retrieval. **D,** The fracture bed on the radial carpal bone has been debrided (above), and the apposing surface of radius is visible (below).

The medial corner of the proximal margin of the intermediate carpal bone can also be fractured, and although these fractures can sometimes migrate proximally into the inaccessible fossa on the palmar intraarticular surface of the radius, a few can be retrieved (see Fig. 4-57). The palmaromedial pouch approach to the antebrachiocarpal joint is used. However, once the arthroscope is in position, the joint may need more extension to expose the fracture fragment. Removal requires a rongeur reaching across the entire palmar margin of the radial carpal bone from the palmaromedial pouch entry. Up-biting rongeurs are often useful.

The proximal lateral compartment of the antebrachiocarpal joint permits arthroscopic removal of fragmentation of the proximal articular margin of the accessory carpal bone. This is indicated when fragmentation at this site is the sole lesion (Fig. 4-58). Lesions at this site may present as both acute injuries and long-standing lesions. Most are identified in LM, flexed LM, and DL-PaMO radiographic projections. There may be varying degrees of size and displacement, with comminuted fractures involving articular and nonarticular surfaces. Fragmentation of the proximal articular margin is seen also in comminuted fractures of the accessory carpal bone (Fig. 4-59). In this instance, acute removal is generally contraindicated, with later removal of only the nonhealing mobile intraarticular portion. Some fractures of the proximal articular surface can extend palmar outside the articular confines. These will involve varying degrees of insertion of the accessorio radial ligament from which the fragments will require dissection. The arthroscope is generally placed proximally within the palmarolateral outpouching of the antebrachiocarpal joint in order to permit a distal instrument portal adjacent to the articular margins. Removal of fragments and debridement of fracture beds is then performed in the conventional manner. Fractures of the accessory or ulnar carpal bones can occur in close proximity and may be difficult to determine the exact site of origin (Fig. 4-60). Entry to the midaccessory pouch can be done from the proximal access portal in chronically distended cases, although visualization of the ulnar carpal bone is limited to a proximal palmar rim (see Fig. 4-59).

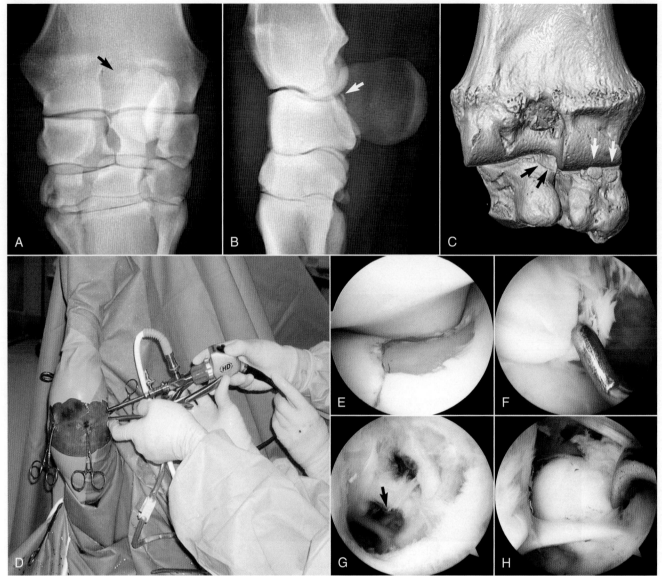

Figure 4-57 A, Dorsopalmar and **B,** lateromedial radiographs of an 11-year-old Quarter Horse that had been lame since purchase 5 months before surgery. The fractures on radiographs *(arrows)* were not clearly associated with any bone, and the dorsomedial to palmarolateral oblique was normal. **C,** Computed tomography shows a large fracture originating from the proximo-medial corner of the intermediate carpal bone *(black arrows)* and two smaller fractures from the radial carpal bone *(white arrows).* **D,** Arthroscopic retrieval showing difficult access and triangulation to the palmaromedial pouch of the left antebrachiocarpal joint. **E,** Examination using dorsal approach shows concurrent cartilage erosion over the distomedial surface of the radius, examined before palmar approaches. **F,** Palmaromedial approach to ABC joint showing probe in one of the radial carpal chip fractures. **G,** Examination more laterally using the palmaromedial entry to the ABC joint shows a large partially obscured fragment *(arrow)* originating from the intermediate carpal bone and residing in the caudal fossa of the radius. **H,** A probe exposes the fragment for removal by rongeurs.

Palmar Fractures in the Middle Carpal Joint

Fragments in the palmar compartments of the antebrachiocarpal and middle carpal joints can originate from the palmar articular margins, or for the middle carpal joint particularly, fragments can originate from the dorsal regions and migrate to the palmar recesses. There is no substantial interosseous or periarticular space in the antebrachiocarpal joint through which such fragments can move. Excoriation of articular surfaces of varying degrees is thus an inevitable consequence as fragments are forced from dorsal to palmar. Fragments can originate at any site but most commonly lodge palmarolaterally. These are profiled in DL-PaMO radiographs (Fig. 4-61) in the distal palmarolateral outpouching of the middle carpal

joint over the fourth carpal bone. Retrieval necessitates ipsilateral arthroscope and instrument portals into the palmarolateral pouch of the middle carpal joint, which necessarily are close together. Regulation of fluid flow/pressure is important to maintain adequate distension while minimizing extravasation. Surgery in the palmar compartments should precede dorsal procedures, again to optimize distension and visibility. Although by definition loose bodies (see Fig. 4-60), migrated fragments quickly become adherent to the palmar synovium from which they are removed with appropriately sized arthroscopic rongeurs.

Fragmentation of the distal palmar margin of the radial carpal bone can occur as a solitary lesion with clinical signs

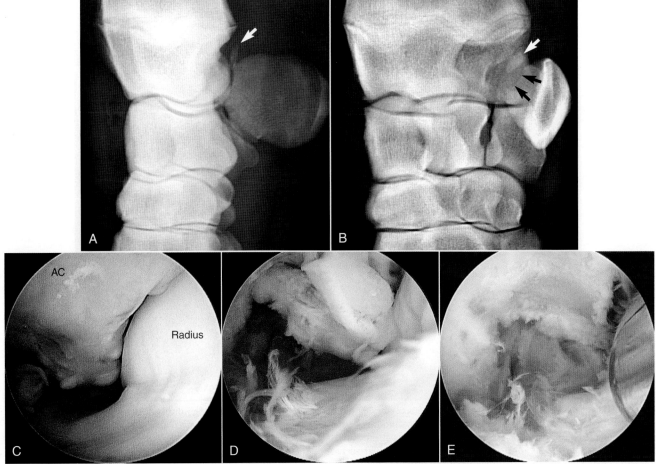

Figure 4-58 A, Lateral and **B,** dorsolateral to palmaromedial oblique radiographs, showing a solitary chip fracture *(white arrows)* from the proximal articular facet of the accessory carpal bone *(black arrows)* of a 2-year-old Quarter Horse/Thoroughbred mix with a 3-month history of lameness. **C,** Arthroscopic view using a proximal entry to the palmarolateral joint pouch of the antebrachiocarpal joint, showing the radius and chronic fracture of the accessory carpal bone articular facet (AC). **D,** Fragment is more exposed by synovial resection and probing. **E,** Fracture bed after fragment removal.

similar to those observed with dorsodistal fragmentation of this bone (Fig. 4-62). It is an uncommon injury and is usually recognized only in DM-PaLO radiographs. Fragments at this site are unstable but are usually minimally displaced. The palmaromedial middle carpal joint is not voluminous. The arthroscopic portal should be made as far palmar as possible in order to permit instrument entry dorsal to this site. Fragments are then managed in a conventional manner.

Fractures of the palmar surfaces of the ulnar and fourth carpal bone are similarly uncommon (Fig. 4-63). Access for removal is through the palmarolateral pouch of the middle carpal joint. This pouch is relatively voluminous compared with the palmaromedial pouch. Identification of the lesion requires synovial resection. Arthroscope and instrument portals are close, and triangulation can often be difficult.

Fractures of the distal palmar surface of the intermediate carpal bone have also been described (Dabareiner et al, 1993). Large palmar fractures that extend to the antebrachiocarpal joint may need removal via the carpal canal or lag screw fixation using similar approaches. Small, more distal fractures can be removed from the middle carpal joint using a combination of dosal and palmarolateral approaches to the intermediate carpal bone with extensive shaving (Fig. 4-64).

A detailed paper identifying sites for arthroscopic access to the palmar aspects of both the middle carpal and antebrachial carpal joints and a detailed description of the visible carpal bone surfaces for each approach has been published (Cheetham and Nixon, 2006). Also, another publication has reported a retrospective study evaluating palmar carpal osteochondral fragments predominantly originating from sites other than the palmar margins of the bones and determining whether the fragments were indicators of the severity of pathologic joint changes or prognosis (31 cases) (Getman et al, 2006). Thirty-one horses met the selection criteria. Multiple palmar fragments were diagnosed in 58% of horses with small fragments (<3 mm in diameter; dust) being the most common (52% of horses). Fifty-two percent of horses returned to racing with 48% earning money and 32% of those having at least five starts. Horses with multiple fragments had significantly less earnings per start and lower performance index values after surgery than those with one fragment. Horses with multiple small fragments were less likely to successfully return to racing than horses with only dorsally located carpal fragments or horses with one or two large palmar fragments. The authors concluded that when possible, removal of palmar carpal osteochondral fragments should be considered. The same group also did another study describing the anatomy of the equine palmar lateral outpouching of the middle carpal joint by comparing its arthroscopic and magnetic resonance (MR) contrast arthrography appearance to define the structures that can be assessed arthroscopically (Getman et al, 2007). MR arthrography was a useful tool for helping to define the

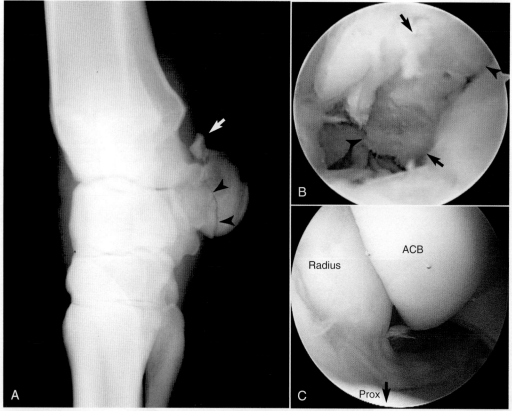

Figure 4-59 **A,** Multiple fractures of the accessory carpal bone in a horse that fell during jumping. An articular fracture fragment has been dislodged from the proximodorsal aspect of the accessory carpal bone *(white arrow)*. A longitudinal fracture of the accessory carpal bone has also occurred that does not involve the articular surface *(black arrow)*. **B,** Arthroscopic approach to the proximal articular surface of the accessory carpal bone with the arthroscope portal placed in the proximal regions of the proximal palmarolateral cul-de-sac of the antebrachiocarpal joint. The fracture fragment is identified by arrows. **C,** A normal arthroscopic appearance to the proximal palmar region of the antebrachiocarpal joint for orientation, using a palmarolateral approach. The articulation of the accessory carpal bone *(ACB)* with the radius is labeled. The horse is in dorsal recumbency with the proximal aspects lower in both **B** and **C.**

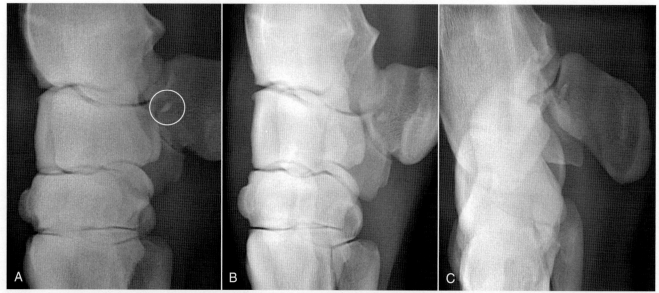

Figure 4-60 **A,** Solitary fracture from the proximal palmar surface of the ulnar carpal bone shown on lateromedial radiographic projection *(circle),* **B,** dorsolateral-palmaromedial oblique, and **C,** proximal (50 degrees) medial to distolateral elevated oblique view showing fragment association with ulnar carpal bone.

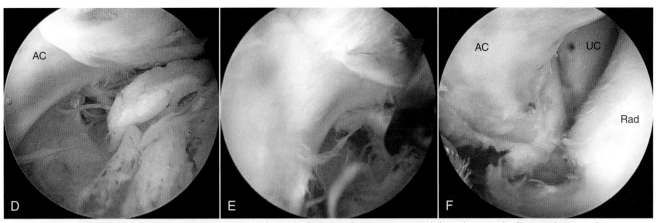

Figure 4-60, cont'd D, Arthroscopic access through the central accessory portal directly over the lesion, showing the fracture fragment. **E,** After removal. **F,** On wider exploration of the central accessory articulation with the radius and ulnar carpal bone.

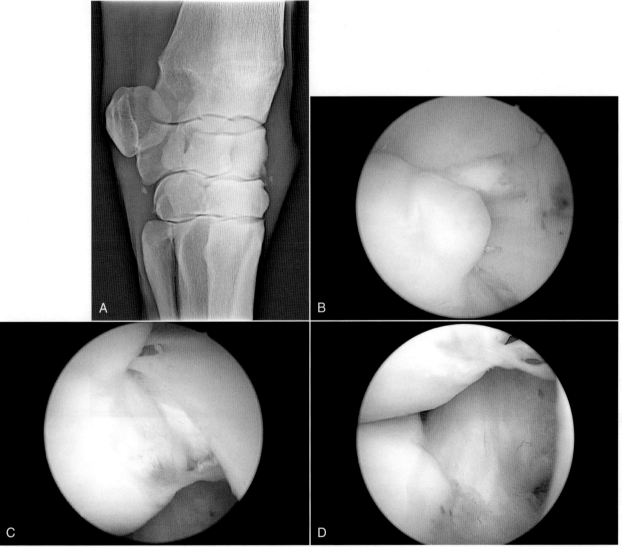

Figure 4-61 A, Radiograph of palmarolateral fragment associated with the distal aspect of the ulnar carpal bone and arthroscopic views before **(B)** and after **(C** and **D)** removal of fragment. Note that there is also a fragment on the distal dorsal aspect of the radial carpal bone.

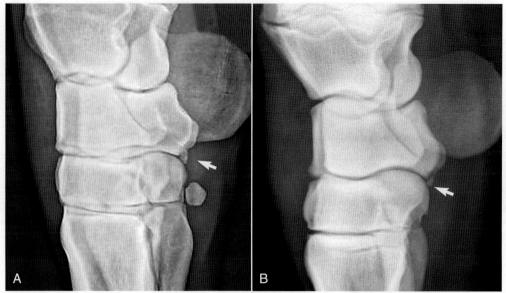

Figure 4-62 A, Fracture of the palmaromedial surface of the distal perimeter of the radial carpal bone in a 12-year-old Warmblood with a 2-year history of chronic low grade lameness. **B,** Fracture in the same region in a Thoroughbred yearling with effusion but no lameness. Both were removed with resolution of symtoms.

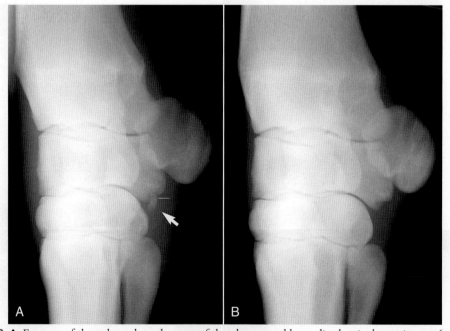

Figure 4-63 A, Fracture of the palmarolateral corner of the ulnar carpal bone distal articular perimeter *(white arrow)*. **B,** Same horse after arthroscopic removal.

anatomy of the palmar lateral outpouching. The authors noted that identification of the articular anatomy could be confusing and that motorized arthroscopic resection of synovial tissue was necessary to view all the structures. Portions of the ulnar carpal bone, fourth carpal bone, fourth metacarpal bone, lateral palmar intercarpal ligament, and lateral collateral ligament of the carpus could be identified within the palmar lateral outpouching of the middle carpal joint in all limbs. In three of seven limbs of the cadaveric study, areas of the third carpal bone and intermediate carpal bone could be seen. It is important to emphasize that synovial and capsular resection is required to see the fourth metacarpal bone, lateral palmar

intercarpal ligament, and the lateral collateral ligament of the carpus, and this may have negative consequences. More extensive resection outside of the normal confines of the palmarolateral pouch is necessary to evaluate the palmarolateral portions of the third and intermediate carpal bones and is not recommended.

ARTHROSCOPIC SURGERY FOR SUBCHONDRAL BONE DISEASE

These lesions were initially described in the proximal aspect of the third carpal bone. A number of radiographic changes may

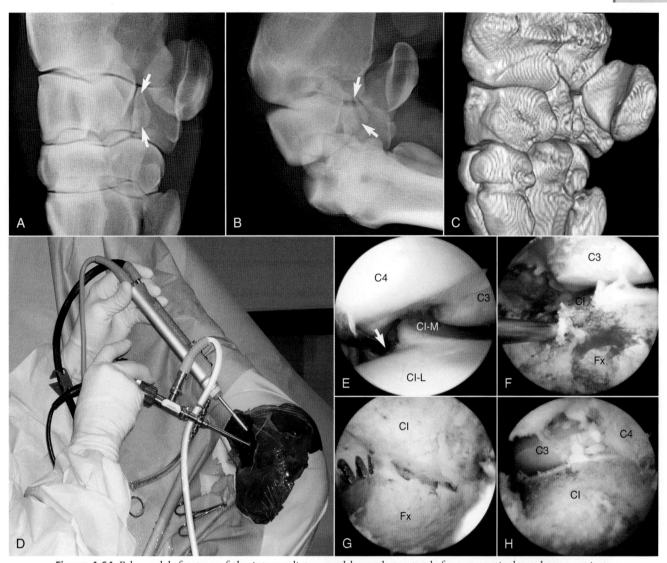

Figure 4-64 Palmar slab fracture of the intermediate carpal bone that extends from nonarticular palmar margin to the distal articular surface in the middle carpal joint. **A,** Dorsolateral-palmaromedial oblique radiographs show the lesion *(arrows)*. **B,** Flexed dorsolateral-palmaromedial oblique radiographs indicate significant mobility, and **C,** computed tomography (CT) shows fracture fragment size, articular involvement in middle carpal joint, and best route for removal. **D,** Palmarolateral approach to the intermediate carpal bone with knee flexed 30 degrees and instrument entry more distal to allow motorized burring of the fracture fragment. **E,** Initial approach using standard dorsolateral portal reveals minor additional cartilage damage, and only the tip of the fracture can be palpated *(arrow)*. The palmar surfaces of the fourth carpal *(C4)*, third carpal *(C3)*, and medial *(CI-M)* and lateral *(CI-L)* facets of the intermediate carpal bones are exposed. A needle and subsequent arthroscope cannula with obturator were introduced from the palmarolateral portal while viewing from the dorsal approach. **F,** Probing the fracture *(Fx)* mobility using a distal palmarolateral instrument portal. **G,** Removal requires burring in situ, with thinning and gradual proximal reduction in the fracture fragment adjacent to the parent intermediate carpal bone *(CI)*. **H,** After complete removal, showing smooth surface of CI and exposed original articulation with third and fourth carpal bones.

be evident on tangential "skyline" views of the third carpal bone, including densification (sclerosis), lytic lesions, or linear defects variously interpreted as incomplete fractures or "pre-slab" lesions. Sclerosis of the radial facet is a well-recognized change, and some authors suggest that it is a primary lesion, often preceding more serious change, such as cartilage damage or gross fracture (DeHaan et al, 1987). These authors also suggest that early recognition of sclerosis of the third carpal bone may help to prevent the occurrence of more serious changes (DeHaan et al, 1987). Sclerosis is considered to arise with training and racing. However, whether this leads to articular cartilage lesions or the same forces that can cause sclerosis also cause articular

cartilage lesions directly has yet to be ascertained. Arthroscopy of a small number of joints that had sclerosis as the only radiographic sign revealed wide variability in the gross appearance of the overlying cartilage (Richardson, 1988).

So-called third carpal bone disease presents as a persistent carpal problem that does not respond to medication and is characterized by lytic change evident on skyline radiographs of the third carpal bone (Fig. 4-65A). Frequently, some degree of surrounding sclerosis accompanies the lytic changes. Most lesions occur on the radial facet; they may be single or multiple and range from linear to circular in outline on skyline radiographs (Richardson, 1988). The proximal subchondral

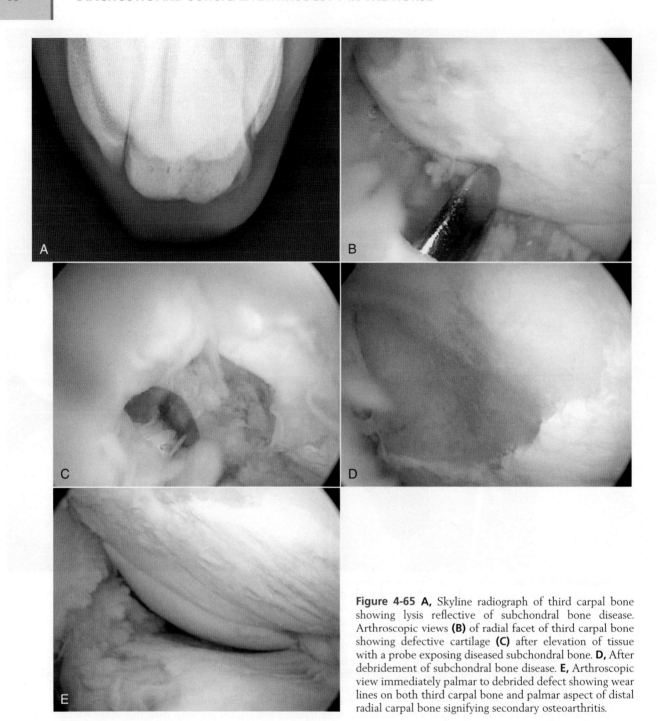

Figure 4-65 A, Skyline radiograph of third carpal bone showing lysis reflective of subchondral bone disease. Arthroscopic views **(B)** of radial facet of third carpal bone showing defective cartilage **(C)** after elevation of tissue with a probe exposing diseased subchondral bone. **D,** After debridement of subchondral bone disease. **E,** Arthroscopic view immediately palmar to debrided defect showing wear lines on both third carpal bone and palmar aspect of distal radial carpal bone signifying secondary osteoarthritis.

bone is particularly thick and dense, so damage and lysis in this area results in dramatic radiolucency in tangential projections.

Arthroscopically, these lesions manifest as an area of defective subchondral bone, with the overlying cartilage absent, a depression in the articular cartilage, an undermined cartilage flap, or fragmented cartilage (see Fig. 4-65B and C). In some cases there is overt fragmentation of the subchondral bone, which, because it is nondisplaced and cannot be imaged in profile, is not recognized radiographically. Loose tissue is removed, and the lesion is debrided with a curette. The defective bone is often granular in nature. A rim of intact tissue on the dorsal margin of the third carpal bone usually remains, although in some cases the defective tissue extends out through this margin. Also, if the remaining rim is narrow, this may be removed to the level of the defect.

It is now recognized that subchondral bone disease can occur at other locations and may be the precursor to exercise/work-induced osteochondral fragmentation. Clinical signs associated with subchondral bone diseases are similar to animals with osteochondral fragmentation. However, presurgical diagnosis (at locations other than the third carpal bone) is difficult; the disease is rarely demonstrable radiographically. The best example is the distal radial carpal bone, where lesions can consistently be found arthroscopically (Fig. 4-66).

Subchondral bone disease has also been seen on the distal radial, proximal third, proximal radial, intermediate carpal bones and on the distal radius (lateral and medial) (see Fig. 4-66). Figure 4-66H illustrates subchondral bone disease on the more palmar areas of the second and radial carpal bone.

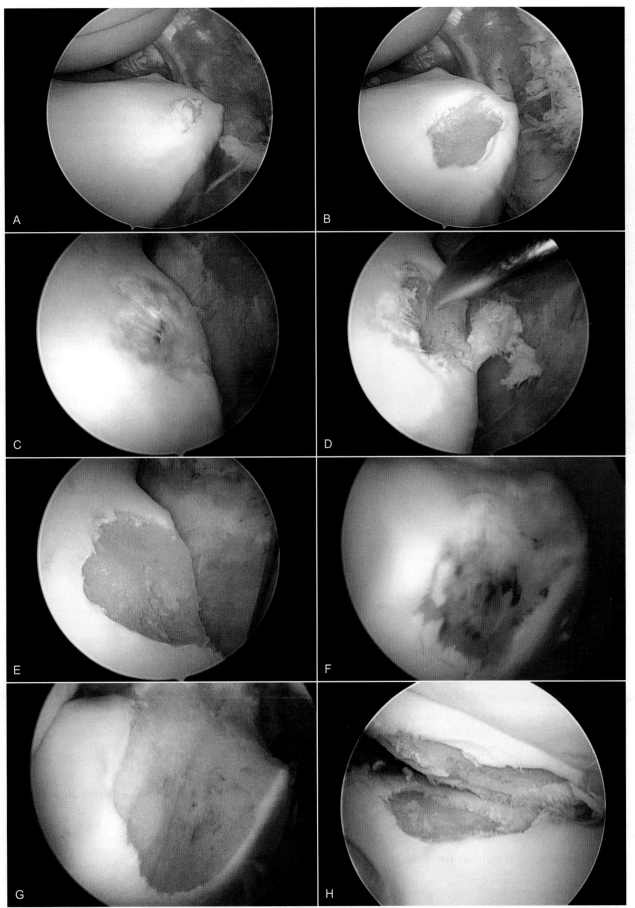

Figure 4-66 Arthroscopic views of subchondral bone disease involving distal radial carpal bone **(A** and **B)**, the distal radius **(C** to **E)**, the proximal intermediate carpal bone **(F** and **G)**, and the palmar areas of the second and radial carpal bones **(H)**. None of these lesions had any associated signs visible on preoperative radiographs.

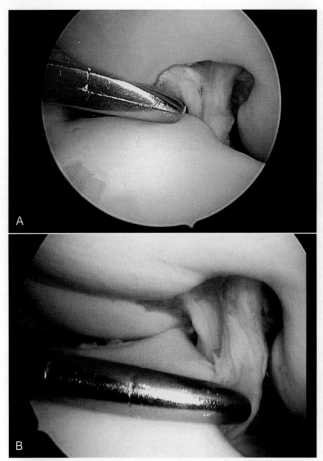

Figure 4-67 Normal arthroscopic view of medial palmar intercarpal ligament **(A)** and palpation of lateral portion of ligament **(B)**.

The postsurgical protocol is determined by the degree of articular compromise, using criteria similar to other carpal arthroscopic procedures. In one report of 13 Standardbred cases involving the third carpal bone, 8 returned to racing, 6 of these in their original class (Ross et al, 1989).

The relationship between increased bone density in the third carpal bone and racing has been investigated (Young et al, 1991). Regional variations in trabecular bone density and stiffness have been implicated in the pathogenesis of third carpal bone fractures (Young et al, 1991). In addition, subchondral lucency, commonly in combination with sclerosis of the third carpal bone radial fossa, has been associated with acute, moderate to severe lameness referable to the middle carpal joint in Standardbred racehorses (Ross et al, 1989). Investigators in Sweden have looked at subchondral sclerosis and subchondral lucency in the third carpal bone in Standardbred horses diagnosed with traumatic carpitis and related it to clinical appearance and prognosis for racing. Subchondral lucency was found significantly to influence the degree of lameness and the time to start, but did not significantly affect the chance of racing within 30 months postexamination (Uhlhorn & Carlsten, 1999). However, it was also recognized that there was a low number of third carpal bones with severe sclerosis and, with no arthroscopic evaluation, this limits what can be concluded from this study.

Lesions of the Medial Palmar Intercarpal Ligament

The medial palmar intercarpal ligament originates on the distal palmarolateral surface of the radial carpal bone. This can be viewed from a dorsolateral arthroscopic portal in the middle carpal joint if the carpus is flexed to not less than 70 degrees and while the joint is maximally distended (Fig. 4-67). At arthroscopy, the body of the ligament is most commonly viewed as two arms. The lateral inserts in the palmar fossa of the third carpal bone and the medial arm on the palmarolateral surface of the second carpal bone (Phillips & Wright, 1994) (see Fig. 4-67). However, there is considerable variation in the dorsal, arthroscopically visible morphology of the ligament. This includes variation in the relative sizes of the two branches ranging from agenesis of the lateral insertion to lack of distinction between the two arms (see Fig. 4-67). The arthroscopic appearance varies also in the degree of carpal flexion.

Tearing of the medial palmar intercarpal ligament has been reported by several authors (Kannegieter & Burbidge, 1990; Kannegieter & Colgan, 1993; McIlwraith, 1992; Moore & Schneider, 1995; Phillips & Wright, 1994). Tearing of the dorsal portions of the ligament usually results in extrusion of disrupted fibrils into the synovial cavity (Fig. 4-68). Lesions invariably involve the lateral (radial–third carpal) arm (McIlwraith, 1992; Phillips & Wright, 1994). Injuries of the medial (radial–second carpal) portion are rare. Fibers of the lateral arm are aligned among the medial-lateral plane of movement of the radial and third carpal bones during flexion/extension of the carpus, and this has been muted in the aetiopathogenesis of these lesions (Phillips & Wright, 1994). The degree of tearing varies from disruption of surface fibrils to complete loss of continuity (see Fig. 4-68).

McIlwraith (1992) reported tears of the medial palmar intercarpal ligament identified at arthroscopy of 45 middle carpal joints in 42 horses. Tearing was unilateral in 39 and bilateral in 3 horses. Twenty-three (55%) animals had concurrent carpal fragmentation. Phillips & Wright (1994) identified damage to the medial palmar intercarpal ligament in 47 of 67 (70%) middle carpal joints undergoing arthroscopic surgery predominantly for treatment of osteochondral lesions. There was no association between the severity of ligament disruption and presence of fragmentation or degree of cartilage damage, but there was a relationship with remodeling or plastic deformation, or both, of the dorsodistal radial carpal bone. Fragmentation of the radial carpal bone at the site of origin of the medial palmar intercarpal ligament has also been recognized in cases with destabilizing slab fractures of the third carpal bone (McIlwraith, 1992).

Removal of disrupted fibrils is advocated on the basis of the rationale outlined in Chapter 3. This is most efficiently done using a motorized synovial resector in oscillating mode. Use of suction is critical. This draws torn tissue into the blades, which is an important safeguard against excessive debridement and subsequent ligament compromise. The blade can then be positioned adjacent to rather than pressed against the ligament.

No studies involving tears of the medial palmar intercarpal ligament only have been reported. Determination of the lesions contribution to case outcome is thus not confidently possible as most horses have concurrent injuries. However, evidence has been presented to suggest that this injury has a negative prognostic influence on case outcome when severe (McIlwraith, 1992).

Lesions of the Lateral Palmar Intercarpal Ligament

The lateral palmar intercarpal ligament originates primarily on the distal palmaromedial surface of the ulnar carpal bone with a smaller attachment to the lateral margin of the intermediate carpal bone. It inserts primarily on the palmaromedial fourth carpal bone with a smaller insertion on the palmarolateral surface of the third carpal bone (Phillips & Wright, 1994; Whitton et al, 1997). The dorsal margin of the ligament is visible in the middle carpal joint. There is some degree of variation in its

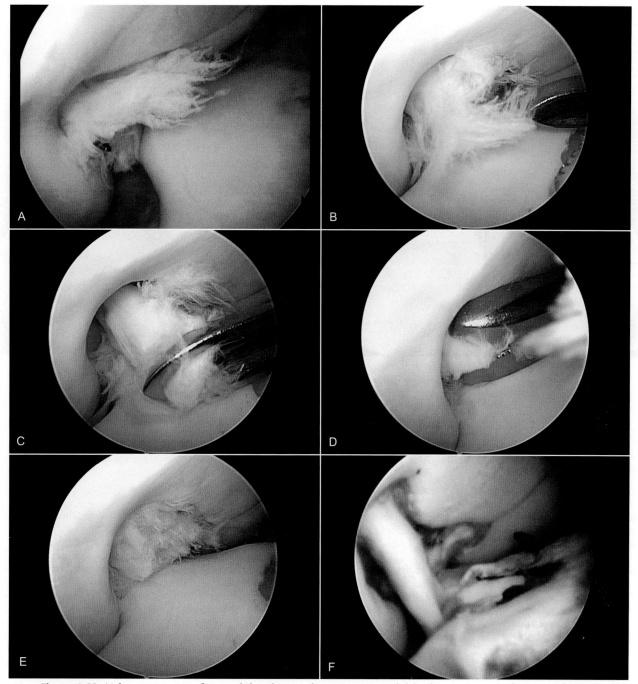

Figure 4-68 Arthroscopic view of minor **(A)** and more obvious tearing and debridement **(B** to **E)** of lateral portion of medial palmar intercarpal ligament. **F,** Avulsion fracture of third carpal bone at insertion of medial palmar intercarpal ligament.

appearance; in some horses it almost fills the space between these bones, whereas in others a small proximal portal of communication to the palmar aspect of the joint may be seen. The ligament is usually covered by non-villous synovium through which a variably twisting fiber alignment can be seen. In chronically inflamed joints, surface vasculature can be seen in the synovium and occasionally this may also be sparsely villous.

Frank tears of the lateral palmar intercarpal ligament, as seen with its medial counterpart, are rare (Kannegieter & Burbidge, 1990; Kannegieter & Colgan, 1993; Phillips & Wright, 1994). Beinlich & Nixon (2005) described avulsion injury in 37 horses. These are predicted by identification of localized osteolysis and/ or fragmentation in the ulnar carpal bone in DL-PaMO and dorsopalmar radiographic projections, which helps separate

these fractures from cyst formation in the ulnar carpal bone (Beinlich & Nixon, 2005) (Fig. 4-69). Such lesions are axially located on the ulnar carpal bone. This appears to differentiate avulsions from osseous cystlike lesions of the ulnar carpal bone, which are a common incidental finding in young Thoroughbreds (Kane et al, 2003a & b). In the reported series, all horses were lame and avulsion of the lateral palmar intercarpal ligament was the only identifiable lesion in 12 cases, of which 5 were bilateral.

Dorsolateral arthroscope and instrument portals are usually employed. Following routine arthroscopic entry, access is aided by increasing carpal flexion. Fragments are embedded to varying degrees within the lateral palmar intercarpal ligament, frequently requiring palpation with a probe for delineation (see Fig. 4-69). They require concomitant amounts of

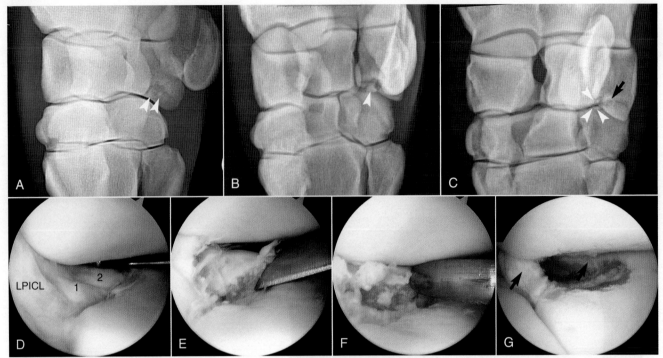

Figure 4-69 Avulsion fragmentation of the lateral palmar intercarpal ligament (LPICL) origin from the ulnar carpal bone in the right carpus. **A,** Dorsolateral-palmaromedial oblique (DLPMO) radiograph shows cystic appearance in ulnar carpal bone with tell-tale osseous fragments *(arrows)* in cavity. **B,** Radiographic projection between DLPMO and dorsoproximal shows the larger fragment **(C)**. Dorsopalmar projection reveals the cystic origin of the fracture *(black arrow)*, with fragments adjacent to avulsion bed. **D,** Arthroscopic view using standard dorsolateral portal (between ECR and CDE tendons) shows two fragments along palmar surface of the ulnar carpal bone *(1,2)* and a small residual intact medial portion of the LPICL. **E,** Dissection of fragment form LPICL using small ⅛" AO elevator. **F,** Fragment retrieval can be done with small rongeur, ethmoid rongeur, or mosquito hemostats. **G,** Residual medial and lateral portions of the LPICL *(arrows)* after avulsion removal.

dissection before removal. This is best done with a sharp, fixed blade knife. Varying degrees of osseous and ligament debridement are necessary in line with general surgical principles.

In the series reported by Beinlich & Nixon (2005), 26 of the 37 horses that had avulsions of the lateral palmar intercarpal ligament underwent surgery, including 7 of the 12 in which this was the sole lesion. Twenty of 21 horses with follow-up returned to work, including 6 of 7 in which avulsion of the lateral palmar intercarpal ligament was the only identifiable lesion. The authors (correctly) conclude that avulsion of the lateral palmar intercarpal ligament can occur without clinical signs and emphasize the importance of establishing significance before surgery is contemplated or advised.

ARTHROSCOPIC SURGERY FOR OSTEOCHONDRITIS DISSECANS

Osteochondritis dissecans can occur in the carpus, but it is uncommon. The diagnosis has been based on similarities in radiologic and arthroscopic appearance to osteochondritic lesions in other locations. Affected animals have all been unbroken and are younger than 2 years old. Although histologic features support the diagnosis, confident differentiation in the pathogenesis between osteochondritis dissecans and juvenile trauma is not possible. Cases present with forelimb lameness or carpal effusion, or both. Lesions have been identified on the distal margins of the radius and radial and intermediate carpal bones and on the proximal surface of the fourth carpal bone (axially at its articulation with the third carpal bone). Radiographs reveal subchondral defects (Fig. 4-70A), and arthroscopic examination demonstrates separation or

osteochondral disease consistent with osteochondritis dissecans (see Fig. 4-70B and C).

Arthroscopic approaches to these lesions are made in an identical manner to removal of traumatic fragmentation. The extent and depth of lesions are assessed with a blunt probe. Detached, unstable, and nonviable tissues are removed with arthroscopic rongeurs. Debridement is performed cautiously and should be conservative. In young animals, the subchondral bone plate is soft and thin, and differentiation between defective tissue and viable, immature bone with the capacity to heal is difficult.

Further fragmentation has been seen postoperatively and is likely to represent continuation of the pathologic process of osteochondrosis. Currently, an adequate number of cases have not been diagnosed or treated to issue confident prognostic decisions.

ARTHROSCOPIC SURGERY FOR SUBCHONDRAL CYSTIC LESIONS

Small, subchondral cystic lesions are occasionally identified in the distal ulnar carpal bone (where they are differentiated from lateral palmar intercarpal ligament avulsion by DP radiographs) and occasionally in other locations. The ulnar carpal bone cysts are common findings in yearling survey or sales radiographs, do not progress, and are invariably of no clinical consequence. Their principal importance is differentiation from avulsion injuries of the lateral palmar intercarpal ligament (see earlier). Large radiolucent zones are occasionally found on the cuboidal bones of the carpus or distal radial epiphysis. Typically, there is a small defect in the subchondral

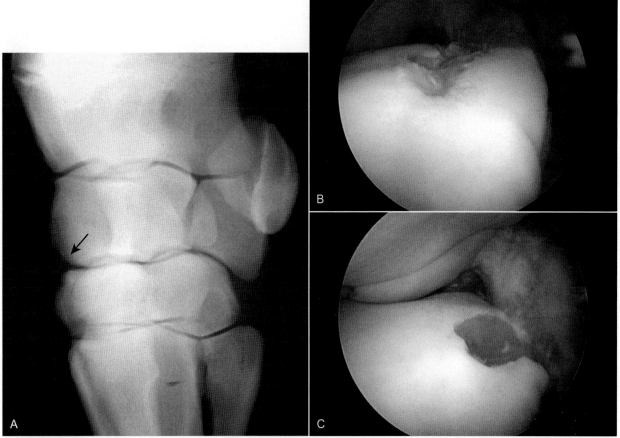

Figure 4-70 Radiographic view of defect *(arrow)* **(A)** and arthroscopic views **(B** and **C)** of osteochondritis dissecans involving the distal radial carpal bone.

bone indicative of an articular communication (cloaca), but the principal part of the "cyst" lies within the cuboidal or epiphyseal spongiosa. Arthroscopic evaluation of the adjacent joint will usually confirm the presence of a small cloaca. Cysts can be evacuated under arthroscopic guidance by enlargement of this communication, but the articular deficit created is substantial (Fig. 4-71). For this reason, two of the authors currently recommend arthroscopically guided infusion of the fibromyxoid cyst lining with corticosteroid as the initial line of therapy. If clinical response is unsatisfactory, then consideration may be given to evacuation and debridement with or without packing techniques either through the enlarged articular communication or by an extraarticular approach. Debridement of cysts in the second and radial carpal bone followed by grafting with bone substitute and stem cells has yielded varying success for one of the authors (A.J.N.). The benefit of grafting in this location has not been proven.

▶ ARTHROSCOPIC SURGERY FOR TREATMENT OF CARPAL SLAB FRACTURES

From surgical and pathogenic perspectives the third carpal bone is usually described with respect to the middle carpal joint as comprising dorsal radial and intermediate facets and a palmar body that lies principally behind the latter. By definition, slab fractures extend from proximal to distal articular surfaces. Incomplete slab fractures involve only one (invariably the proximal) subchondral bone plate and extend varying distances into the cuboidal spongiosa. Fractures that exit the dorsal surface of the bone are more correctly termed *chip fractures*, although management is similar.

Schneider et al (1988) identified, described, and classified 157 slab fractures in a series of 371 fractures of the third carpal bone in 313 horses. Ninety-three (59.2%) were in the frontal plane and confined to the radial facet, and 35 (22.3%) were frontal plane and involved both radial and intermediate facets; 17 (10.8%) were sagittal and situated on the medial side of the radial facet. Nine (5.7%) were frontal and 3 (1.9%) were sagittal fractures involving the intermediate facet. Additionally, these authors identified 39 incomplete fractures involving the proximal subchondral bone of the radial facet only. Of these, 59.5% were identified only in flexed dorsoproximal-dorsodistal oblique projections of the distal row of carpal bones.

Comprehensive radiographic review is mandatory in all horses in which a carpal fracture is possible or suspected (Fig. 4-72). The projections in which individual slab fractures of the third carpal bone are usually recognized are given in Table 4-2. Slab fractures of both radial and intermediate facets are usually situated further palmar in lateromedial projections than their single facet counterparts.

Sagittal fractures are inherently more stable than fractures in the frontal plane. There may be displacement of comminuted fragments, but there is invariably little or no displacement of the principal fracture fragments. Dorsal displacement of complete frontal plane fractures is common. This is usually, at least partially, rotational with greater dorsal displacement of the proximal articular surface. Most displaced fractures are reduced, at least in part by flexion. Flexed lateromedial projections are thus a useful presurgical guide to the ease of intraoperative reduction and thus repair.

Radiographs of frontal plane slab fractures should be scrutinized carefully for the presence of proximal palmar

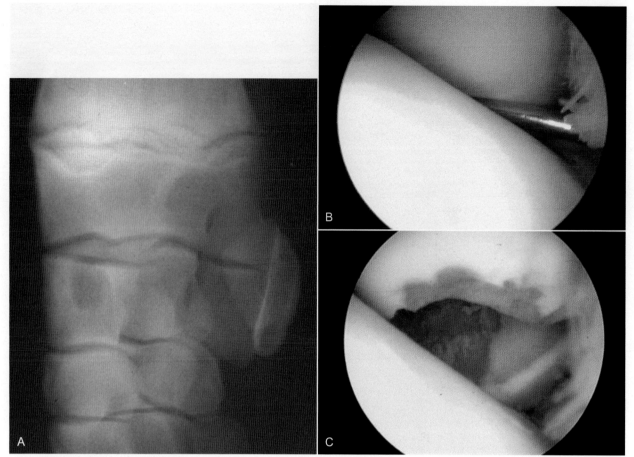

Figure 4-71 **A,** Subchondral cyst of the radial carpal bone. **B** and **C,** Arthroscopic views in the antebrachiocarpal joint before and after debridement.

Table • 4-2

Projections in Which Individual Slab Fractures of the Third Carpal Bone Are Most Usually Recognized

FRACTURE	PROJECTION					
	DPa	LM	Flexed LM	DL-PaMO	DM-PaLO	Flexed DPr-DDiO
Frontal radial facet		✓	✓	✓		✓
Frontal radial and intermediate facets		✓	✓	✓	✓	✓
Sagittal radial facet	✓					✓
Frontal intermediate facet		✓	✓		✓	✓
Sagittal intermediate facet	✓					✓

DL-PaMO, Dorsolateral-palmaromedial oblique; *DM-PaLO,* dorsomedial-palmarolateral oblique; *DPa,* dorsopalmar; *DPr-DDiO,* dorsoproximal-dorsodistal oblique; *LM,* lateromedial.

comminution. This is usually identified as a wedge-shaped fragment(s) in DL-PaMO projections. If irreparable, these can leave substantial articular deficits that influence negatively the prognosis. Such fragmentation is frequently reduced on carpal flexion and may not therefore be so readily visible in flexed LM and DPr-DDiO projections, although in the latter multiple fracture lines and/or a lack of definition of the palmar fracture line are suspicious radiologic indicators.

▶ Removal of Slab Fractures of the Third Carpal Bone

The authors' general philosophy is that whenever articular surfaces can accurately and safely be reconstructed, this should be the primary treatment goal. However, because of small size, removal of small slab fragments arthroscopically is sometimes appropriate (and usually dictated by

inability to screw because of comminution). Standard dorsolateral arthroscopic and dorsomedial instrument portals are employed. Removal of the fragment necessitates sharp dissection from the dorsal joint capsule and associated transverse dorsal intercarpal ligaments. This is most effectively achieved with a fixed-blade knife and use of straight and curved elevators. A motorized synovial resector is useful during dissection in order to maximize visibility. Once the fragment is loose, it is manipulated proximally in order that it may be grasped with large arthroscopic rongeurs. These are then twisted in order to free the last remaining soft tissue attachments before the fragment is removed. Enlargement of the skin incision is frequently necessary at this point. Debridement of the fracture bed follows and, in addition, limited debridement of the joint capsule and dorsal intercarpal ligaments is appropriate.

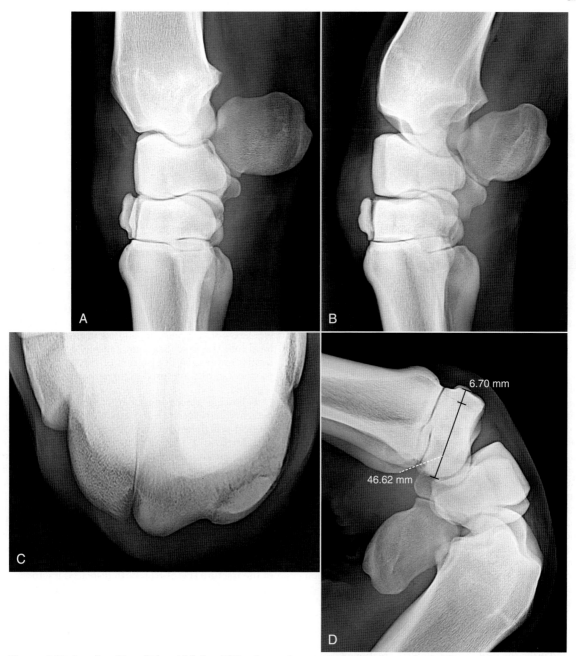

Figure 4-72 Standing **(A** and **B)** and "skyline" **(C)** radiographic views of slab fracture of radial facet of third carpal bone. **D,** Measurement of slab thickness and third carpal bone depth have been made on the radiograph digitally.

Lag Screw Fixation of Frontal Slab Fractures of the Radial Facet

These fractures are defined with a complete set of carpal radiographs (see Fig. 4-72). The technique described and recommended is a variation on that originally developed by Richardson (1986 & 2002) (Figs. 4-73 to 4-78). Preoperative planning is important. The surgeon should ascertain the distance from the dorsal surface of the bone to the fracture and full dorsopalmar thickness of the bone, both of which are most reliably determined from lateromedial radiographs. Fractures can be repaired with AO/ASIF cortex screws of either 3.5-mm or 4.5-mm diameter. This is determined principally by overall fragment size, but generally fragments measuring less than 10 mm in the dorsopalmar plane will require smaller implants. Surgery can be performed with horses in dorsal or lateral

recumbency. The former offers greater versatility of limb positioning and also permits bilateral surgical procedures. The limb should be suspended in a manner that permits movement between the standard position for arthroscopy of the middle joint and full carpal flexion.

The middle carpal joint is evaluated using the dorsolateral arthroscopic portal. In acute injuries there is usually marked hemarthrosis, and lavage will be necessary to permit visibility. The dorsal compartment of the joint should then be evaluated completely and any additional lesions assessed. There is a wide range of arthroscopic fracture morphology. The most common configuration is curved and centered in the middle of the radial facet. Some are more angular adjacent to the dorsal margin of the bone. Less commonly, fractures can have an almost straight configuration. These are the most difficult to reduce because there is little inherent mediolateral stability. Simple,

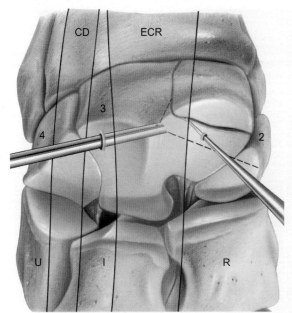

Figure 4-73 Diagram of arthroscope position and instrument entry for debridement of fracture.

nondisplaced fractures can have little articular disruption, but this is highly variable. Some fractures, which on radiographic examination appear nondisplaced, are found to be unstable at arthroscopic evaluation. Comminution of the dorsal margins can be seen in all but is most common with displaced fractures and usually takes the form of marginal fragmentation. Palmar comminution is again most common with, but is not confined to, displaced fractures. In some cases fragments can be present right through the fracture plane, and without prior removal these can confound reduction. The most common form of palmar comminution is a wedge involving various depths of subchondral bone. Full-thickness cartilage loss adjacent to the palmar fracture margin is another frequent finding.

Reduction (when necessary) is effected by progressive carpal flexion. Any fragments that preclude complete reduction should be removed. Surgical opinion is divided on the fate of large palmar fragments. If these can be retained and stabilized in the repair, some surgeons prefer this option to removal and consequent creation of a large proximal articular deficit. If necessary, minor, particularly mediolateral, incongruity can be corrected using the drill sleeve following creation of a glide hole in the fragment.

The proximal medial and lateral margins of the fracture are marked by arthroscopically guided percutaneous insertion of hypodermic needles (see Figs. 4-74 and 4-75). It is important that these are placed perpendicular to the dorsal surface of the carpus in order to accurately delineate the fracture width. An 18-gauge spinal needle is then placed midway between these two needles close and parallel to the proximal articular surface and directed across the midpoint of the fracture as close to 90 degrees as possible. This needle is the most important directional guide for implant placement. The configuration of most frontal plane slab fractures of the radial facet is such that the tip of the needle usually lodges in the palmar fossa of the bone. It can be pushed into the nonarticular surface at this point to stabilize the needle sufficiently during the repair process to provide confident implant trajectory. It is important that the needles at the medial and lateral margins of the fracture are used to determine the position of this needle. The eccentric position of the arthroscope and its inclined lens angle create a "fish-eye" view such that accurate determination

of the midpoint of the fracture from the arthroscopic image alone is not possible. Once the spinal needle has been placed, a further needle is inserted into the carpometacarpal joint directly distal to its point of entry. If required, radiographs can be made at this time to check needle location and direction (see Fig. 4-75).

At this stage the arthroscope can be held by a surgical assistant to confirm stable location of the marker needles and to monitor the repair process. A short (stab) incision is made midway between the spinal needle and the needle in the carpometacarpal joint using a No. 10 or No. 11 blade. The incision should extend to the dorsal face of the bone, which at this point has a strongly convex dorsal protuberance. A glide hole is drilled in the fragment parallel to the spinal needle (see Fig. 4-76). Once this has reached the fracture plane, an insert sleeve is positioned in the glide hole. In most cases in which a small amount of articular incongruity persists, limited fracture manipulation can be performed under arthroscopic guidance at this time. The thread hole is then drilled in the body of the bone to a depth checked against preoperative measurements (see Fig. 4-77). A countersink is used to create an appropriately sized bed for the screw head. The strongly convex dorsal surface of the third carpal bone means that this is important for all screw sizes in order to avoid point contact, maximize efficiency of compression, and avoid protrusion of the screw head into the overlying joint capsule, dorsal intercarpal ligaments, and tendon of insertion of extensor carpi radialis. The process can be monitored using radiography or fluoroscopy as required.

Following repair, unstable comminuted fragments and detached cartilage are removed in line with basic arthroscopic surgical principles and the joint is lavaged. Skin portals only are closed in a routine manner, and a padded dressing is applied for the immediate postoperative period. Follow-up radiographs of a repaired frontal slab fracture are presented in Figure 4-78, and the arthroscopic appearance is depicted in Figure 4-79.

Undisplaced fractures of the radial facet of the third carpal bone are managed in the same fashion with regard to fixation. However, sometimes they may only be visible on skyline radiographs and the articular defects are minor (Fig. 4-80). Follow-up radiographs are recommended to ascertain healing of the fracture (Fig. 4-81). With displaced fractures, one is frequently left with significant defects at the articular surface. There is usually a defective subchondral bone wedge or multiple pieces, and after removal a large size defect remains (Fig. 4-82). Figure 4-82D illustrates grafting this residual gap with chondrocytes in a PRP vehicle to allow improved restoration of the articular surface.

Occasionally, frontal plane slab fractures of the radial facet are complicated by concurrent sagittal fractures. This can take a number of forms. The first is as described later for simple sagittal fractures with a common dorsal exit point. The second is sagittal fractures that extend palmarly from the frontal plane fracture, and the third divide the frontal plane fragment. Most are predicted by careful scrutiny of radiographs, but occasionally sagittal fractures palmar to the frontal plane fragment are found only at surgery. Fractures with the first configuration are managed by repairing the two fractures independently but staggering the screws proximodistally to avoid impingement. The second type are repaired by avoiding, as far as possible, the plane(s) of the sagittal fracture(s). Repair of the third configuration necessitates two (usually 3.5-mm) screws; one placed on each side of the sagittal fracture.

Use of a titanium, headless variable-pitched, tapered, cannulated compression screw for repair of frontal plane slab fractures of the third carpal bone has been reported by Hirsch et al (2007). The authors documented a number of theoretic advantages of the implant over use of AO/ASIF cortical lag

Text continued on page 103

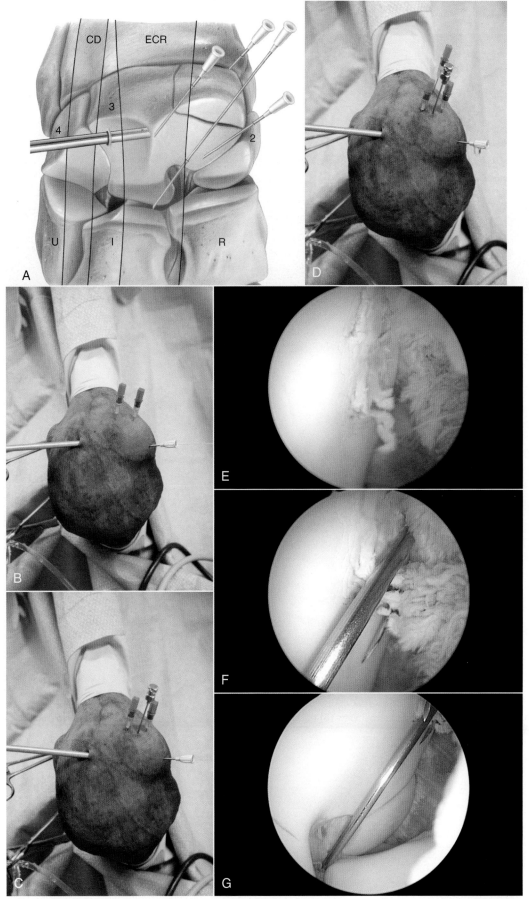

Figure 4-74 Diagram **(A)** and external view **(B)** demonstrating position of arthroscope and placement of needles during fixation of a frontal plane slab fracture of the third carpal bone under arthroscopic visualization. **C** and **D,** Demonstration of position of arthroscope and placement of needles during fixation of a frontal plane slab fracture of the third carpal bone under arthroscopic visualization. **E,** Arthroscopic view of slab fracture prior to the placement of needles. **F** and **G,** Arthroscopic view of needle at medial aspect limit of fracture and placement of spinal needle. Note in **G** how spinal needle is embedded at MPICL fossa.

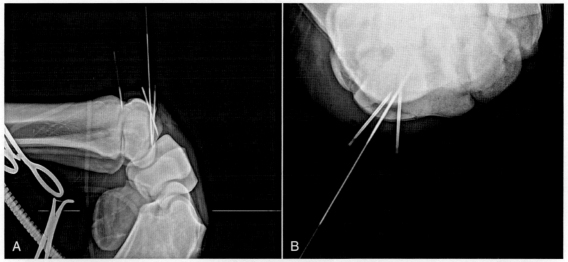

Figure 4-75 **A** and **B,** Radiograph showing needles in position during fixation of carpal slab fracture.

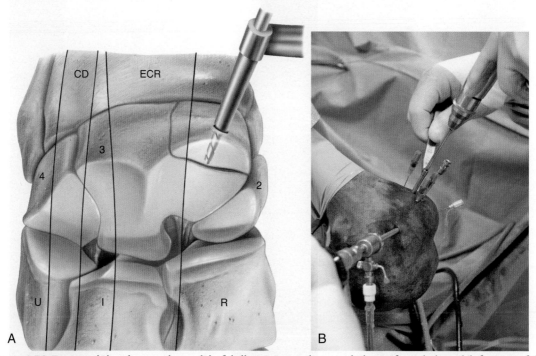

Figure 4-76 Diagram **(A)** and external view **(B)** of drilling 3.5-mm diameter hole in a frontal plane slab fracture of the third carpal bone.

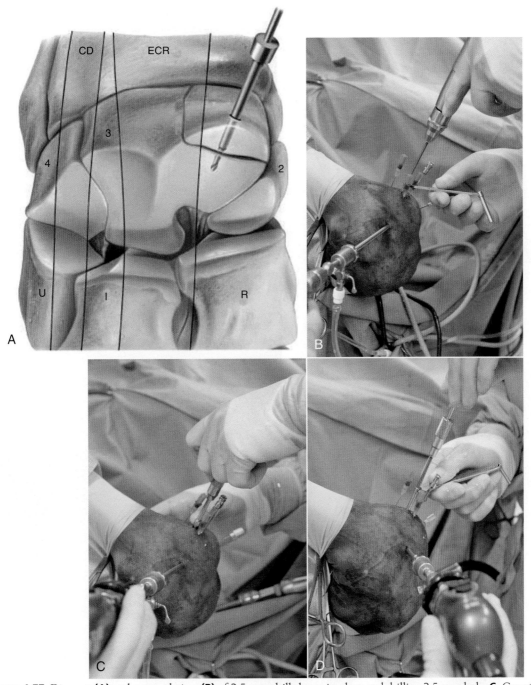

Figure 4-77 Diagram **(A)** and external view **(B)** of 2.5-mm drill sleeve in place and drilling 2.5-mm hole. **C,** Countersinking. **D,** Tapping.

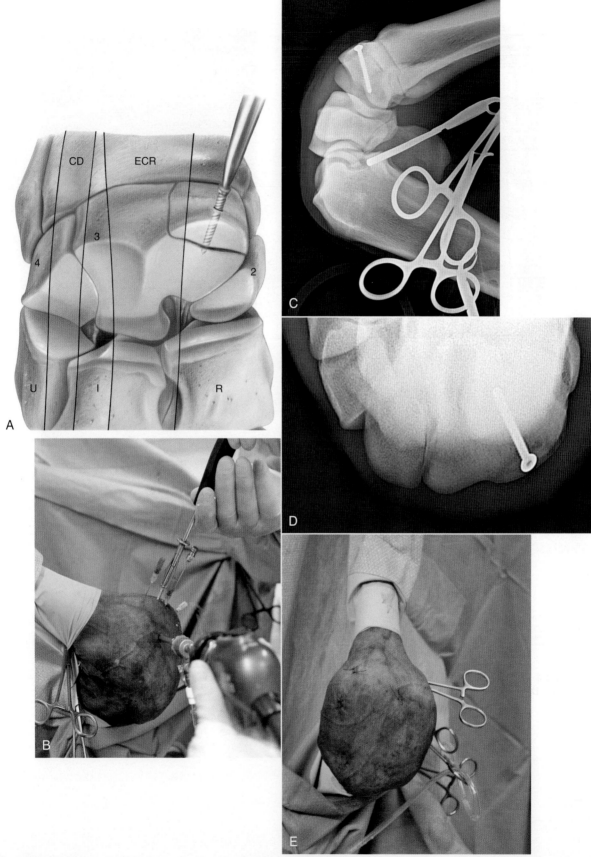

Figure 4-78 Diagram **(A)**, external view of screw placement **(B)** and radiographs confirming appropriate screw placement **(C** and **D)** sutures placed at completion of surgery. **E,** Sutures placed at completion of surgery.

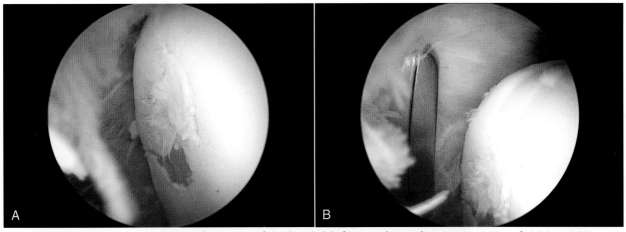

Figure 4-79 Arthroscopic views after repair of displaced slab fracture depicted in Figures 4-72 and 4-74 to 4-78. **A,** Articular defect with preservation of a wedge of cartilage and bony defect more medially and **B,** dorsodistal aspect of repaired fracture.

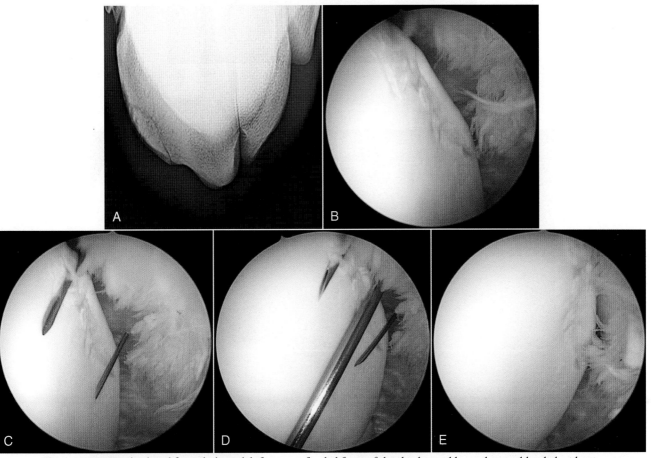

Figure 4-80 Nondisplaced frontal plane slab fracture of radial facet of the third carpal bone that could only be identified on a flexed dorsoproximal-dorsodistal oblique radiographic projection **(A)** with arthroscopic images during repair procedure **(B to E).** Note the minor articular surface defect associated with this fracture.

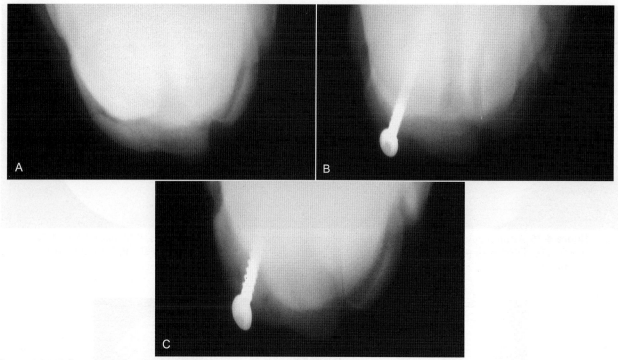

Figure 4-81 Follow-up skyline (DPrDDiO) radiographs illustrating fracture healing at 0 **(A)**, 3 **(B)**, and 6 **(C)** months postoperatively.

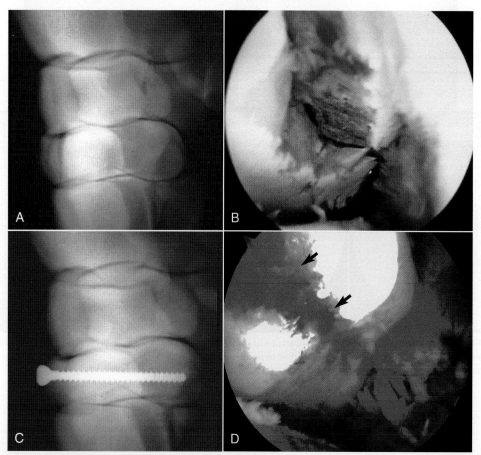

Figure 4-82 **A,** Third carpal bone frontal slab fracture in 4-year-old Thoroughbred. **B,** Intraoperative view shows more expected damage with wedge-shaped bone loss on the palmar side of the primary fracture line. **C,** A 4.5-mm lag screw has been placed to repair the primary fracture. **D,** The residual gap is grafted *(arrows)* with chondrocytes in a PRP vehicle.

screws and results in 17 horses, which suggests that it is a reasonable alternative. However, no major clinical advantages were established. The screw insertion technique is more technically demanding and time consuming and there have been reported risks of drill breakage. It has not therefore been widely adopted. The technique of alignment for insertion under arthroscopic guidance is identical to that for standard lag screw fixation.

Frontal Plane Fractures Involving Radial and Intermediate Facets

There are two principal configurations of slab fractures involving both radial and intermediate facets of the third carpal bone. The first commences dorsally at approximately the midpoint of the radial facet and then curves laterally and palmarly to exit the intermediate facet through its articulation with the fourth carpal bone. The second is a straighter configuration that extends from the articulation of the radial facet with the second carpal bone directly to the articulation between the intermediate facet and fourth carpal bone. Varying degrees of displacement are encountered, although in general this is less than with slab fractures of individual facets. The basic principles of fracture management are similar to those described above for frontal plane fractures of the radial facet. In most cases two implants are necessary (Fig. 4-83). These are inserted at the junctions of the first and second, and third and fourth

quadrants with implant location determined (as described earlier) with percutaneous needles. The wedge shape of the third carpal bone necessitates a degree of palmar implant convergence, which will be predicted by the trajectories of the spinal needles. Implant size is determined by the individual fracture configuration but is usually a pair of 4.5-mm screws.

Frontal plane slab fractures of the radial and intermediate facets can be complicated by sagittal comminution as described for fractures involving the radial facet only. These are managed in a similar manner.

▶ Sagittal and Parasagittal Fractures of the Radial Facet

Arthroscopic evaluation usually reveals a fracture line commencing in the dorsal margin of the radial facet at the junction of its middle and medial one thirds (Fig. 4-84). The fractures can be straight or curved, and most are seen to exit through the articulation with the second carpal bone. The fractures do not displace, which probably accounts for the less marked clinical signs that accompany the injury compared with fractures in the frontal plane. Most are simple, but dorsolateral comminution is sometimes encountered. There may also be loss of cartilage adjacent to the fracture.

The joint and fracture are assessed through a standard dorsolateral arthroscopic portal. The dorsal margin of the fracture and the junction between the second and third carpal bones

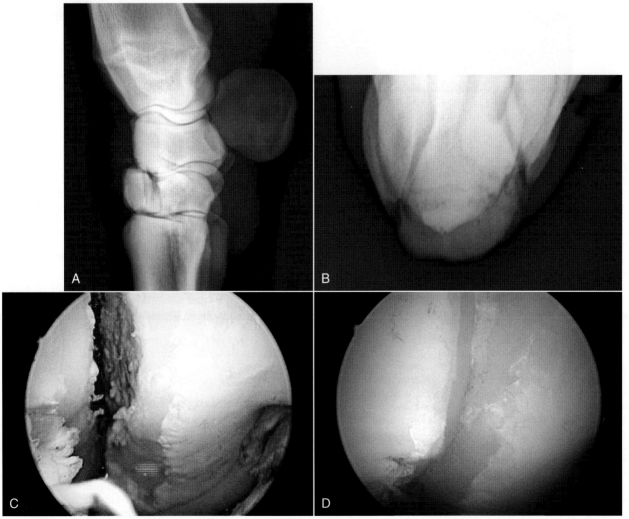

Figure 4-83 Preoperative radiographs (**A** and **B**) and arthroscopic views before (**C**) and (**D**) after fixation of frontal plane slab fracture involving both the radial and intermediate facets of the third carpal bone repaired with two screws.

Continued

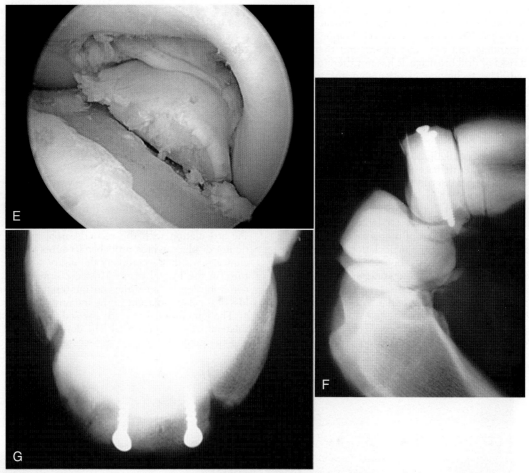

Figure 4-83, cont'd E, Arthroscopic view of avulsion fracture of third carpal bone, which is typical in these cases. **F and G,** Intraoperative radiographs showing reduction in fixation of the slab fracture.

are demarcated by arthroscopically guided percutaneous needles (see Fig. 4-84). Both must be placed perpendicular to the skin in order to accurately demarcate this narrow dorsomedial segment of the third carpal bone. The trajectory of the implant is determined by percutaneous placement of an 18-gauge spinal needle. In order to effectively compress the fracture, this will be close to medial to lateral and requires that the screw is inserted close to, but not impinging on, the dorsal surface of the second carpal bone. There is little margin for error, and meticulous placement of marker needles is critical. Once this has been determined, a needle is placed in the carpometacarpal joint immediately distal to the spinal needle. A short (stab) incision is then made with a No. 10 or No. 11 blade midway between the middle and carpometacarpal margins of the third carpal bone.

All sagittal and parasagittal fractures of the radial facet are repaired with 3.5-mm AO/ASIF cortex screws in order that a small head of these implants can be safely located in the dorsal medial margin of the bone without impingement on the second carpal bone (see Fig. 4-84). Sagittal and parasagittal fractures of the radial facet of the third carpal bone are all narrow and do not require larger implant diameter. Standard insertion technique is employed. The dorsal surface of the radial facet is convex, and use of a countersink is necessary and recommended. As in other sites, preoperative planning is important and includes determination of the desired length of the glide and thread holes.

Parasagittal fractures can be radiologically silent for more than 2 weeks. Serial radiographs are therefore necessary when horses exhibit clinical signs consistent with their presence.

Conservative management has been reported (Fischer & Stover, 1987). In this series half of the cases managed conservatively healed. Additionally, the authors have seen clinically active delayed and nonunion fractures at this site. Usually, minimal debridement is necessary aside from fragment removal in the minority of cases with dorsolateral comminution.

Slab Fractures of the Intermediate Facet of the Third Carpal Bone

Both frontal and sagittal fractures of the intermediate facet are uncommon. The latter are usually incomplete and are not considered to be surgical candidates. Frontal plane slab fractures are approached with a dorsomedial arthroscopic portal, which optimizes evaluation of the intermediate facet and guidance for repair. This aside, the fractures are managed in a manner identical to frontal plane slab fractures of the radial facet, although they are usually smaller and require only a 3.5-mm screw.

Incomplete Slab Fractures

Proximodistally incomplete slab fractures of the third carpal bone are, by definition, stable and can heal with conservative management. When present in horses with other articular lesions, principally fragmentation of other (commonly the radial) carpal bones, such fractures have been repaired as a "safety first" procedure principally to protect the fracture in recovery from general anesthesia. This has been effected by insertion of small (2.7-mm or 3.5-mm) AO/ASIF cortex screws inserted just distal to the subchondral bone plate in a lag technique. This has resulted in radiologic evidence of compression

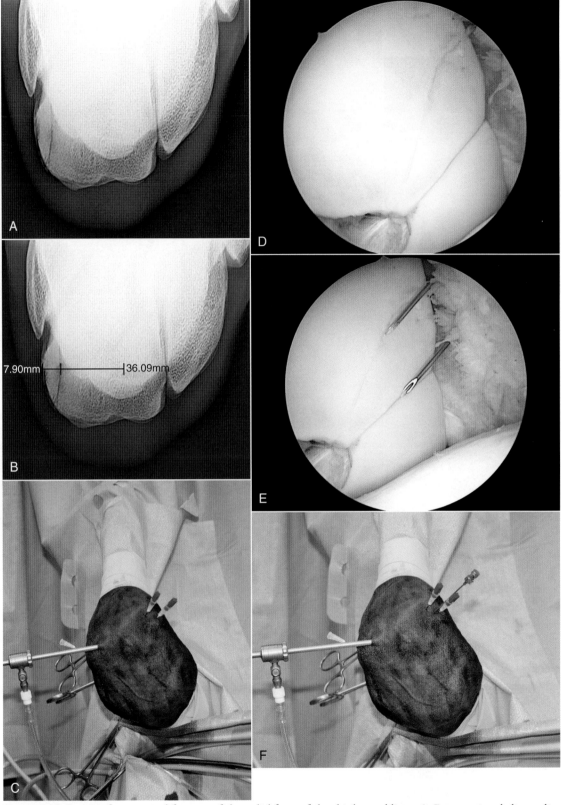

Figure 4-84 Repair of parasagittal fracture of the radial facet of the third carpal bone. **A,** Preoperative skyline radiograph showing parasagittal fracture. **B,** Radiograph with measurements made to define width of fracture and to give indication for screw length in third carpal bone. **C,** External view with arthroscope inserted through a dorsolateral portal and hypodermic needles placed at junction of second and third carpal bone, as well as at fracture line. **D,** Arthroscopic view of fracture before needle placement. **E,** Arthroscopic view of needles in that position. **F,** External view of placement of spinal needle in postion desired for screw placement.

Continued

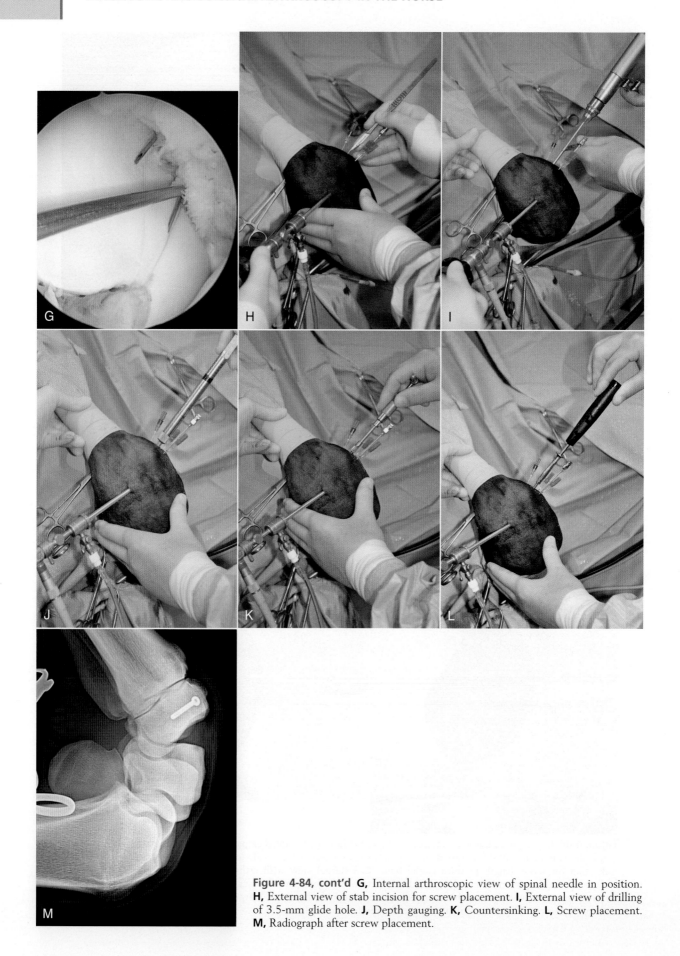

Figure 4-84, cont'd **G,** Internal arthroscopic view of spinal needle in position. **H,** External view of stab incision for screw placement. **I,** External view of drilling of 3.5-mm glide hole. **J,** Depth gauging. **K,** Countersinking. **L,** Screw placement. **M,** Radiograph after screw placement.

and timely fracture healing. Repair is a logical elective option in the management of simple incomplete fractures. However, this should be considered and undertaken only with caution as, in some cases, fractures may not be arthroscopically visible (i.e., the overlying articular cartilage is intact). In such instances, safe fracture repair is precluded. When the fracture can be identified, its medial and lateral margins are delineated with percutaneous needles and its midpoint is marked with percutaneous spinal needles. The implant is placed in line with the spinal needle at the level of the capsular reflection, which places the screw just distal to the proximal subchondral bone plate. Technique of insertion is as described earlier.

ARTHROSCOPIC SURGERY FOR TREATMENT OF OTHER CARPAL SLAB FRACTURES

Slab fractures of other carpal bones are uncommon but can also be assessed, reduced, and repaired under arthroscopic guidance. Frontal plane slab fractures of the radial carpal bone are assessed arthroscopically through dorsolateral portals in both middle and antebrachiocarpal joints. The fracture margins and implant trajectory are determined by arthroscopically guided percutaneous needles in a manner similar to that employed in corresponding fractures of the third carpal bone. The fracture configuration will determine the size and number of implants necessary.

ARTHROSCOPIC SURGERY FOR TREATMENT OF COMPLEX CARPAL SLAB FRACTURES

Most complex fractures involve the medial aspect of the carpus and can result in varying degrees of collapse. The most common is centered on unstable fractures involving both radial and intermediate facets of the third carpal bone with sufficient loss of osseous support that the radial and/or intermediate carpal bones are displaced distally. Commonly, such injuries will also involve lesions of these bones. If the fractures can be reduced and reconstruction effected sufficiently to provide osseous support, then arthroscopically guided repair is appropriate and indicated. If this cannot be achieved, then partial carpal arthrodesis is necessary as a salvage procedure. Even when reconstruction is possible, there is usually gross damage to articular surfaces both as a result of direct fragmentation and from milled osteochondral debris, which is usually scattered throughout the joint. Fractures are reduced and reconstructed as described for the individual configurations. Displaced and unstable fragments are removed in such cases, external support is also necessary, and a sleeve cast from proximal antebrachium to distal metacarpus should be fitted with the limb in extension for recovery from general anesthesia and for the immediate postoperative period.

Postoperative Care for Slab Fractures

Following repair, most carpal slab fractures require only dressings as used following arthroscopic removal of fragmentation. Complex injuries and fractures that exhibit evidence of collapse recover from general anesthesia in a sleeve cast. Surgeons vary widely in use and choice of perioperative antimicrobial and analgesic agents. Exercise is determined on an individual case basis with periods of stall rest varying between 2 and 6 weeks according to the severity of the injury. A protracted period of controlled exercise follows, usually involving a 6- to 8-week period of increasing amounts of walking exercise first in hand and later, if required, on a mechanical walker. Manual flexion exercise is encouraged as soon as bandages are removed and should continue until a full and unresented range of flexion (no painful response to flexion) is consistently obtained. At the end of the walking period, progressive increase in exercise is permitted. This may involve continued controlled exercise, such as ridden trotting or free exercise in a small paddock. Swimming may also be beneficial at this point. The average convalescent period is generally considered to be approximately 6 months for return to training.

With appropriate screw placement, complications are uncommon. A further fracture extending to the screw or the creation of a chip fracture, or both, at this site have been recognized. Unless there is good clinical and radiologic evidence to implicate the implant(s) in lameness, screws are not removed.

Results

Martin et al (1988) and Stephens et al (1988) reported follow-up on horses that had sustained frontal plane slab fractures of the third carpal bone. Combining their data provides a pool of 114 horses in which fractures were repaired with lag screw fixation by arthrotomy. These comprise 77 Thoroughbreds and 37 Standardbreds with follow-up on 104 horses. Seventy-five (72%) raced postsurgery, of which 49 (68%) were Thoroughbreds and 26 (79%) Standardbreds. The mean time to the first race reported by Martin et al (1988) was 9.5 months and by Stephens et al (1988) 10.4 months in Thoroughbreds and 11.5 months in Standardbreds. Stephens et al (1988) compared performance of horses in which fractures were repaired with those by rest alone or by fragment removal, although the severity of the injury was a major determinant of the selected treatment modality. Nonetheless, when using earnings as an indicator of performance, horses in which fractures were repaired had less loss of athletic ability than the other groups (increased mean earnings postsurgery in Standardbreds and reduced mean earnings postsurgery in Thoroughbreds). The series reported by Martin et al (1988) were all Thoroughbreds, and these also had reduced postfracture performance measured by reduced mean claiming value in 50% of horses postinjury.

Conservative management of 12 horses with sagittal slab fractures of the third carpal bone was reported by Fischer and Stover (1987). All received periods of rest of up to 1 year. None were repaired, but one was surgically debrided via arthrotomy. Seven (58%) horses returned to work, including 5 of 10 racehorses. Further data was provided by Kraus et al (2005) who compared the preinjury and postinjury performance of 32 racehorses following sagittal slab fractures of the third carpal bone. These comprised 19 Thoroughbreds, 11 Standardbreds, and 2 Arabians. Seven horses also had osteochondral fragmentation at other sites (6 radial and 1 intermediate carpal bones). Cases were treated by arthroscopic debridement (9), lag screw fixation by arthrotomy (7), or rest alone (16). All 7 horses in which fractures were repaired, 8 of 9 with fracture debridement, and 7 of 16 conservatively managed raced postsurgery. Additionally, the postinjury earnings of horses in which fractures were repaired were greater than those that were managed conservatively.

There are limited published results for arthroscopically guided repair of slab fractures of the third carpal bone. Richardson (1986), in describing the technique for arthroscopic repair of slab fractures of the third carpal bone, reported results in 23 horses. Seventeen had follow-up of at least 6 months, and of these 10 (59%) raced postsurgery. Analysis of data from one author (I.M.W.) of the last 50 slab fractures of the third carpal bone in Thoroughbreds with greater than 1-year follow-up, all repaired under arthroscopic guidance, has yielded the following information. Thirty-six (72%) horses raced postsurgery. Thirty-four horses had raced prefracture, and of these 29 raced after surgery. This group had a total of 302 runs presurgery and 314 postsurgery for 41 and 39 wins, 79 and 76 places, respectively. Seven of the 16 horses that were unraced presurgery ran postrepair for a total 22 runs, including 1 win and 2 places. These fractures have not been classified by configuration, and all horses ran under United Kingdom racing legislation (Wright, unpublished data).

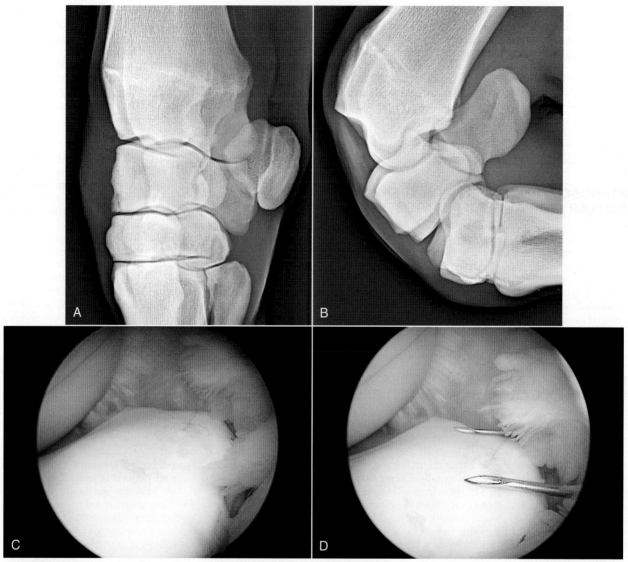

Figure 4-85 Repair of osteochondral fracture of the dorsodistal radial carpal bone using a 2.7-mm screw. **A,** Dorso-lateral-palmaromedial oblique and **B,** flexed lateromedial radiographic projection. **C,** Arthroscopic appearance of the fracture depicted in **A** and **B. D,** Medial and lateral margins of the fracture demarcated with percutaneous needles.

ARTHROSCOPIC SURGERY FOR THE REPAIR (WITH SCREW FIXATION) OF CARPAL CHIP FRACTURES

Chip fractures of the carpal bones that are of sufficient size and infrastructure can be repaired by arthroscopically guided internal fixation. Wright & Smith (2011) described the technique and results obtained with 35 fractures in 33 Thoroughbred racehorses, including the dorsodistal radial carpal bone (*n* = 25), dorsoproximal third carpal bone (*n* = 9), and dorsodistal radius (*n* = 1).

The prognosis following arthroscopic removal of carpal chip fractures deteriorates as the size of the resultant articular deficit increases (McIlwraith et al, 1987 & 2005). Reconstruction aims to preserve articular congruency. The depth of the lesion will determine the location of screws, but in all chip fractures implants are placed in or adjacent to the subchondral bone. This has a number of important implications for the surgeon. The first is that avoiding inadvertent protrusion into the joint leaves little margin for error. Particular care is necessary in placing the guide needle immediately adjacent to the articular surface. When drilling, the surgeon must remain either parallel to or diverging from this, as determined by the

fracture configuration. The second is that subchondral bone is dense, and undue pressure on the small drill bits used can result in breakage. Additionally, the dorsodistal articular surface of the radial carpal bone is convex, which determines the maximal length of the subchondral screw to avoid emergence and impingement on the third carpal bone. This distance is predetermined in flexed lateromedial radiographs before surgery. The flat proximal articular surface of the third carpal bone does not create such limitation. The dorsodistal articular surfaces of the radius are concave, but the concavity is shallow compared with the depth of most fragments so that the implant length and trajectory are less critical.

The technique is a modification of that described for repair of slab fractures of the third carpal bone (Fig. 4-85A-H). The horse is positioned, and joint evaluated as described earlier for each fracture location. Suitable fractures are generally not displaced or minimally displaced. When necessary, reduction can be effected by increasing joint flexion or by manipulation using the (2-mm) drill sleeve after creation of the glide hole, or both. The medial and lateral margins of the fracture are defined by placement of percutaneous needles (23-gauge × 25 mm) (see Fig. 4-85D). It

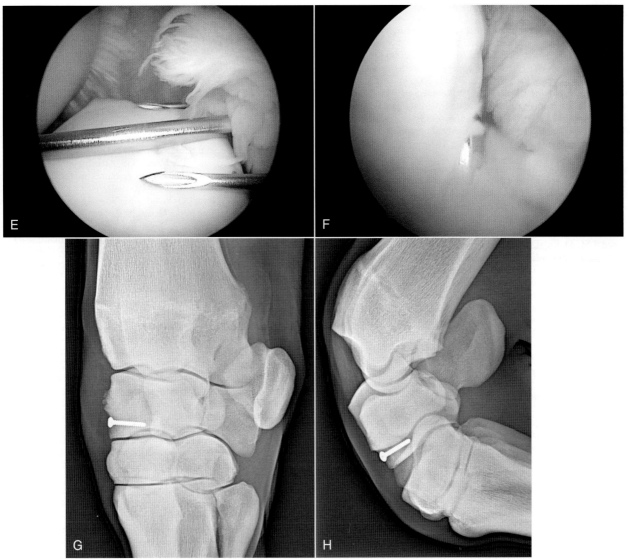

Figure 4-85, cont'd E, Mediolateral midpoint and distal margin of the fracture identified by passage of a spinal needle midway between the two needles depicted in **D** along the distal articular surface of the radial carpal bone and a trajectory chosen for the implant. **F,** Head of 2.7-mm screw in the dorsal surface of the fracture fragment adjacent to the capsular reflection. **G,** Dorsolateral-palmaromedial oblique and **H,** flexed lateromedial radiographic projections taken 18 weeks postsurgery.

is important that these are inserted perpendicular to the skin to avoid erroneous assessment of fracture size and location. These are followed by an 18-gauge × 89-mm spinal needle placed midway between the marker needles and parallel to the articular surface of the fractured bone (see Fig. 4-85E). This acts as a guide for drill trajectory. A further needle (19-gauge × 38 mm) is then used to mark the proposed site of screw placement immediately adjacent to the capsular attachment. This places the screw close to the endosteal side of the subchondral bone plate and means that the repair process is visualized arthroscopically (see Fig. 4-85F). A stab incision is made at this point with a No. 11 blade and a 2.7-mm glide hole created through the fracture fragment to a radiographically predetermined depth. Following confirmation of fragment depth, the 2-mm drill guide (insert) is located in the hole and the 2-mm hole is drilled into the parent bone to the radiographically predetermined distance to permit a cortical screw to be inserted using the lag principle. The hole is countersunk, measured, and then tapped to cut a thread before a 2.7-mm AO/ASIF cortical screw, of selected length, is inserted and tightened. An appropriate (usually LM) radiograph

is then taken to confirm appropriate implant placement (Fig. 4-85G-H). Small, unstable, or loose osteochondral fragments and detached cartilage flaps can be removed, but debridement is generally kept to a minimum. Skin portals are closed, and the leg is dressed as described previously.

Convalescence and postoperative exercise should be determined on an individual case basis. In the series described by Wright & Smith (2011), horses were confined to their stable for 1 to 4 (mean 2) weeks followed by 4 to 12 (mean 8) weeks of walking and a similar period (mean 6 weeks) of trotting exercise.

The fractures reported by Wright & Smith (2011) represented 10% of their cases which underwent arthroscopic surgery for carpal fragmentation in the 4-year study period. Fractures healed in 18 of 19 horses with radiologic follow-up. Twenty-three of 28 (82%) of horses with clinical follow-up returned to racing, with 19 (68%) racing at a level equal to or better than presurgery and 4 at a reduced level. The mean time between surgery and the first race was 10 (range 3 to 22) months.

REFERENCES

Beinlich CP, Nixon AJ: Prevalence and response to surgical treatment of lateral palmar intercarpal ligament avulsion in horses: 37 cases (1990-2001), *J Am Vet Med Assoc* 226:760–766, 2005.

Cheetham J, Nixon AJ: Arthroscopic approaches to the palmar aspect of the equine carpus, *Vet Surg* 35:227–231, 2006.

Dabareiner RM, Sullins KE, Bradley W: Removal of a fracture fragment from the palmar aspect of the intermediate carpal bone in a horse, *J Am Vet Med Assoc* 203:553–555, 1993.

DeHaan CE, O'Brien TR, Koblik PD: A radiographic investigation of third carpal bone injury in 40 racing Thoroughbreds, *Vet Radiol* 28:88–92, 1987.

Finerman GAM, Noyce FR, editors: *Biology and biomechanics of the traumatized synovial joint: The knee as a model*, Rosemount IL, 1992, American Academy of Orthopedic Surgeons.

Fischer AT, Stover SM: Sagittal fractures in the third carpal bone in horses: 12 cases (1977–1985), *J Am Vet Med Assoc* 191:106–108, 1987.

Getman LM, McKnight AL, Richardson DW: Comparison of magnetic resonance contrast arthrography and arthroscopic anatomy of the equine palmar lateral outpouching of the middle carpal joint, *Vet Radiol Ultrasound* 48:493–500, 2007.

Getman LM, Southwood LL, Richardson DW: Palmar carpal osteochondral fragments in racehorses: 31 cases (1994–2004), *J Am Vet Med Assoc* 228:1551–1558, 2006.

Hirsch JE, Galuppo LD, Graham LE, Simpson EL, Ferraro GL: Clinical evaluation of a titanium, headless variable-pitched tapered cannulated compression screw for repair of frontal plane slab fractures of the third carpal bone in Thoroughbred racehorses, *Vet Surg* 36:178–184, 2007.

Johnson LL: *Arthroscopic surgery principles and practice*, St Louis, 1986, Mosby.

Kane AJ, McIlwraith CW, Park RD, Rantanen NW, Morehead JP, Bramlage LR: Radiographic changes in Thoroughbred yearlings. Part II: Associations with racing performance, *Equine Vet J* 35:366–375, 2003.

Kane AJ, Park RD, McIlwraith CW, Rantanen NW, Morehead JP, Bramlage LR: Radiographic changes in Thoroughbred yearlings. Part I: Prevalence at the time of the yearling sales, *Equine Vet J* 35:354–365, 2003.

Kannegieter NJ, Burbidge HM: Correlation between radiographic and arthroscopic findings in the equine carpus, *Aust Vet J* 67:132–133, 1990.

Kannegieter NJ, Colgan SA: The incidence and severity of intercarpal ligament damage in the equine carpus, *Aust Vet J* 70:89–91, 1993.

Kawcak CE, McIlwraith CW, Norrdin RW, Park RD, Steyn PS: Clinical effects of exercise on subchondral bone of carpal and metacarpophalangeal joints, *Am J Vet Res* 61:1252–1258, 2000.

Kawcak CE, McIlwraith CW, Norrdin RW, Park RD, James SP: The role of subchondral bone in joint disease: a review, *Equine Vet J* 33:120–126, 2001.

Kraus BM, Ross MW, Boston RC: Surgical and nonsurgical management of sagittal slab fractures of the third carpal bone in racehorses: 32 cases (1991-2001), *J Am Vet Med Assoc* 226:945–950, 2005.

Lucas JM, Ross MW, Richardson DW. Post operative performance of racing Standardbreds treated arthroscopically for carpal chip fractures: 176 cases (1986-1993), *Equine Vet J* 31:48–52, 1999.

Martin GS, Haynes PF, McClure JR: Effect of third carpal slab fracture and repair on racing performance in Thoroughbred horses: 31 cases (1977–1984), *J Am Vet Med Assoc* 193:107–110, 1988.

Martin GS, McIlwraith CW: Arthroscopic anatomy of the intercarpal and radiocarpal joints of the horse, *Equine Vet J* 17:373–376, 1985.

McIlwraith CW: *Arthroscopic surgery-athletic and developmental lesions. Proceedings of the 29th Annual Meeting of the American Association of Equine Practitioners*, 1983.

McIlwraith CW: Experiences in diagnostic and surgical arthroscopy in the horse, *Equine Vet J* 16:11–19, 1984.

McIlwraith CW: *Diagnostic and surgical arthroscopy in the horse*, ed 2, Philadelphia, 1990, Lea & Febiger, pp 33–84.

McIlwraith CW: Tearing of the medial palmar intercarpal ligament in the equine midcarpal joint, *Equine Vet J* 24:367–371, 1992.

McIlwraith CW, Bramlage LR: Surgical treatment of joint disease. In McIlwraith CW, Trotter GW, editors: *Joint disease of the horse*, Philadelphia, 1996, WB Saunders, pp 292–317.

McIlwraith CW, Yovich JV, Martin GS: Arthroscopic surgery for the treatment of osteochondral chip fractures in the equine carpus, *J Am Vet Med Assoc* 191:531–540, 1987.

McIlwraith CW, Nixon AJ, Wright IM, Boening KJ: *Diagnostical and Surgical Arthroscopy in the Horse*, 2005.

Moore RM, Schneider RK: Arthroscopic findings in the carpal joints of lame horses without radiographically visible abnormalities: 41 cases (1986-1991), *J Am Vet Med Assoc* 206:1741–1746, 1995.

Palmer SE: Prevalence of carpal fractures in Thoroughbred and Standardbred racehorses, *J Am Vet Med Assoc* 188:1171–1173, 1986.

Phillips TJ, Wright IM: Observations on the anatomy and pathology of the palmar intercarpal ligaments in the middle carpal joints of Thoroughbred racehorses, *Equine Vet J* 26:486–491, 1994.

Pool RR, Meagher DM: Pathologic findings and pathogenesis of racetrack injuries, *Vet Clin North Am Equine Pract* 6:1–30, 1990.

Richardson DW: Technique for arthroscopic repair of third carpal bone slab fractures in the horse, *Am Vet Med Assoc* 188:288–291, 1986.

Richardson DW: *Proximal surface lesions of the third carpal bone. Proceedings of the 1st Advanced Arthroscopy Course*, Colorado State University, 1988.

Richardson DW: Arthroscopically assisted repair of articular fractures, *Clin Techn Equine Pract* 1:211–217, 2002.

Ross MW, Richardson DW, Beroza GA: Subchondral lucency of the third carpal bone in Standardbreds racehorses: 13 cases (1982–1988), *J Am Vet Med Assoc* 195:789–794, 1989.

Schneider RK, Bramlage LR, Gabel AA, Barone LM, Kantrowitz BM: Incidence, location and classification of 371 third carpal bone fractures in 313 horses, *Equine Vet J Suppl* 6:33–42, 1988.

Stephens PR, Richardson DW, Spence PA: Slab fractures of the third carpal bone in Standardbreds and Thoroughbreds: 155 cases (1977–1984), *J Am Vet Med Assoc* 193:353–358, 1988.

Uhlhorn H, Carlsten J: Retrospective study of subchondral sclerosis and lucency in the third carpal bone in Standardbred trotters, *Equine Vet J* 31:500–505, 1999.

Whitton RC, McCarthy PH, Rose RJ: The intercarpal ligaments of the equine midcarpal joint, Part I: The anatomy of the palmar and dorsomedial intercarpal ligaments in the midcarpal joint, *Vet Surg* 26:359–366, 1997.

Wilke M, Nixon AJ, Malark J, Myhre G: Fractures of the palmar aspect of the carpal bones in horses: 10 cases (1984–2000), *J Am Vet Med Assoc* 219:801–804, 2001.

Wright IM: Ligaments associated with joints, *Vet Clin N Am* 11:249–291, 1995.

Wright IM, Smith MRW: The use of small (2.7 mm) screws for arthroscopically guided repair of carpal chip fractures, *Equine Vet J* 43:270–279, 2011.

Young DR, Richardson DW, Markel MD, Numamaker DM: Mechanical and morphometric analysis of the third carpal bone of Thoroughbreds, *Am J Vet Res* 52:402–409, 1991.

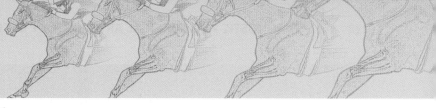

CHAPTER 5

Diagnostic and Surgical Arthroscopy of the Metacarpophalangeal and Metatarsophalangeal Joints

Arthroscopy has proven to be a most valuable technique in the metacarpophalangeal and metatarsophalangeal (fetlock) joints. Its original use was principally in arthroscopic surgery in the dorsal aspect of the joint but then extended into the palmar/plantar aspect. Arthroscopic surgery in the dorsal aspect of the fetlock joint is probably the best equine example of what can be achieved with joint distension.

The same advantages that have been discussed in the carpus hold for arthroscopic surgery in the fetlock. The indications for arthroscopic surgery in the metacarpophalangeal and metatarsophalangeal joints include the following conditions:

1. Osteochondral fragments of the dorsal aspect of the proximal phalanx
2. Erosions of articular cartilage and subchondral bone disease on the dorsal margin of the proximal phalanx
3. Synovial pad fibrotic proliferation (villonodular synovitis) of the metacarpophalangeal joint
4. Other forms of proliferative synovitis
5. Osteochondritis dissecans of the third metacarpal or metatarsal bones (McIII/MtIII)
6. Osteochondral fragments in the dorsal plica
7. Subchondral cystic lesions of McIII
8. Impact and chondral fractures
9. Tears and avulsions of the fibrous joint capsule
10. Osteochondral fragments associated with the palmar or plantar aspect of the proximal phalanx
11. Removal of apical fragments of the proximal sesamoid bone
12. Removal of abaxial fragments of the proximal sesamoid bones
13. Removal of basilar fragments of the proximal sesamoid bones
14. Axial osteitis of the proximal sesamoid bones and lesions of the intersesamoidean ligament
15. Avulsions of the suspensory ligament insertions
16. Repair of fractures of the McIII/MtIII condyles
17. Repair of fractures of the proximal phalanx
18. Repair of proximal sesamoid bone fractures

DIAGNOSTIC ARTHROSCOPY OF THE FETLOCK JOINTS

Arthroscopic examination of the fetlock joint may be indicated specifically as a diagnostic procedure or as a prelude to arthroscopic surgery (McIlwraith, 1984). The latter situation is more common, although diagnostic arthroscopy is indicated in cases involving lameness that has localized to the fetlock but for which the radiographic and other diagnostic imaging features are equivocal. The procedure is most valuable if synovial effusion is present or if the area of lameness has been identified as intraarticular, on the basis of a response to intraarticular analgesia and when there has not been a response to conservative treatment.

A complete arthroscopic examination of the metacarpophalangeal or metatarsophalangeal joint is not possible. Two arthroscopic approaches give an effective examination of both the dorsal and palmar (plantar) compartments. Vanderperren et al (2009) quantified the amount of the articular surfaces of the metacarpal and metatarsal condyles that could be visualized

in cadaver limbs (positioned in lateral recumbency). Dorsal and palmar/plantar arthroscopic portals were used. The former was placed approximately 1 cm further distad than that described later (and used as routine by the authors) in order to maximize distal evaluation when the joint is flexed. A conventional proximal palmar/plantar arthroscopic portal was employed together with a distal palmar/plantar portal as described later for access to the palmar/plantar processes of the proximal phalanx and bases of the proximal sesamoid bones. The joints were evaluated in extension and flexion. The flexion angles possible in this study varied between 110 and 130 degrees in the forelimbs and between 92 and 127 degrees in the hindlimbs. In the forelimbs 235 degrees (83%) of the condyles could be visualized. This comprised 105 degrees (45%) dorsally, 60 degrees (25%) proximopalmar, and 30 degrees (13%) palmarodistal. In the hindlimbs 225 degrees of visualization was obtained. This comprised 130 degrees (58%) of the condyles dorsally, 50 degrees (22%), with a proximoplantar portal and 20 degrees (9%) from a distoplantar arthroscopic portal. Thirty-nine degrees (17%) and 25 degrees (11%) of the metacarpal and metatarsal condyles, respectively, could not be visualized. The authors concluded that more of the dorsal condyles could be visualized in hindlimbs and more of the palmar condyles in the forelimbs. The nonvisualized areas of the condyles were palmar/plantarodistal in both fore and hind joints.

Each diagnostic examination is described. Because the dorsal approach is performed most commonly on the metacarpophalangeal joint, it is described for that joint. The only difference in examination of the metatarsophalangeal joint is that it may be more difficult because of the decreased ability to maintain extension of the joint. The plantar (palmar) examination is facilitated by flexion, and this is especially convenient in the hind limb.

Arthroscopic examination can be performed with the horse in dorsal or lateral recumbency. If lateral recumbency is used, the horse should be positioned so that the site for arthroscopic entry is up. For the same reason of versatility mentioned in Chapter 4 with regard to the carpal joints, the use of dorsal recumbency is preferred. While the leg is being surgically prepared and draped, it is held by an assistant or is suspended by a mechanical device (the authors use the latter technique) (Figs. 5-1 and 5-2). Draping can be completed with the fetlock resting back on the elbow or appropriately suspended so that the joint remains extended or flexed depending on the procedure.

Arthroscopic Examination of the Dorsal Metacarpophalangeal Joint
Insertion of the Arthroscope

The metacarpophalangeal joint is distended with fluid (Fig. 5-3) before making the arthroscopic portal. In this joint, distension facilitates the recognition of the correct place for the arthroscopic portal and minimizes the risk of iatrogenic trauma to the joint on entry of the arthroscopic sleeve. There are no tendon sheaths to avoid as in the carpus, and the surgeon does not have to be concerned with exact localization of structures before distension.

Distension is achieved with approximately 35 mL of fluid after inserting a needle dorsally or into the palmar pouch adjacent to the proximal sesamoid bone (Misheff & Stover, 1991)

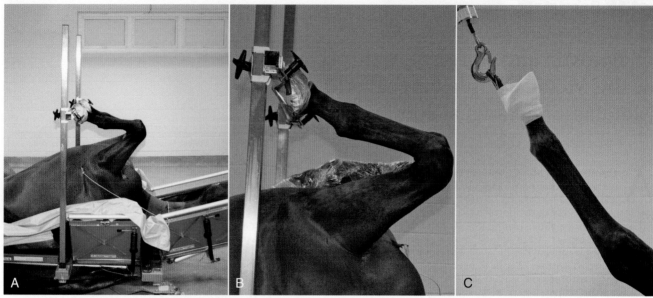

Figure 5-1 Both forelimbs **(A)** and single forelimb **(B)** positioned for arthroscopy of the dorsal metacarpophalangeal joint. **C,** Hindlimb secured by a hoist for arthroscopy of the dorsal metatarsophalangeal joint.

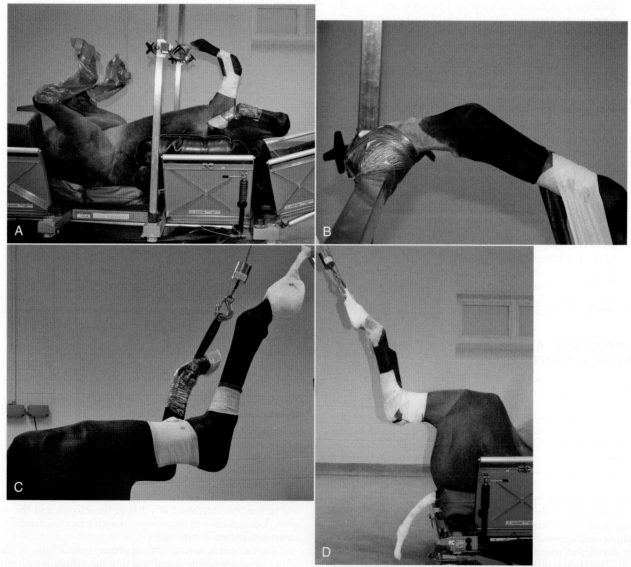

Figure 5-2 Limbs positioned for palmar **(A and B)** and plantar **(C and D)** arthroscopy of the metacarpophalangeal and metatarsophalangeal joints.

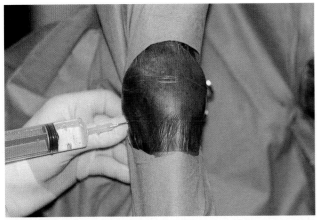

Figure 5-3 Draping is complete and distention of the metacarpophalangeal joint is performed.

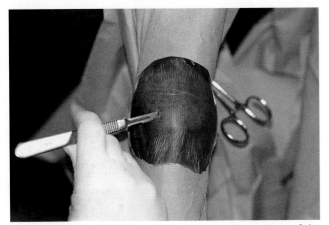

Figure 5-4 A No. 11 blade is inserted at site for insertion of the arthroscope into the dorsal pouch.

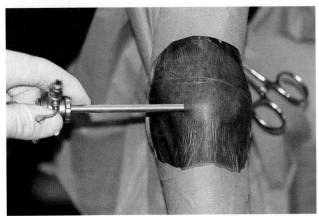

Figure 5-5 Insertion of the arthroscopic sheath and conical obturator in the proximal portion of the dorsal metacarpophalangeal joint. Note that the sheath is directed perpendicular to the limb (90 degrees) to avoid damage to the sagittal ridge of the metacarpus.

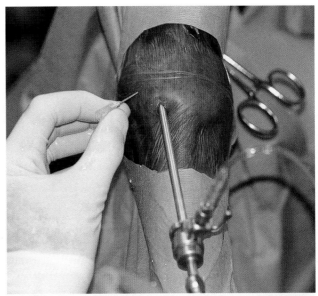

Figure 5-6 The arthroscope is redirected with the end now distad and directed toward the lateral dorsal eminence of the proximal phalanx. A needle is inserted to determine the position of a lateral instrument portal.

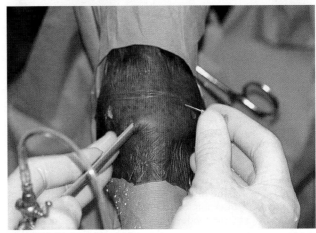

Figure 5-7 Use of a needle to ascertain an approximate position for a medial instrument portal.

(see Fig. 5-3). Adequate distension can be recognized easily with bulging of the joint capsule on either side of the common digital extensor tendon. The outpouching of the distended joint is more prominent lateral to the common digital extensor than it is medial to it, despite the insertion of the lateral digital extensor tendon, which ramifies over the joint capsule and is penetrated when the lateral portal is created.

The site for the laterally placed arthroscopic portal is in the proximolateral quadrant created by distending the joint maximally (see Fig. 5-3). This site reduces the risk of iatrogenic damage to the sagittal ridge of the third metacarpal bone and provides the best overall view of the joint. A No. 11 blade is used to incise the skin and stab through the joint capsule (Fig. 5-4). The arthroscopic sleeve containing a conical obturator is then inserted through the joint capsule, initially perpendicular to the skin and then parallel to the articular surface of McIII to avoid iatrogenic damage to this area (Fig. 5-5). Entry is completed by advancing the sheath proximad to avoid damage to the midsagittal ridge of McIII (see Fig. 5-5). The sheath can then be directed distad once over the sagittal ridge. When the arthroscopic sleeve is inserted so that its tip touches the medial capsule, the arthroscope is inserted and the examination can begin.

As in the carpus, creation of an instrument portal and insertion of an egress cannula or probe are the next steps. A useful measure is to insert a needle at the proposed instrument portal location to check if a site is appropriate (Figs. 5-6 and 5-7). The use of a needle to ascertain ideal positioning for instrument portals represents a departure from what was previously

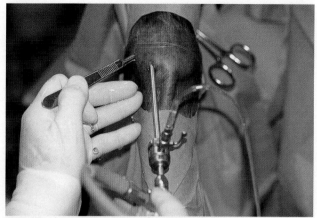

Figure 5-8 Making lateral instrument portal through the joint capsule using a No. 11 scalpel blade.

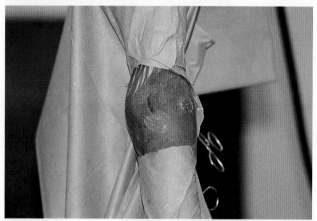

Figure 5-9 Skin portals are closed with single sutures at the end of arthroscopic procedure.

described in the carpus. However, the carpus is unique and the skin incisions for the instrument portal are made before joint distension and insertion of the arthroscope merely to avoid entering an extensor tendon sheath. There are no such issues in the fetlock joint, or most other joints for that matter. The practice of inserting a needle to ascertain the ideal position for instrument insertion and surgical maneuverability is common to all joints other than the carpus. By making a skin incision with a scalpel and No. 11 blade, the surgeon creates the instrument portal through the joint capsule (Fig. 5-8). The small egress cannula can then be inserted through this portal without the trocar. An arthroscopic examination can then commence. At the completion of arthroscopy, the skin incisions only are closed (Fig. 5-9).

▶ Diagnostic Arthroscopy of the Dorsal Pouch of the Fetlock Joint

With slight retraction of the arthroscope and looking across the joint, the first area visualized is the proximal portion of the dorsal joint proximal to the articular cartilage of the distal McIII, where the synovial membrane forms a reflection (Fig. 5-10). At this transition zone, the synovium has a flap, plica, or pad that varies in size and the surgeon must be familiar with the normal range (see Fig. 5-10). Synovial pad fibrotic proliferation (villonodular synovitis) manifests as an enlargement of this flap. Apart from the flap, the synovial membrane in the remainder of this area is nonvillous.

The articular surface of the medial condyle and midsagittal ridge of McIII can then be examined by rotating the arthroscope so that the lens is angled distad (see Fig. 5-10). The tip of the

arthroscope is then moved distad (eyepiece moving proximad) to inspect the dorsomedial articular margin of the proximal phalanx (see Fig. 5-10). The synovial membrane of the dorsal joint capsule is also evaluated during these maneuvers. The synovial membrane is notably more villous as one progresses distad, and villi can sometimes obscure the view of the dorsal rim of the proximal phalanx. The synovial membrane attaches immediately adjacent to this rim; use of instruments (including the egress cannula) to elevate the joint capsule improves inspection of the proximal phalanx and is common practice during both diagnostic and surgical arthroscopy. Withdrawing the tip of the arthroscope further and moving it across the sagittal ridge laterally (eyepiece moving medially) permits inspection of the lateral condyle of McIII, as well as the proximal lateral aspect of the proximal phalanx (see Fig. 5-10).

The examination described previously enables recognition and characterization of synovial pad fibrotic proliferation (villonodular synovitis), other forms of synovitis, fragments off the proximal dorsal aspect of the proximal phalanx, wear lines and erosions on the distal articular surface of McIII, osteochondritis dissecans of the midsagittal ridge and condyles of McIII, tears of plicae and joint capsule, articular components of fractures of McIII and proximal phalanx, and subchondral cystic lesions of McIII.

▶ Arthroscopic Examination of the Palmar or Plantar Metacarpus/Metatarsophalangeal Joints

This examination can be performed with the horse in dorsal or lateral recumbency, but the authors prefer dorsal recumbency for all evaluations/conditions in the palmar/plantar compartment. Although flexion from an assistant is sometimes necessary, advantages include less hemorrhage, convenient operating position, ability to use medial and/or lateral instrument portals, and the option of arthroscope/instrument portal interchange.

Insertion of the Arthroscope

The joint is prepared for surgery and distended by placing the needle in the palmar pouch using the approach described by Misheff & Stover (1991). A skin incision is then made with a No. 11 blade in the proximal part of the bulging capsule (Fig. 5-11). The arthroscopic sheath and conical obturator are inserted perpendicular to the skin initially and then are directed distad (Fig. 5-12). The fetlock is in 30- to 45-degree flexion at this time to facilitate passage between the distal metacarpus/metatarsus and the proximal sesamoid bones. The degree of flexion varies depending on the area being examined (for instance, increased flexion is used to bring the proximal phalanx into view).

Diagnostic Arthroscopy of Palmar (Plantar) Pouch of the Fetlock Joint

Examination of the metacarpophalangeal or metatarsophalangeal joint commences with the arthroscope perpendicular to the skin and the lens oriented proximad (Fig. 5-13). Here, the unusual highly villous, interlacing synovial membrane of the proximal recess of the joint can be visualized. Rotation of the arthroscopic lens palmad allows inspection of the apices of the sesamoid bones and the fibrocartilaginous scutum in which they are partially embedded (see Fig. 5-13).

The tip of the arthroscope is then advanced distad (this can be done safely if the joint is flexed and distension is maintained) to examine the articular surfaces of the sesamoid bones and the intersesamoidean ligament palmad and the articular surface of the distal palmar McIII dorsad (see Fig. 5-13). Advancement of the arthroscope continues until the base of the sesamoids is visualized (see Fig. 5-13) and, with increased flexion, the palmar rim of the proximal phalanx can be evaluated (see Fig. 5-13).

Diagnostic arthroscopy of the palmar or plantar pouch of the fetlock joint is now a commonly used procedure.

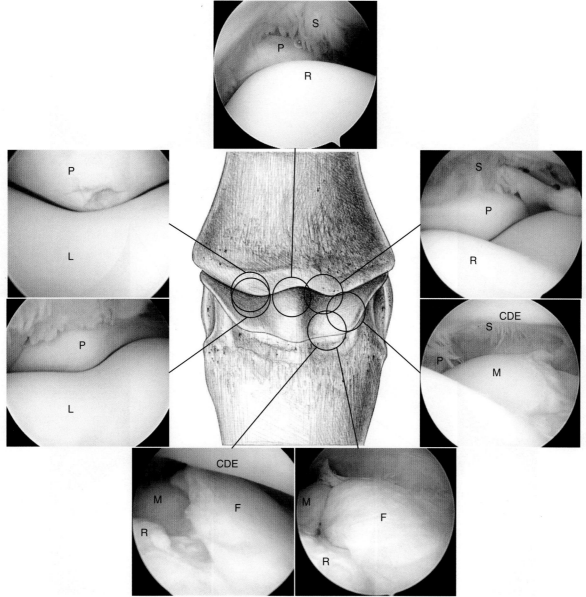

Figure 5-10 Composite of arthroscopic images obtained from dorsal metacarpophalangeal joints using a dorsolateral arthroscopic approach. Note that there can be variations in the normal dorsal synovial pad. *CDE*, Common digital extensor tendon; *F*, dorsal synovial fold; *LDE*, lateral digital extensor tendon; *M*, medial condyle of McIII; *L*, lateral condyle of McIII; *P*, dorsal margin of proximal phalanx; *R*, proximal sagittal ridge of McIII; *S*, villous synovium.

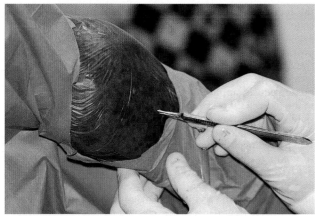

Figure 5-11 Incision into the palmar pouch of fetlock for insertion of the arthroscope.

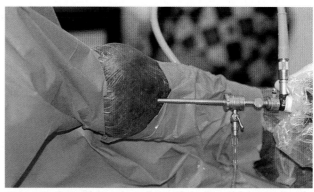

Figure 5-12 Arthroscope positioned for diagnostic examination of the palmar pouch of the metacarpophalangeal joint. The fetlock is slightly flexed to facilitate examination of the distal aspect of the joint.

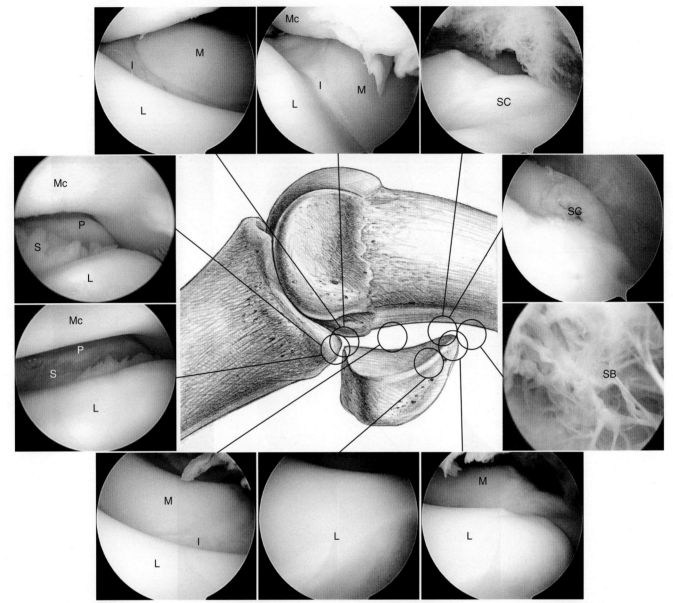

Figure 5-13 Composite of arthroscopic images illustrating examination of the palmar pouch of a metacarpophalangeal joint. *SB*, Characteristic synovial bands in proximal recess. *I*, Intersesamoidean ligament; *L*, lateral and *M*, medial sesamoid bones; *Mc*, McIII condyle; *P*, proximal palmar rim of the proximal phalanx; *S*, synovium; *Sc*, scutum proximal to the sesamoid bones.

Indications for arthroscopic surgery include fragments off the palmar/plantar processes of proximal phalanx, apical, abaxial, and basilar fractures of the proximal sesamoid bones, osteitis of the axial portion of the sesamoid bones and tearing of the intersesamoidean ligament, avulsion injuries of the suspensory ligament branches, as well as adjunctive visualization for assessment and reduction of lateral condylar fractures of McIII/MtIII and management of associated damage. When diagnostic examination of both dorsal and palmar/plantar compartments is to be performed, the former is generally performed first.

ARTHROSCOPIC SURGERY OF THE FETLOCK JOINTS
▶ Removal of Osteochondral Fragments from the Dorsal Margin of the Proximal Phalanx

Before the advent of arthroscopy, surgical removal of these fragments was not routine because some surgeons questioned the benefits of surgical invasion of this area with arthrotomy (Raker,

1973, Meagher, 1974). Now, a horse with problems referable to the fetlock joint and radiographically evident fragments associated with the proximal dorsal aspect of the first phalanx is a candidate for arthroscopic surgery. Arthroscopic surgery can provide a faster return to full function and help to minimize the degenerative changes that can result. All the advantages of arthroscopic surgery discussed in Chapter 4 relative to the carpus are equally applicable when discussing arthroscopic surgery in the fetlock. Of probably increased importance is the need for skillful atraumatic surgery. The dorsal joint capsule and proximal first phalanx tend to be less forgiving to trauma.

The radiographic and arthroscopic manifestations of dorsoproximal fragmentation of the proximal phalanx vary (Figs. 5-14 to 5-19). Fragments can be acute and sharply margin-ated or rounded when more chronic, of varying sizes, single or multiple, and with varying amounts of displacement. The location of these fragments, as represented by one of the author's (C.W.M.) publications reporting on 439 fetlock joints in 336 horses, is given in Tables 5-1 and 5-2. The typical fragment

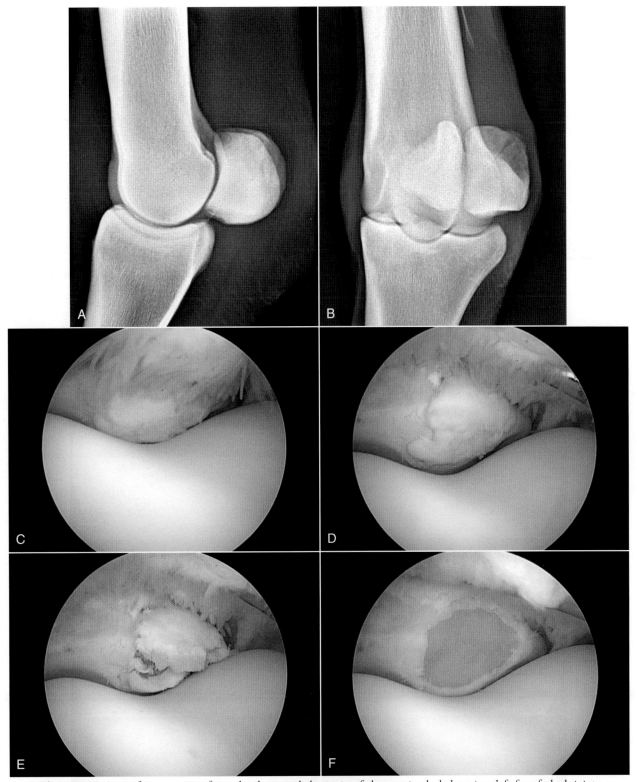

Figure 5-14 Acute fragmentation from the dorsomedial margin of the proximal phalanx in a left fore fetlock joint. **A,** Lateromedial and **B,** Dorsolateral-palmaromedial oblique radiographs of fresh fragment. **C,** Initial arthroscopic view of the fragmentation prior and **D,** after elevation of the joint capsule. **E,** Fragmentation after elevation. **F,** Site following fragment removal and debridement of defect.

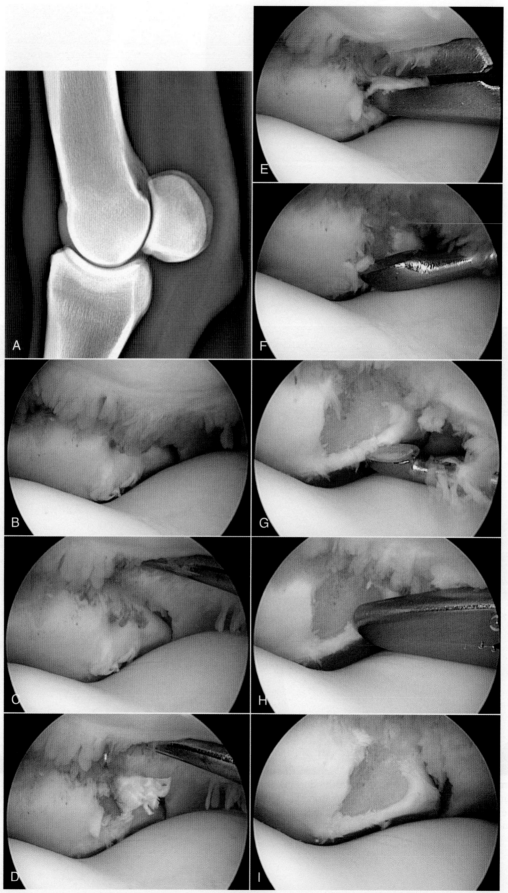

Figure 5-15 Small, acute fragment from the dorsomedial margin of the proximal phalanx in a left forelimb. **A,** Lateromedial radiograph. Arthroscopic views before **(B)** and after **(C)** elevation of joint capsule. **D,** Arthroscopic view of fragment after elevation. **E,** Removal of fragment with arthroscopic rongeurs. **F-G,** Curettage of fragment site. **H,** Removal of small remaining fragments and **I,** Appearance at end of surgery.

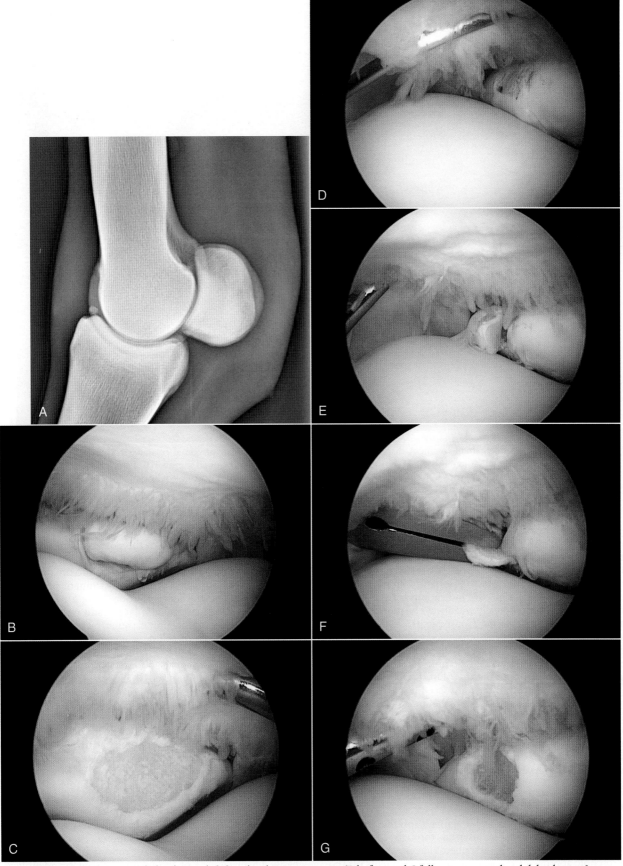

Figure 5-16 Lateromedial radiograph (**A**) and arthroscopic views (**B** before and **C** following removal and debridement) of chronic fragmentation of the proximal dorsomedial aspect of the proximal phalanx. **D,** Small fragment in another fetlock joint that was not detectable radiographically at initial diagnosis, **E,** after elevation, **F,** removal, **G,** after debridement of defect.

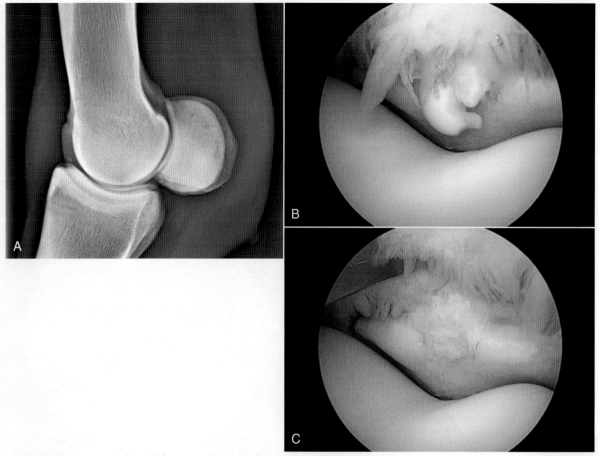

Figure 5-17 Rounded small fragment displaced from dorsomedial margin of proximal phalanx in right fore fetlock joint. **A,** Lateromedial radiograph. **B,** Arthroscopic appearance of fragment prior to removal. **C,** Parent bone following removal demonstrating mature fibrous tissue beneath the fragmentation, which was not debrided.

involves the proximal articular margin, but in some situations (more typical in the racing Quarter Horse), the fragments extend distad into fibrous joint capsule attachments (see Fig. 5-19). Large chip fractures appropriate for internal fixation are considered separately later. Most importantly, all fragments, if accompanied by clinical signs, are indications for surgery. The damage evident arthroscopically will always be more extensive than that seen on radiographs. Consequently, many referred cases are often ones with persistent evidence of synovitis and capsulitis (despite medical therapy) but with relatively minor fragmentation or with only a radiographic defect in the proximal phalanx (see Figs. 5-15 and 5-16D-G). Occasionally the fragment will be free within the joint (see Fig. 5-18). Uncommonly, the fragment is embedded in the dorsal joint capsule, and this may be difficult to ascertain from the radiographs. Sometimes the fragment can be recognized only as a roughening of the proximal phalanx. The neophyte arthroscopist should try initially to limit his or her cases to those involving fresh acute chips that are both loosely attached to the bone and accessible.

Technique

For all cases of dorsoproximal fragments of the proximal phalanx, the arthroscope is inserted through a proximal lateral portal as previously described. The instrument and arthroscopic approach for operating on chip fragments off the lateral and medial eminences, respectively, are represented diagrammatically in Figures 5-20 and 5-21. The authors recommend performing all arthroscopic surgery in the dorsal

pouch of the fetlock joint with the same arthroscopic portal in the proximal lateral aspect of the dorsal pouch. After a complete diagnostic arthroscopy, the osteochondral fragments are removed. If a fragment is present on the proximal lateral eminence, it is removed first. A lateral instrument portal is made after ascertaining the ideal position using a needle (see Fig. 5-6). The needle placement is lateral and midway down the distended portion of the joint capsule. If it is too proximal, the curved joint surfaces preclude adequate access to the palmar margins of lesions. After ascertaining the ideal position for the portal, a No. 11 blade is used to make a stab incision and the instruments are then inserted. If a medial fragment is present, a medial instrument portal is created after using a needle in the same fashion as laterally (see Figs. 5-7 and 5-22). If synovial pad fibrotic proliferation exists concomitantly, it can usually be removed through the same instrument portals.

As the instrument portal is created, the tip of the arthroscope must be located sufficiently proximad to avoid any damage to the arthroscope. By using the proximal arthroscopic portal, the arthroscope is rotated to angle down (distad) on to the lesion. The lesion is initially evaluated with a probe (or the egress cannula), as in the carpal joints. The arthroscopic manifestations of the fragments vary considerably and cannot usually be predicted from the radiographs. Fresh chips are usually attached only at the joint capsule reflection and can be moved easily. Displacement of the fragment facilitates identification and removal. Figure 5-15 illustrates the sequence of events in removing a small acute fragment, including elevation, removal with Ferris-Smith rongeurs, curetting of the defect, removal

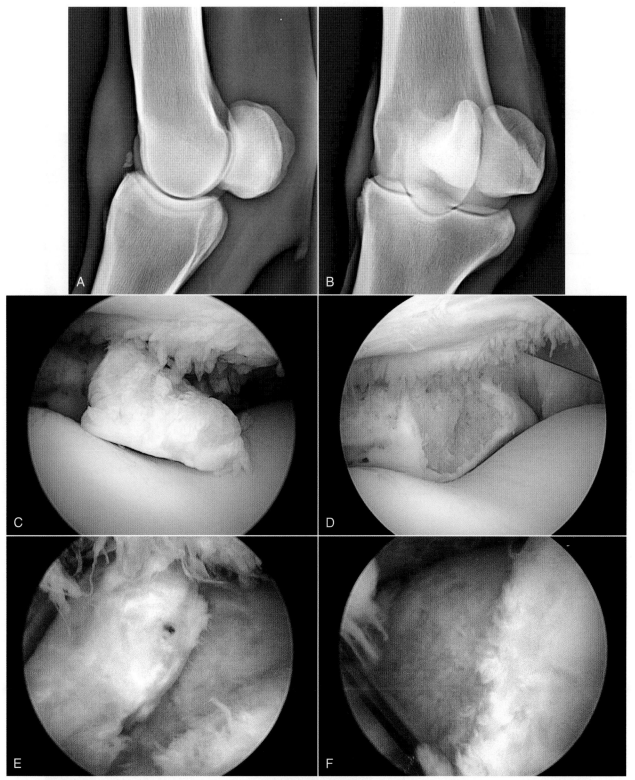

Figure 5-18 A large displaced chip fracture of the dorsomedial margin of the proximal phalanx in a left metacarpophalangeal joint. **A,** Lateromedial and **B,** Dorsolateral-palmaromedial oblique radiographs. Note capsular new bone associated with dorsal surface of the proximal phalanx. **C,** Large loose osteochondral fragment displaced to lie adjacent to medial condyle of the third metacarpal bone. **D,** Arthroscopic appearance following fragment removal and debridement of the fracture bed. **E** and **F,** Arthroscopic views of different case in which a free fragment has caused secondary articular cartilage damage on distal McIII.

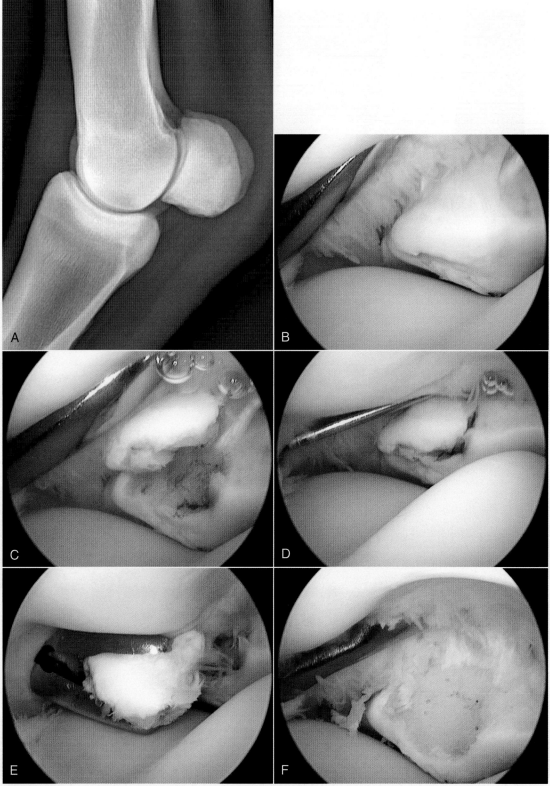

Figure 5-19 A Lateromedial radiograph and **B,** Arthroscopic appearance of a large dorsomedial fragment attached to the joint capsule. **C,** After elevation. **D,** Use of a sharp fixed blade knife to cut fibrous joint capsule attachments. **E,** During removal of fragment. **F,** After debridement of defect. This is more typical of the racing Quarter Horse.

Table • 5-1

Limbs and Sites of Osteochondral Fragmentation of the Dorsoproximal Aspect of the Proximal Phalanx in 336 Horses

FETLOCK JOINTS	PROXIMOMEDIAL	PROXIMOLATERAL	BOTH	TOTAL
Left fore	96	9	22	127
Right fore	65	6	22	93
Both fores	40	0	57	97
Left hind	2	1	0	3
Right hind	13	1	0	14
Both hinds	1	0	0	1
All four limbs	0	0	1	1
Total	217	17	102	336

From Kawcak CE, McIlwraith CW. Proximodorsal first phalanx osteochondral chip fragmentation in 336 horses. *Equine Vet J* 26:392–396,1994.

Table • 5-2

Incidence of Fetlock and Carpal Lesions

LESION	OVERALL (%)	RH (%)	TB RH (%)	QH RH (%)	OTHERS (%)
Fragments only	96 (28.6)	87 (28.0)	62 (33.0)	25 (21.0)	9 (36.0)
Fragments + other fetlock lesions	140 (41.7)	124 (39.9)	93 (22.7)	27 (22.7)	16 (64.0)
Fragment + carpal arthroscopy	63 (18.7)	63 (20.3)	19 (10.1)	44 (37.0)	—
Fragment + carpal arthroscopy + other fetlock lesions	37 (11.0)	37 (11.8)	14 (7.4)	23 (19.3)	—
Total	336	311	188	119	25

TB, Thoroughbred; *QH*, Quarter Horse, *RH*, racehorse.
From Kawcak CE, McIlwraith CW. Proximodorsal first phalanx osteochondral chip fragmentation in 336 horses. *Equine Vet J* 26:392–396,1994.

of small pieces with ethmoid forceps, and lavage. In other cases the cartilage over the fragment is intact and elevation is required to define the fragment. With larger fragments, the attachments of the fragment at the joint capsule may well be more extensive (see Fig. 5-19). With more chronic chips, the fragments tend to be rounded (see Figs. 5-16A-C and Fig 5-17). Some fragments have deep attachments in the joint capsule and require more separation (proximal Fig. 5-19). In some cases, the dorsoproximal rim of the first phalanx may only show a defect on lateromedial radiographs, but an oblique radiograph will show a small fragment. Occasionally, fragments are embedded in the joint capsule. This situation can be recognized if the fragment projects into the joint. Otherwise, such a density will probably not be found, and the final diagnosis of a capsular mass is based on the absence of a fragment on arthroscopic examination despite its presence on radiographs.

Most fragments are removed using Ferris-Smith arthroscopic rongeurs. Low-profile 4 × 10 mm Ferris-Smith rongeurs have the ideal combination of strength and ability to access the fragment. As in the carpus, the use of forceps that can enclose the fragment minimizes the risk of leaving fragments in the joint. Twisting of the instrument to ensure breakdown of soft tissue attachments is carried out before withdrawal of the fragment.

The surgical manipulations to remove the fragment will depend on the arthroscopic features described earlier. A 10-× 4-mm Ferris-Smith low-profile rongeur forceps is used to remove a totally free chip. If a fragment is small, fresh, and has minor soft tissue attachments as ascertained by manipulation, then direct removal with forceps is appropriate. For all chips with significant attachments, the fragment is initially freed by using an elevator. For chips that have a strong fibrous union, the elevator is used to pry the fragment off the bone. The elevator or a curette can be used to break down capsular

attachments to the dorsal aspect of the fragment but sharp dissection is less traumatic. Additionally, because of suspected sensitivity of the dorsoproximal area of the fetlock joint, the surgeon should limit debridement beyond the fibrous joint capsule (Fig. 5-23).

If a fracture line extends distad deep into the capsular attachment area and it is not displaced, then surgical removal is not indicated. Fixation with a small fragment screw is sometimes appropriate (see later).

After removal of the fragment, the defects remaining in the proximal phalanx and adjacent joint capsule are inspected (see Figs. 5-14 to Fig. 5-19) to ensure that no fragments remain. This latter inspection must involve palpation and visualization because the fragments can merge into the capsule. The defect commonly has some tags or raised edges of cartilage that can be removed with a pair of ethmoid or 2 × 10 mm Ferris-Smith rongeurs (the pointed nose enables these forceps to enter the narrow areas where the fragment was removed). Alternatively, a curette may be used. Debridement of the bone is done carefully with a small (2–0) curette taking care not to cause damage to the fibrous joint capsule (see Figs. 5-18 and 5-23).

Variable degrees of articular cartilage damage on the distal metacarpal or metatarsal condylar surfaces may be noted. In many cases no damage is apparent, but in others varying degrees of wearline formation (see Fig. 5-23C) and full-thickness erosions may be seen (see Fig. 5-23D). When these lesions are more severe, the prognosis is not as favorable (Kawcak & McIlwraith, 1994).

Unless a capsular mass projects into the joint, it is not removed. Also, it is not considered necessary or beneficial to then perform an arthrotomy to remove the mass. The benefit of arthroscopy in such a case has been to ascertain the location of the radiographically apparent mass. If the remainder

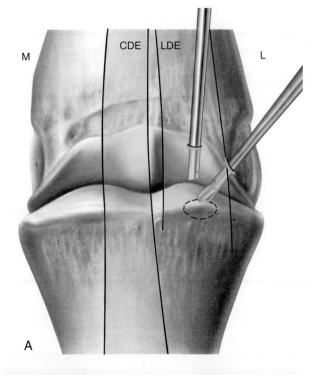

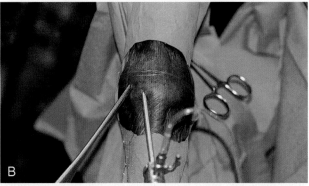

Figure 5-20 Diagram **(A)** and photograph **(B)** of the positioning of the arthroscope and instrument during operations involving a chip fracture off the lateral eminence of the proximal phalanx.

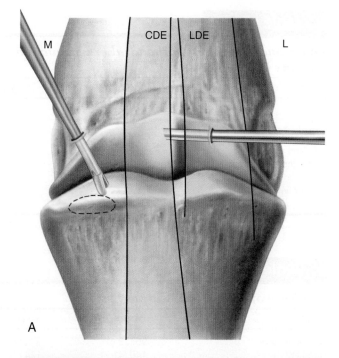

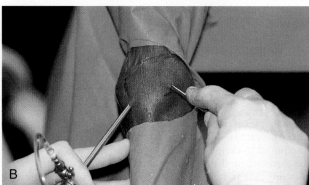

Figure 5-21 Diagram **(A)** and photograph **(B)** of the positioning of the arthroscope and instrument during operations involving a chip fracture off the dorsomedial eminence of the proximal phalanx.

of the joint is in satisfactory condition, then a mineralized mass remaining in the joint capsule may not adversely affect prognosis.

As in the carpus, the size or number of fragments that can be removed is limitless, but that fact does not mean that every patient should undergo surgery. The surgeon must consider the amount of subchondral bone being removed, the amount of cancellous bone exposed in the joint, and the amount of capsular trauma caused by fragment isolation and removal.

At the end of the surgery, the joint is flushed with fluid by moving an open egress cannula around the whole dorsal compartment. The skin portals are sutured and the leg is bandaged. The bandages are maintained for at least 2 weeks after surgery. Hand walking commences after 1 week. With simple acute fragments, the horses can be put into training after 6 to 8 weeks. For horses with more extensive involvement, the convalescence time is increased for a variable period up to 6 months. Specific postoperative recommendations are discussed in Chapter 17 including intraarticular medication, but some veterinarians favor its use. As discussed in Chapter 4, the most important factor to the patient's recovery is removing the fragment.

Results

The results with arthroscopic surgery for uncomplicated cases of proximal phalangeal fragmentation have been excellent. If fractures are associated with severe capsulitis, wear lines, osteoarthritis, or extensive fragmentation of the proximal first phalanx, the prognosis decreases accordingly. As with the carpus, surgical intervention can still improve the status of these patients, but communication to owner and trainer is important to ensure that no one is disappointed.

The results of arthroscopic surgery in 74 fetlock joints of 63 horses (35 Thoroughbreds and 28 Quarter Horses) over a 2-year period were initially reported by Yovich & McIlwraith (1986). Larger numbers have replaced these data. The results of arthroscopic surgery were reported in 1994 in 336 horses with 572 osteochondral fragments removed from 439 fetlock joints (Kawcak & McIlwraith, 1994). Of these horses, 311 were racehorses, including 188 Thoroughbreds, 119 Quarter Horses, 2 Standardbreds, 1 racing Arabian, and 1 racing Appaloosa. There were 25 nonracehorses. A single metacarpophalangeal joint was operated on in 220 horses, and both metacarpophalangeal joints were operated on in 97 horses, a single metatarsophalangeal joint in 17 horses, both metatarsophalangeal joints in one horse, and all 4 fetlock joints in 1 horse.

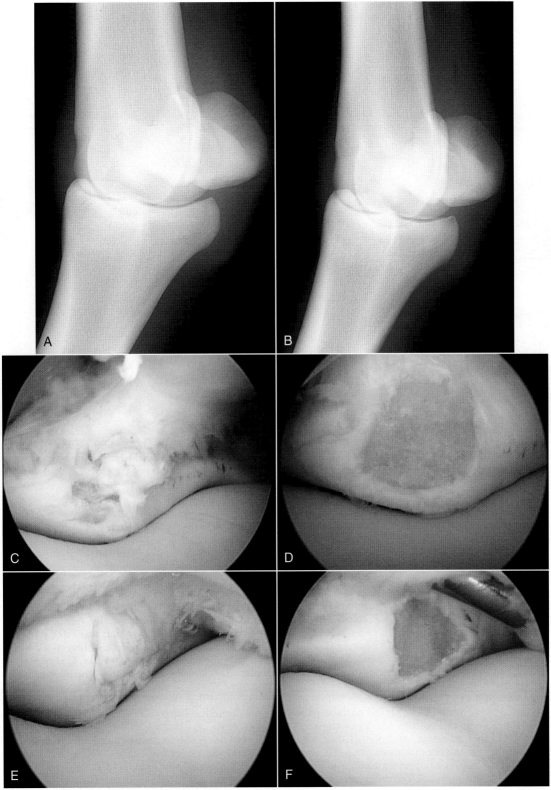

Figure 5-22 Oblique radiographs showing normal lateral eminence **(A)**, a fragment of the medial eminence **(B)**, and arthroscopic views of the same joint with a fragment on lateral eminence before **(C)** and after **(D)** removal; proximal medial fragment before **(E)** and after **(F)** removal and debridement.

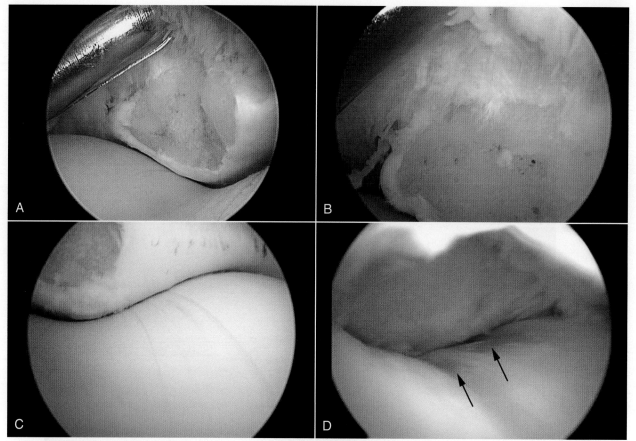

Figure 5-23 A and **B,** Arthroscopic views of defects after debridement. The junction of the fibrous joint capsule and bone can be visualized, and debridement of bone should not extend beyond this. **C,** Wear lines associated with proximal lateral and proximal medial proximal phalanx fragmentation and **D,** erosions *(arrows)* of the articular cartilage of the distal McIII in association with proximal dorsal phalanx fragmentation.

Fragmentation of the proximal phalanx was the only lesion in the fetlock joints of 96 horses. Along with fragmentation, 140 horses had other lesions in the fetlock, comprising 64 with wear lines, 11 with articular cartilage erosion, 15 with chronic proliferative synovitis, 4 with osteochondritis dissecans, and 45 with a combination of the previously mentioned lesions. Carpal arthroscopy for the removal of osteochondral chips was performed concomitantly in 100 horses (Table 5-2).

Follow-up was available for 286 horses (85.1%): 208 (73%) returned to their previous use, of which 153 horses (73.6%) returned to the same level of performance and 55 (26.4%) returned to work, but at a lower class; 18 horses (6.3%) developed another fragment and 60 (21%) horses did not return to their previous use. Of the 270 racehorses with follow-up, 196 (72%) returned to racing and 141 (51.7%) of these raced at the same or a higher level. Eighteen (6.6%) of the racehorses developed another fragment, and 56 (21.0%) were in the failure category. Of the nonracehorse group, 12 of 16 (75%) returned and 4 (25%) did not return to their previous use at the same level of performance. The difference of return to previous use between racehorses and nonracehorses was not significant. The overall success rate in horses with fragments only returning to use was 85.9%; with fragments and other fetlock lesions it was 75%; with fetlock fragments and concomitant carpal arthroscopy it was 68.6%; and with fragments plus carpal arthroscopy and other fetlock lesions it was 80.6%.

In a third study done to examine the longevity of postoperative careers and quality of performance of 461 Thoroughbred racehorses after arthroscopic removal of dorsoproximal osteochondral fragments from the proximal phalanx, 659 chip fragments were removed from 574 joints (Colon et al, 2000). It was found that 89% of the horses (411/461) raced after surgery and 82% (377/461) did so at the same or a higher class; 68% of the horses raced in a stakes or allowance race postoperatively.

Horses that raced before and after surgery (258) had an average of 8.4 starts (median = 6) before surgery and 13 (median = 11) after surgery. The average time between surgery and first postoperative start was 189 days (median = 169); 87% of the horses racing before surgery (224/258) returned to race at the same or higher class. The average earnings per start after surgery was less than the average earnings before surgery in 61% of these horses and greater in 32%. This paper confirmed that the quantity and quality of performance was not diminished after arthroscopic treatment of dorsoproximal fragments, and that surgical removal of a chip fragment preserved the economic value of a racing Thoroughbred, allowing a rapid and successful return to racing at the previous level of performance (Colon et al, 2000).

Colon et al (2000) considered the 11% postoperative failure rate to be due to various factors. It was noted that horses that did not race after surgery tended to be older at the time of surgery and had raced more times preoperatively. They concluded that the lack of return to racing was not related to chip incidence, location, or size because these did not differ between the raced and unraced group. They carefully measured fragment size and concluded that it did not affect postsurgical racing prognosis: 48% of the surveyed horses had at least one fragment larger than the mean and 87% of these raced after surgery. They concluded that the hypothesis that

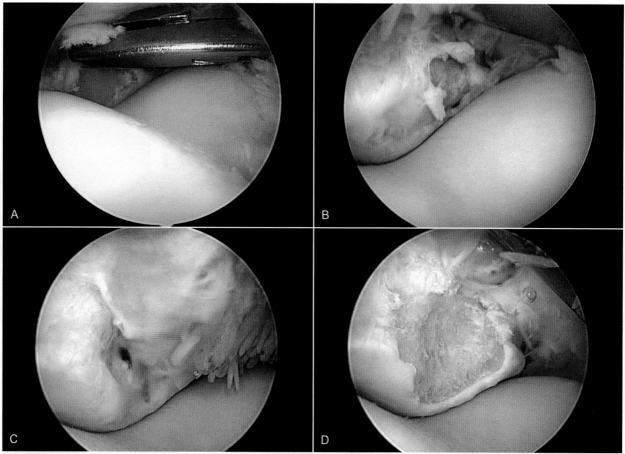

Figure 5-24 Arthroscopic view of articular cartilage separation **(A)**, articular cartilage erosion **(B)**, and subchondral bone disease before **(C)** and after **(D)** debridement on the proximal dorsomedial eminence of the proximal phalanx.

"the smaller the chip fragment, the better the prognosis" was rejected by these findings. The authors noted that it was not possible, in their study, to compare postoperative racing performance with arthroscopic assessment of articular cartilage health or associated intraarticular lesions but pointed out, appropriately, that articular cartilage damage is usually not severe and can be managed medically.

Arthroscopic Removal of Dorsoproximal Chip Fractures of the Proximal Phalanx in Standing Horses

This technique has been described and reported in 104 horses (Elce & Richardson, 2002). With skilled technique and in appropriate circumstances, it is feasible to perform arthroscopic surgery in the dorsal aspect of the fetlock in this fashion. However, the authors only recommend it if, for some reason, general anesthesia is not possible or cannot be undertaken with reasonable safety. Throughout this textbook, the authors recommend surgery under general anesthesia to optimize intraarticular evaluation and surgery with due regard to (morbidity and mortality) risks versus benefits on an individual case basis.

Erosions of Articular Cartilage and Subchondral Bone Disease on the Dorsal Margin of the Proximal Phalanx

As seen at sites in the carpus, there is a spectrum of disease on the dorsoproximal margin of the proximal phalanx ranging from separation and/or loss of articular cartilage, to degenerative disease of the subchondral bone. Previously discussed osteochondral fragments are considered to be pathologic fractures and are the end result of a gradation of microdamage,

microfractures, and cellular death (Kawcak et al, 2000). This range of lesions occurs in the same locations as previously described for osteochondral fragments, and the surgical management is the same.

The referring clinical signs are also similar, but radiographically there may only be a suspicion of disease. However, on arthroscopic examination, the various manifestations of articular cartilage separation (Fig. 5-24A), articular cartilage erosion (Fig. 5-24B), and subchondral bone disease (Fig. 5-24C and D) are encountered. Separated cartilage and bone are removed. Defective bone is debrided (larger pieces removed), and the joint lavaged. The resultant articular defects are often of a similar area, and the prognosis is comparable with completely separated osteochondral fragments in this area.

Treatment of Frontal Fractures of Dorsal Margin of the Proximal Phalanx Using Lag Screw Fixation

Frontal fractures of the dorsal aspect of the proximal phalanx occur regularly. The clinical signs are similar to other osteochondral fragments on the proximal dorsal rim, and radiographs are used to make the definitive diagnosis (Fig. 5-25). The authors have encountered cases in the hindlimbs bilaterally and, because of the consistent location of these fractures involving both the proximal medial eminence and sagittal groove, a developmental predisposition may be present.

Although some of these fractures can heal (McIlwraith, 1990a), others that did not heal and continued to cause clinical signs have been encountered. The recommendation now is to provide compression of these fractures with 2.7-mm AO/ASIF cortical screws.

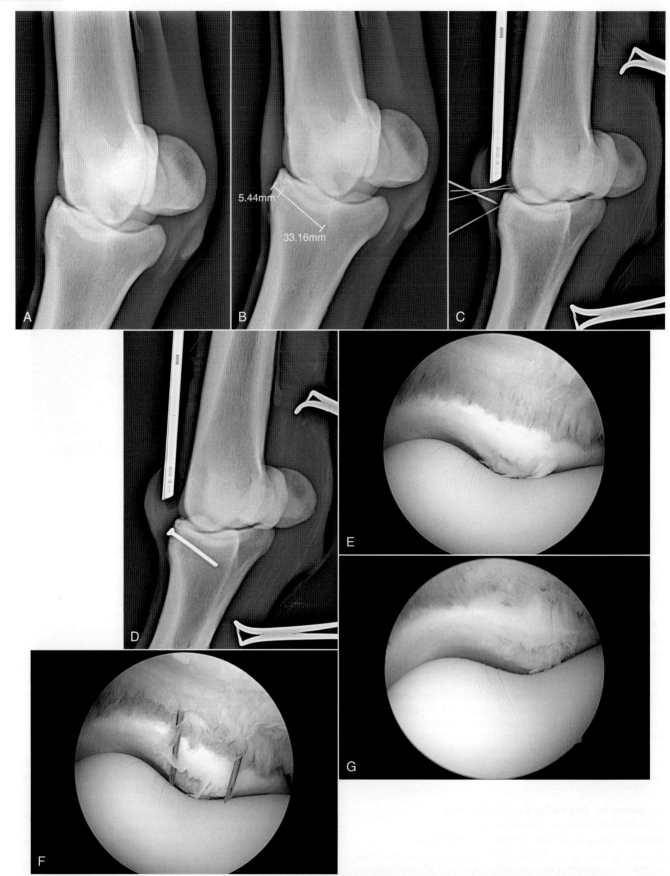

Figure 5-25 Radiographs of large nondisplaced fracture of the dorsal margin of the proximal phalanx. **A** and **B,** Preoperative radiographs with measurements for screw length in **B. C** and **D,** Intraoperative radiographs. **E,** Arthroscopic view of fracture. **F,** Needles placed on either side of fracture. **G,** Postoperative view after internal fixation.

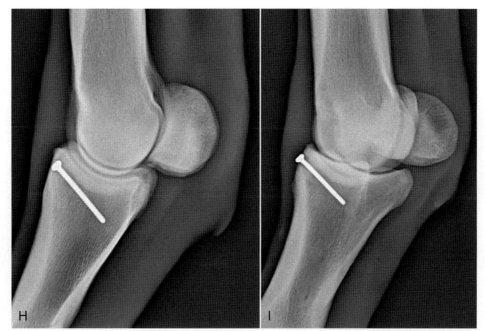

Figure 5-25, cont'd H and **I,** Radiographic appearance 3 months postsurgery.

Arthroscopic surgery is performed with the normal approach to the dorsal pouch and with the limb(s) in extension. Examination of the joint will confirm the presence of the fracture (see Fig. 5-25). Needles are placed to ascertain ideal positioning of the screw and, after a stab incision is made in the appropriate location, a 2.7-mm hole is drilled obliquely down through the fracture fragment. The hole is generally perpendicular to the fracture line. Radiographs are made to confirm appropriate positioning and that the glide hole is beyond the fracture line. A 2-mm hole is continued beyond this. After countersinking, a 2.7-mm diameter, 36-mm long cortical bone screw is inserted to compress the fracture. If appropriate, debridement is then performed in the fracture line. The manifestations at the fracture site will vary, and sometimes no tissue needs to be removed (see Fig. 5-25); other times, debridement in a comparable fashion to a carpal slab fracture is required.

▶ Treatment of Synovial Pad Fibrotic Proliferation (Villonodular Synovitis)

The condition initially designated as villonodular synovitis (Nickels et al, 1976) and later described as chronic proliferative synovitis (van Veenendaal & Moffatt, 1980; Kannegieter, 1990) is seen in the metacarpophalangeal joint. It involves a proliferative response from the synovial pad (plica) in the proximal dorsal aspect of the joint and, therefore, the term *synovial pad fibrotic proliferation* (Dabereiner et al, 1996) is preferred.

The term *pigmented villonodular synovitis* was originally used to describe pedunculated growths forming in the synovial linings of tendon sheaths and joints in man (Jaffe et al, 1941). These fibrous masses were polyp-like formations that originated from the synovial membrane and were often pigmented with hemosiderin. Villonodular synovitis in humans, therefore, should not be confused with enlargement of the synovial pads of the equine metacarpophalangeal joint.

Originally the condition was demonstrated with contrast arthrography and treated with arthrotomy (Nickels et al, 1976; Haynes, 1980). Neither contrast arthrography nor arthrotomy are used anymore because of the development of ultrasound examination in diagnosis (Steyn et al, 1989) and arthroscopic surgery for treatment.

The synovial pad of the metacarpophalangeal (and metatarsophalangeal) joint is a fold (plica) of fibrous connective tissue located in the proximal recess of the dorsal compartment at the joint capsule attachment to McIII. The synovial pad is normally 1 to 2 mm in thickness medially and laterally with a thinner midline isthmus adjacent to the sagittal ridge of McIII. It tapers to a thin edge at its distal border, which aligns with commencement of the articular cartilage on the McIII condyles. Proximal to this, beneath the palmar surface of the plica, the McIII is covered by thin and frequently rather irregular periosteum. Its function is unknown, but it has been suggested that the pad acts as a contact interface or cushion between the dorsal rim of the proximal phalanx and distal McIII during full extension of the fetlock joint (White, 1990; Dabareiner et al, 1996). Repetitive trauma during fast exercise can result in irritation and enlargement of the synovial pad and development of clinical signs of lameness and chronic joint effusion that often resolves temporarily with rest and intraarticular medication. There is commonly radiographic evidence of bone remodeling, with a concavity at the distal dorsal aspect of McIII, and this is suggestive of synovial pad proliferation (Figs. 5-26A and 5-28A). Ultrasound is now the method of choice to identify and further define the soft tissue changes (Steyn et al, 1989) (Figs. 5-26B and 5-28B). Although this condition is commonly seen in the racehorse, it has been seen in other horses not subjected to fast athletic exercise (LoSasso & Honnas, 1994).

The medical records, radiographs, and ultrasound examinations have been reported in 63 horses with metacarpophalangeal joint synovial pad proliferation (Dabareiner et al, 1996). All the horses had lameness, joint effusion, or both of these clinical signs, associated with one or both metacarpophalangeal joints. Bony remodeling and concavity of the distal dorsal aspect of McIII immediately proximal to the metacarpal condyles was identified by radiography in 71 joints (93%); 24 joints (32%) had radiographic evidence of a chip fragment from the dorsal margin of the proximal phalanx. Fifty-four joints (71%) were examined by ultrasound. The mean ± SD sagittal thickness of the synovial pad was 11.3 ± 2.8 mm. (The authors also reported that the synovial pad was considered abnormal if the thickness was greater than 4 mm on the sagittal view,

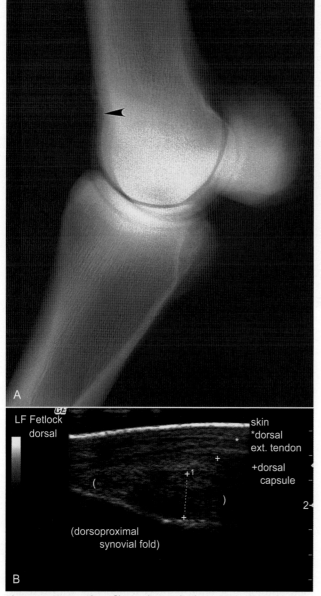

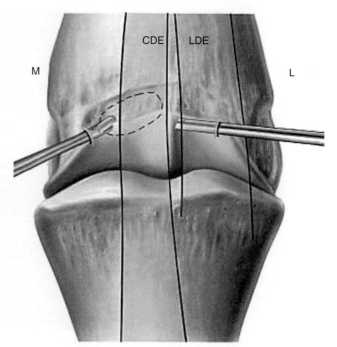

Figure 5-27 Diagram of positioning of arthroscope and instrument to remove synovial pad fibrotic proliferation by a single instrument approach.

Figure 5-26 A, Plain film radiograph showing an irregular concave defect *(arrowhead)* with capsular new bone adjacent. **B,** Ultrasound image of synovial pad fibrotic proliferation. *(Courtesy Dr. Wade Byrd.)*

the distal margin was rounded, or hypoechoic regions were observed within the pad.) Seventy-nine percent of the horses had single joint involvement, with equal distribution between the right and left forelimbs. In addition to presurgical diagnosis of this condition, it is also quite common to encounter thickened and enlarged synovial pads at arthroscopic surgery (usually for removal of dorsal fragments from the proximal phalanx) (McIlwraith, 2002).

The surgical approach used when operating on horses with this condition arthroscopically is illustrated in Figure 5-27. The authors in most cases use a single instrument approach. A two-instrument approach has also been described (McIlwraith, 1990a, 2002). With the arthroscope in the lateral portal, the instrument portal is made medially. Dabareiner et al (1996) considered excision of a portion of the synovial pad to be necessary if it was enlarged and inelastic when probed during surgery or if hard nodules could be felt within the pad. The mass can sometimes be torn off by using grasping forceps that have

a cutting edge. Alternatively, and more commonly, the mass is severed at its base by using a flat knife or arthroscopic scissors (see Chapter 2). Disposable scalpel blades should not be used because they may break within the joint. After severing the base, the proliferated pad is removed with Ferris-Smith rongeurs (see Fig. 5-28D) and the base trimmed with basket forceps or a motorized resector. Proliferation of the synovial pad is more common medially than laterally and, consequently, surgery often involves removal of the medial portion alone. However, examination should be made to ensure that there is not similar proliferation of the lateral portion. If there is, then portals are interchanged so that the arthroscope is placed medially and instruments are placed laterally to remove the lateral portion. In one report in the literature, complete or partial excision of both medial and lateral synovial pads was achieved in 42/68 joints (Dabareiner et al, 1996). The medial synovial pad only was excised or trimmed in 21 joints, and 5 joints had removal limited to the lateral pad.

Once the pad is removed, there may be some full-thickness erosion with minor debris where debridement is indicated. More commonly, the bone is left alone (see Fig. 5-28E), but if there are any elevated cartilage tags, these are trimmed. As has been previously noted, enlarged, thickened pads will sometimes be noted when the indication for arthroscopic surgery was originally the removal of fragments. Conversely, fragments from the dorsal margin of the proximal phalanx may be encountered at the time of arthroscopic surgery for removal of a proliferated pad when the fragments were not visible on presurgical radiographs. This emphasizes the importance of a complete examination of the dorsal pouch at the commencement of all arthroscopic procedures so that lesions can be appropriately dealt with.

In a report of 68 joints in 55 horses treated by arthroscopic surgery, 60 joints (88%) had debridement of chondral or osteochondral fragmentation from the dorsal surface of the distal McIII beneath the synovial pad (more frequently done than by the authors) and 30 joints (44%) had fragments removed from the dorsal margin of the proximal phalanx (Dabareiner et al, 1996).

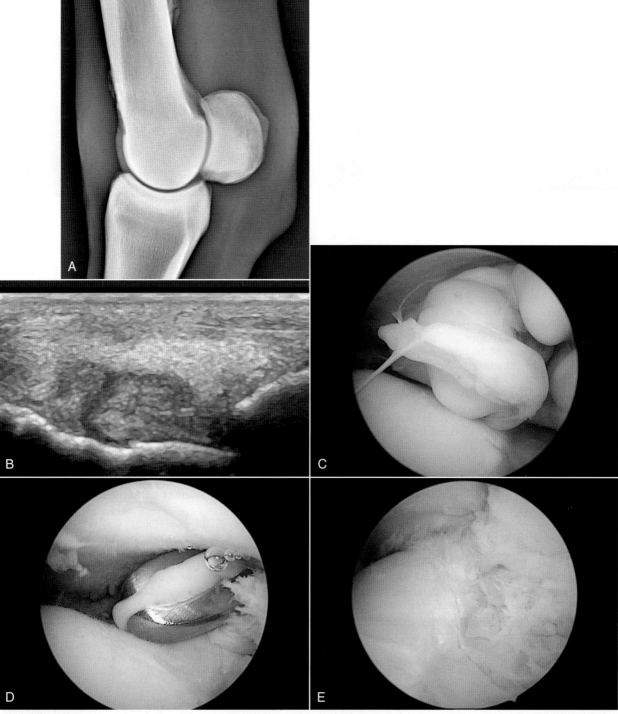

Figure 5-28 Arthroscopic removal of proliferative fibrotic synovial pad **A,** Lateromedial radiograph demonstrating irregular new bone on the dorsodistal surface of the third metacarpal bone with an irregular zone of bone loss between this and the sagittal ridge/dorsal condyles of the third metacarpal bone. **B,** Longitudinally oriented ultrasonograph demonstrating a large mass of echogenic material filling the dorsal compartment of the joint. **C,** Marked proliferation of the dorsal plica obscuring the entire dorsomedial portion of the joint. **D,** Removal of portions of the proliferative dorsal plica with arthroscopic rongeurs. **E,** Site of resection of the dorsal plica proximal to the medial condyle of the third metacarpal bone.

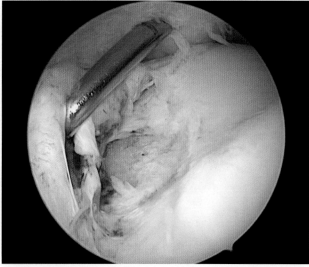

Figure 5-29 Acute tearing/avulsion of synovial plica in a right metacarpophalangeal joint. The arthroscopic probe is in the tear.

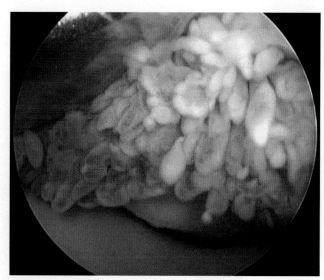

Figure 5-30 Proliferated synovial membrane in the dorsal pouch of a fetlock that was treated with synovectomy.

Postoperative management in cases involving proliferative synovitis treated arthroscopically is similar to those with fragmentation of the proximal phalanx. Horses that have synovial pad proliferation without articular cartilage loss or proximal phalangeal fragments can return to racing in 8 weeks, whereas horses with more extensive cartilage damage or more significant dorsal fragmentation of the proximal phalanx should get 3 to 4 months before training is resumed.

Follow-up on 50/55 horses was reported by Dabareiner et al (1996): 43 (86%) horses returned to racing, with 34 (68%) racing at an equivalent or better level than before surgery. Horses that returned to racing, at a similar or equal level of performance, were significantly younger than horses returning at a lower level or not racing. Eight horses (8 joints) with synovial pad proliferation and remodeling of the distal dorsal aspect of McIII were treated medically with intraarticular hyaluronan and systemic nonsteroidal antiinflammatory medication. Three (38%) of these horses returned to racing, and only 1 horse raced better than the preinjury level.

Arthroscopically guided CO_2 or an Nd:YAG laser extirpation of metacarpophalangeal synovial pad proliferation has been described in 11 horses (Murphy and Nixon, 2001). Mean synovial pad thickness, measured ultrasonographically, was 9 mm, and 7 (64%) of the horses had radiographic evidence of remodeling of the dorsal cortex of distal McIII; 3 horses (27%) had concurrent dorsal fragmentation of the proximal phalanx. All 11 horses returned to training within 90 days of surgery without recurrence of the lesion. Nine horses (82%) sustained race training and apparently improved their performance following surgery. The use of the CO_2 laser requires gas distension of the joint. The authors cited advantages with the laser technique that included the ability to be used arthroscopically, better visualization of the joint, better access to lesions on both sides of the sagittal ridge, reduced convalescence time, and better cosmetic and functional results. However, with current (conventional) arthroscopic techniques, it is questionable if these advantages exist anymore.

Acute Tearing/Avulsion of the Dorsal Synovial Plica

Acute tearing/avulsion of the dorsal synovial plica from its attachment to the third metacarpal bone has been seen at diagnostic arthroscopy (Fig. 5-29). When this is found it should be treated with appropriate resection of the torn portion.

Treatment of Other Forms of Proliferative Synovitis

Occasionally, forms of proliferative synovitis that are not localized to the dorsoproximal aspect of the joint are seen (see Chapter 3). Typically, these cases present as chronic synovitis and capsulitis that is nonresponsive to symptomatic intraarticular or systemic antiinflammatory treatments. In some cases, diagnostic arthroscopy has revealed proliferated, thickened, and enlarged synovial villi in the dorsal compartment of the metacarpophalangeal joint (Fig. 5-30). The treatment has been resection of these villi and, in the limited case numbers available, overall results have been good.

▶ Treatment of Osteochondritis Dissecans of the Dorsal Aspect of McIII/MtIII

There is a divergence of opinion as to what is considered osteochondritis dissecans (OCD) within the fetlock joint and also those entities that might be considered to be appropriate to include in the term *developmental orthopedic disease* (McIlwraith, 1993). However, it is generally agreed that osteochondral defects of the dorsal aspect of the distal McIII and MtIII are manifestations of OCD; this is the condition described later. The lesion was initially described as OCD of the sagittal ridge of the third McIII/MtIII (Yovich et al, 1985), but this term has been modified after recognition that the disease process commonly extends onto the condyles of the bones (McIlwraith & Vorhees, 1990). In one radiographic study, OCD changes on the dorsal aspect of the sagittal ridge of McIII or MtIII were seen in 118/753 yearling Standardbred trotters with 61 forelimbs and 147 hindlimbs affected (Groendahl, 1992).

Fragments from the proximal palmar/plantar margin of the proximal phalanx have also been reported as osteochondrosis (Foerner, 1987; Nixon, 1990), but it is not now generally accepted that osteochondrosis is the pathogenesis. The treatment of this condition is described later in this chapter.

The third condition described as OCD is proximal dorsal fragments of the proximal phalanx in young horses. Although most of these fragments, at least in racehorses in training, are the result of work-related trauma or failure of adaptation, there is evidence that some fragments have an osteochondrosis

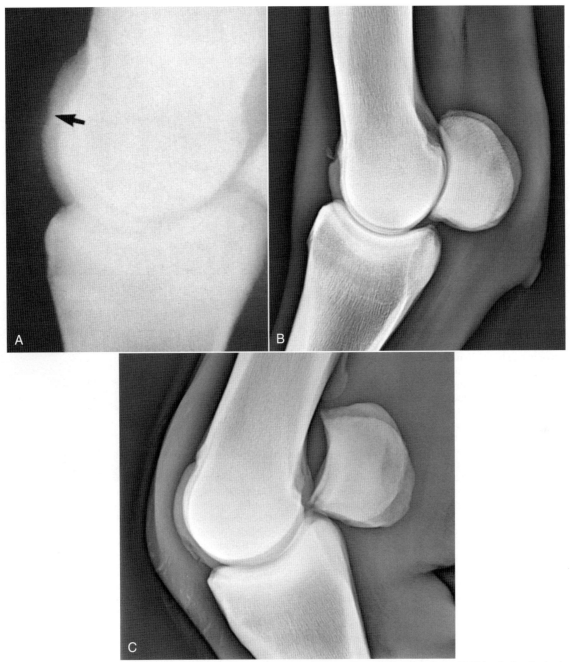

Figure 5-31 Examples of the radiographic appearance of osteochondritis dissecans (OCD) of the fetlock joint. **A,** Type I OCD of the midsagittal ridge of the metacarpophalangeal joint. **B,** Type II OCD on the proximal aspect of the dorsal sagittal ridge of the third metacarpal bone. **C,** Type II OCD of the distal sagittal ride of the third metacarpal bone.

basis, at least when they present in yearlings. Such fragments were diagnosed in 36 (4.8%) of 753 yearling Standardbred trotters on a radiographic survey (Groendahl, 1992) and were seen in 34 forelimbs and 14 hindlimbs.

A fourth condition initially described as OCD of the palmar metacarpus (Hornoff et al, 1981) is now accepted to be a traumatic entity, not part of the syndrome of osteochondrosis, and is not considered further here.

OCD of the distal dorsal aspect of the McIII/MtIII can occur in both metacarpophalangeal and metatarsophalangeal joints, but it is more common in the latter. The lesions vary in their radiographic manifestations, from a subchondral concavity to defects associated with fragments (Fig. 5-31). In some cases, fragments break away completely from the primary lesion and become loose bodies. The presenting clinical signs include synovial effusion of the fetlock joint with or without lameness. The horses are usually yearlings (Yovich et al, 1986). In most instances, the patients are weanlings to yearlings and quite often are presented for treatment before sale. In some instances, training and racing may have occurred before the symptoms develop. Although the degree of lameness varies, a positive response to a fetlock flexion test is usually elicited and radiographs confirm the presence of lesions associated primarily with the sagittal ridge of McIII/MtIII.

For purposes of treatment decisions and prognosis, the lesions have been divided into three types:

- Type I is that in which a defect or flattening is the only visible radiographic lesion.
- Type II is that in which fragmentation is associated with the defect.
- Type III is that in which there is a defect or flattening with or without fragmentation plus one or more loose bodies.

Oblique radiographs should be taken, as well as dorsopalmar (plantar) and lateromedial radiographs for the purpose of discerning the medial or lateral condyles of McIII/MtIII (McIlwraith & Vorhees, 1990). On the basis of an initial study (Yovich et al, 1985), it was believed that type II and type III OCD lesions should be treated surgically and many type I lesions would resolve. In a second study of 15 cases with type I lesions that were treated conservatively, 12 resolved clinically and 8 of these showed remodeling of the lesions with improvement on radiographic examination (McIlwraith & Vorhees, 1990). In 3 cases the clinical signs persisted: In 2 of these, the radiographs showed no change and the horses eventually underwent surgery, whereas, in the other case, the clinical and radiographic signs progressed and the horse was not operated on.

In eight cases of type II lesions where owners requested conservative management, two eventually underwent surgery because of the persistent clinical signs. Clinical signs persisted in five others, but surgery was not performed. The clinical signs improved in only one horse. In most of these cases where clinical signs persisted, the fragmentation also progressed radiographically. It was also clear in this study that clinical signs of effusion may appear before definitive radiographic changes. Progression of some type I lesions was noted: Such cases do not develop osseous fragmentation, but the lesions progress to become larger defects, particularly on the condyles (seen on oblique view radiographs). Some cases of type II lesions improved radiographically. These were generally cases with small fragments that fused to the parent-bone such that a spur resulted.

On the basis of the previously described findings, arthroscopic surgery is considered the appropriate treatment if fragments are present (type II and III lesions). In other cases in which a defect only is detectable radiographically, the decision for surgery is based on the degree of clinical signs, size and location of the defect, and planned use of the horse.

The arthroscopic approach is the same as that for fragments off the proximodorsal aspect of the proximal phalanx or synovial pad proliferation, using a proximally or distally placed instrument portal, depending on the location of the fragment or loose body (Fig. 5-32). When operating on metatarsophalangeal joints, an effort must be made to achieve complete extension. In some cases, the OCD lesion manifests as a defect within the sagittal ridge (Fig. 5-33) and curettage is performed. More commonly, osteochondral fragments may be within the defect or have loose attachments to the area (see Figs. 5-33 to 5-34). These fragments can be in the proximal aspect of the sagittal ridge (see Fig. 5-33A), central in the sagittal ridge, or distal in the sagittal ridge (Fig. 5-34). In all cases, the fragments are removed and any defective articular cartilage is debrided (Figs. 5-34 and 5-35). Loose fragments are located and removed (usually with Ferris-Smith rongeurs). When undermined cartilage extends medially and/or laterally from the sagittal ridge of McIII and MtIII, it is also debrided. OCD can also occur on the metacarpal or metatarsal condyles above. Type III lesions are treated with fragment removal and debridement (see Fig. 5-35).

Osteochondritis dissecans lesions can also be found distally in the sagittal ridge of McIII or MtIII, although these are most common in the former. Lesions are most readily identified in flexed lateromedial radiographs (see Fig. 5-31C) and also in dorsopalmar projections (see Fig. 5-34). Their distal location usually precludes recognition in standing (extended) lateromedial radiographs. In dorsopalmar projections lesions can be confused with subchondral bone cysts but are differentiated by their appearance

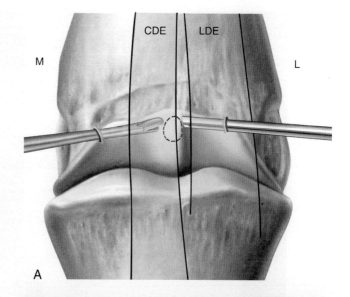

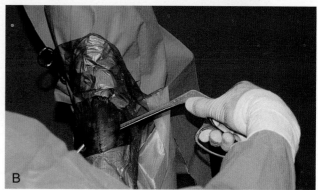

Figure 5-32 A, Diagram of positioning of arthroscope and instrument to operate on an osteochondritis dissecan (OCD) lesion of the proximal sagittal ridge of McIII; M, medial; L, lateral; CDE, common digital extensor tendon; LDE lateral digital extensor tendon. **B,** External view of the technique in a hindlimb.

in flexed lateromedial views. Lesions may be accompanied by fragmentation or can be predominantly of osteolytic nature.

Lesions are accessed by arthroscopy of the dorsal compartment of the joint but require a modified technique (see Fig. 5-34). The initial arthroscopic portal should be made just distal to the proximodistal midpoint when the dorsal outpouching of the joint is maximally distended. The arthroscopic cannula with the conical obturator in situ is then inserted cautiously to avoid impacting on and causing iatrogenic damage to the sagittal ridge of McIII. Once the arthroscope has been inserted, the joint is flexed in order to bring into view the distal portion of the sagittal ridge of McIII. Lesion morphology is similar to that seen in other sites of OCD and can vary from crevices in the articular cartilage overlying defective subchondral bone to frank subchondral fragmentation. The site for an appropriate instrument portal is made with percutaneous needle guidance as described previously. The portal site is generally further axial than appropriate for other lesions and usually involves penetration of the common digital extensor tendon. This does not appear to be of clinical consequence. Attached fragments and affected osteochondral tissues are removed and lesions debrided in the conventional manner. At the end of these procedures, the surgeon should lavage both dorsal and palmar compartments of the joint because debrided debris can be shed on both sides of the joint.

In a series of 42 horses that were operated on with arthroscopic surgery, there were few type I lesions (usually operated on because they had not responded to conservative treatment or if an individual horse being treated for a type II

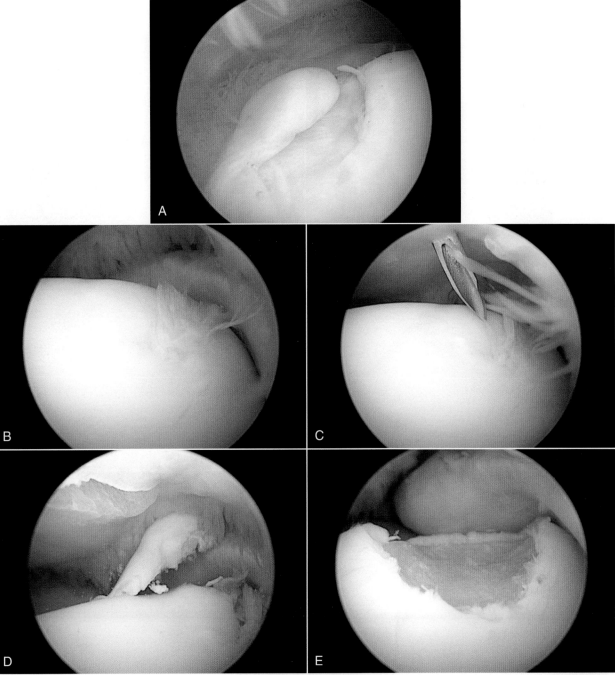

Figure 5-33 Arthroscopic views of type II OCD fragments. **A,** depicted radiographically in Figure 5-31B) of the proximal aspect of the sagittal ridge of the McIII and B-D, OCD of the aspect of the sagittal ridge of McIII (case depicted radiographically in Figure 5-31C. **B,** Arthroscopic appearance of the lesion with the joint in a flexed position. Tufts of fibrillated cartilage protrude from a punctate subchondral defect. The dorsal contour of the sagittal ridge is distorted over the lesion. **C,** Determination of a suitable instrument portal with a needle passed close to the midline through the common digital extensor tendon. **D,** Elevation of the fragment before removal. **E,** Lesion following fragment removal and completion of debridement.

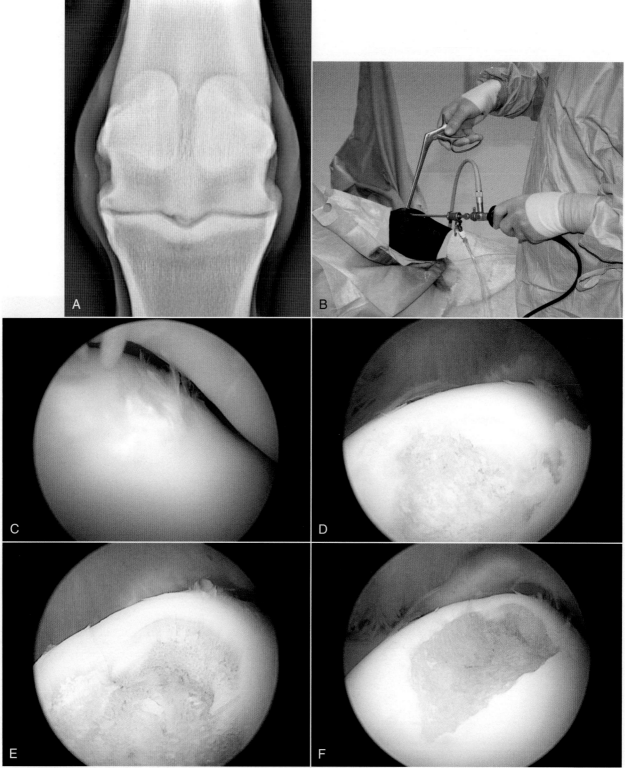

Figure 5-34 Osteochondritis dissecans of the distal sagittal ridge of McIII. A, Dorsopalmar radiographic projection demonstrating fragmentation of the distal margin of the sagittal ridge. There is also remodeling of the abaxial margins of both condyles **(B).** Arthroscopic surgery with the joint in flexion, the arthroscope in the central one third of the dorsal outpouching and a vertical instrument portal being necessary to access the lesion. **C,** Initial arthroscopic appearance of fibrillated cartilage adjacent to a crevice in the surface of the sagittal ridge. **D,** Appearance following fragment removal. **E,** Distal margin of the lesion during debridement illustrating the junction of hyaline cartilage and mineralized cartilage interfaced with the subchondral bone. This is well organized distally and disorganized proximally (which has not yet been debrided). **F,** Lesion at completion of debridement.

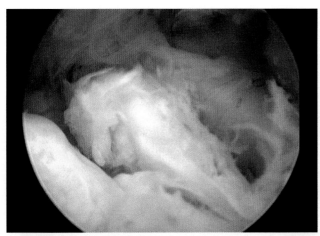

Figure 5-35 Arthroscopic view of type III osteochondritis dissecans (OCD) of distal dorsal McIII.

or type III lesion happened to have a type I lesion in another joint). The horses included 20 Thoroughbreds, 8 Quarter Horses, 7 Arabians, 4 Warmbloods, 1 Standardbred, 1 Percheron, and 1 Appaloosa (McIlwraith & Vorhees, 1990). Forelimbs were involved in 10, hindlimbs were involved in 15, and both forelimbs and hindlimbs were involved in 17 horses. One fetlock joint was operated in 10, 2 fetlocks in 17, 3 fetlocks in 1, and 4 fetlocks in 14 horses. Forty-eight cases involved the proximal 2 cm of the sagittal ridge, and 11 extended distal to this point. In 44 joints, lesions involved the lateral and/or medial condyles of McIII/MtIII, with or without lesions of the sagittal ridge.

Follow-up was obtained in 28/42 horses that had surgery, 8 horses were convalescing, and in 6 follow-up was unavailable. Surgery was successful in 16 (57.1%) cases and 12 (42.8%) were unsuccessful. Of the unsuccessful cases, 7 were still considered to have a problem in the fetlock joint (25%): 3 were unsuccessful for other reasons; 1 was unsuccessful for unidentified reasons but was considered to be normal in the fetlock joint; and 1 horse died. The success rate was also found to be related to other factors. There was a trend for the success rate to be higher for surgery in hindlimbs compared with forelimbs. On the one hand, in the forelimbs only 2 cases were successful and 6 were unsuccessful, whereas in the hind limb 7 were successful and 3 were unsuccessful. When both forelimbs and hindlimbs were involved, there were 7 successes and 3 failures. Type III lesions had 4 successes and 4 failures, whereas type II lesions had 10 successes and 4 failures (difference not statistically significant). Only 3/12 cases with erosions or wear lines present at arthroscopy were successful, whereas 13/16 with no erosions were successful ($p = 0.0029$). Probably related to that, there was a significantly inferior result when a defect was visible on the condyle on oblique radiographs. When a defect was visible, 6/13 were successful, whereas if a defect was not visible, 10/15 were successful ($p = 0.0274$). Osteophytes were also negative prognosticators; 3/9 with osteophytes on the proximal phalanx were successful, whereas 13/19 with no osteophytes were successful.

It was concluded that surgical management of type II and type III lesions will allow athletic activity in a fair number of cases, but clinical signs will persist in 25%. Whether the surgery will be successful or not will be affected by the extent of the lesions, as evident arthroscopically (and in some instances, radiographically), as well as by the presence of osteophytes, erosions, and wear lines. Since the McIlwraith & Vorhees (1990) paper was published, the first author feels that the success rate has improved further because of earlier intervention, particularly when treating horses radiographed at a young age to ensure clean joints at yearling sales.

Osteochondritis Dissecans Fragments of the Dorsal Margin of the Proximal Phalanx

Disease and fragmentation of the dorsoproximal margin of the proximal phalanx typical of OCD is seen quite commonly in young horses. The radiographic manifestations are of a smooth and usually small fragment on the proximal dorsal aspect of the proximal phalanx (Fig. 5-36). The arthroscopic manifestations can vary, as illustrated in Figure 5-36. In some instances, there will be a flap with diseased bone underneath, typical of OCD (see Fig. 5-36B). But in most instances, there will be a rounded fragment (see Fig. 5-36C and D). Rarely, extensive fragmentation may be present (see Fig. 5-36E to G).

Aftercare in these cases is the same as for traumatic fragments off the proximal dorsal aspect of the proximal phalanx. Many of these horses are young and therefore have long periods for convalescence before being put into training. The prognosis is consequently very good.

The prognosis is based on the appearance of the joint during surgery, as well as on the age of the horse. If there is no other damage or only a minimally sized defect in the sagittal ridge, the prognosis is good. Declercq et al (2009) reported fragmentation of the dorsal margin of the proximal phalanx in 117 young Warmblood horses. One-hundred and fifty joints (67 metacarpophalangeal and 83 metatarsophalangeal) underwent arthroscopy. Eighty-eight horses had 1, 25 had 2, and 4 had 3 joints operated on. Only 8 horses were lame; the remainder underwent surgery for prophylactic reasons and/or to remove radiologic blemishes. Ninety-five percent of the fragments were located dorsomedially; there was no difference between forelimbs and hindlimbs. Histopathologic evaluation of 45 fragments revealed consistent findings. None of the findings had the appearance of chip fractures, but evaluation failed to provide etiologic differentiation between osteochondrosis and juvenile/neonatal traumatic fragmentation. The authors concluded that they were a form of developmental orthopedic disease.

Osteochondral Fragments in the Dorsal Plica

In addition to fragmentation of the proximal dorsal margin of the sagittal ridge of McIII/MtIII, which is considered to be a manifestation of osteochondrosis and is described earlier, surgeons have been aware that fragments or foci of dystrophic mineralization, or both, are also found attached to or embedded within the adjacent dorsal plica. These have been described by Declercq et al (2008). The relationship (if any) between the two conditions has not yet been determined. Declercq et al (2008) reported fragments in the dorsal plica (proximal synovial pad) of 127 joints in 104 Warmblood horses; 20 horses had 2, 1 horse had 4, and the remainder had 1 joint affected. Fifty (40%) were in forelimbs and 77 (60%) were in hindlimbs. Only 2 horses were lame. Fifty-two (37%) of the fragments were medial, 47 (33%) central, and 43 (30%) lateral. Histologic examination of 24 fragments revealed a tissue organization that was not considered consistent with osteochondrosis or traumatic fragmentation, and the etiology remains unknown. Radiographs predict presence and location of fragments and implicate the dorsal plica by location. Confirmation of an intraplical location can be made before surgery by ultrasonography. Figure 5-37 illustrates the radiographic appearance and arthroscopic surgery for such a lesion.

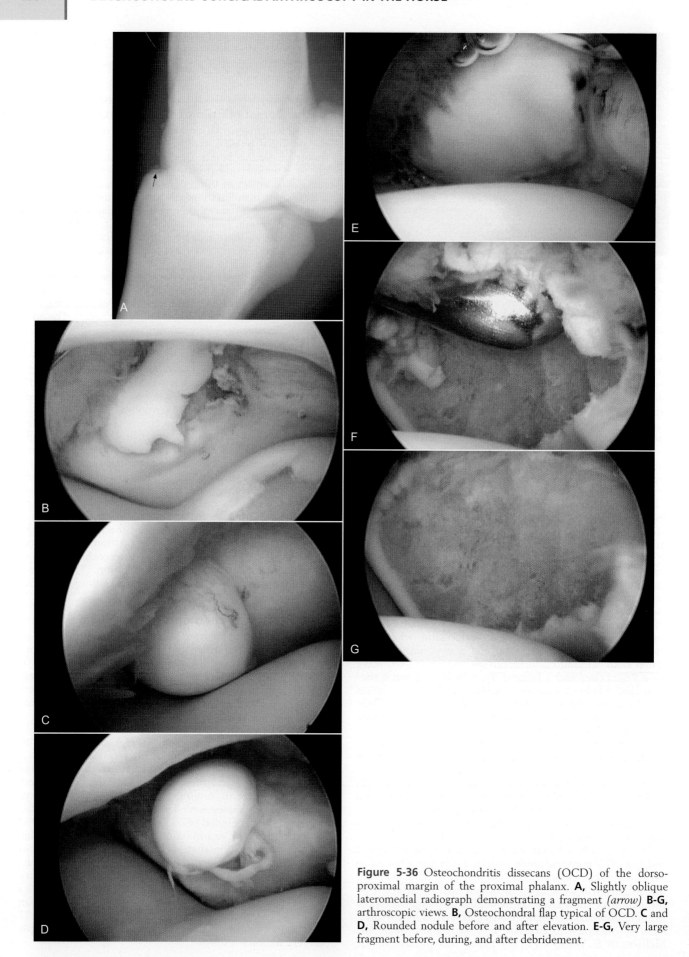

Figure 5-36 Osteochondritis dissecans (OCD) of the dorso-proximal margin of the proximal phalanx. **A,** Slightly oblique lateromedial radiograph demonstrating a fragment *(arrow)* **B-G,** arthroscopic views. **B,** Osteochondral flap typical of OCD. **C** and **D,** Rounded nodule before and after elevation. **E-G,** Very large fragment before, during, and after debridement.

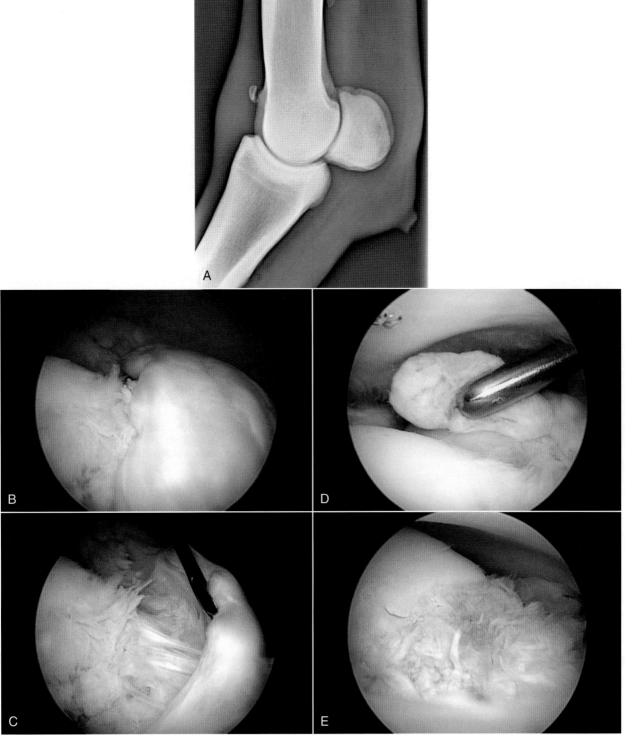

Figure 5-37 Osteochondral fragmentation in the dorsal plica. A, Lateromedial radiograph demonstrating a smoothly marginated radiodensity with definable infrastructure adjacent to the dorsoproximal margin of the sagittal ridge of the third metacarpal bone. There are no identifiable defects in the latter. **B,** Arthroscopic appearance. **C,** Dorsal plica and mineralized focus lifted with 19-gauge needle. **D,** Fragment grasped with Ferris-Smith rongeurs following isolation by sharp dissection. **E,** Arthroscopic appearance following fragment removal.

Debridement of Subchondral Cystic Lesions of the Third Metacarpal Bone

The distal McIII is one of the less common locations for sub-chondral cystic lesions (SCLs), but they do occur with relative regularity (Nixon, 1990; McIlwraith, 1990b). Most horses are aged 2 years old or younger when clinical signs become apparent, and they usually have a history of recently increased physical activity (such as entering athletic training). The diagnosis is confirmed with radiographs (Fig. 5-38A and B). As with most SCLs, they occur in a location subject to maximal weight bearing during the support phase of the stride. Once a cystic lesion becomes clinically apparent, the prognosis for athletic soundness is variable and appears to be dependent on several factors, including the anatomic location of the lesion, presence of any associated degenerative changes in the joint, and treatment regimen (surgical or conservative) chosen (Bramlage, 1993).

Before the use of arthroscopic surgery, most cases were managed conservatively and empirically and with limited success (McIlwraith, 1982). If conservative therapy was not successful, a dorsal arthrotomy was recommended to surgically debride the lesion and this technique has been more recently replaced by arthroscopic surgery. The technique is less invasive and provides the advantage of clear visual assessment of the articular surfaces of the joint.

The arthroscopic approach depends on the location of the cystic lesion. The majority of lesions are on the medial condyle of McIII, in which case the arthroscope and the instrument are both placed medially (see Fig. 5-38). In order to expose the opening of the SCL, flexion is required, so having the arthroscope on the same side obviates the potential problem that flexion creates (sagittal ridge interfering with the arthroscopic position). The arthroscope is placed laterally for an SCL on the lateral condyle or the sagittal ridge. With flexion, the opening of the cystic lesion can be visualized (see Fig. 5-38). A needle is used to ascertain the ideal position for an instrument portal; this tends to be distal and axial over the cystic lesion. The SCL is then debrided with a curette and pieces are removed with forceps. The cartilaginous edges are trimmed and debris is removed by flushing. Osteostixis (drilling) of SCLs is no longer performed.

A 4- to 6-month lay-up period is recommended with these cases. The initial 2 months involve stall confinement with a program of hand walking. A series of cases have been reported (Hogan et al, 1997) and serve as a basis for prognosis. SCLs in the distal McIII were surgically treated in 15 horses. The median age at presentation was 18 months (range 10 months to 12 years) with 10/15 horses younger than 2 years old. The SCLs were confined to the front limbs in all cases, with two horses having bilateral lesions. Lesions were isolated to the medial condyle of McIII in 13/15 horses; a cystic lesion occurred in the lateral condyle in 1 horse and in the sagittal ridge in another. One horse with bilateral lesions had an additional SCL lesion in the right medial femoral condyle. Fourteen of 15 horses had a history of moderate lameness attributable to the metacarpophalangeal joint; the lesion was an incidental finding in 1 horse. Duration of lameness ranged from 4 weeks to 8 months and was either acute in onset or occurred intermittently and was associated with exercise. Fetlock flexion significantly exacerbated the lameness in all cases. Synovial effusion was absent in 8 (53%) cases.

Cystic lesions were curetted arthroscopically in 12 horses, and through a dorsal pouch arthrotomy in 3 horses. Concurrent osteostixis of the cystic cavity was performed in 7 horses. In follow-up periods of 1-6 years following surgery, 12/15 horses (80%) were sound for intended use, 2 horses did not regain soundness, and follow-up information was unavailable in 1 horse. Follow-up radiographs were available for 9 horses. Mild periarticular osteophyte formation and enthesophyte formation at the dorsal joint capsular attachments were present in 5 horses. Bony infilling of the SCL was detectable in 8 horses, and enlargement of the cystic cavity was observed in 1 horse. On the basis of this study, it appears that surgical treatment of SCLs in the distal McIII should result in a favorable outcome for athletic use (Hogan et al, 1997).

More recently, SCLs in the distal McIII have been treated with intralesional injection of triamcinolone acetonide as described in Chapter 6 for medial femoral condyle SCLs (Wallis et al, 2008). When cases are managed by this means the convalescence time is considerably shorter. Insufficient numbers are available at this stage for accurate prognostic figures.

Byron & Goetz (2007) reported arthroscopic debridement of a subchondral bone defect in the distal palmar medial condyle of the third metacarpal bone in a Standardbred racehorse. A conventional proximal arthroscopic portal was employed, and visibility of the lesion was enhanced by use of an arthroscope with a 70-degree lens. Such lesions are more accessible using a distal arthroscopic portal when a standard 25-degree or 30-degree arthroscope can be employed. More cases are necessary before confident prognostic guidelines can be issued.

Impact and Chondral Fractures

Full-thickness cartilage fractures and compressive fractures of the subchondral bone have been seen in the distal metacarpal condyles similar to the impact fracture of the proximal phalanx described by Cullimore et al (2009). The horses have the clinical commonality of acute-onset, severe lameness localizing to the metacarpophalangeal joint, which is distended. The authors' cases have all involved the medial condyle of the third metacarpal bone, and most have been seen in jumping horses. In the acute and subacute phases, there are usually no radiologic abnormalities. Later, degrees of subchondral bone resorption may be evident and in chronic cases there may be narrowing of the joint space and incongruity between the sagittal ridge of the third metacarpal bone and corresponding groove of the proximal phalanx. Arthroscopic evaluation quantifies the articular insult, which in turn determines prognosis. Treatment is effected along the lines of general arthroscopic principles. Joint flexion can aid access to distal portions of the lesions, but this may still not be adequate to visualize the most distal/palmar margins.

Tears and Avulsions of the Fibrous Joint Capsule

Disruption of the fibrous joint capsule is seen in both dorsal and palmar/plantar compartments as discussed in Chapter 3 (Wright & Minshall, unpublished data). In the former tears are most commonly abaxial and may extend from the level of the dorsal plica to the proximal phalanx. They can occur medially, laterally, or biaxially. Sometimes when the joint is maximally distended before creation of an arthroscopic portal, the presence of such tears will be signaled by an abnormal outpouching on the affected site. Arthroscopically the edges of the tear are usually extruded into the synovial space and are readily identifiable. Some, particularly biaxial tears, can extend proximally increasing markedly the volume of the dorsal compartment. Tears can be seen as sole injuries in horses with lameness localizing to the metacarpophalangeal/metatarsophalangeal joint or in conjunction with other lesions. The tears are usually irregular and frayed, and they do not appear amenable to repair. Treatment to date has therefore consisted of arthroscopic removal of flaps and extruded torn tissue with a goal of reducing synovial irritation and promoting second intention healing. In the palmar/plantar compartment two forms of tearing have been identified: (1) abaxial tears similar to those seen dorsally and (2) tears with the appearance of avulsions from the palmar/plantar surface of the third metacarpal/third metatarsal bone. These are usually biaxial and result in the arthroscopic exposure of increased amounts of the palmar/plantar supracondylar fossae.

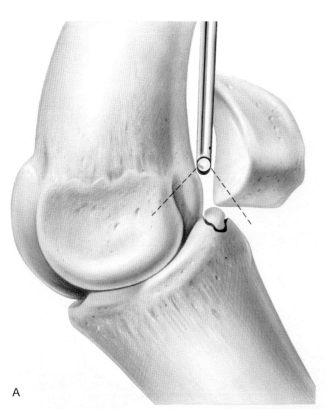

A

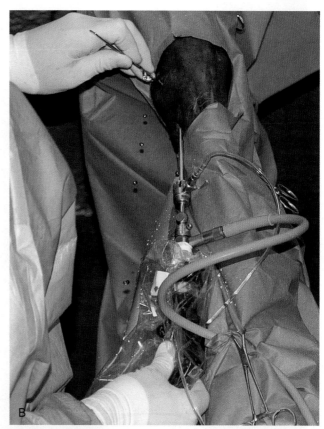

B

Figure 5-40 Diagram **(A)** and photograph **(B)** of positioning of arthroscope (and instrument in **B**) during operations involving a fragment from the proximal plantar aspect of the proximal phalanx.

radiographically demonstrable fragment (see Fig. 5-39). The fragment can be identified on the lateral and flexed lateral views. Dorsoplantar radiographs taken with the fetlock flexed have also been recommended (Birkeland, 1972). Optimal definition of lesion location is achieved with oblique views with the tube at a 30-degree proximal to distal angle (see Fig. 5-39B). Both oblique views (DPrL-DiMO and DPrM-DiLO) are essential because lesions can be biaxial.

Nonsurgical treatment usually lowers the horse's performance (Barclay et al, 1987). Arthroscopic surgery is now the standard technique. Dorsal or lateral recumbency can be used. The authors prefer dorsal recumbency because the instrument portal can conveniently be made laterally or medially. However, flexion of the joint is necessary and a suitable limb support system or an assistant, or both, will be required. If the surgery is done in lateral recumbency, the side where the fragment is located should be up and the arthroscope and instrument approaches will be made from the same side. The arthroscope is placed in the plantar or palmar joint pouch, as previously described, and is positioned to visualize the distal part of the joint; if necessary an assistant can facilitate this step by placing flexion on the joint (Fig. 5-40). An instrument portal is made distal to the base of the proximal sesamoid bone (PSB) and collateral sesamoidean ligament (see Figs. 5-40 and 5-41). This enables instruments to pass transversely between the PSB and proximal phalanx, perpendicular to the long axis of the limb. This position is ascertained by prior placement of a percutaneous needle. Often, the fragment can be visualized; if not, a probe is used to ensure its location. Local synovial resection can aid visualization. The fragment is then separated from the soft tissue with a fixed blade knife and removed by using a

Ferris-Smith arthroscopic rongeurs (Fig. 5-41). Removal of this fragment leaves a defect within the joint capsule and short-digital sesamoidean ligaments, and any loose tags of tissue are removed from this area. Debridement of the plantar defect in the proximal phalanx is sometimes appropriate but is not usually necessary. Multiple fragments can occasionally be present.

This condition is one of the few in equine arthroscopic surgery for which the use of sharp dissection is essential. Different instruments have been used, including a tenotomy knife, a banana knife, a narrow bistoury, and an Arthro-Lok™ retractable blade. The authors prefer a broad, flat blade. The disposable No. 11 blade should not be used because of the risk of breakage. Electrocautery probes have also been used for this dissection (Simon et al, 2004). The authors demonstrated its efficacy as an alternative to conventional arthroscopic dissection techniques. It has hemostatic advantages, but with horses in dorsal recumbency or with use of an Esmarch bandage and tourniquet, or both, intraoperative hemorrhage is not a limiting factor to surgery. The immediate postoperative care is the same as for other arthroscopic procedures in the fetlock joint. A period of 2 to 3 months rest before training resumes is recommended.

There have been two reports of treatment of these osteochondral fragments with follow-up. Whitton & Kannegieter (1994) reported on 21 horses, of which 16 returned to racing: 12 had improved performance, while 3 showed no improvement, and 1 horse was retired for other reasons. Degenerative changes within the fetlock joint were detected at surgery in 8 horses. Four horses were treated conservatively: 1 horse returned to its previous level of performance temporarily after intraarticular medication, 1 horse showed no improvement, and 2 horses were resting at the time of the report.

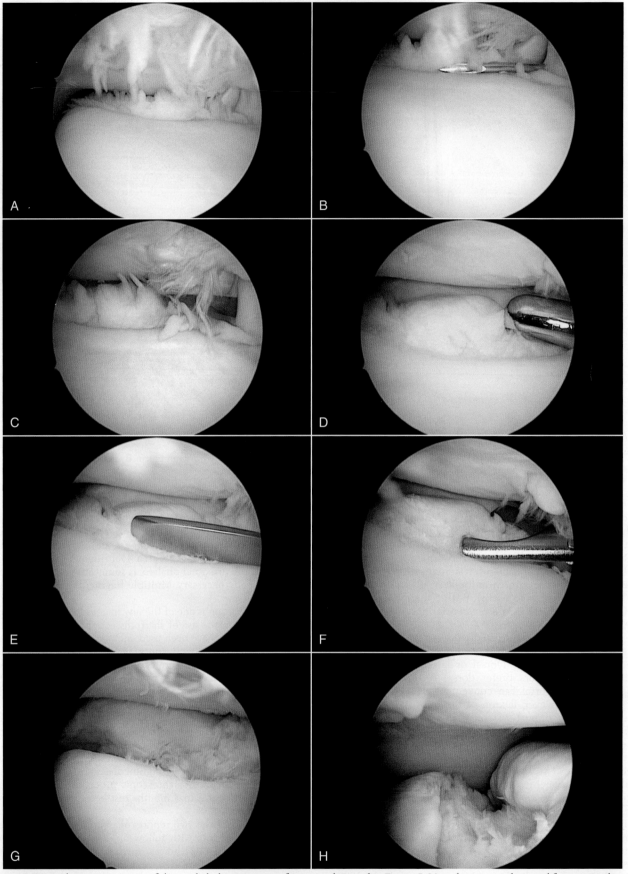

Figure 5-41 Arthroscopic images of the medial plantar process fragment depicted in Figure 5-39 and its removal viewed from an ipsilateral arthroscopic portal. **A,** Initial arthroscopic image with proliferative synovium overlying the fragment. **B,** Determination of a suitable instrument portal by passage of a 19-gauge needle adjacent to the collateral sesamoidean ligament and parallel with the base of the proximal sesamoid bone. **C,** Creation of an instrument portal with a number 11 blade. **D,** Removal of proliferative synovium with a motorized resector to delineate the fragment. **E,** Dissection of the fragment from the short distal sesamoidean ligament with a fixed blade menisectomy knife. **F,** Completion of dissection using curved (menisectomy) scissors. **G,** Appearance following fragment removal. **H,** Insertion of the arthroscope into the instrument portal to ensure complete fragment removal and appropriate debridement.

In a larger series of 119 horses (109 Standardbreds), 55/87 (63%) racehorses and 100% of 9 nonracehorses, performance returned to preoperative levels after surgery (Fortier et al, 1995). Fragment numbers or distribution and concurrent OCD of the distal intermediate ridge of the tibia or tarsal osteoarthritis were not significantly associated with outcome. Abnormal surgical findings, consisting of articular cartilage fibrillation or synovial proliferation, were significantly ($p < 0.001$) associated with adverse outcome.

Removal of Fragments from the Proximal Sesamoid Bones

Osteochondral fractures amenable to removal occur at the apical, abaxial, and basal margins of the proximal sesamoid bones. Arthroscopic techniques for the removal of these fragments have been developed. Previous dogma had proposed limitations of fragment removal on the basis of the size of the fragment and degree of attachment to the suspensory and distal sesamoidean ligaments. However, current follow-up on the first author's cases that have been treated arthroscopically suggest that limitations should be redefined. As a generalization, the hypothesis that the prognosis will decrease with greater involvement of both bone and soft tissue attachments is still valid, but the actual proportions are higher than previously thought.

The diagnosis of sesamoid fractures is made radiographically with ultrasonography used to assess the degree of suspensory apparatus compromise (Fig. 5-42). Special views are used to clearly delineate abaxial involvement. Arthroscopic surgery for the removal of sesamoid fragments is performed with the horse in either lateral or dorsal recumbency; the latter is preferred. The technique for an apical sesamoid fragment is illustrated in Figure 5-43. The arthroscope is placed in the most proximal portion of the palmar or plantar pouch of the fetlock joint in all cases. With partial flexion of the joint, a needle is used to ascertain the ideal placement for the instrument portal. The arthroscope portal can be ipsilateral or contralateral, and both techniques are illustrated in Figures 5-44 and 5-45, respectively. Sharp dissection is used to separate the apical fragment from the suspensory ligament using a flat blade, before a curved blade (Foerner-Scanlan elevator) is used to dissect the fragment from the intersesamoidean ligament and to continue dissection from the abaxial attachment (see Fig. 5-44). After isolation of the fragment, it is removed with Ferris-Smith rongeurs (see Fig. 5-44). Soft tissue attachments are trimmed with basket forceps or a motorized resector. The bone is debrided with a curette. Fractures involving more than one third of the articular surface are not considered good candidates for arthroscopic removal, and reconstruction techniques should be considered. Apical sesamoid fragments in foals can be treated in the same fashion.

The same arthroscopic approach is used for surgery on abaxial fragments. Case selection can sometimes be a challenge because there are a few fragments that are nonarticular. If conventional radiographs (Fig. 5-46) do not clearly delineate an abaxial fracture as articular, then a "skyline" (PrLDiMO/PrMDiLO) view should be taken (Palmar, 1982). The arthroscopic approach is illustrated in Figures 5-46 to 5-48. There are advantages and disadvantages to both ipsilateral and contralateral arthroscopic portals, and in some cases both can be used to advantage. Sharp dissection with the flat blade is limited to severing the suspensory ligament attachments (see Fig. 5-47B). It is important that the instrument portal is made appropriately distal so that the knife can sever the suspensory ligament attachments from the abaxial fragment. After removal, the bone and cartilage are debrided with a curette. A motorized resector is used to debride the suspensory ligament tags.

Fragmentation of both the apical and abaxial regions of the sesamoid bone can occur concomitantly (Fig. 5-49). The arthroscopic technique for these fragments is the same as for removing them independently. Generally, the abaxial fragment is removed first, followed by the apical fragments (see Fig. 5-49).

Intraarticular basal sesamoid fragments can be removed arthroscopically when implicated in lameness (Figs. 5-50 and 5-51). A reasonable number of fragments are of sufficiently small size that their removal does not compromise the distal sesamoidean ligament attachments; the exact size limitations have been defined by Southwood et al (1998). The technique is illustrated in Figure 5-52. Both ipsilateral and contralateral arthroscope and instrument positions are possible. The arthroscope is placed in the same fashion as for surgery on apical and abaxial fragments. The instrument is brought in below the base of the sesamoid bone as described earlier for removal of fragments from the palmar/plantar processes of the proximal phalanx. Sharp dissection is used to sever the fragments from the capsular and distal sesamodian ligament attachments. Following fragment removal, the defects are debrided (bone and soft tissue) and the joints lavaged (see Figs. 5-50 and 5-51). In some cases visualization of the palmar/plantar margins of the fracture can be compromised. In this situation insertion of the arthroscope into the instrument portal provides confident assessment of complete fragment removal and appropriate debridement.

Results following arthroscopic removal of apical, abaxial, and basal sesamoid fragments have been documented in the literature. On reviewing the results of 82 cases of apical fractures of the proximal sesamoid bones, follow-up data were obtained for 54 racehorses: 36/54 (67%) horses returned to racing, 28 (52%) in the same class and 8 (15%) in a lower class. Fragments were also grouped by size. Small fragments were classified with a proximodistal length less than 10 mm or less than 25% of the sesamoid bone, and large fragments had a proximodistal length more than 10 mm or more than 25% of the sesamoid bone (Southwood et al, 2000). Among the horses with small apical fractures, 14/18 (78%) returned to racing, 11 in the same class and 3 in a lower class. Although 11/19 (58%) with large apical fractures returned to racing and all raced in the same class, 11/17 (65%) horses with apical-abaxial fractures returned to racing, 6 in the same class and 5 in a lower class. Of the horses that had raced before surgery, 33/40 (83%) horses raced after surgery.

In a series of 47 cases of abaxial fragments of the proximal sesamoid bones, follow-up information was obtained for 41 horses (35 racehorses, 6 nonracehorses). Twenty-five of 35 (71%) racehorses were able to return to racing (16 in the same class, 9 in a lower class); all 6 nonracehorses were able to return to performance at the same level. Horses with small fracture fragments or fractures involving the abaxial surface of the proximal sesamoid bone only had a more favorable outcome compared with horses with large apical-abaxial fractures (Southwood et al, 1998). There were 10 (21%) grade 1 fractures, 23 (49%) grade 2 fractures, and 14 (30%) grade 3 fractures. All 5 horses with grade 1 fractures returned to racing (4 in the same class and 1 in a lower class). Twelve of 18 horses with grade 2 fractures returned to racing (9 in the same class and 3 in a lower class). Eight horses with grade 3 fractures returned to racing (3 in the same class and 5 in a lower class). Four racehorses had not raced before surgery; 2 of these horses raced after surgery, and 2 did not race before or after surgery. Compared with horses with large fragments, horses with small fragments returned to racing in the same class more often; however, the differences were not significant.

Subsequently, Schnabel et al (2006 & 2007) reported the results of arthroscopic removal of apical sesamoid fracture fragments in Thoroughbred racehorses. Of Thoroughbreds 2 years of age or older, 65 out of 84 (77%) started a mean of 12 times after surgery. Of those that had raced previously,

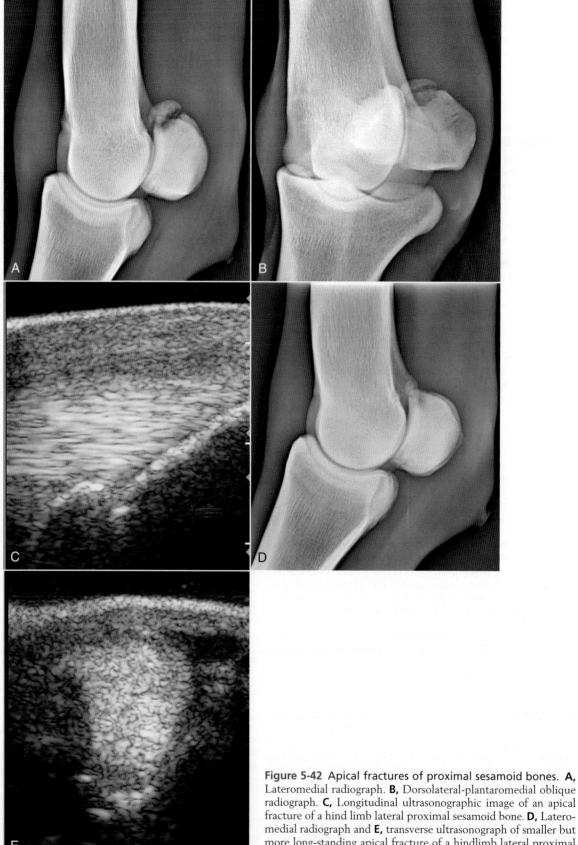

Figure 5-42 Apical fractures of proximal sesamoid bones. **A,** Lateromedial radiograph. **B,** Dorsolateral-plantaromedial oblique radiograph. **C,** Longitudinal ultrasonographic image of an apical fracture of a hind limb lateral proximal sesamoid bone. **D,** Latero-medial radiograph and **E,** transverse ultrasonograph of smaller but more long-standing apical fracture of a hindlimb lateral proximal sesamoid bone.

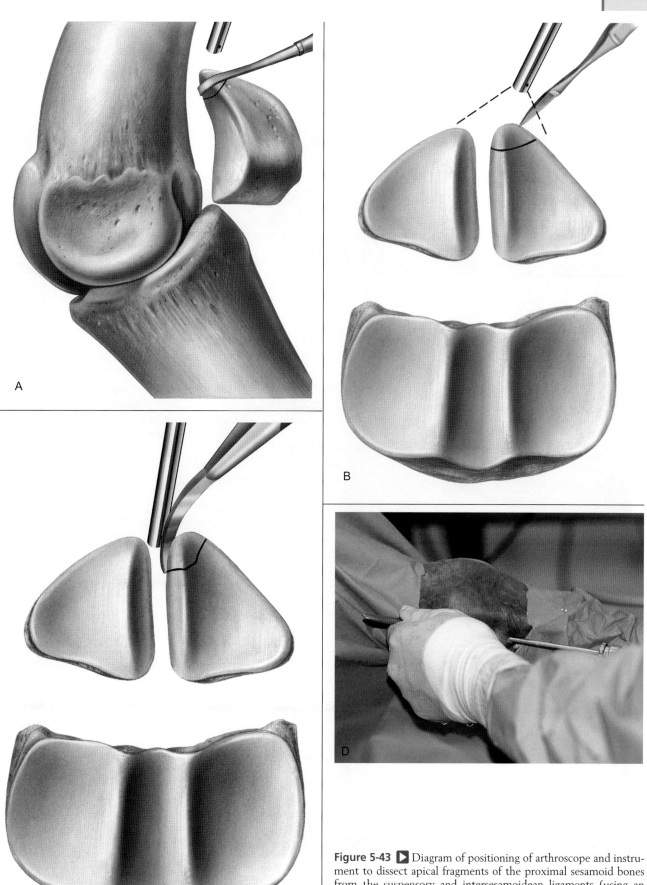

Figure 5-43 ▶ Diagram of positioning of arthroscope and instrument to dissect apical fragments of the proximal sesamoid bones from the suspensory and intersesamoidean ligaments (using an ipsilateral approach). **A,** Lateral view. **B,** Dorsal view incising the suspensory ligament. **C,** Incising intersesamoidean ligament dorsal view. **D,** Photograph of ipsilateral approach.

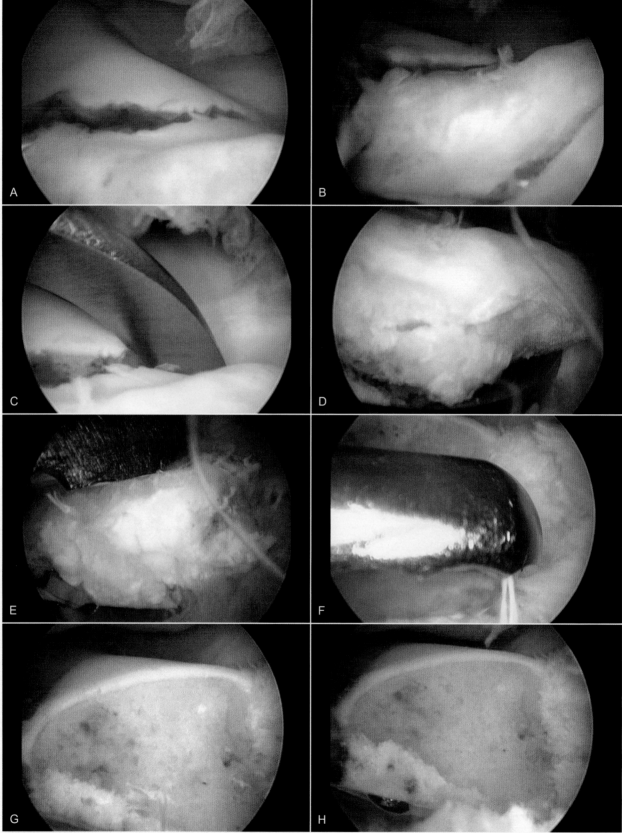

Figure 5-44 Arthroscopic views **(A-H)** of removal of an apical sesamoid fragment using an ipsilateral approach. **A,** Initial appearance, **B,** incising suspensory attachment, **C,** incising intersesamoidean ligament attachment, **D,** completing dissection, **E,** removing fragment with Ferris-Smith rongeurs, **F,** debriding suspensory ligament tags with motorized resector, **G,** Fracture site after subridement, and **H,** final lavage.

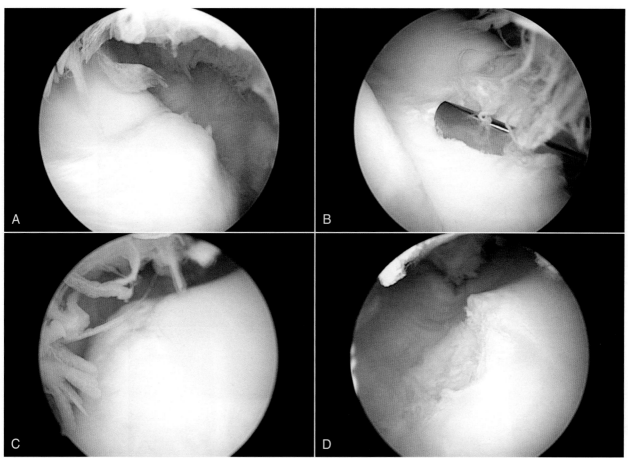

Figure 5-45 Arthroscopic images of removal of apical sesamoid fragments using a contralateral arthroscope portal. **A,** Arthroscopic image of fracture depicted in Figure 5-46A to C before removal. **B,** Fixed-blade menisectomy knife being used to section the intersesamoidean ligament and adjacent fibrocartilagenous scutum. **C,** Arthroscopic appearance of fracture depicted in Figure 5-46D and E before removal and **D,** following fragment removal. The fracture bed is covered by mature scar tissue/fibrous tissue and required no further debridement.

31 out of 38 (82%) ran at the same or at an improved level (Schnabel et al, 2006). Horses with medial proximal sesamoid bone fractures were less likely (26 out of 40; 65%) to race postoperatively than those with lateral fractures (35 out of 39; 90%). Analyzed further, these comprised 9 of 19 (47%) forelimb and 17 of 21 (81%) hindlimb medial proximal sesamoid bone fractures. Horses with apical fractures of forelimb medial proximal sesamoid bones are thus less likely to race following fragment removal than fractures in other locations. All 10 of 10 horses with forelimb lateral proximal sesamoid bone fractures raced after surgery. The presence of suspensory desmitis in the affected limb also has a negative association with postoperative performance; 63% of horses with identified suspensory desmitis raced postsurgery compared with 77% without. In a second paper (Schnabel et al, 2007) these authors assessed the racing performance of 151 Thoroughbreds that had apical sesamoid fragments removed arthroscopically when younger than 2 years of age. Among these horses, 123 out of 147 (84%) raced postoperatively and there was no difference between their performance and maternal siblings. However, horses with apical sesamoid fractures in the forelimbs were less likely to race than those in the hindlimbs (55% vs. 86%, respectively). Similar to their older counterparts, animals with fractures of a forelimb medial proximal sesamoid bone were less likely to race and had poorer performance than those with proximal sesamoid bone fractures in other locations.

Kamm et al (2011) evaluated the influence of size and geometry of apical sesamoid fracture fragments on the prognosis for racing following removal in Thoroughbreds. Data from 166 horses were reported. These included 110 weanlings and yearlings that had not begun training and 56 horses in training. No relationships between fragment size or shape and racing performance were identified. Woodie et al (1999) also found that there was no association between the length of the abaxial surface involved and racing outcome in Standardbreds with apical sesamoid fractures. Although the results of these studies are counterintuitive, they are important when counseling connections before surgery is undertaken.

Southwood and McIlwraith (2000) reported the results of arthroscopic removal of fracture fragments involving a portion of the base of the proximal sesamoid bone in 24 racehorses and 2 nonracehorses. Twelve (50%) racehorses returned to racing and started in at least 2 races; 8/14 of horses with grade I fractures (≤25% of the base involved) and 4/10 with grade II fractures (>25%, but <100% of the base involved) had successful outcomes; 10/16 without associated articular disease had successful outcomes compared with 2/8 with associated articular disease. However, fragment size and presence of associated articular disease were not significantly associated with outcomes (probably related to the relatively low numbers). It was concluded that horses with a fracture fragment involving a portion of the base of the bone removed arthroscopically have a fair prognosis for return to racing.

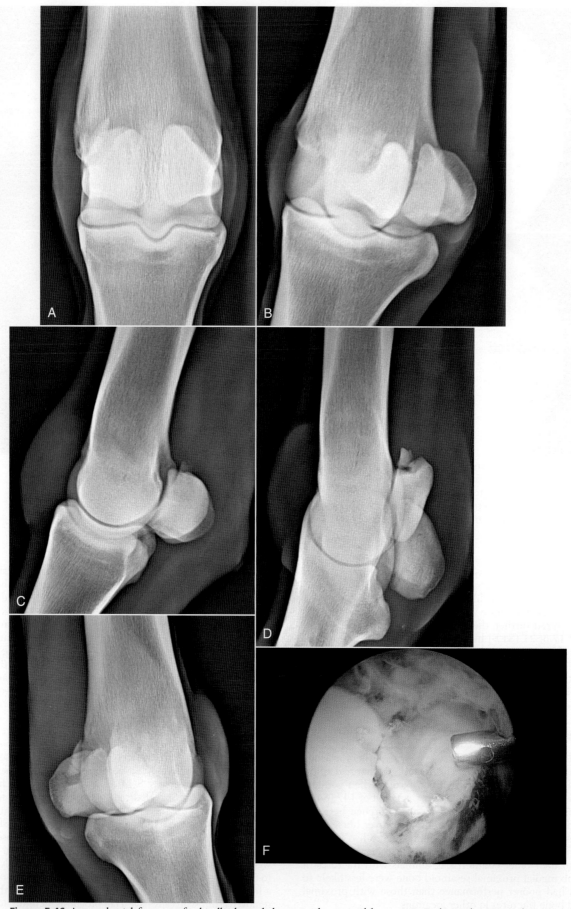

Figure 5-46 Acute abaxial fracture of a hindlimb medial proximal sesamoid bone. **A-E,** Radiographs. **F-P,** Arthroscopic images illustrating the fracture, removal, and debridement using contralateral arthroscope and ipsilateral instrument portals.

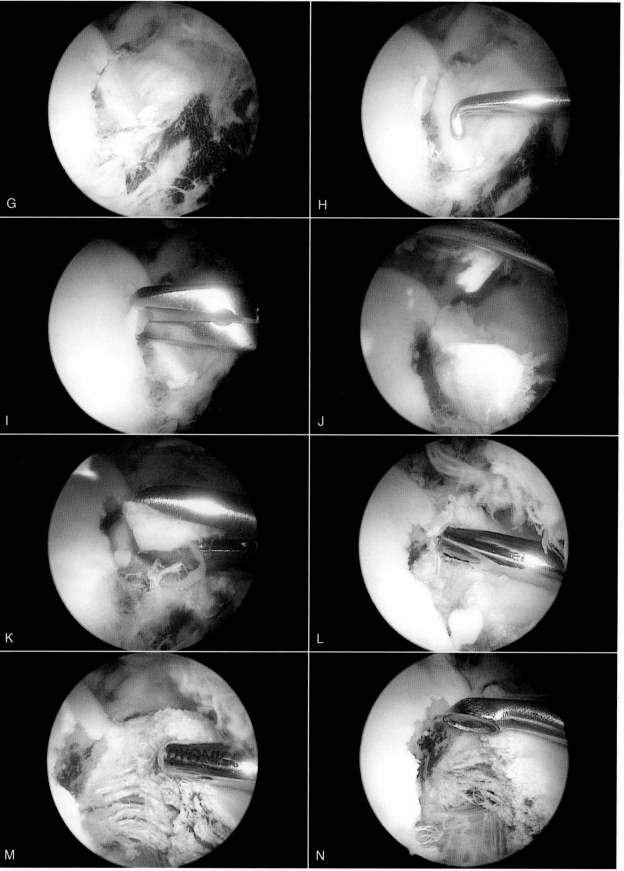

Figure 5-46, cont'd

Continued

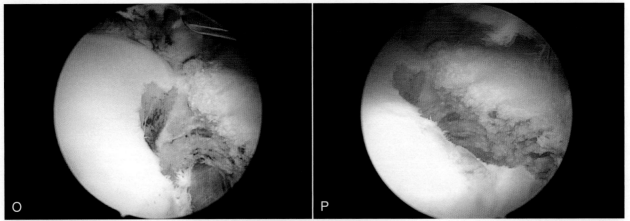

Figure 5-46, cont'd

There has also been a report of the use of electrocautery probes in arthroscopic removal of apical sesamoid fracture fragments in 18 Standardbred horses (Bouré et al, 1999). Distension of the joints was achieved using a 1.5% glycine solution, and the suspensory and intersesamoidean ligament attachments to the abaxial and axial margins of the apical fragment were transected using a hook electrocautery probe. Subsequently, the palmar (plantar) soft tissue attachments were transected with a loop electrocautery probe. After being freed of soft tissue attachments, the apical fragment was removed with Ferris-Smith intervertebral disk rongeurs. It was reported that the electrocautery probe made an easy and precise dissection of all soft tissue attachments; 10/14 horses returned to racing (7/9 horses that raced before surgery raced again and 3/5 horses that had not raced before surgery raced afterwards).

Avulsions of the Suspensory Ligament Insertions

Approximately 30% of the branches of insertion of the suspensory ligament are subsynovial in the metacarpophalangeal/metatarsophalangeal joints (Minshall & Wright, 2006). Tears involving the dorsal surface of the suspensory ligament branches can result in articular deficits and extrusion of disrupted ligaments fibers into this synovial cavity. Most occur at or close to the abaxial margins of the proximal sesamoid bones and appear to be avulsion injuries. Minshall & Wright (2006) described 18 cases with equal distribution between forelimbs and hindlimbs and between medial and lateral branches. All affected joints were distended. Defects involving the dorsal (articular) surface of the suspensory ligament branches are identifiable ultrasonographically (Fig. 5-53).

The arthroscopic appearance varies. In some cases, flaps of avulsed suspensory ligament insertion are readily identifiable. In others, bundles of torn fibers suspended in irrigating fluid can overlie substantial defects in suspensory ligament insertion (see Fig. 5-53). Treatment involves removal of torn ligament with the intention of promoting second intention healing. Large flaps or bundles of tissue are sectioned using arthroscopic scissors and removed with rongeurs before defects are debrided with a motorized synovial resector. Smaller masses of torn tissue can be removed with the resector alone.

In the reported series, 15 of 18 horses were sound postsurgery with 13 returning to work at levels equal to or greater than those achieved preinjury.

Axial Osteitis of the Proximal Sesamoid Bones and Lesions of the Intersesamoidean Ligament

Eight cases of osteitis of the axial margin(s) of the proximal sesamoid bones that were evaluated arthroscopically were described by Dabareiner et al (2001). All were unilateral; five were in hindlimbs and three in forelimbs. The horses presented because of lameness and six of eight cases had synovial effusion. Two cases had diffuse cellulitis and effusion of the digital flexor tendon synovial sheath. All horses had osteolysis of the axial border of the proximal sesamoid bone on radiographs. In five horses, arthroscopy of the palmar or plantar pouch of all the metacarpophalangeal or metatarsophalangeal joint and of the digital sheath was performed. In the remaining three horses, only the palmar or plantar pouch of the metacarpophalangeal or metatarsophalangeal joint was examined. Damage to the intersesamoidean ligament was seen in all horses and consisted of discoloration, fraying, and detachment from the associated proximal sesamoid bone. Osteochondral fragmentation and osteomalacia involving the axial borders of the proximal sesamoid bone were also seen and removed in all joints. After debridement, the palmar or plantar pouch of the affected joint communicated with the digital flexor tendon sheath through the disrupted ligament. Figure 5-54 illustrates the radiographic and arthroscopic manifestations of such a case.

Three cases were considered to be infected and five noninfected, but all exhibited similar histopathologic features of chronic degenerative inflammation. A vascular etiology resulting from avulsion of the intersesamoidean ligament was suggested. A further case report identified fungal osteomyelitis at this site (Sherman et al, 2006).

At follow-up, all five horses without evidence of sepsis returned to their previous use with the median recovery time of 9 months. However, one of these horses remained grade 1/5 lame and radiographs obtained 1 year after surgery revealed secondary osteoarthritis of the affected metacarpophalangeal joint. Two horses were radiographed 12 months after surgery revealing remodeling of the sesamoid bones with a smooth contour to the axial margins of the sesamoid bone.

The authors have encountered lesions of the intersesamoidean ligament and adjacent axial margins of the proximal sesamoid bones, which appear morphologically consistent with avulsion injury. These generally involve substantially less bone loss than lesions described by Dabareiner et al (2001) such that this may be radiologically silent. The lesions have been managed by removal of detached and apparently nonviable tissue in line with standard arthroscopic principles.

Text continued on p. 160

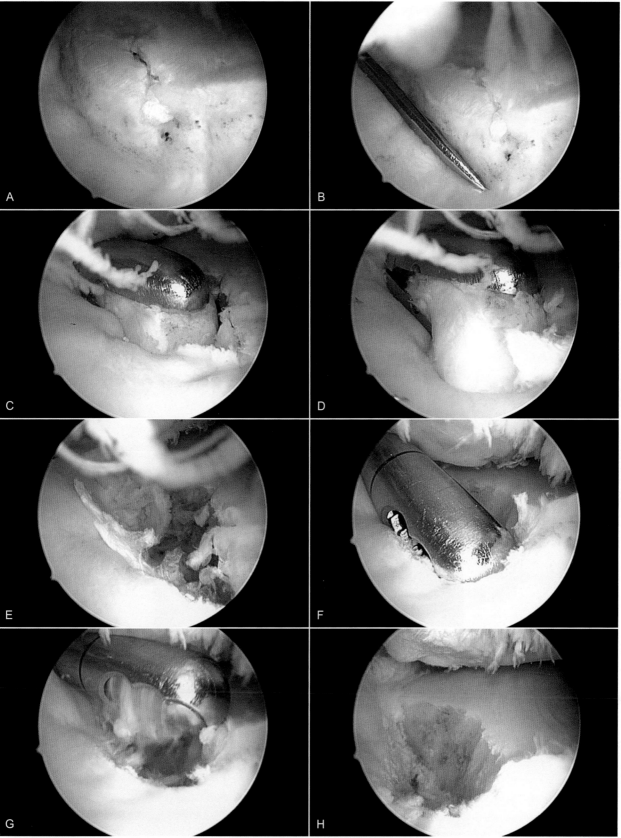

Figure 5-47 ▶ Arthroscopic views of removal of an abaxial fracture fragment of a proximal sesamoid bone using an ipsilateral approach. **A,** Evaluation of fracture, **B,** severing of a suspensory ligament attachment with flat knife, **C,** grasping of fragment with Ferris-Smith rongeurs, **D,** twisting of fragment free using Ferris-Smith rongeurs, **E,** defect in bone after removal of fragment and before debridement, **F** and **G,** resection of suspensory ligament tags with synovial resector, and **H,** view of defect in sesamoid bone and suspensory ligament after curettage and lavage.

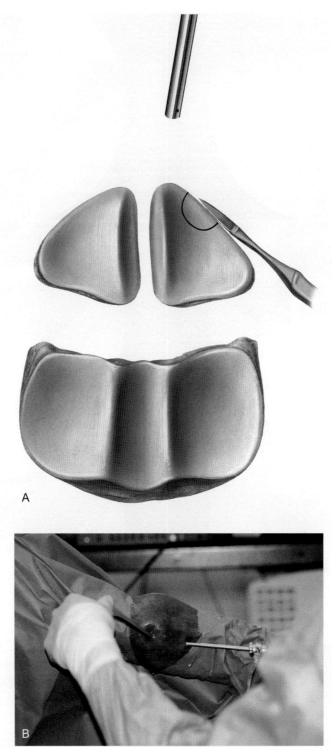

Figure 5-48 Diagram of the positioning of the arthroscope and instrument **(A)** and external photograph **(B),** to operate on an abaxial sesamoid bone fracture (ipsilateral approach).

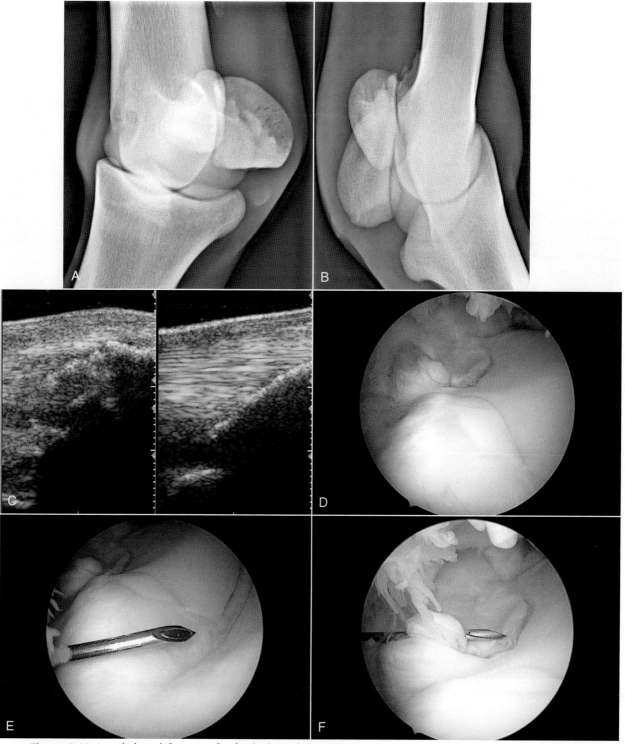

Figure 5-49 Apical/abaxial fracture of a forelimb medial proximal sesamoid bone. **A,** Dorsomedial-palmarolateral oblique radiograph. **B,** Lateral proximal distomedial oblique radiograph. **C,** Longitudinal ultrasonographs of the medial (left) and lateral (right) suspensory branch insertions. **D-K,** Arthroscopic images depicting fractures, removal and debridement using a contralateral arthroscopic portal. **L,** Arthroscope inserted into the ipsilateral instrument portal at the end of the procedure to ensure complete fragment removal and appropriate debridement.

Continued

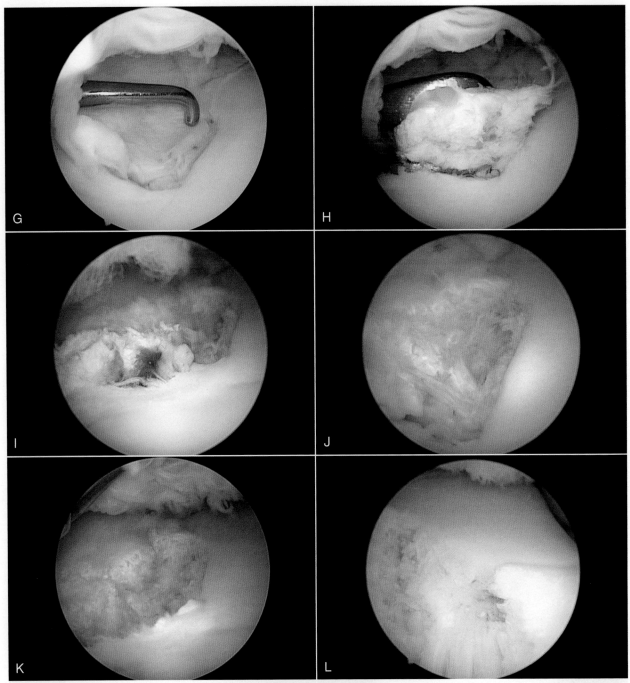

Figure 5-49, cont'd

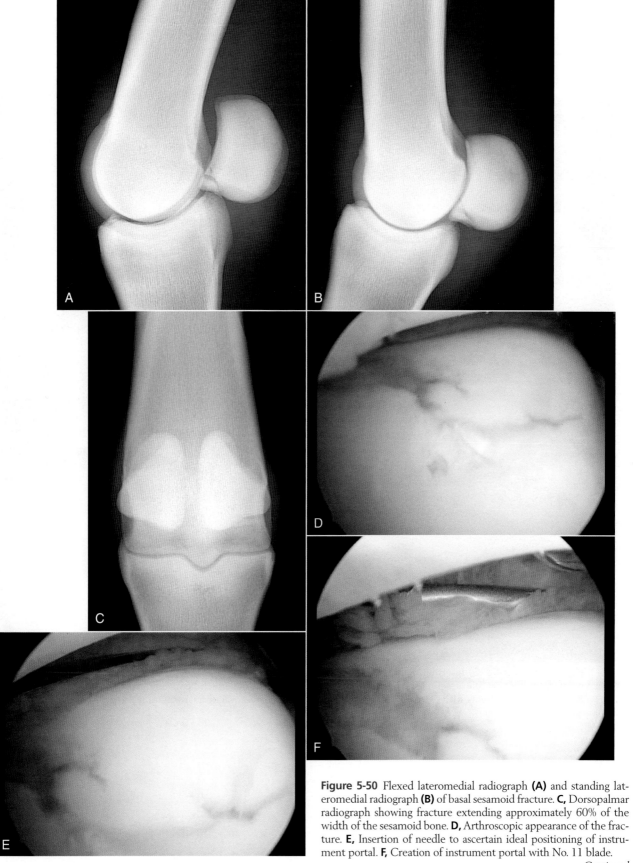

Figure 5-50 Flexed lateromedial radiograph **(A)** and standing lateromedial radiograph **(B)** of basal sesamoid fracture. **C,** Dorsopalmar radiograph showing fracture extending approximately 60% of the width of the sesamoid bone. **D,** Arthroscopic appearance of the fracture. **E,** Insertion of needle to ascertain ideal positioning of instrument portal. **F,** Creation of instrument portal with No. 11 blade.

Continued

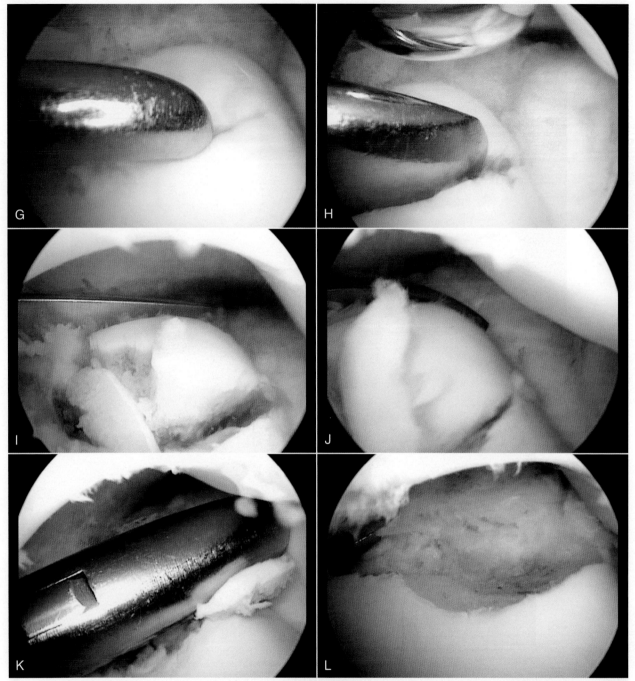

Figure 5-50, cont'd G, Insertion of probe in fracture line. **H,** Elevation of fragments. **I,** Sharp dissection of fragments from joint capsule attachments. **J,** Completion of dissection of axial attachments using curved Foerner elevator. **K,** Removal of fragments with Ferris-Smith rongeurs. **L,** Defect after removal of fragmentation and debridement.

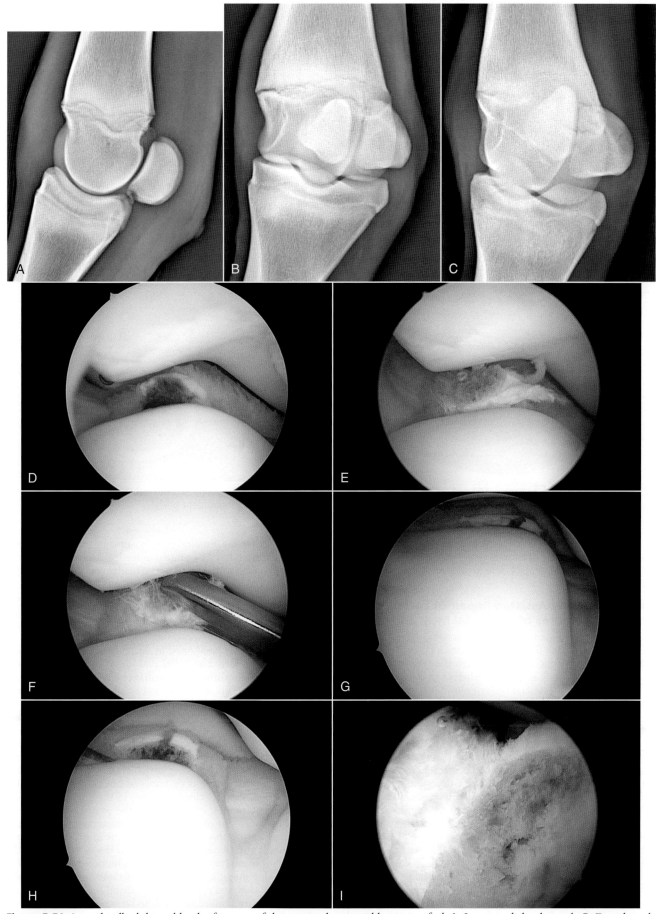

Figure 5-51 Acute hindlimb biaxial basilar fractures of the proximal sesamoid bones in a foal. **A,** Lateromedial radiograph. **B,** Dorsolateral-planataromedial oblique radiograph. **C,** Dorsomedial-plantarolateral oblique radiograph. **D-F,** Medial fracture viewed from a contralateral instrument portal. **G** and **H,** Lateral fracture viewed from an ipsilateral instrument portal. **I,** Arthroscope inserted into the lateral instrument portal in order to inspect the fracture site following fracture removal and debridement.

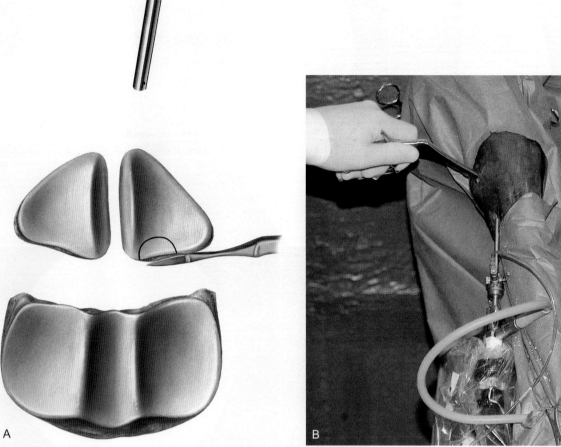

Figure 5-52 ▶ Diagram **(A)** and external view **(B)** of the positioning of the arthroscope and instrument to operate on a basal fragment of a proximal sesamoid bone using ipsilateral arthroscope and instrument portals.

Instances of focal subchondral bone disease involving the sesamoid bones have been seen elsewhere and have been treated with debridement of defective tissue (Fig. 5-55). The pathogenesis is unknown.

Arthroscopically Assisted Repair of Lateral Condylar Fractures of the Distal McIII and MtIII

Fractures of the metacarpal and metatarsal condyles are the commonest long bone fracture of racehorses (Wright & Nixon, 2013; Jacklin & Wright, 2013), although they are encountered in other horses working at speed (Misheff et al, 2010). Fractures of the metacarpal/metatarsal condyles have recently been classified (Jacklin & Wright, 2013). In all cases, articular congruency is critical to outcome. The authors recommend repair under arthroscopic guidance for all complete fractures of the lateral condyle. Experiences of such have demonstrated the inability of all current imaging techniques and open surgical evaluation, including arthrotomy, to identify and accurately reduce articular deficits. Once articular congruency is assessed or achieved, then repair can be effected using either percutaneous insertion of implants or following an open extraarticular approach.

A complete preoperative radiographic evaluation is mandatory. This should include flexed dorsopalmar/plantar projections (flexed dorsal distal 35 degrees—proximal palmar/oblique is the technique of choice) to image the palmar/plantar subchondral bone without superimposition (Jacklin & Wright, 2012) (Fig. 5-56). Radiographs should be evaluated closely for the presence of complicating lesions such as comminution and fractures of the axial margin of the lateral proximal sesamoid bone. The latter is seen only with displaced fractures. Comminution may be articular or extraarticular. Comminution of the palmar/plantar subchondral bone is of major prognostic significance; this often has a pyramidal or wedgelike form and may or may not be displaced. Dorsal intraarticular comminution is usually recognized as small displaced fragments, which may be scattered throughout the joint. Extraarticular comminution is most common at the proximal margin of the fracture and, although recognition is important in determining technique and implant size, this is generally of less prognostic significance.

Horses may be positioned in dorsal or lateral recumbency; the latter is preferred by A.J.N. and I.M.W. Use of an Esmarch bandage and tourniquet can enhance visibility and increase surgical speed. This should always be placed just distal to the carpus; more proximal placement will interfere with extension of the metacarpophalangeal/metatarsophalangeal joint and thus be a limitation to reduction. Occasionally, the presence of a tourniquet distal to the metacarpus can also limit mobility and may require intraoperative removal in order to permit reduction. The precise order in which the joint is evaluated and location for implants determined can be varied according to individual surgical circumstances, in theater imaging facilities and equipment, etc. However, the principles are consistent. Displacement of fractures of the lateral condyle of the third metacarpal/third metatarsal bone is invariably proximal and usually rotational with abaxial and dorsal rotation of the proximal portion of the fragment. Reduction requires extension of the metacarpophalangeal/metatarsophalangeal joint with adduction and rotation of the distal limb. These manipulations in turn require the limb to be supported in a manner that allows such movements while allowing the surgeon to orient the drill (and therefore implants) perpendicular to the third metacarpal/third metatarsal bone.

Text continued on p. 164

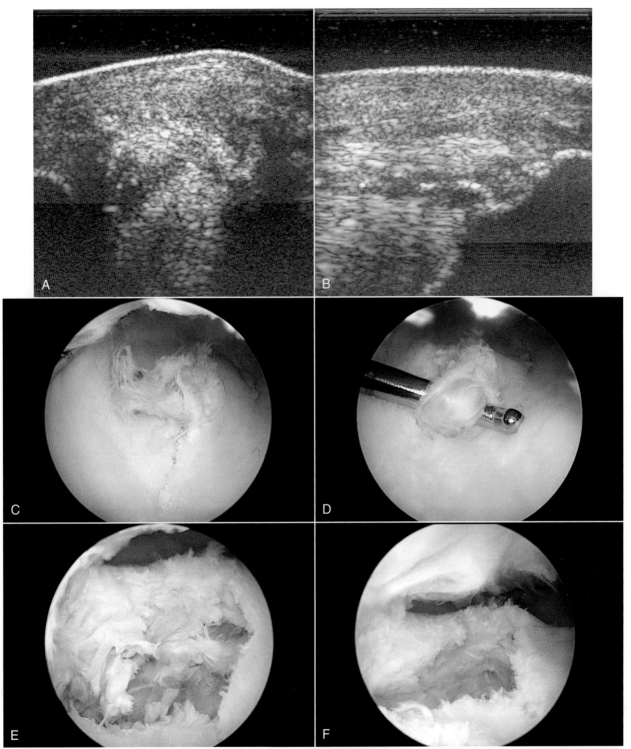

Figure 5-53 Ultrasonographic images **(A** and **B)** and arthroscopic images **(C-F)** of intraarticular tearing/avulsion of the medial branch of insertion of a hind limb suspensory ligament. **C,** Arthroscopic image from a contralateral portal. A linear defect is seen abaxial to the proximal sesamoid bone with torn fibers extruded into the synovial space. **D,** Arthroscopic probe placed under a large bundle of torn fibers. **E,** Defect in the suspensory branch exposed. **F,** Lesion at the end of debridement.

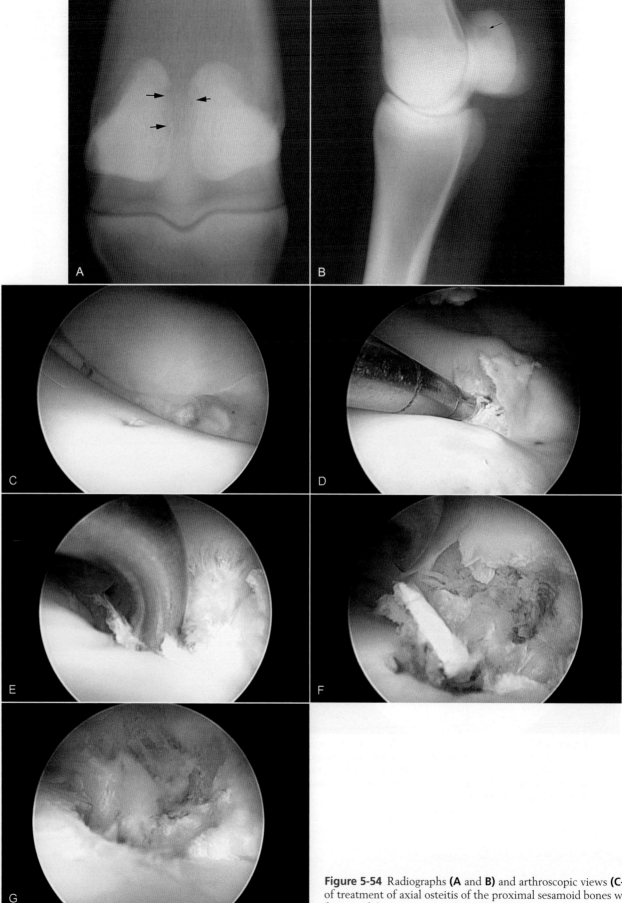

Figure 5-54 Radiographs (**A** and **B**) and arthroscopic views (**C-G**) of treatment of axial osteitis of the proximal sesamoid bones with fraying of the intersesamoidian ligaments.

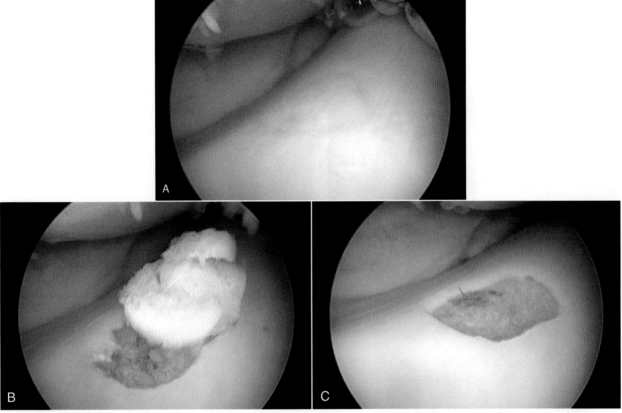

Figure 5-55 A, Arthroscopic views of a case of a focal bone disease in the central articular area of the sesamoid bone prior to debridement. **B,** During debridement. **C,** Following debridement.

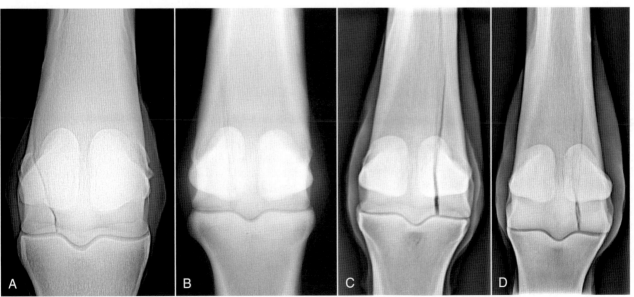

Figure 5-56 Dorsopalmar radiograph **(A)** of an undisplaced fracture of the lateral condyle of McIII requiring one screw for fixation. **B,** Dorsopalmar radiograph of an undisplaced fracture of the lateral condyle of the McIII that was repaired with two screws. **C,** Dorsopalmar radiograph and **(D)** flexed dorsopalmar radiograph of a displaced fracture of the lateral condyle of the McIII.

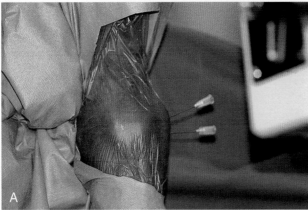

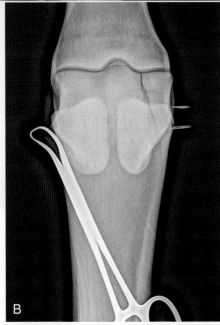

Figure 5-57 A, External view of surgery to repair an undisplaced lateral condylar fracture: placement of needles. **B,** Radiograph using needles to locate site for screw placement in and proximal to the condylar fossa.

Figures 5-57 to 5-61 illustrate fixation of an undisplaced fracture of the lateral condyle of the McIII. A stab incision is made over the lateral condylar fossa and a 4.5-mm hole drilled through to the fracture line. A 3.2-mm hole is drilled beyond this and after countersinking and tapping. A 52-mm or 54-mm cortical bone screw is placed to compress the fracture. Reduction and the condition of the fracture are monitored with arthroscopy, but no reduction is necessary. Repair of nondisplaced fractures is usually done with one or two screws (as illustrated in Figs. 5-57 to 5-61).

The same principles of lag screw fixation through stab incisions are used for the repair of displaced fractures of the lateral condyle of the distal metacarpus. Evaluation of the dorsal compartment of the joint is most important for reduction; this is performed through a standard dorsolateral arthroscopic portal. The technique for repair of a displaced lateral condylar fracture is illustrated in Figures 5-62 and 5-63. Immediate lavage is necessary to clear hemorrhage. Reduction can be effected by two techniques, and sometimes a combination of these is required. The most useful technique is to manipulate the limb as described earlier and, when the fracture is accurately reduced to fix it in this position, by application of large AO/ASIF reduction forceps

laterally and medially at the level of the epicondylar eminence (physeal scar) (Richardson, 2002). The second technique, which may be employed if the first technique alone is inadequate, involves prior creation of the distal glide hole. The location in the epicondylar fossa is made under radiographic guidance, and a 4.5-mm hole is drilled to the fracture plane but not beyond. A 3.2-mm insert sleeve is placed in the hole, and a 3-mm Steinmann pin is inserted. This can then be used as leverage for further reduction. When this is achieved, large AO/ASIF reductions forceps are applied as described earlier. Standard lag screw repair follows (Richardson, 2002; Wright & Nixon, 2013).

Two of the authors (C.W.M. and I.M.W.) use 4.5-mm AO/ASIF cortical screws at all available sites; one author (A.J.N.) uses a 5.5-mm AO/ASIF cortical screw as the distal implant. Fractures that narrow proximally to less than 10-mm depth require 3.5-mm AO/ASIF cortical screws. Use of a countersink is necessary at all locations (Wright & Nixon, 2013).

In some cases, comminution within the fracture plane can preclude reduction. In this instance, an instrument portal is made dorsally directly over the fracture. Instruments are then introduced to effect distraction and removal of obstructing fragments. This can include fragmentation extending throughout the full dorsopalmar/plantar thickness of the bone, including comminution of the palmar/plantar subchondral bone. Once this has been removed, the fracture can be reduced using the techniques described earlier.

Arthroscopy also permits identification and removal of radiologically silent articular comminution in both dorsal and palmar/plantar compartments. When wedge-shaped comminuted fragments of the palmar/plantar subchondral bone are nondisplaced, the authors' preference is conservation and incorporation in fracture repair. In some instances, reduction of the principal fracture will result in expulsion of such fragments. Removal is then inevitable. Displaced fractures are commonly associated with lesions of the lateral proximal sesamoid bone. Some axial fractures can be identified by preoperative radiographs (Barclay et al, 1985; Ellis, 1994; Greet, 1987), but others can be identified only by arthroscopic examination. The authors have also encountered fractures of the basal axial margin of the lateral proximal sesamoid bone and cartilage erosions to the lateral proximal sesamoid bone, which are only identified arthroscopically; both are of therapeutic and prognostic importance.

For further details regarding fracture management and a contemporaneous review of results, the reader is referred to Wright & Nixon (2013). It is not yet possible to determine the contribution of arthroscopy to case outcome from results published to date.

Fractures of the Proximal Phalanx

Sagittal fractures of the proximal phalanx are the second most common long bone fracture in racehorses. Arthroscopy has illustrated the inadequacy of radiography at detecting proximodistal and dorsopalmar/plantar displacement (Fig. 5-64). The authors now consider that it is indicated as part of the evaluation and treatment of all complete parasagittal fractures of the proximal phalanx (i.e., those in which there is any potential for displacement). As with fractures of the lateral condyle of the third metacarpal/metatarsal bone, reduction can be effected by limb manipulation or use of the 3.2-mm sleeve with a 3-mm Steinmann pin inserted, or both. Large AO/ASIF reduction forceps are then applied to fix the fracture, which is compressed with lag screws in a standard technique.

The authors have also used arthroscopy to guide reduction and removal of intraarticular comminution from fractures of the palmar/plantar processes before lag screw repair.

Text continued on p. 172

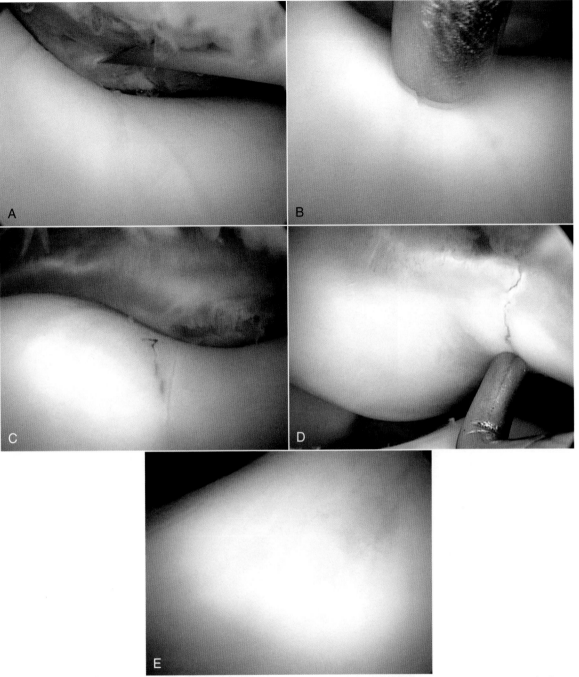

Figure 5-58 Arthroscopic monitoring of condylar fractures. Undisplaced fracture depicted in Figure 5-56A before fixation (**A**) and after fixation (**B**) (note the presence of a fragment off the proximal lateral eminence of the proximal phalanx in **A**). **C,** Arthroscopic view of fracture depicted in Figure 5-56B as screw is tightened with a small amount of blood coming from fracture line. **D,** View in palmar compartment of same fracture after reduction and fixation. **E,** Small superficial lesion on lateral sesamoid bone associated with lateral condylar fracture.

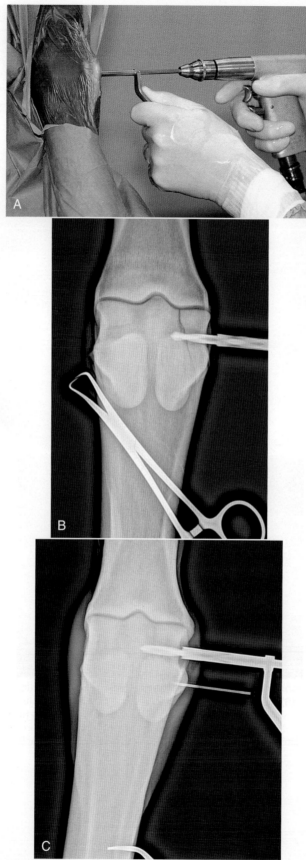

Figure 5-59 A 4.5-mm glide hole is drilled in the lateral condylar fossa. **A,** External view. **B** and **C,** Radiographic views of cases depicted previously in Figure 5-56A and B.

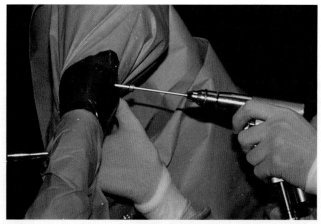

Figure 5-60 A 3.2-mm hole is drilled through the remaining portion of the McIII.

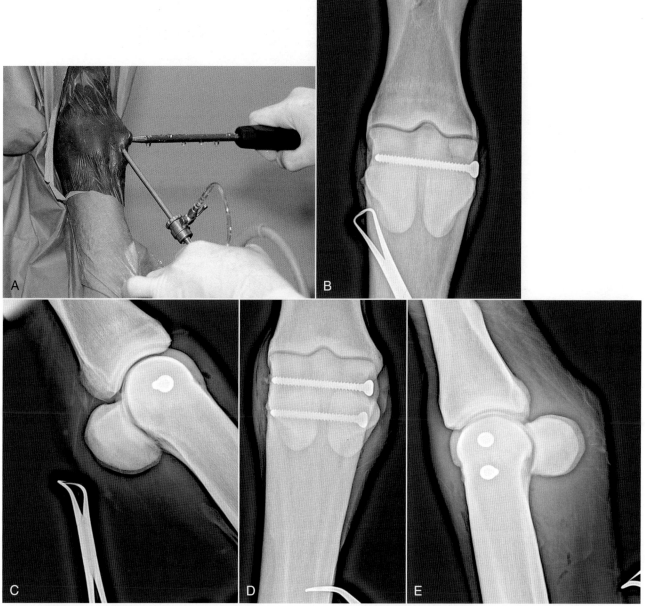

Figure 5-61 Placement of screws to compress undisplaced fracture. **A,** External view. **B** and **C,** Dorsopalmar and lateromedial radiographic views of case depicted in Figure 5-56A. **D** and **E,** Dorsopalmar and lateromedial views of case presented in Figure 5-56B.

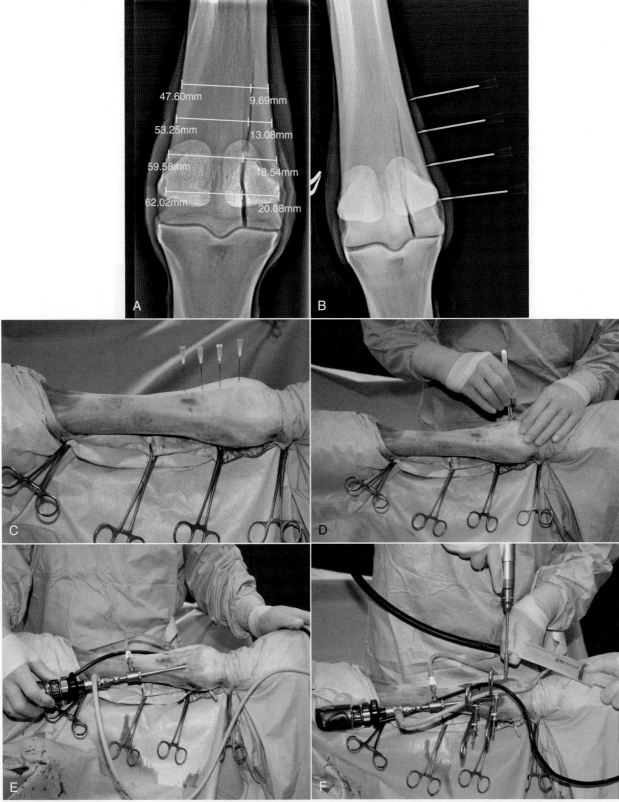

Figure 5-62 ▶ **A,** Dorsopalmar radiograph of a displaced fracture of the lateral condyle of the left McIII depicted in Figure 5-56C and D with a preoperative plan. **B,** Intraoperative radiograph with percutaneous needles at proposed implant site. **C,** External view illustrating needles placed at proposed implant sites. **D,** Making stab incision for distal screw in lateral condylar fossa. **E,** Arthroscope placed in the proximal lateral aspect of the dorsal pouch to assess fracture. **F,** Drilling 4.5-mm glide hole for distal screw.

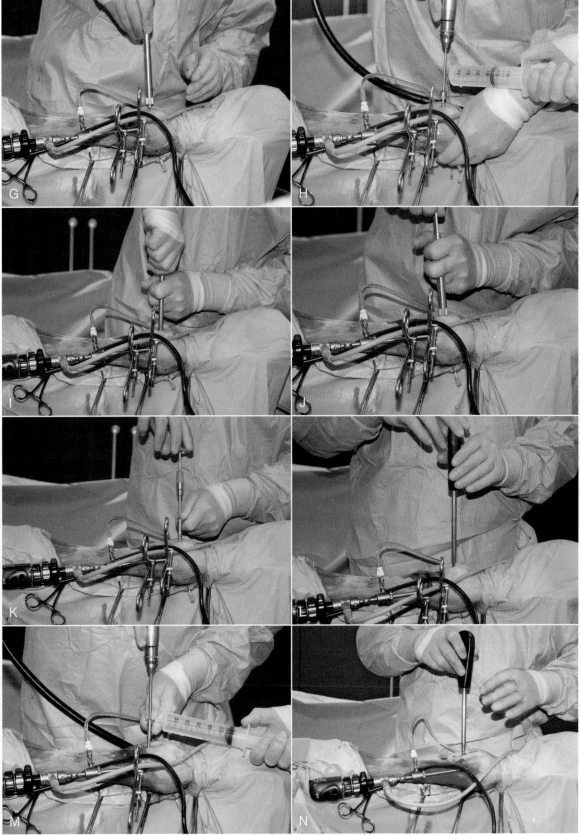

Figure 5-62, cont'd G, Measuring depth of glide hole to ensure it is past fracture site (the other option is to take a radiograph). **H,** Drilling 3.2-mm hole through remaining bone. **I,** Countersinking. **J,** Use of the depth gauge. **K,** Tapping. **L,** Placing screw. **M,** Drilling a second hole. **N,** Placing second screw.

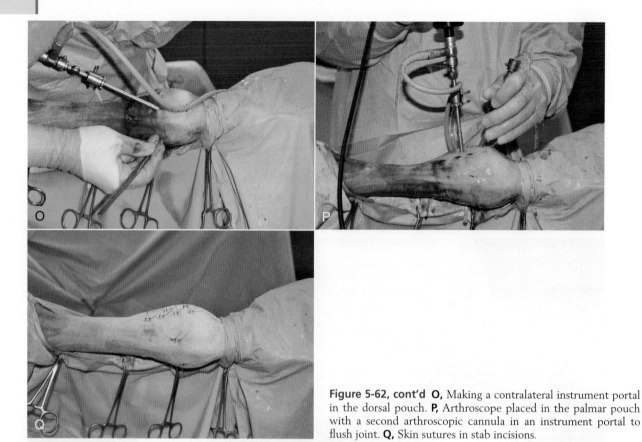

Figure 5-62, cont'd O, Making a contralateral instrument portal in the dorsal pouch. **P,** Arthroscope placed in the palmar pouch with a second arthroscopic cannula in an instrument portal to flush joint. **Q,** Skin sutures in stab incisions.

Figure 5-63 Arthroscopic images of the fracture illustrated in Figures 5-56C and D and 5-62. **A,** Appearance of the fracture from the dorsal aspect following lavage of the joint to remove intraarticular hemorrhage. **B,** Appearance of the dorsal surface of the fracture following reduction by manipulation and application AO/ASIF large reduction forceps. **C,** Dorsal appearance of the fracture at completion of repair. **D,** Palmar aspect of the fracture after completion of repair illustrating a full-thickness defect in the adjacent lateral proximal sesamoid bone.

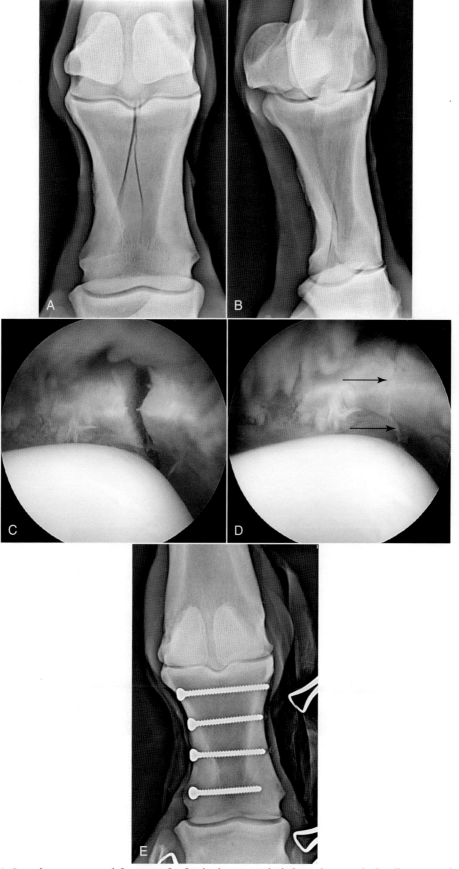

Figure 5-64 Complete parasagittal fracture of a forelimb proximal phalanx that spirals distally to exit through the lateral articular surface. **A** and **B,** Dorsopalmar and dorsolateral-palmaromedial oblique radiographs. **C,** Arthroscopic image demonstrating proximodistal and dorsopalmar displacement that was not detected radiographically. **D,** Arthroscopic image following reduction by manipulation and repair (*arrows* indicate reduced fracture). **E,** Dorsopalmar radiograph at completion of surgery.

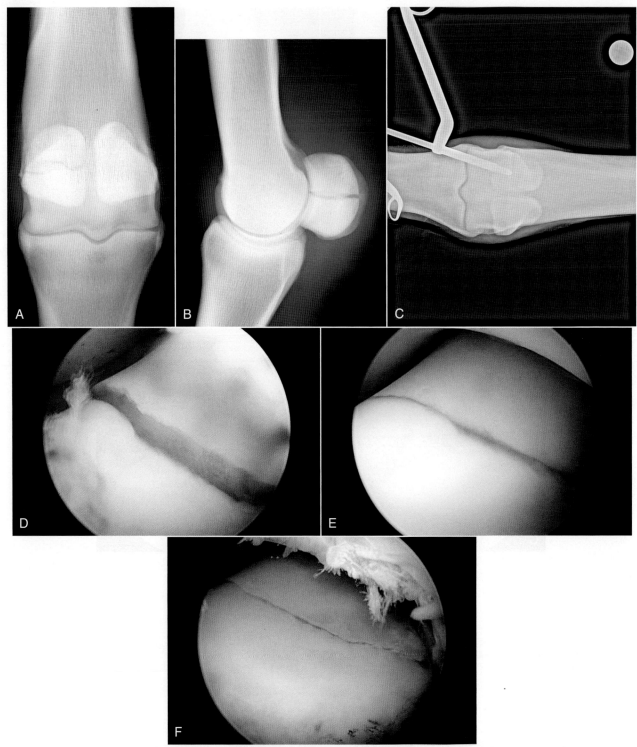

Figure 5-65 Lag screw fixation of midbody fracture of a medial proximal sesamoid bone under arthroscopic visualization. **A,** Dorsopalmar radiograph and **B,** lateromedial radiograph of fracture. **C,** Dorsopalmar radiograph with 4.5-mm drill in the glide hole. Arthroscopic views before **(D),** after reduction with manipulation **(E),** and after placement of a lag screw **(F).**

Repair of Proximal Sesamoid Bone Fractures

A technique for arthroscopically guided repair of midbody proximal sesamoid bone fractures has been reported by Busschers et al (2008), who described insertion of a single 4.5-mm AO/ ASIF cortical screw with a distal to proximal trajectory. The technique is illustrated in Figure 5-65. The center of the base of the proximal sesamoid bone is located, and drill trajectory determined by a percutaneous needle (18 gauge/1.2 mm × 3.5 inch/85 mm) past palmar/plantar to the neurovascular bundle through the distal sesamoidean ligaments. This position is assessed and modified by radiographic/fluoroscopic examinations in dorsopalmar/plantar and lateromedial planes. A short (stab) incision is then made along this line at the base of the bone before a 4.5-mm drill guide is passed and, if required, its position also confirmed radiographically. A glide hole is then created to the fracture plane, a 3-mm Steinmann pin inserted,

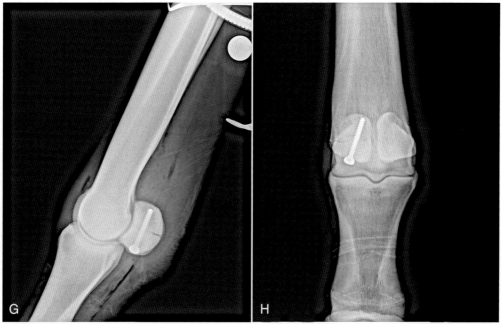

Figure 5-65, cont'd Postoperative lateromedial **(G)** and lateromedial and dorsopalmar **(H)** radiographs.

and a 3.2-mm sleeve passed over the pin. A long sleeve is necessary because the skin to fracture plane distance in horses of more than 400-kg body weight is usually greater than 50 mm. The articular surface is evaluated from an ipsilateral proximal arthroscopic portal. Removal of comminuted fragments and debridement of the fracture can be performed as needed through an instrument portal created at the level of the fracture. Fracture reduction is achieved by a combination of joint flexion and manipulation using the 3.2-mm sleeve and contained Steinmann pin. Once satisfactory, the pin is withdrawn and a 3.2-mm hole drilled in the apical fragment, taking care to minimize protrusion of the drill bit into the suspensory ligament insertion. Additional stability for this process can be provided by prior application of large AO/ASIF reduction forceps. Standard lag screw insertion follows. The base of the proximal sesamoid bone is concave dorsal to palmar/plantar and is centrally concave mediolaterally. The authors did not report or discuss the desirability of countersinking screw heads. This is necessarily a balance between optimizing the conditions for the implant and minimizing trauma to the distal sesamoidean ligaments. The authors favor judicious use. The depth of soft tissue precludes accurate use of the depth gauge. In nondisplaced fractures the length of the affected proximal sesamoid bone and in displaced fractures the length of its intact contralateral counterpart along the trajectory of the implant are the best determinants of screw size. Intraoperative radiographic monitoring is essential throughout. The authors describe use of this technique in 10 horses and a further 6 repaired by arthrotomy. Eleven of 16 (44%) of horses raced after surgery.

The authors have used a modification of this technique for the repair of basilar fractures of the proximal sesamoid bones using 4.5-mm and 3.5-mm AO/ASIF cortical screws. Some apical/abaxial fractures of proximal sesamoid bones can also be reduced and repaired under arthroscopic guidance with 3.5-mm or 2.7-mm AO/ASIF cortical screws, or both.

REFERENCES

Barclay WP, Foerner JJ, Phillips TN: Axial sesamoid injuries associated with lateral condylar fractures in horses, *J Am Vet Med Assoc* 186:278–279, 1985.

Barclay WP, Foerner JJ, Phillips TN: Lameness attributable to osteochondral fragmentation of the plantar aspect of the proximal phalanx in horses: 19 cases (1981-1985), *J Am Vet Med Assoc* 191:855–857, 1987.

Birkeland R: Chip fractures of the first phalanx in the metatarsophalangeal joint of the horse, *Acta Radiol (Suppl)* 29:73–77, 1972.

Bouré L, Marcoux M, Laverty S, Lepage OM: Use of electrocautery probes in arthroscopic removal of apical sesamoid fracture fragments in 18 Standardbred horses, *Vet Surg* 28:226–232, 1999.

Bramlage LR: Osteochondrosis-related bone cysts, *Proc AAEP* 39:83–85, 1993.

Busschers E, Richardson DW, Hogan PM, Leitch M: Surgical repair of mid-body proximal sesamoid bone fractures in 25 horses, *Vet Surg* 37:771–780, 2008.

Byron CR, Goetz TE: Arthroscopic debridement of a palmar third metacarpal condyle subchondral bone injury in Standardbred, *Equine Vet Educ* 19:344–347, 2007.

Carlsten J, Sandgren B, Dalin G: Development of osteochondrosis in the tarsocrural joint and osteochondral fragments in the fetlock joints of Standardbred Trotters. 1. A radiological survey, *Equine Vet J Suppl* 16:42–47, 1993.

Colon JL, Bramlage LR, Hance SR, Embertson RM: Qualitative and quantative documentation of the racing performance of 461 Thoroughbred racehorses after arthroscopic removal of dorsoproximal first phalanx osteochondral fractures (1986–1995), *Equine Vet J* 32:475–481, 2000.

Cullimore AM, Finnie JW, Marmion WJ, Booth TM: Severe lameness associated with an impact fracture of the proximal phalanx in a filly, *Equine Vet Educ* 21:247–251, 2009.

Dabareiner RM, Watkins JP, Carter GK, et al.: Osteitis of the axial border of the proximal sesamoid bones in horses: eight case (1993-1999), *J Am Vet Med Assoc* 219:82–86, 2001.

Dabareiner RM, White NA, Sullins KE: Metacarpophalangeal joint synovial pad fibrotic proliferation in 63 horses, *Vet Surg* 25:199–206, 1996.

Dalin G, Sandgren B, Carlsten J: Plantar osteochondral fragments in the metatarsophalangeal joints in Standardbred trotters; result of osteochondrosis or trauma? *Equine Vet J* 16(Suppl):62–65, 1993.

Declercq J, Martens A, Bogaert L, Boussauw B, Forsyth R, Boening KJ: Osteochondral fragmentation in the synovial pad of the fetlock in Warmblood horses, *Vet Surg* 37:613–618, 2008.

Declercq J, Martens A, Maes D, Boussauw B, Forsyth R, Boening KJ: Dorsoproximal proximal phalanx osteochondral fragmentation in 117 Warmblood horses, *Vet Comp Orthop Traumatol* 22:1–6, 2009.

Elce Y, Richardson DW: Arthroscopic removal of dorsoproximal chip fractures of the proximal phalanx in standing horses, *Vet Surg* 31:195–200, 2002.

Ellis DR: Some observation in condylar fractures of the third metacarpus and third metatarsus in young Thoroughbreds, *Equine Vet J* 26:178–183, 1994.

Foerner JJ: Osteochondral fragments of the palmar and plantar aspects of the fetlock joint, *Proceedings of the 33rd Annual Meeting of the American Association of Equine Practitioners* 739–744, 1987.

Fortier LA, Foerner JJ, Nixon AJ: Arthroscopic removal of axial osteochondral fragments of the plantar/palmar proximal aspect of the proximal phalanx in horses: 119 cases (1988-1992), *J Am Vet Med Assoc* 206:71–74, 1995.

Greet TRC: Condylar fracture of the cannon bone with axial sesamoid fracture in three bones, *Vet Rec* 120:223–225, 1987.

Haynes PF: Diseases of the metacarpophalangeal joint, *Vet Clin North Am (Large Anim Pract)* 2:37–49, 1980.

Hogan PM, McIlwraith CW, Honnas CM, Watkins JP, Bramlage LR: Surgical treatment of subchondral cystic lesions of the third metacarpal bone: results in 15 horses (1986-1994), *Equine Vet J* 29:477–482, 1997.

Hornof WH, O'Brien TR, Poole RR: Osteochondritis dissecans of the distal metacarpus in the adult racing Thoroughbred horse, *Vet Radiol* 22:98–106, 1981.

Jacklin B, Wright IM: Frequency distributions of 174 fractures of the distal condyles of the third metacarpal and metatarsal bones in 167 Thoroughbred racehorses (1999-2009), *Equine Vet J* 44:707–713, 2012.

Jaffe HL, Lichtenstein L, Sutro CS: Pigmented villonodular synovitis, bursitis, and tenosynovitis, *Arch Pathol* 31:731–765, 1941.

Kamm JL, Bramlage LR, Schnabel LV, Ruggles AJ, Embertson RM, Hopper SA: Size and geometry of apical sesamoid fracture fragments as a determinant of prognosis in Thoroughbred racehorses, *Equine Vet J* 43:412–417, 2011.

Kannegieter NJ: Chronic proliferative synovitis of the equine metacarpophalangeal joint, *Vet Rec* 127:8–10, 1990.

Kawcak CE, McIlwraith CW: Proximodorsal first phalanx osteochondral chip fragmentation in 336 horses, *Equine Vet J* 26:392–396, 1994.

Kawcak CE, McIlwraith CW, Norrdin RW, Park RD, Steyn PS: Clinical effects of exercise on subchondral bone of carpal and metacarpophalangeal joints in horses, *Am J Vet Res* 61:1252–1258, 2000.

LoSasso MB, Honnas CM: Chronic proliferated synovitis in a horse, *Equine Pract* 16:29–32, 1994.

McIlwraith CW: Subchondral cystic lesions (osteochondrosis) in the horse, *Comp Cont Educ Pract Vet* 4:282S–291S, 1982.

McIlwraith CW: Experience in diagnostic and surgical arthroscopy in the horse, *Equine Vet J* 16:11–19, 1984.

McIlwraith CW: *Diagnostic and surgical arthroscopy in the horse*, ed 2, Philadelphia, 1990a, Lea & Febiger.

McIlwraith CW: Subchondral cystic lesions in the horse – the indications, methods, and results of surgery, *Equine Vet Educ* 2:75–80, 1990b.

McIlwraith CW: Osteochondritis dissecans of the metacarpophalangeal and metatarsophalangeal (fetlock) joints. Proceedings 39th AAEP Convention. 63–67, 1993.

McIlwraith CW: Arthroscopic surgery for osteochondral chip fragments and other lesions not requiring internal fixation in the carpal and fetlock joints of the equine athlete: What have we learned in 20 years? *Clin Tech Equine Pract* 1:200–210, 2002.

McIlwraith CW, Vorhees M: *Management of osteochondritis dissecans of the dorsal aspect of the distal metacarpus and metatarsus. Proceedings 35th AAEP Annual Convention.* 547–550, 1990.

Meagher DM: Joint surgery in the horse: the selection of surgical cases and consideration of the alternatives. Proceedings of the 20th Annual Meeting of the American Association of Equine Practitioners, 1974, Las Vegas.

Minshall GM, Wright IM: Arthroscopic diagnosis and treatment of intra-articular insertional injuries of the suspensory ligament branch in 18 horses, *Equine Vet J* 38:10–14, 2006.

Misheff MM, Alexander GR, Hirst GR: Management of fractures in endurance horses, *Equine Vet Educ* 22:623–630, 2010.

Misheff MM, Stover SM: A comparison of two techniques for arthrocentesis of the equine metacarpophalangeal joint, *Equine Vet J* 23:273–276, 1991.

Murphy DJ, Nixon AJ: Arthroscopic laser extirpation of metacarpophalangeal synovial pad proliferation in 11 horses, *Equine Vet J* 33:296–301, 2001.

Nickels FK, Grant BD, Lincoln SD: Villonodular synovitis of the equine metacarpophalangeal joint, *J Am Vet Med Assoc* 168:1043–1046, 1976.

Nixon AJ: Osteochondrosis and osteochondritis dissecans of the equine fetlock, *Compend Cont Educ Pract Vet* 12:1463–1475, 1990.

Nixon AJ, Pool RR: Histologic appearance of axial osteochondral fragments from the proximoplantar/proximopalmar aspect of the proximal phalanx in horses, *J Am Vet Med Assoc* 207:1076–1080, 1995.

Pettersson H, Ryden G: Avulsion fractures of the caudoproximal extremity of the first phalanx, *Equine Vet* 14:333–335, 1982.

Raker CW: Orthopedic surgery: errors in surgical evaluation and management. Proceedings of the 19th Annual Meeting of the American Association of Equine Practitioners, 1973, Denver.

Richardson DW: Arthroscopically assisted repair of articular fractures, *Clin Tech Equine Pract* 1:211–217, 2002.

Sandgren B, Dalin G, Carlsten J: Osteochondrosis in the tarsocrural joint and osteochondral fragments in the fetlock joints in Standardbred Trotters. 1, *Epidemiology. Equine Vet J Suppl* 16:31–37, 1993.

Schnabel LV, Bramlage LR, Mohammed HO, Embertson RM, Ruggles AJ, Hopper SA: Racing performance after arthroscopic removal of apical sesamoid fracture fragments in Thoroughbred horses age >2 years: 84 cases (1989-2002), *Equine Vet Educ* 38:446–451, 2006.

Schnabel LV, Bramlage LR, Mohammed HO, Embertson RM, Ruggles AJ, Hopper SA: Racing performance after arthroscopic removal of apical sesamoid fracture fragments in Thoroughbred horses age <2 years; 151 cases (1989-2002), *Equine Vet Educ* 39:64–68, 2007.

Sherman KM, Myhre GD, Heymann EI: Fungal osteomyelitis of the axial border of the proximal sesamoid bones in a horse, *JAVMA* 229:1607–1611, 2006.

Simon O, Laverty S, Boure L, Marcoux M, Scoke M: Arthroscopic removal of axial osteochondral fragments of the proximoplantar aspect of the proximal phalanx using electrocautery probes in 23 Standardbred racehorses, *Vet Surg* 33:422–427, 2004.

Southwood LL, McIlwraith CW: Arthroscopic removal of fracture fragments involving a portion of the base of the proximal sesamoid bone in horses: 26 cases (1984-1997), *J Am Vet Med Assoc* 217:236–240, 2000.

Southwood LL, McIlwraith CW, Trotter GW, et al.: Arthroscopic removal of apical fractures of the proximal sesamoid bone in horses: 98 cases (1989-1999), *Proc AAEP* 46:100–101, 2000.

Southwood LL, Trotter GW, McIlwraith CW: Arthroscopic removal of abaxial fracture fragments of the proximal sesamoid bones in horses: 47 cases (1989-1997), *J Am Vet Med Assoc* 213:1016–1021, 1998.

Steyn PF, Schmidt D, Watkins J, et al.: The sonographic diagnosis of chronic proliferative synovitis in the metacarpophalangeal joint of a horse, *Vet Radiol* 3:125–138, 1989.

van Veenendaal JC, Moffatt RE: Soft tissue masses in the fetlock joint of horses, *Aust Vet J* 56:533–536, 1980.

Vanderperren K, Martens Haers H, Duchateau L, Saunders JH: Arthroscopic visualization of the third metacarpal and metatarsal condyles in the horse, *Equine Vet J* 41:526–533, 2009.

Wallis TW, Goodrich LR, McIlwraith CW, Frisbie DD, Hendrickson DA, Trotter GW, Baxter GM, Kawcak CE: Arthroscopic injection of corticosteroids into the fibrous tissue of subchondral cystic lesions of the medial femoral condyle in horses: a retrospective study of 52 cases (2001-2006), *Equine Vet J* 40:461–467, 2008.

White NA: Synovial pad proliferation in the metacarpophalangeal joint. In White NA, Moore JN, editors: *Current practice of equine surgery*, Philadelphia, 1990, Lippincott, pp 550–558.

Whitton RC, Kannegieter J: Osteochondral fragmentation of the plantar/palmar aspect of the proximal phalanx in racing horses, *Aust Vet J* 71:318–321, 1994.

Woodie JB, Ruggles AJ, Bertone AL, Hardy J, Schneider RK: Apical fractures of the proximal sesamoid bone in Standardbred horses: 43 cases (1990-1996), *J Am Vet Med Assoc* 214:1653–1656, 1999.

Wright IM, Nixon AJ: Fractures of the condyles of the third metacarpal and metatarsal bones. In Nixon AJ, editor: *Equine Fracture Repair*, ed 2, Philadelphia, 2013, WB Saunders.

Yovich JV, McIlwraith CW: Arthroscopic surgery for osteochondral fractures of the proximal phalanx of the metacarpophalangeal and metatarsophalangeal (fetlock) joints in horses, *J Am Vet Med Assoc* 188:273–279, 1986.

Yovich JV, McIlwraith CW, Stashak TS: Osteochondritis dissecans of the sagittal ridge of the third metacarpal and metatarsal bones in horses, *J Am Vet Med Assoc* 186:1186–1191, 1985.

CHAPTER 6

Diagnostic and Surgical Arthroscopy of the Femoropatellar and Femorotibial Joints

During the genesis of previous editions of this text, arthroscopy became a most important technique for diagnosis, as well as for surgery in the femoropatellar and femorotibial joints (Foland et al, 1992; Lewis, 1987; Martin & McIlwraith, 1985; McIlwraith & Martin, 1984; Moustafa et al 1987; Nickels & Sande, 1982; Walmsley, 2002; Walmsley et al 2003). This progress has continued with development and refinement of techniques and increased clinical experience (Barrett et al, 2012; Cohen et al, 2009; Hendrix et al, 2010; Muurlink, et al 2009; McNally et al, 2011; Sparks et al, 2011b; Vinardell et al, 2008; Wallis et al, 2008; Watts and Nixon, 2006). Diagnostic and surgical arthroscopy techniques for each joint are presented in this chapter.

DIAGNOSTIC ARTHROSCOPY OF THE FEMOROPATELLAR JOINT

Insertion of the Arthroscope into the Femoropatellar Joint

The horse is positioned in dorsal recumbency with the leg in extension. If both legs are involved, each leg should remain flexed when not being examined. This positioning reduces the chance of postoperative femoral nerve paresis or quadriceps myopathy. Alternatively, the legs may be elevated and tied back so that tension is not concentrated on the quadriceps muscles.

The skin incision for the usual arthroscopic portal is located between the middle and lateral patellar ligaments and halfway between the tibial crest and the distal aspect of the patella (Fig. 6-1). This arthroscopic portal allows a complete diagnostic

examination of the femoropatellar joint, as well as fulfilling all needs for observation during surgical manipulations. An 8-mm stab incision is made through the skin, superficial fascia, and deep fascia into the femoropatellar fat pad (see Fig. 6-1B). The sleeve and conical obturator are manipulated through the stab incision in the skin and fascia and then angled 45 degrees to the skin in a proximal direction (Fig. 6-2). The femoropatellar joint space is entered by gently manipulating the obturator and arthroscope sleeve under the patella and over the femoral trochlea. This maneuver may be facilitated by elevation of the distal limb. If resistance is encountered, the sleeve and obturator are not forced but are directed more laterally to lie under the lateral part of the patella facet and over the lateral trochlear ridge (LTR) of the femur. At this location, the patella can be displaced further from the trochlear ridge, which allows the sleeve to slide proximally more easily.

When the sleeve is positioned to the hilt, the obturator is removed and replaced with the arthroscope. The light cable and ingress fluid line are attached and the joint is distended. Figure 6-3 demonstrates the position of the arthroscopic sheath at the completion of insertion, and the diagrams in Figure 6-4 show the position of the arthroscope at the beginning of the diagnostic examination.

▶ Normal Arthroscopic Anatomy

The suprapatellar pouch is the first area of the joint visible when the arthroscopic sleeve is situated beneath the patella and rests in the intertrochlear groove (see Fig. 6-4). This is capacious, but the lining synovial membrane can be visualized on all surfaces of the pouch (Fig. 6-5). The proximal extent

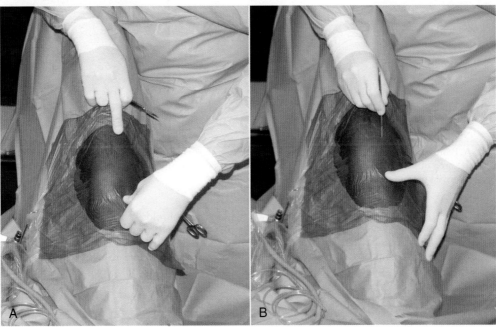

Figure 6-1 **A,** Adhesive drape is in place and landmarks are identified with surgeon's right finger indicating junction of middle patellar ligaments and proximal tibia and left thumb indicating distal patella junction with middle patellar ligament in left femoropatellar joint. **B,** Skin incision for arthroscopic portal is made midway between these points.

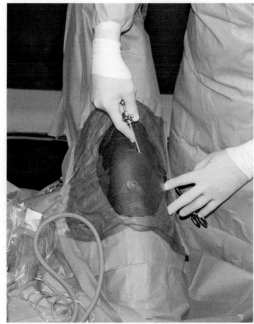

Figure 6-2 Manipulation of the arthroscopic sleeve and blunt obturator under the patella.

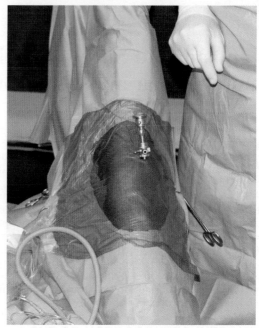

Figure 6-3 Completion of insertion of the arthroscopic sheath in the femoropatellar joint.

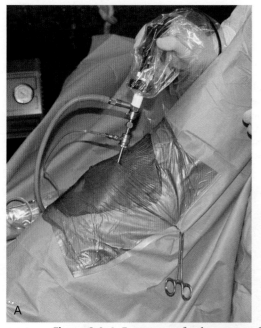

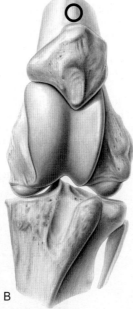

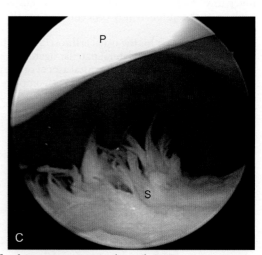

Figure 6-4 A, Positioning of arthroscope in femoropatellar joint with tip of arthroscope in proximal pouch. **B,** Diagram showing visual area of arthroscope. **C,** Arthroscopic view of circled area of proximal pouch of femoropatellar joint. *P,* Patella; *S,* synovial membrane.

of the suprapatellar pouch may be poorly illuminated with low-output light sources.

The articular surface of the patella and intertrochlear groove can be visualized by withdrawing the arthroscope from this position (see Fig. 6-5). Specific examination of each area can be achieved by rotating the arthroscope. The suprapatellar pouch disappears from view as the arthroscope is withdrawn, and eventually the tension of the patellar ligaments abruptly forces the arthroscope out from beneath the patella. At this stage, the distal apex of the patella is visualized resting in the intertrochlear groove (see Fig. 6-5). A fringe of villous synovium usually overhangs the distal margin of the patella.

Longitudinal folds or ridges are often observed in the central part of the intertrochlear groove and are apparently normal, particularly in the more distal regions of the groove.

The medial trochlear ridge (MTR) and the medial aspect of the distal patella can be visualized by rotating the arthroscope and directing the angled field of view toward the medial aspect of the joint (see Fig. 6-5). Despite joint distention, the patella and MTR are more closely apposed than their lateral counterparts. The MTR is examined by moving the distal end of the arthroscope carefully along the length of the ridge (the eyepiece of the arthroscope is moving proximally during this maneuver) (see Fig. 6-5). This will also visualize the medial

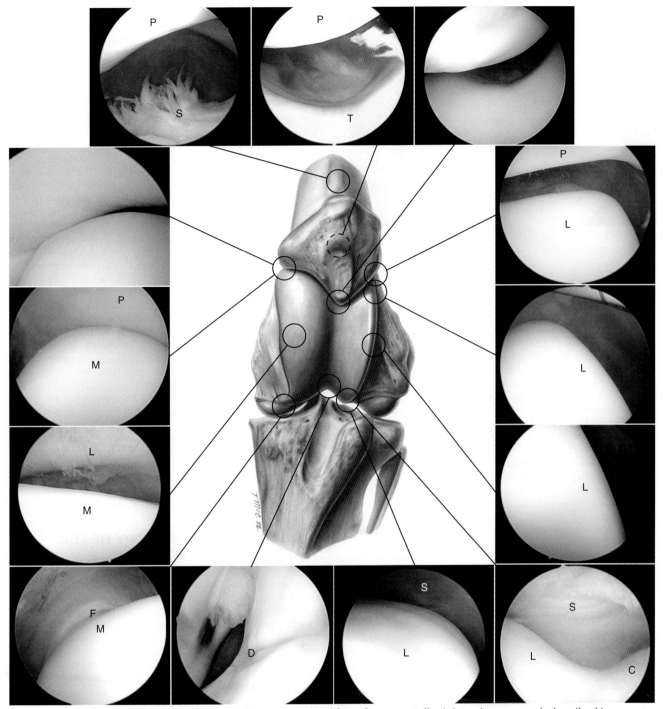

Figure 6-5 Composite of arthroscopic images obtained from femoropatellar joint using approach described in Figure 6-4. *F,* Fossa between distal aspect of medial trochlear ridge and medial femoral condyle; *L,* lateral trochlear ridge of femur; *M,* medial trochlear ridge of femur; *P,* patella; *S,* synovial membrane; *T and TG,* trochlear groove of femur.

patellar fibrocartilage and conjoined medial patellar ligament. Advancing the arthroscope over the MTR and viewing caudally, one can view the synovial recess beyond the MTR. In some cases, a fold of synovial membrane overlies the distal extremity of the MTR (see Fig. 6-5). If this fold is elevated, a communication into the medial femorotibial joint may be apparent: This communication can permit the passage of the arthroscope and visualization of the cranial aspect of the medial condyle.

The arthroscope is returned to the proximal aspect of the MTR and is rotated laterally and across the intertrochlear groove to the LTR (see Fig. 6-5). With fluid distention, the patella is separated from the LTR. This facilitates examination of the proximal aspect of the LTR, as well as the undersurface of the patella, and also allows advancement of the arthroscope proximally into the suprapatellar pouch without risk of damage to the articular surfaces (as mentioned previously, this is the reason why moving the arthroscope sleeve

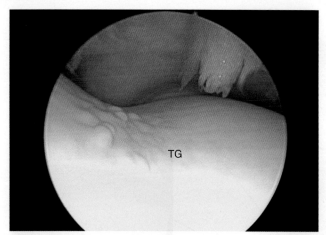

Figure 6-6 Arthroscopic views of commonly seen raised areas in distal aspect of trochlear groove of femur.

laterally facilitates initial entry of the arthroscope into the joint). The synovial membrane in the lateral aspect of the joint adjacent to the area of articulation of the LTR and distal patella is smooth and nonvillous (see Fig. 6-5), but it becomes quite villous distal to this point. The entire length of the LTR is then explored by moving the distal end of the arthroscope distad and advancing the arthroscope further into the joint as needed (see Fig. 6-5). This maneuver involves moving the eyepiece of the arthroscope medially and proximally. The synovial membrane is villous adjacent to the distal one-half of the LTR (see Fig. 6-5), and fluid distention is often critical to allow a clear view of this area. The trochlear ridge is examined until the synovial reflection of the distal extremity is encountered (see Fig. 6-5). In the event of the view being obscured by hypertrophied synovial villi, viewing of a specific area of the trochlear ridges can be improved with gradual flexion. As the arthroscope is moved axially from the LTR, the distal aspect of the intertrochlear groove can be examined. Irregular cartilaginous protuberances and creases are commonly seen and are considered normal (Fig. 6-6).

An arthroscopic approach has been described for the equine suprapatellar pouch (SPP) (Vinardell et al, 2008). An experimental study with 24 cadaveric equine femoropatellar joints and a retrospective clinical study in five horses concluded that the optimal arthroscopic portal was located approximately 10 cm lateral to the longitudinal patellar axis and 2 cm proximal to the patellar base corresponding to the intermuscular septum between the biceps femoris and vastus lateralis muscles. The approach allowed arthroscopic observation of the proximal aspect of the lateral and medial femoral trochlear ridges, the intertrochlear groove, the patella base, and the synovial recess of the SPP. Additional arthroscopic and instrument suprapatellar portals were used in 5 of 25 horses to complete lavage or debridement, or both, in osteochondritis dissecans (OCD) and septic arthritis. The authors concluded that suprapatellar arthroscopy improved arthroscopic observations of structures located proximally in the femoropatellar joint and facilitated surgical access to the SPP. The authors also considered it a safe and complementary approach to the traditional distal arthroscopic portal and could be helpful for inspection and removal of free fragments/debris/fibrin located in the SPP, for OCD lesions extending proximally, and for fractures involving the proximal aspect of the patella.

It should be noted that a suprapatellar instrument portal has been used regularly for removal of large fragments and debris located in the SSP, usually after debridement of OCD lesions (McIlwraith et al, 2005). A more recent paper has described placing a 10-mm diameter laparoscopic cannula and

trocar unit in this portal to make removal of debris or loose fragments easier (McNally et al, 2011). The use of this portal will be revisited when discussing arthroscopic surgery for OCD. It has also been recognized by one of the authors (AJN) that this portal is more prone to fibrosis after surgery, which generally self-resolves but can be alarming for several months.

Diagnostic Arthroscopy of Clinical Conditions

The primary indication for arthroscopy of the femoropatellar joint has been in cases of OCD. Surgical intervention for this condition is discussed in a separate section. Arthroscopic surgery also has value in cases of distal patellar fragmentation and patellar fractures. Diagnostic arthroscopy of the femoropatellar joint is also performed in cases of persistent femoropatellar effusion in which the radiographic changes are equivocal or absent. Ultrasound has also been proposed as a useful adjunct to radiography for diagnosing OCD lesions in the femoropatellar joint, especially in cases of high clinical suspicion but equivocal radiographic findings (Bourzac et al, 2009). In some cases of diagnostic arthroscopy, cartilage lesions may be seen on the articular surface of the patella; these cannot be imaged ultrasonographically. Some appear to be cases of OCD, but in others the changes are consistent with what is described as chondromalacia in the human knee. The pathogenesis and significance of such an entity in the horse is still uncertain. If such changes in the articular cartilage are visualized, the pathologic area is debrided (chondroplasty) and clinical improvement has occurred after such treatment in equine patients.

The use of the probe in evaluating all cartilage lesions, particularly those of OCD, cannot be overemphasized. The portal for a probe can be made virtually anywhere in the femoropatellar joint because there are no adjacent tendon sheaths and bursae. The usual locations for instrument portals when operating on lesions at various positions within the femoropatellar joint are presented subsequently. These portals are also sites for probe entry. Surgeons can ascertain optimal sites for probe penetration by inserting an 18-gauge 1.5-inch needle into the joint to determine if the site and angle are satisfactory.

DIAGNOSTIC ARTHROSCOPY OF THE FEMOROTIBIAL JOINTS

The femorotibial articulation has two noncommunicating compartments: medial and lateral femorotibial joints, each divided into a communicating cranial and caudal pouch by the articulation of the femur, tibia, and the fibrocartilagenous menisci. The caudal pouch of the lateral femorotibial joint is further divided into a proximal and distal pouch by the tendon of the popliteal muscle (Edwards and Nixon, 1996; Trumble et al, 1994). Because of its small size and considerable extraarticular soft tissue stability, there are limitations to arthroscopic exploration compared with the human knee. Because of these limitations, arthroscopic approaches to both cranial and caudal pouches of the femorotibial joints have been developed. The central part of the joint remains essentially inaccessible unless the collateral ligaments are disrupted (Desjardins and Hurtig, 1991).

Insertion of the Arthroscope into the Cranial Pouch of the Medial Femorotibial Joint

The horse is positioned in dorsal recumbency with the leg in flexion (approximately 90 degrees at hock and stifle). The leg is surgically prepared and draped. Three approaches have been used for diagnostic arthroscopy of the medial femorotibial joint: cranial (Moustafa et al, 1987), lateral (Lewis, 1987), and craniolateral (Nickels & Sande, 1982). All approaches provide an effective examination of the cranial part of the medial femorotibial joint. The authors use the first two approaches, and they are described. The cranial approach allows more consistent examination of the intercondylar (cruciate) area. On the

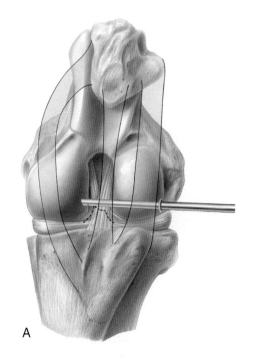

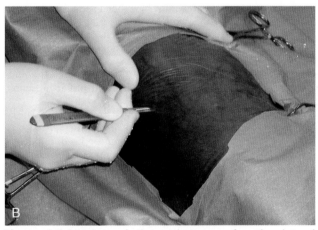

Figure 6-7 Position of the arthroscope for the lateral approach to the medial femorotibial joint. **A,** Diagram and **B,** external view showing location of arthroscope portal.

other hand, the lateral approach leaves a clear area cranially for instrument placement when operating on medial condylar lesions.

Lateral Approach. The site of the arthroscopic portal is caudal to the lateral patellar ligament, cranial to the long digital extensor tendon, and 2 cm proximal to the tibial spine (Lewis, 1987) (Fig. 6-7). The arthroscopic cannula with conical obturator in place is then directed medially and slightly caudad to penetrate the synovial membrane in the lateral aspect of the medial femorotibial joint (Fig. 6-8A). The obturator is removed and the arthroscope is inserted. After checking that the arthroscope is in the cranial compartment (Fig. 6-8B), the joint is distended, and the examination begins (see Fig. 6-9).

▶ *Cranial Approach.* The medial femorotibial joint may be distended with sterile fluid through an 18-gauge needle inserted cranially, but the authors generally find this unnecessary. A skin incision is made and continued through the fascia between the middle and medial patellar ligament about 2 cm proximal to the tibial crest. The arthroscopic sleeve containing the conical obturator is then inserted through the fat pad in a slightly proximad, caudad, and axial direction until it penetrates the medial femorotibial joint capsule (Fig. 6-10). The arthroscope is then inserted and the examination can begin (Fig. 6-11).

Approach to the Cranial Pouch of the Medial Femorotibial Joint from the Femoropatellar Joint

This technique was originally described by Boening (1995) and subsequently reported in the United States by Peroni & Stick (2002). A longer arthroscope is preferred for this technique. The femoropatellar joint is entered through the normally described portal between the lateral and middle patellar ligaments, midway between the patellar and tibial crests. The slitlike openings communicating with the medial femorotibial and, in some cases, the lateral femorotibial joints can be dissected open with a knife or arthroscopic scissors to create a window between the respective femorotibial joint and the femoropatellar joint. This allows arthroscopic access to the femorotibial joints. This approach provides a good view of the axial aspect of the femorotibial joints, but examination further laterally and medially is limited. It is not used by the authors.

Normal Arthroscopic Anatomy of the Cranial Compartment of the Medial Femorotibial Joint

Whether using a lateral or cranial arthroscopic approach, the medial intercondylar eminence of the tibia and axial side of

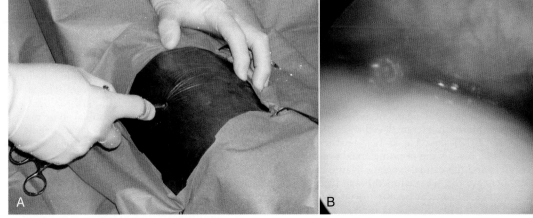

Figure 6-8 A, Manipulation of the arthroscopic sleeve and conical obturator into the medial femorotibial joint. **B,** Confirmation of entry into joint before distention.

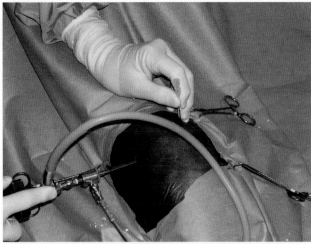

Figure 6-9 Positioning of the arthroscope in the medial femorotibial joint (lateral approach) and use of spinal needle to ascertain ideal position for cranial instrument portal.

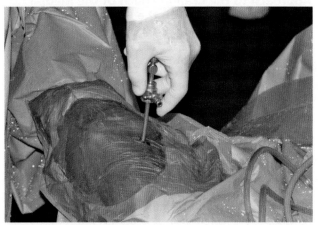

Figure 6-10 Manipulation of the arthroscopic sleeve and blunt obturator into the medial femorotibial joint using a cranial approach.

the medial condyle of the femur can be easily located in the distal medial aspect of the joint and used as reference points (Fig. 6-12). The cranial ligament of the medial meniscus and the cranial portion of the medial meniscus are visible by moving the arthroscope medially along the distal aspect of the medial condyle of the femur (see Fig. 6-12).

The tip of the arthroscope is retracted to the center of the joint, and the arthroscope is rotated upward to visualize the central weight-bearing area of the medial condyle of the femur (see Fig. 6-12). Visualization of the medial and cranial aspects of the medial condyle of the femur may be facilitated by some extension of the joint (see Fig. 6-12). Visualization of the medial collateral ligament is usually possible (consistently possible with a cranial arthroscopic approach) (Barrett et al, 2012) (see Fig. 6-12). Further retraction of the arthroscope reveals the proximal axial portion of the medial condyle and the caudal cruciate ligament running proximodistal beneath the synovial membrane (see Fig. 6-12). The cranial cruciate ligament is subsynovial and axial (lateral) to the medial tibial eminence. A better view of the cruciate ligaments can be obtained with the cranial approach, but a more complete examination can be done

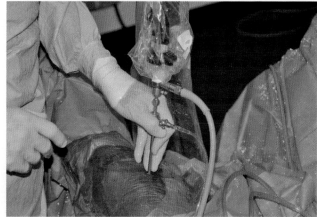

Figure 6-11 Positioning of the arthroscope in the medial femorotibial joint (cranial approach).

with either approach following resection of the interarticular septum.

Insertion of the Arthroscope into the Cranial Compartment of the Lateral Femorotibial Joint

Medial approaches to this joint have been described by both Nickels & Sande (1982) and Moustafa et al (1987) and are favored over a cranial or a lateral approach. Attempts to create a direct lateral portal are inhibited by the lateral collateral ligament and the lateral patellar ligament and by the tendon of origin of the long digital extensor. A portal between the middle and lateral patellar ligaments can be used, but arthroscopic manipulation is limited.

If evaluation of the cranial compartment of the lateral femorotibial joint follows evaluation of the medial femorotibial joint using a lateral portal, this can be used. Fluids are switched off, and the arthroscope and cannula are withdrawn into the intraarticular septum. The scope is then replaced by a conical obturator, and this is withdrawn a further few millimeters before the operator's hand is moved axially to direct the arthroscopic cannula and conical obturator caudally into the cranial compartment of the lateral femorotibial joint. This position offers good evaluation of the lateral tibial eminence, cranial horn of the lateral meniscus and its cranial ligament, intraarticular portion of the long digital extensor tendon, lateral condyle of the femur, and cranial cruciate ligament in its subsynovial position. The latter can be evaluated by further resecting the overlying intraarticular septum.

For the medial approach to the lateral femorotibial joint (Moustafa et al, 1987), the arthroscope (after approaching the medial femorotibial joint using the cranial approach) is returned to the intercondylar reference point in the medial femorotibial joint and then directed to view the synovial septum cranial to the intercondylar eminence of the tibia. In this position, the arthroscope is replaced by the conical obturator and the sleeve is inserted caudolaterally behind the long digital extensor tendon, to the far side of the joint. The arthroscope is then placed in the sleeve and the arthroscopic examination commences. The lateral femorotibial joint may be predistended with fluid through an 18-gauge needle inserted between the lateral patellar ligament and the lateral collateral ligament, but this is not necessary.

Alternatively, the lateral femorotibial joint may be approached directly without prior arthroscopic examination of the medial femorotibial joint. The lateral femorotibial joint is distended as described previously, and an 8- to 10-mm skin incision is made medial to the middle patellar ligament. The arthroscopic sheath and trocar is then advanced caudolaterally

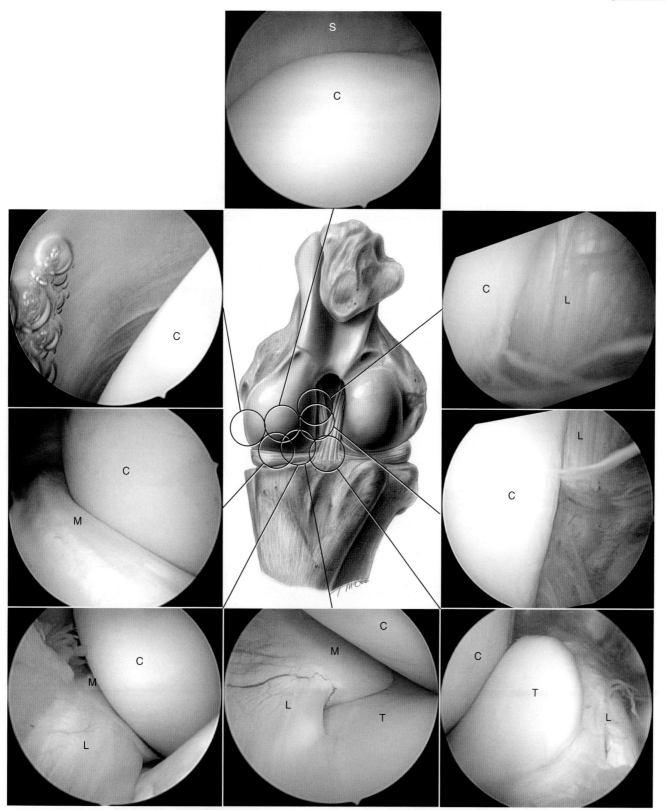

Figure 6-12 Composite of arthroscopic images obtained from cranial compartment of medial femorotibial joint using a lateral arthroscopic approach. *C,* Medial condyle of femur; *CCL,* cranial cruciate ligament (beneath synovial membrane); *CLM,* cranial ligament of medial meniscus (medial menisco-tibial ligament); *M,* cranial aspect of medial meniscus; *MCL,* medial collateral ligament; *ME,* medial intercondylar eminence of the tibia; *T,* proximomedial condyle of tibia.

to penetrate the joint capsule on the cranial side and advanced to the lateral side of the joint.

Normal Arthroscopic Anatomy of the Cranial Compartment of the Lateral Femorotibial Joint

After entry, the initial view should include the lateral aspect of the lateral femoral condyle, as well as the popliteal tendon within its synovial diverticulum (Fig. 6-13). Withdrawal of the arthroscope reveals the lateral femoral condyle and lateral meniscus (see Fig. 6-13). Further medial, the cranial ligament of the lateral meniscus and the lateral tibial condyle may be visualized, as well as the long digital extensor tendon under the synovial membrane and within the sulcus muscularis of the tibia (see Fig. 6-13). With further withdrawal and rotation of the arthroscope, the lateral aspect of the cranial cruciate ligament can be seen axially under the median septum (see Fig. 6-13). A small area of tibial condyle is visible axial to these structures.

Cranial Intercondylar Approach to the Caudal Pouch of the Medial Femorotibial Joint

A cranial approach to the caudal pouch of the medial femorotibial joint has been described (Muurlink et al, 2009). It provides assessment of unique regions, including extensive portions of the caudal cruciate ligament body and insertion, and axial attachments of the medial meniscus. However, successful entry does not occur in 100% of cases and the range of visibility is limited. The authors therefore prefer the conventional approach (described next) to the caudal compartment of the medial femorotibial joint. A further advantage is being able to have caudal instrument access without interference from the arthroscope.

Insertion of the Arthroscope into the Caudal Pouch of the Medial Femorotibial Joint

Arthroscopy of the caudal pouches of both the medial and lateral femorotibial joints is technically more demanding than their cranial partners, and the synovial membrane and capsule

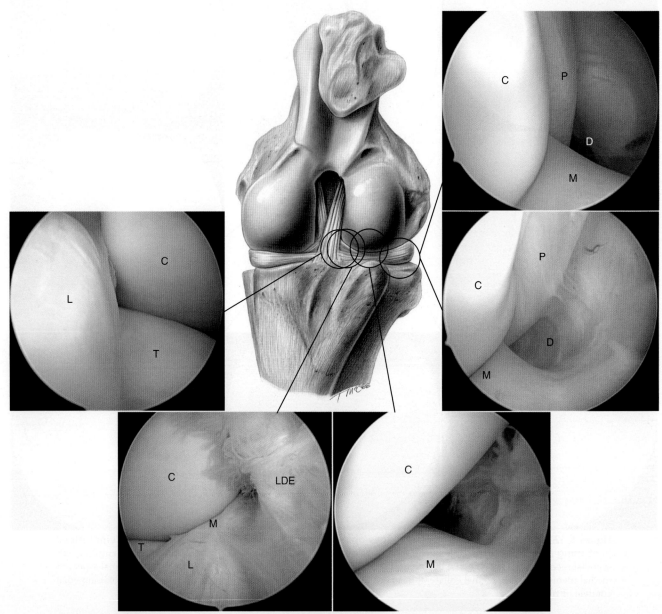

Figure 6-13 Composite of arthroscopic images obtained from cranial compartment of lateral femorotibial joint using dorsomedial approach. *D,* Synovial diverticulum within sulcus muscularis of tibia; *LDE,* long digital extensor tendon with overlying villus synovial membrane; *M,* lateral femoral condyle; *P,* popliteous tendon running into diverticulum laterally; *T,* lateral tibial condyle.

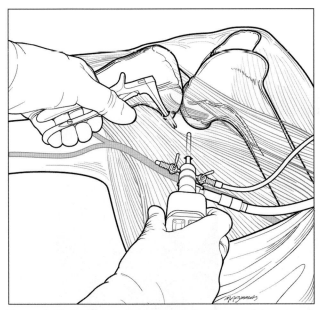

Figure 6-14 Arthroscopic approach to the caudal compartment of the medial femorotibial joint. The arthroscope sleeve enters 6 to 8 cm caudal to the medial collateral ligament, 1 cm proximal to the level of a line between the tibial tuberosity and the tibial condyle and immediately cranial to the medial saphenous vein. The instrument portal is made after appropriate needle verification, 2 to 4 cm cranial to the arthroscope entry. *(Reproduced with permission from Watts and Nixon, 2006.)*

are extremely thin. This provides little tactile feedback that the arthroscope sleeve has penetrated the joint cavity. The stifle is positioned at approximately 120 degrees of flexion (i.e., less than for cranial approaches). The authors usually do this examination following examination of the cranial pouch. Some authors prefer to enter this joint compartment first, in which case the joint is distended with 50 to 60 mL of fluid using a spinal needle placed just proximal to the most caudal palpable medial eminence of the tibia and caudal to the medial collateral ligament (Fig. 6-14) (Walmsley, 2002). A number of positions for the arthroscopic portal have been described, including (1) on the same plane as the medial eminence of the tibia but 3 cm caudally, 2.5 cm proximal to the distal level of the medial meniscus, and 3 cm caudal to the medial collateral ligament (Trumble et al, 1994) and (2) 3 cm more proximad to allow for a distal instrument portal (Hance et al, 1993). More recently an approach has been described by Watts and Nixon (2006) where the arthroscopic portal is located 6 to 8 cm caudal to the medial collateral ligament, 1 cm proximal to the level of the line between the palpable tibial tuberosity and tibial condyle, 1 to 2 cm cranial to the medial saphenous vein and cranioproximal to the palpable gracilis muscle. The more caudal approach allows better examination of the caudal horn of the medial meniscus and insertion of the caudal cruciate ligament, as well as leaving more room for instrument entry. Additionally, during insertion it directs the arthroscope sleeve and obturator toward the surface of the medial condyle, rather than across the caudal articulation, where the popliteal artery and vein are at risk of inadvertent injury. An instrument portal can be created 2.5 to 4 cm cranial to the arthroscopic portal after using the spinal needle to define access and direction (see Fig. 6-14).

The first author uses a simple technique of making the arthroscopic portal 2 cm caudal and 2 cm proximal to the caudal medial eminence of the tibia. This examination is routinely done after the joint is left distended from cranial pouch arthroscopy and has proved predictable. The caudal cruciate ligament can be visualized, but there is less room for instrument portals compared

with the technique of Watts and Nixon (2006). This becomes an issue if shavers and rongeurs are necessary to debride the caudal horn of medial meniscus and caudal surface of the medial condyle because the deeply inserted arthroscope sleeve and instruments markedly interfere. However, if a diagnostic examination confirms the need for an instrument portal, the arthroscope can be inserted more caudally with the aid of a switching stick, and the existing portal is perfectly positioned for instrument access to the meniscus and caudal surface of the condyle.

▶ Normal Arthroscopic Anatomy of the Caudal Pouch of the Medial Femorotibial Joint

The caudal medial femoral condyle and caudal medial meniscus are initially visualized (Fig. 6-15). It is possible to view completely the caudal portion of the medial femoral condyle, the caudal horn of the medial meniscus from the medial collateral ligament to the axial termination, and the intrasynovial portion of the caudal cruciate ligament (see Fig. 6-15). In addition, horizontal synovial folds or invaginations with a variable synovial frond covering can be identified in the caudoaxial aspect of the medial compartment (see Fig. 6-15).

Insertion of the Arthroscope into the Caudal Compartment of the Lateral Femorotibial Joint

This approach is based on the initial description of Trumble et al (1994) and described in more detail by Watts and Nixon (2006). It is important to be aware that the peroneal nerve lies 7 cm caudal to the lateral collateral ligament, so no portal should be made this far caudally. Additionally, the nerve is closer to the caudal joint pouch with the limb extended, so flexion aids in avoiding peroneal nerve injury. The popliteal tendon divides the caudal lateral femorotibial joint. Distention is performed with a spinal needle placed caudal to the collateral ligament. For examination proximal to the popliteal tendon, the portal is placed 2.5 cm proximal to the tibial plateau and 3 cm caudal to the collateral ligament (Fig. 6-16). Structures seen through this portal are limited to the lateral femoral condyle and the proximal border of the popliteal tendon. To view the pouch distal to the popliteal tendon, the portal is located at the level of the tibial plateau, 1.5 cm caudal to the lateral collateral ligament, and the arthroscope is placed through the popliteal tendon to allow examination of the more caudal articulation of the joint. It was noted by Trumble et al (1994) that the popliteal tendon being contiguous with the joint capsule makes arthroscopic exploration of this pouch particularly difficult.

Normal Arthroscopic Anatomy of the Caudal Compartment of the Lateral Femorotibial Joint

With the proximal arthroscopic portal, it is possible to view the proximal border of the popliteal tendon and the lateral femoral condyle (Fig. 6-17). Using the distal portal through the popliteal tendon it is possible to examine the caudal lateral meniscus, part of the caudal aspect of the lateral femoral condyle, the intraarticular portion of the popliteal tendon, and the lateral tibial condyle, but this examination is limited and difficult.

Diagnostic Arthroscopy of Clinical Conditions in the Femorotibial Joint

The initial indication for arthroscopy of the femorotibial joint was in cases of cystic lesions of the medial condyle of the femur (Lewis, 1987). Surgical intervention for this condition is discussed in a separate section. Recently, femorotibial arthroscopy has been performed more frequently for diagnostic purposes to define a clinical problem localized to the femorotibial joint (Lewis, 1987; McIlwraith, 1990; Prades et al, 1989; Scott et al 2004; Walmsley, 1995, 2002). Lewis (1987) described the arthroscopic findings in 20 cases of unilateral lameness, with a positive response to intraarticular anesthesia of the medial femorotibial joint but without major radiographic abnormalities. A consistent finding was abnormality of the articular surface of

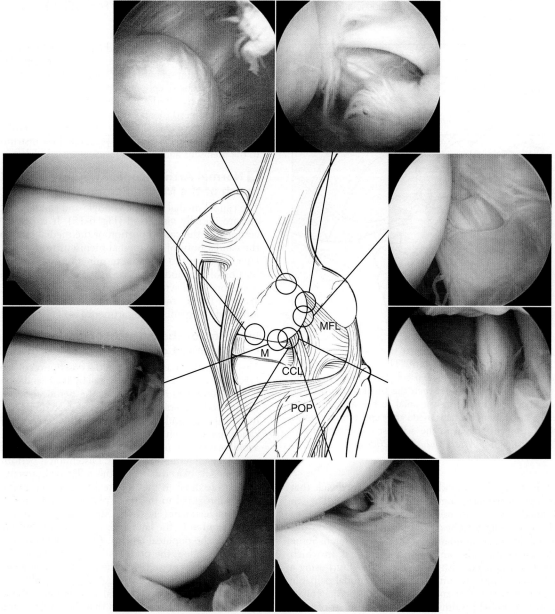

Figure 6-15 Composite of arthroscopic images obtained from the caudal compartment of the medial femorotibial joint using the approach illustrated in Figure 6-14. *CCL,* Caudal cruciate ligament, normal horizontal fold; *M,* meniscus; *MFC,* medial femoral condyle; *MFL,* meniscofemoral ligament. *(Reproduced from Watts and Nixon, 2006.)*

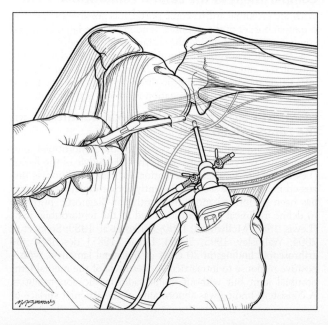

Figure 6-16 Arthroscopic approach to proximal pouch of the caudal compartment of the lateral femorotibial joint. The arthroscope enters 3 cm caudal to the lateral collateral ligament and 2 cm proximal to the tibial plateau for entry proximal to the popliteal muscle. *(Reproduced with permission from Watts and Nixon, 2006.)*

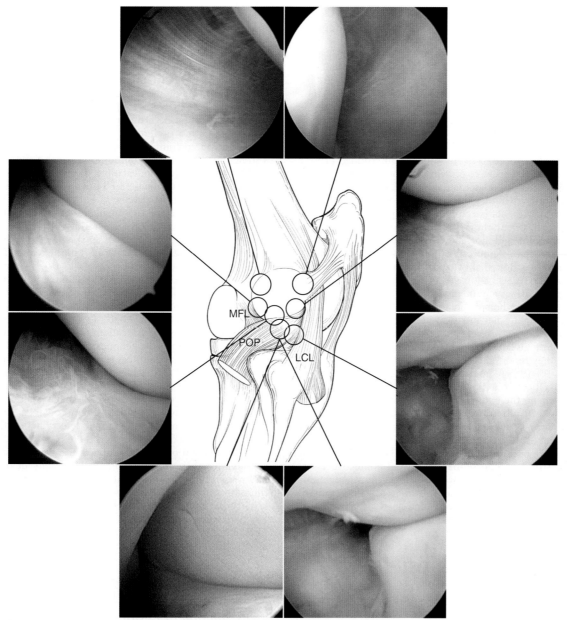

Figure 6-17 Composite of arthroscopic images obtained from the caudal compartment of the lateral femoro-tibial joint proximal and distal to the popliteal muscle and tendon. The partially grayed-in circles represent anatomic location to obtain images from the distal pouch. *LFC,* Lateral femoral condyle; *MFL,* meniscofemoral ligament; *POP,* popliteal muscle. *(Reproduced with permission from Watts and Nixon, 2006.)*

the distal weight-bearing portion of the medial femoral condyles: Abnormalities included fibrillation of the articular cartilage; partial- to full-thickness erosion, sometimes accompanied by subchondral bone lysis; and, in some cases, full-thickness cartilage flaps. Abnormalities of the medial meniscus were evident in 9 cases, including mild to marked fibrillation and degeneration of the proximal surface. A meniscal laceration was noted in 3 cases, and a partial avulsion/rupture of the cranial ligament of the medial meniscus was seen in 1 case. Examination of the menisci was limited in all cases, and Lewis (1987) noted a lack of ability to adequately evaluate the body and caudal segments of the meniscus. Of the 20 cases in which arthroscopic examination revealed articular cartilage change or meniscal damage, only 6 horses were still usable as intended. All 20 had the benefit of extended rest, intraarticular medication, nonsteroidal antiinflammatory agent therapy, or a combination of therapeutic measures.

Prades et al (1989) reported on injuries to the cranial cruciate ligament (CCL) and associated structures in 10 horses.

Arthroscopic examination of the affected femorotibial joints was performed in 5 horses, and this confirmed the presumptive diagnosis of cranial cruciate ligament injury or rupture. The authors reported the following abnormalities in all 5 horses: disruption of the septum surrounding the cruciate ligaments, which separates the medial and lateral compartments; increase in the joint space due to ligamentous laxity; inflammation of the synovial membrane; and areas of hemorrhage in the CCL. Other individual findings included partial longitudinal tear of the CCL body, cranial longitudinal tear of lateral meniscus, desmitis of the CCL at its insertion on the tibial eminence (2 horses), tearing of cranial attachment of lateral meniscus, erosion and fibrillation of articular cartilage of the medial femoral condyle, and complete tear of the CCL.

Walmsley (1995) reported use of arthroscopy to both diagnose and treat vertical tears of the cranial horn of the meniscus and the cranial ligament of the meniscus, and Schneider et al (1997) described the evaluation of cartilage lesions on the medial femoral condyle. Subsequently, Walmsley et al (2003) reported 80 cases of meniscal tears. A more recent paper reported 44 horses with lameness referable to the stifle that were diagnosed with osteoarthritis, meniscal tears, or other intraarticular soft tissue injuries on the basis of arthroscopic examination and documented their long-term outcome (Cohen et al, 2009). The authors examined the femoropatellar joint alone in four limbs, the femorotibial joint in 12 limbs, and both the femoropatellar and cranial femorotibial joints in 33 limbs. The caudal aspect of the femorotibial joint was explored in 3 limbs. Chondral lesions were observed in 37 horses (84%) and graded from 0-3 (using a modification of the human Outerbridge [1961] system); meniscal tears were present in 30 horses (68%). These conditions are discussed later in more detail, separately.

The septum separating the lateral and medial femorotibial joint compartments is commonly disrupted in association with cruciate ligament injury; a cranial approach to the medial femorotibial joint will also allow examination of the cranial pouch of the lateral femorotibial joint in these cases. If both cranial cruciate and medial collateral ligaments are disrupted, the resulting laxity will allow greater visualization of the femorotibial articulations and menisci.

In a series of 44 horses, Cohen et al (2009) reported that an ultrasonographic diagnosis was confirmed at arthroscopic surgery in 11 horses, whereas a false-positive ultrasonographic diagnosis of meniscal tear was made in 4 horses. For horses in that series they reported that diagnostic ultrasound had a sensitivity of 79% (95% confidence interval [CI] = 49% to 95%) and a specificity of 56% (95% CI = 21% to 86%) for identifying meniscal tears in the equine stifle. Since then a detailed comparison between ultrasonographic and arthroscopic boundaries of the normal equine femorotibial joint has been reported (Barrett et al, 2012). Simultaneous arthroscopy and ultrasonography were performed in 10 equine cadaver stifles, as well as bilateral stifles on a horse that underwent nonrecovery surgery. The arthroscopic probe was visualized ultrasonographically, and concurrent video and still images were acquired. It was found that arthroscopy provided good visualization of the cranial meniscal ligaments, the distal portion of the cranial cruciate ligament, proximal portion of the medial collateral ligament within the fibrous tissue of the joint capsule, and a limited view of the abaxial border of meniscus. In this study, ultrasonography allowed for almost complete visualization of the menisci, collateral ligaments, and cranial meniscal ligaments and a portion of the cranial cruciate ligament. It was included that the combination of ultrasonography and arthroscopy provided the most complete diagnostic examination.

ARTHROSCOPIC SURGERY OF THE FEMOROPATELLAR JOINT

▶ Osteochondritis Dissecans

Arthroscopic surgery is the standard surgical technique to treat OCD in the femoropatellar joint. The techniques presented subsequently are based on the experience of the authors with clinical cases of OCD in the femoropatellar joint and the follow-up data that have been generated from these cases (Foland et al, 1992; Martin & McIlwraith, 1985; McIlwraith, 1984; McIlwraith & Martin, 1984, 1985). Although historically, successful results were obtained using arthrotomy, potential complications included seroma formation, local cellulitis and fasciitis, and wound dehiscence (Pascoe et al, 1980, 1984; Trotter et al, 1983).

Preoperative Considerations

Preoperative diagnosis of OCD is based on clinical and radiographic signs. The clinical signs that initially prompt the attention of owners are usually lameness or distension of the femoropatellar joint(s). The disease is not breed specific, but it is a disease of young horses. In some instances, however, no clinical problems are apparent until the horse is in training or has raced (McIlwraith & Martin, 1985). Lesions that manifest at this stage are generally less severe. Clinical examination generally reveals some degree of synovial effusion as a consistent finding. Lameness ranges from nondiscernible through subtle gait changes (shortened anterior phase of stride, low arc of flight, and unusual flight path with the stifle rotated outward and the hock inward) to obvious lameness with a stiff gait and difficulty in getting up. Animals may have difficulty in trotting with a preference to canter or "bunny-hop." Postural or acquired conformational abnormalities manifesting as a straighter, more upright hindlimb(s) are also common.

The radiographic manifestations of the disease vary. Lesions most commonly occur on the LTR but are also seen on the MTR of the femur or on the patella, or both (Box 6-1). The lesions in turn may be localized to a small area or be distributed along the entire length of the trochlear ridge. The most common radiographic manifestation of OCD is a defect (with or without discernible fragments) on the LTR of the femur (Fig. 6-18). Defects can be described as concave (Fig. 6-19), flattened (Fig. 6-20), cystic, or undetermined. Lesions on the MTR (when evident radiographically) usually manifest as a concave defect but often are not visible on radiographs (due to a normal subchondral bone contour) (see Fig. 6-20). Lesions can also be observed (less frequently) in various locations on the patella usually manifesting as some form of subchondral defect (Fig. 6-21).

For many years the authors recommended arthroscopic surgery for all cases of OCD, particularly if an athletic career were planned. However, the study by McIntosh & McIlwraith (1993) shows that, with conservative management (stall or pen confinement for 60 days), a number of femoropatellar OCD cases can heal. On the basis of this study, if defects are less than 2 cm long and less than 5 mm deep and there is no severe lameness, or mineralization or fragmentation of the flap on radiographs, conservative therapy is a viable option. Many of these cases had resolution of lameness and synovial effusion, and 80% of these horses raced. It has also been pointed out by Dik et al (1999) that up to age 8 months it is possible for radiographic lesions on the femoral trochlear ridges to resolve. In a longitudinal study of Dutch Warmblood foals, radiographed at 1 month old and subsequently at 4-week intervals, the midregion

---

| Box • 6-1 | |

Distribution of Lesions as Seen at Surgery in 252 Joints with Femoropatellar Osteochondritis Dissecans

No. of Joints	Location
161	LTR
31	LTR and patella
17	MTR
17	LTR and MTR
4	LTR, patella, and TG
3	LTR, MTR, and patella
3	MTR and patella
3	Patella
3	LTR, MTR, TG, and patella
3	LTR and TG
3	LTR, MTR, and TG
3	MTR and TG
1	TG
252	

LTR, Lateral trochlear ridge; MTR, medial trochlear ridge; TG, trochlear groove.
From Foland et al 1992.

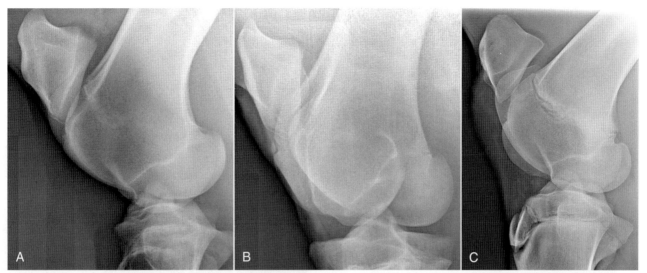

Figure 6-18 A, Lateral to medial radiographic view of osteochondritis dissecans (OCD) with defect and fragment on lateral trochlear ridge. **B,** Cranial caudal medial oblique radiographic view more clearly defining defect in OCD lesion. **C,** Lateromedial radiograph of Thoroughbred yearling with larger OCD lesion of the lateral trochlear ridge of the femur with minor fragmentation within the defect. Soft tissue swelling is consistent with distention of the femoropatellar joint.

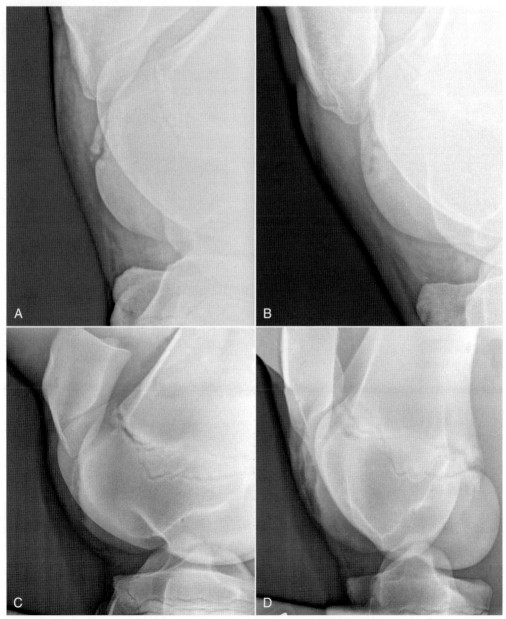

Figure 6-19 A, Larger fragment in defect on lateral trochlear ridge (LTR) of femur. **B,** Osteochondritis dissecans (OCD) of lateral trochlear ridge manifesting as mottling. **C,** Moderate length shallow OCD defect of LTR. **D,** Oblique radiograph of image in **C.**

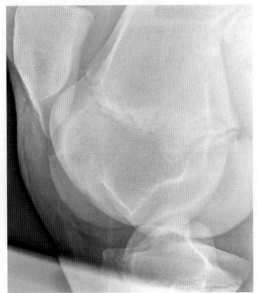

Figure 6-20 Osteochondritis dissecans lesions in both lateral and medial trochlear ridges of femur.

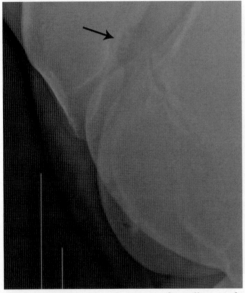

Figure 6-21 Osteochondritis dissecans of patella manifesting as subchondral loss of bone in the central caudal aspect *(arrow)*. (For arthroscopic views, see Fig. 6-38.)

of the lateral femoral trochlear ridge became radiographically abnormal from 3 to 4 months old. Subsequent progression of radiographic abnormalities was usually followed by regression and resolution, with the appearance returning to normal at 8 months old in most cases. At 5 months old, 20% of the stifles were abnormal radiographically, but at 11 months old this percentage had decreased to 3%. Normal and abnormal appearances were permanent from 8 months of age (Dik, 1999).

The authors currently recommend that all lesions greater than 2 cm in length or 5 mm in depth, or any lesion that contains osseous densities in the presence of synovial effusion, be treated with arthroscopic surgery. In some of the cases that can potentially heal conservatively, owner or trainer requests for assurance of correction also leads to early surgical treatment. Persistence of synovial effusion is always an indication for surgery, and in some cases persistent lameness or developing conformational abnormalities, or both, can also necessitate arthroscopic intervention.

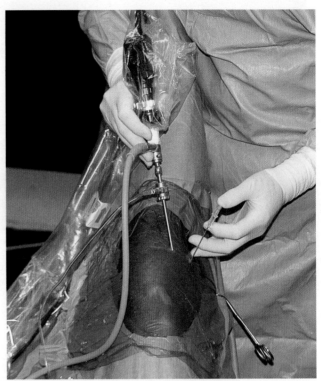

Figure 6-22 The ideal site for the instrument portal used during operations involving the upper part of the lateral trochlear ridge is ascertained by using a spinal needle.

A direct comparative study was done comparing radiographic and arthroscopic findings in the femoropatellar joint (Steinheimer et al, 1995). It is rare to find an arthroscopic lesion less severe than the radiographic insinuation. On the other hand, it is common to find more pathologic change at arthroscopic surgery than predicted by radiographs. Occasionally animals present with marked deformity of the trochlear ridges or patella, or both, secondary to severe OCD; this will not be reversed by surgery.

A comparative study of radiography and ultrasonography for the diagnosis of OCD in the equine femoropatellar joint suggested that ultrasound should be considered as a useful adjunct to radiography, especially in cases of high clinical suspicion but equivocal radiographic findings. In a study of 21 horses, OCD lesions were diagnosed by radiography (30/32 joints) and ultrasound (32/32 joints) (Bourzac et al, 2009). When specific lesions were considered, two LTR and three MTR lesions, not seen on radiographs, were diagnosed by ultrasound and confirmed with arthroscopy or necropsy. The specificity was 100% regardless of the site and imaging procedure except for the distal third of the MTR (94% for ultrasound). The sensitivity varied depending on lesion site.

Technique

A number of different instrument portals are used to perform surgery at various locations in the femoropatellar joint. Previously, six different triangulation approaches were described to operate on the various lesions of OCD in the femoropatellar joint (McIlwraith, 1990). However, exact sites for instrument entry do not need to be rigidly fixed. Rather, the use of an 18-gauge spinal needle is now recommended to ascertain the ideal location for an instrument portal (Fig. 6-22). In all cases, a 1-cm incision is made through the skin and then superficial and deep fasciae before a stab incision with a No. 11 blade completes entry into the joint. Instruments are then inserted through the portal as required (Fig. 6-23). The various surgical approaches are illustrated in Figures 6-24 to 6-29.

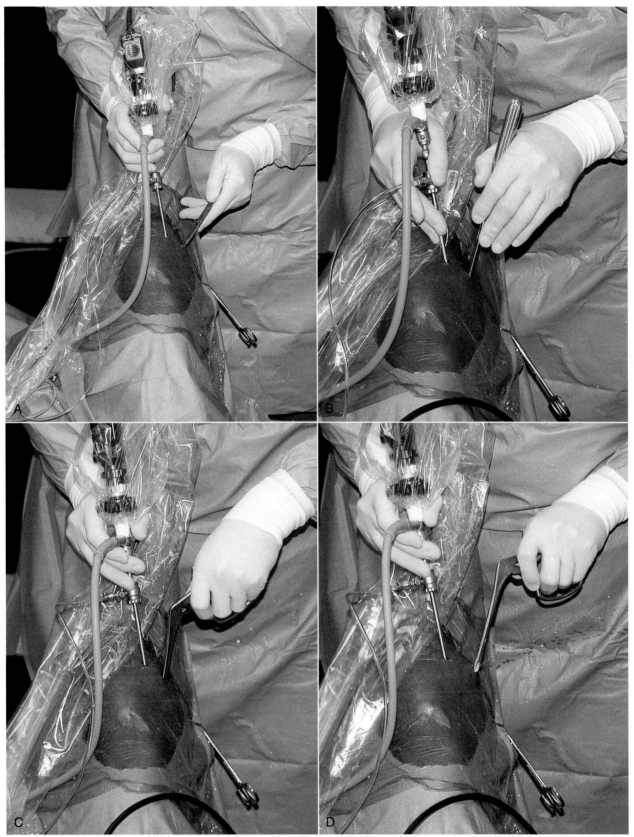

Figure 6-23 Making an instrument portal **(A),** palpating lesion with probe **(B),** and use of Ferris-Smith rongeurs **(C** and **D)** to operate on a lesion on the proximal part of the lateral trochlear ridge of the femur.

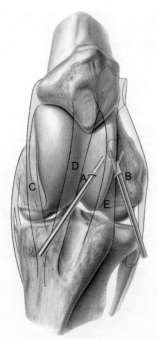

Figure 6-24 Location of the arthroscope and instrument during operations involving lesions in the proximal aspect of the lateral trochlear ridge of the femur. *A,* Arthroscope; *B,* instrument; *C,* medial patellar ligament; *D,* middle patellar ligament; *E,* lateral patellar ligament.

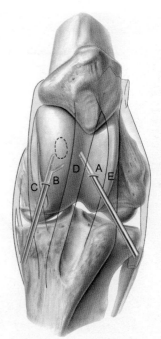

Figure 6-25 Location of the arthroscope and instrument during operations involving lesions on the proximal aspect of the medial trochlear ridge of the femur. *A,* Arthroscope; *B,* instrument; *C,* medial patellar ligament; *D,* middle patellar ligament; *E,* lateral patellar ligament.

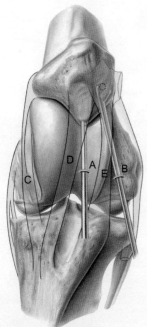

Figure 6-26 Location of the arthroscope and instrument during operations involving lesions on the articular surface of the patella. *A,* Arthroscope; *B,* instrument; *C,* medial patellar ligament; *D,* middle patellar ligament; *E,* lateral patellar ligament.

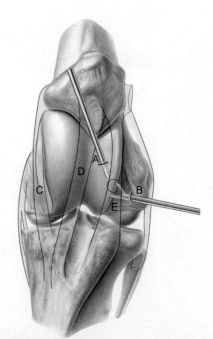

Figure 6-27 Location of the arthroscope and instrument during operations involving lesions on the distal aspect of the lateral trochlear ridge. *A,* Arthroscope; *B,* instrument; *C,* medial patellar ligament; *D,* middle lateral patellar ligament; *E,* lateral patellar ligament.

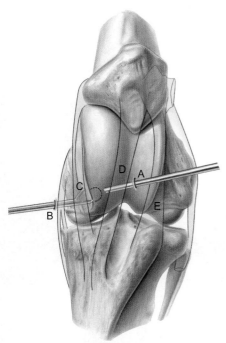

Figure 6-28 Location of the arthroscope and instrument during operations involving lesions on the distal aspect of the medial trochlear ridge. *A,* Arthroscope; *B,* instrument; *C,* Medial patellar ligament; *D,* middle patellar ligament; *E,* lateral patellar ligament.

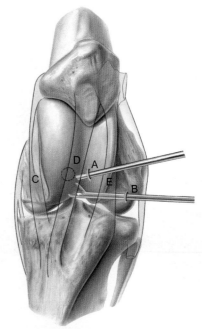

Figure 6-29 Location of the arthroscope and instrument during operations involving lesions on the axial aspect of the distal medial trochlear ridge. *A,* Arthroscope. *B,* instrument; *C,* medial patellar ligament; *D,* middle patellar ligament; *E,* lateral patellar ligament.

In all instances, the authors use the same arthroscopic portal between the lateral and middle patellar ligament, although it is noted that an arthroscopic portal between the middle and medial patellar ligaments has also been used for operations involving LTR lesions (Bramlage personal communication, 1987).

Lesions on the proximal one-half of the LTR are reached through a portal proximolateral to the arthroscopic portal (see Fig. 6-24). The instrument may pass either lateral to or (usually) through the lateral patellar ligament when using this portal. If the entry is too far lateral, the instrument cannot be manipulated up and over the LTR. Passing the instrument through the lateral patellar ligament does not seem to be of any consequence. Lesions of the proximal portion of the MTR are reached by using a portal between the medial and middle patellar ligaments, entering the skin distal to the lesion (see Fig. 6-25).

To effectively operate the underside of the patella, an instrument portal must be level with or distal to the arthroscopic portal and usually 2 cm lateral to the arthroscopic portal (see Fig. 6-26). If this portal is more proximal than the arthroscopic portal, the end of the instrument cannot make contact with the undersurface of the patella. The portal is made lateral to the middle patellar ligament, depending on the position of the lesion on the patella. To operate on lesions on the distal aspect of the LTR, the same arthroscopic portal is used as that chosen for the proximal trochlear ridge, although the arthroscope is directed distad. The instrument portal is made low over the distended femoropatellar joint through or immediately adjacent to the lateral patellar ligament (see Fig. 6-27). For lesions on the distal aspect of the MTR, a distal portal is usually made between the middle and medial patellar ligaments (see Fig. 6-28). If the lesion on the MTR is located on the trochlear groove (axial) side of the distal MTR, however, a medial portal does not always allow the instrument to reach this location. In this instance, a lateral instrument portal, allowing the instrument to pass under the middle patellar ligament, is necessary (see Fig. 6-29).

Manipulations of the surgical instruments vary, but a sequential protocol is generally followed. A number of cases are used to demonstrate the manipulations (Figs. 6-30 to 6-34). In all cases, the lesions are initially evaluated with a probe. The probe is useful in defining the limits of an osteochondral or chondral flap, as well as for assessing its mobility. The probe is also used to evaluate any cracking, wrinkling, or fibrillation in the articular cartilage. If the cartilage is cracked but firmly attached to subchondral bone, it is not removed. Normal-appearing articular cartilage is also probed, particularly if radiographs have revealed lesions in the subchondral bone in that area. If intact cartilage overlies a subchondral defect, the probe breaking through the articular cartilage into the defect locates the lesions and the undermined articular cartilage is then removed.

The most common form of pathologic change encountered on arthroscopic examination of OCD of the LTR of the femur is flap formation or fragmentation within the articular cartilage and subchondral bone (see Figs. 6-30 and 6-31). This situation is common when ossified flaps or fragments have been observed on preoperative radiographs. When the lesions manifest radiographically as subchondral defects in the trochlear ridge, chondral or osteochondral flaps are also commonly found. Gross and histopathologic examinations frequently confirm osseous tissue in the cartilage fragments and flaps, even when they are not discernible on radiographs.

In either situation, the flaps are manipulated and elevated, usually by using a periosteal elevator or rongeurs (see Fig. 6-31). The flaps are then removed by using Ferris-Smith rongeurs or an equivalent instrument (see Figs. 6-23 and 6-31 to 6-34). The flap is removed in successive bites with the rongeurs, leaving it attached at its proximal edge. This technique reduces the chance of the flap slipping from the grasp of the forceps and becoming a loose body. In joints in which the subchondral defect does not contain a distinct flap, the nature of the lesion varies from a dimple to an openly eroded lesion. Fragments of cartilage within a matrix of granulation or

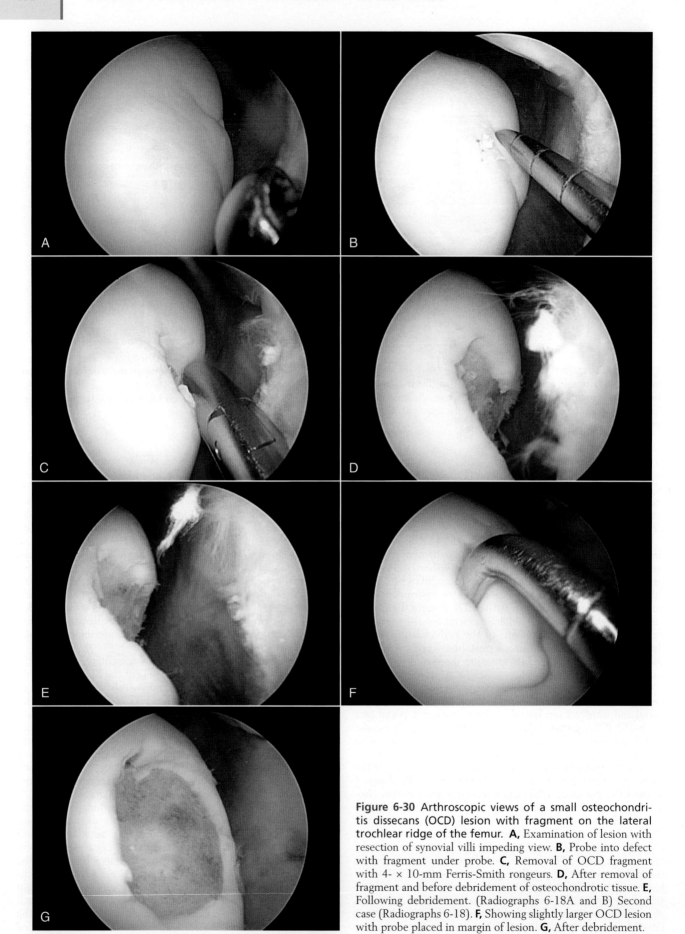

Figure 6-30 Arthroscopic views of a small osteochondritis dissecans (OCD) lesion with fragment on the lateral trochlear ridge of the femur. **A,** Examination of lesion with resection of synovial villi impeding view. **B,** Probe into defect with fragment under probe. **C,** Removal of OCD fragment with 4- × 10-mm Ferris-Smith rongeurs. **D,** After removal of fragment and before debridement of osteochondrotic tissue. **E,** Following debridement. (Radiographs 6-18A and B) Second case (Radiographs 6-18). **F,** Showing slightly larger OCD lesion with probe placed in margin of lesion. **G,** After debridement.

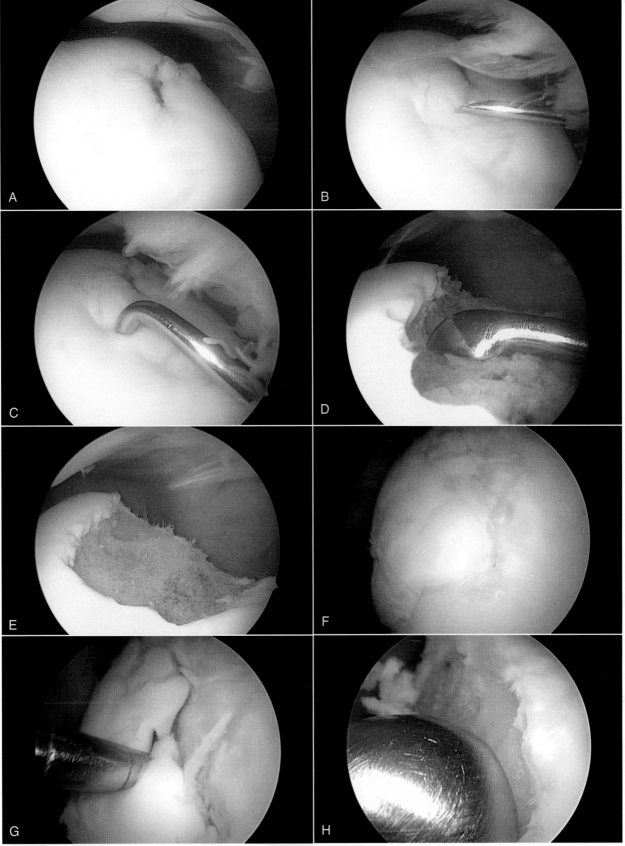

Figure 6-31 Arthroscopic views of medium-sized osteochondritis dissecans (OCD) lesion **(A)** on initial examination. **B,** With spinal needle placed to ascertain instrument portal location and angle. **C,** Probe placed in lesion. **D,** During debridement with a curette (note vertical nature of curetting and removal of defective bone). **E,** At completion of debridement. Arthroscopic views of OCD lesion of LTR, before probing **(F). G,** Manipulation of flap with probe and **H,** during debridement. Arthroscopic manifestation of OCD on LTR that exhibited radiographic mottling (radiograph shown in Fig. 6-19B) with spinal needle inserted to ascertain instrument portal **(I)** and **(J)** after debridement.

Continued

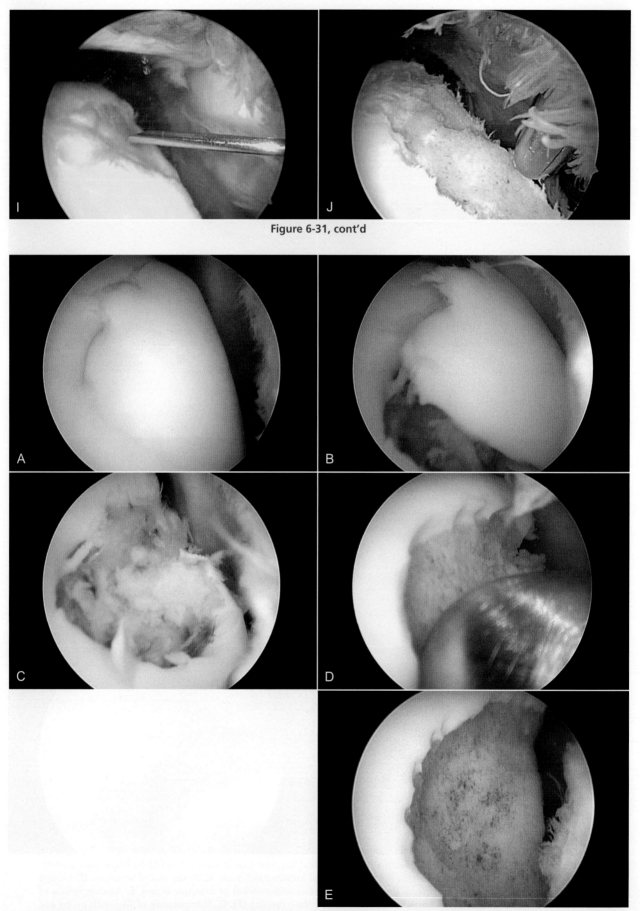

Figure 6-31, cont'd

Figure 6-32 Arthroscopic views of large osteochondritis dissecans flap on lateral trochlear ridge of femur. **A,** Evaluation of flap. **B,** Elevation. **C,** Defect after flap removal. **D,** Debridement. **E,** Completely debrided defect.

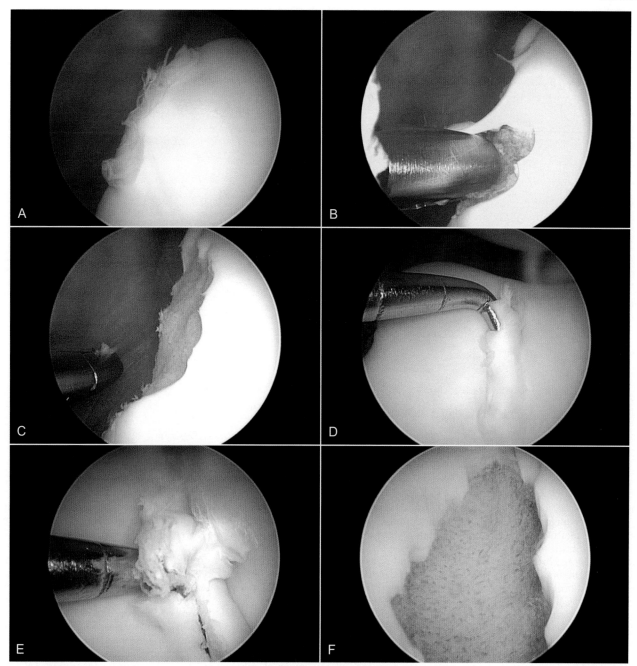

Figure 6-33 Arthroscopic views of osteochondritis dissecans lesions that occurred on the lateral trochlear ridge (LTR), medial trochlear ridge, and central trochlear groove (TG) of the femur in the same femoropatellar joint. **A,** LTR lesion with typical elevated cartilage. **B,** Removal of LTR lesion. **C,** Debridement of LTR defect. **D,** Axial TG lesion. **E,** Debridement of TG lesion. **F,** Defect left in TG.

Continued

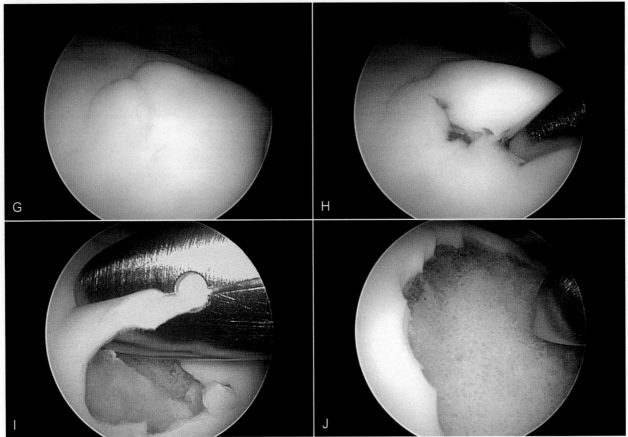

Figure 6-33, cont'd G, Medial trochlear ridge (MTR) lesion. **H** and **I,** Removal of MTR flap. **J,** Defect left after debridement of MTR.

fibrous tissue may be noted within the defect. After removal of the flap or fragments (see Fig. 6-34), undermined articular cartilage unattached to subchondral bone is removed by using Ferris-Smith rongeurs or basket forceps (see Figs. 6-32 and 6-33). More chronic cases of OCD will manifest as more rounded fragments (Fig. 6-35A to C) and secondary articular cartilage fibrillation on adjacent trochlear ridge or patella (see Fig. 6-35C). Multiple loose fragments in the joint are also manifestations (see Fig. 6-35D), and if the lesion is more severe, secondary remodeling can develop in the distal apex of the patella (see Fig. 6-35E).

Debridement of the remaining subchondral defect is then performed. Hand curettage is used in most cases. A motorized burr can be effective in debriding the defects to healthy subchondral bone (Fig. 6-36) but can easily result in excessive loss of tissue. A hand curette is used in most cases (see Figs. 6-31 to 6-33), which allows better definition between normal and pathologic bone. At the completion of subchondral debridement, tags of defective cartilage that commonly remain at the edge of the defect are removed using rongeurs. The important criterion to satisfy at the completion of debridement is that no undermined, unattached articular cartilage remains.

The arthroscopic manifestations of MTR lesions vary but are often found during arthroscopic examination where no lesions were detected radiographically. They commonly occur as raised areas of articular cartilage (see Figs. 6-33 and 6-37), but flap lesions also occur occasionally. They are treated surgically in the same fashion as LTR lesions but with a medial instrument portal (see Figs. 6-25, 6-28, 6-33, and 6-37).

In some instances, lesions exist in surgical distal trochlear area and on the axial sides of the trochlear ridges. It is quite common to see OCD lesions on the axial side of the MTR. The

best access for the instrument approach is gauged by inserting a spinal needle, but generally has to come somewhat laterally because coming over the MTR will not allow access to the lesion. The positioning of arthroscope and instrument is depicted in Figure 6-29. It is to be noted that secondary remodeling on preoperative radiographs indicates severe intraarticular disease and surgery is contraindicated (see Fig. 6-49).

Primary OCD lesions of the patella are uncommon, but they do occur (Fig. 6-38). The surgical technique is similar to that for lesions on the trochlear ridges, with removal of undermined and detached articular cartilage and debridement of subchondral bone. In addition to primary OCD of the patella, degenerative erosive lesions that appear to be secondary to OCD lesions on the trochlear ridge of the femur are also observed. More commonly, proliferative buds of cartilage (with bone sometimes) are seen on the patella in association with LTR OCD (Fig. 6-39). The usual site for these patellar lesions is the lateral facet of the patella at the point at which it articulates with the area of OCD on the LTR. Histologic examination of these buds of cartilage in one author's (A.J.N.) laboratory suggests that these are primary OCD lesions. Spurs are also sometimes noted on the lateral margin of the patella.

Lack of correlation between radiographic lesions and actual pathologic changes found intraoperatively are a feature of OCD of the femoropatellar joint. This lack of correlation takes a number of forms: (1) cartilaginous change more severe than expected, based on the subchondral lesions seen on the radiographs; (2) cartilaginous lesions on the trochlear ridge or patella where no subchondral bone changes were radiographically detectable; or (3) less severe cartilaginous change than expected (usually taking the form of intact articular cartilage

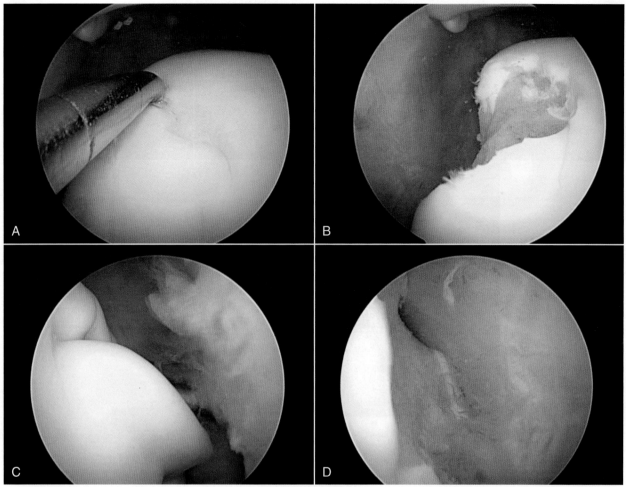

Figure 6-34 A-D, Arthroscopic views of osteochondritis dissecans of both lateral **(A and B)** and medial **(C and D)** before and after debridement (radiographs seen in Fig. 6-20).

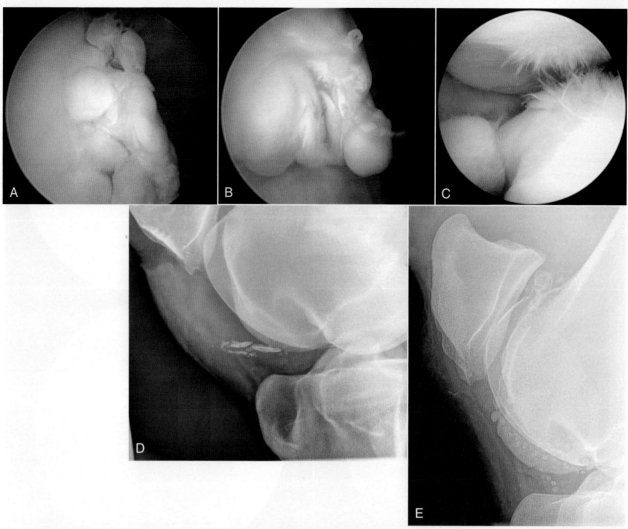

Figure 6-35 Chronic osteochondritis dissecans (OCD) lesions of lateral trochlear ridge (LTR). **A** and **B,** Views of nodular rounded fragments lateral to a defect. **C,** Arthroscopic view of chronic OCD lesion with fragment rounded and lateral to defect with secondary articular fibrillation on both LTR and patella. **D,** Radiograph of chronic case of femoropatellar OCD with multiple loose fragments in distal aspect of joint. **E,** Radiograph of chronic fragmentation of LTR with secondary remodeling developing in distal apex of patella.

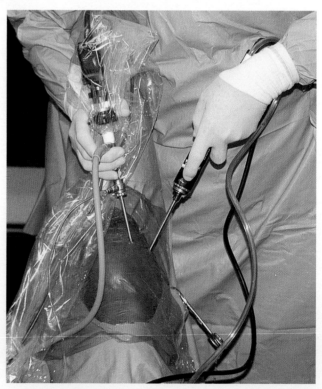

Figure 6-36 Use of a motorized arthroburr to debride a lesion on the lateral trochlear ridge of the femur.

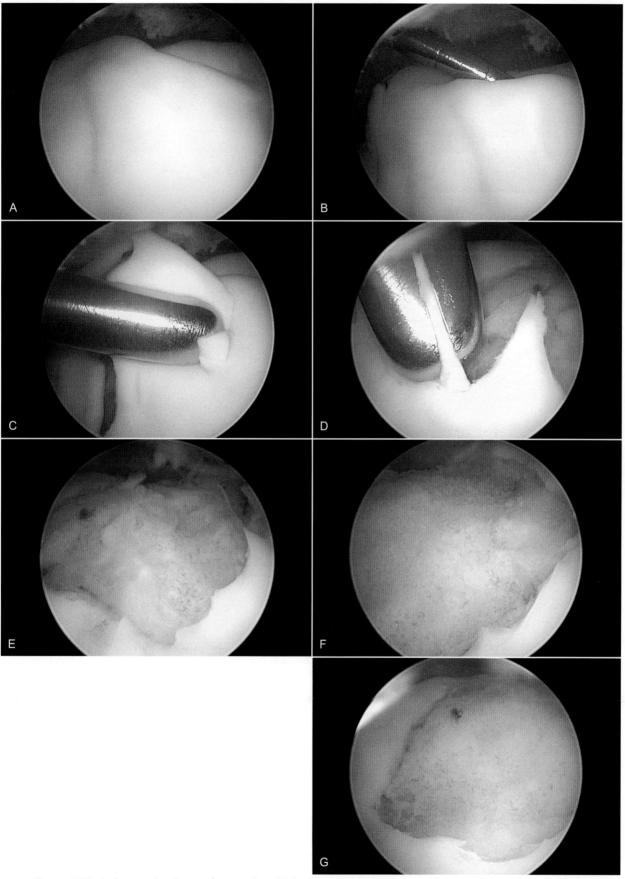

Figure 6-37 Arthroscopic views of osteochondritis dissecans lesion on medial trochlear ridge of femur. **A,** Observation of lesion: note intact cartilage. **B,** Probing of elevated cartilage. **C** and **D,** Removal of separated cartilage. **E,** Debridement of defect. **F** and **G,** Debrided defect.

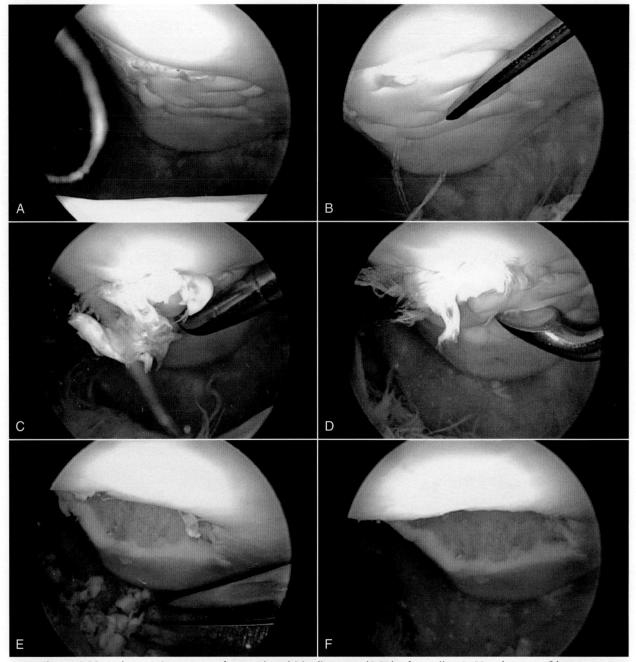

Figure 6-38 Arthroscopic surgery of osteochondritis dissecans (OCD) of patella. **A,** Visualization of lesion in central portion of patella. **B,** Placement of spinal needle to ascertain ideal positioning of instrument portal to allow access and manipulation of lesion. **C,** Placement of probe in defect and elevation of defective tissue. **D,** Use of angled curette to commence debridement. **E,** After curettage of OCD lesion. Note debris proximal to the patella. **F,** Defect after debridement and lavage of joint. (Preoperative radiographic view is depicted in Fig. 6-21.)

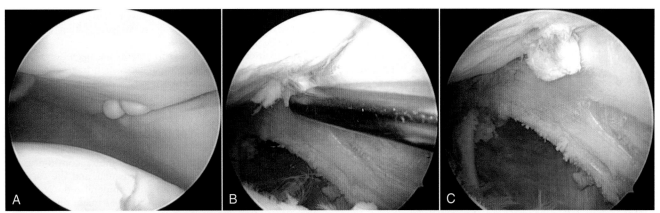

Figure 6-39 Protruding knobs of cartilage off patella that are commonly seen with osteochondritis dissecans of the lateral trochlear ridge. **A,** Small example where need for removal is questioned. **B,** Debridement of a larger protrusion. **C,** After elevation of a protrusion and before removal.

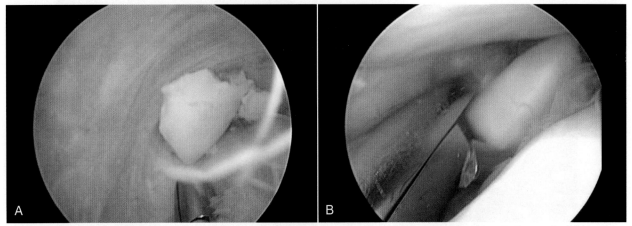

Figure 6-40 A, Arthroscopic view of large fragment in proximal pouch of femoropatellar joint. **B,** Removal of fragment with Ferris-Smith rongeurs.

over radiographically lucent subchondral change). The various radiographic defects manifest in a number of ways during arthroscopic examination. Usually some form of cartilaginous flap or islands of cartilage in a fibrous tissue stroma are present within a concave defect (see Figs. 6-30 and 6-31); other cases involve a dimple-type defect or an area of cartilage fibrillation or loss with or without undermined or detached articular cartilage. In some instances, intact cartilage is separated from the bone (see Figs. 6-31 and 6-33).

Osteochondral bodies that have detached from primary trochlear ridge lesions can be a challenging surgical problem. They may be free within the joint or embedded within the synovial membrane and joint capsule. If these bodies are totally free within the joint, the surgeon must grasp the fragment carefully without pushing it away and causing it to float up into the suprapatellar pouch (Fig. 6-40). Switching off the ingress fluids at this stage can decrease the fluid flow and minimize movement of the loose body.

In instances of large fragments, the skin incision is enlarged to facilitate removal and occasionally the deep fascial incision is also enlarged. However, a proximal instrument portal above the patella into the suprapatellar pouch can be used to remove large fragments with satisfactory results (Fig. 6-41). A spinal needle is used to confirm the correct position before creating a portal through the quadriceps muscle into the suprapatellar pouch. Large fragments are removed more easily through this portal because they do not have to come through the inelastic deep fascia, as occurs with the conventional lateral or medial instrument portals. As in other joints, the skin alone is sutured and no healing problems have been observed. The use of a suprapatellar pouch portal and laparoscopic cannula for removal of debris and loose fragments following arthroscopy of the femoropatellar joint has been recently described in a series of 245 joints in 168 horses (McNally et al, 2011).

It is difficult to make specific recommendations with regard to how to manage osteochondral masses embedded in the synovial membrane or in the fibrous joint capsule. For cases in which the loose body is attached to synovial membrane but is clearly visible within the joint, removal is indicated and can be performed arthroscopically without problems. For a less-visible or less-accessible lesion, arthrotomy can be performed and the first author (C.W.M.) has used this technique in one instance of such a lesion (McIlwraith & Martin, 1985). It is questionable if removal of this mass was necessary, and the authors currently favor leaving alone masses that are embedded completely within the joint capsule. Formation of osseous bodies in the soft tissue has occurred postoperatively, and similar lesions have been noted on radiographs obtained after arthrotomy (Pascoe et al, 1984). Horses with these osseous masses can race, leading to the interpretation that these animals do not need surgery.

Contraindications for surgery include lateral patellar instability owing to excessive loss of the LTR and deformity or extensive secondary remodeling changes of the patella identified radiographically (see Fig. 6-36).

At the completion of the surgical procedures for OCD, the joint is liberally lavaged and vacuumed to ensure removal of small debris released at the time of surgical debridement. A special, larger egress cannula has been developed for this purpose. It is 8 mm in diameter and 20 cm in length. It is inserted until its tip lies within the suprapatellar pouch (see Fig. 6-41A). The suction tubing can be applied directly to the end. A motorized fluid system is critical in flushing this joint. Use of this special egress cannula at the end of the procedure is most appropriate because the debris collects in the suprapatellar pouch and an instrument of large diameter is necessary to allow its removal. An alternative is to insert a large-diameter egress or second arthroscopic cannula into the suprapatellar pouch through a portal proximal to the patella as described previously.

After completion of the procedure and suturing of the incisions, a sterile Ioban® drape or Covaderm Plus® composite dressing is placed over the surgery site in lieu of a bandage (see Fig. 6-41B and C). Alternatively, small gauze "stent" bandages can be sewn over portals.

Pin fixation of large OCD fragments has been described in humans (Guhl, 1984). In human cases such fragments have a rigid bony component, which is rarely present in the equine case. However, a technique for using polydiaxanone (PDS) Orthosorb® pins has been described by Nixon et al (2004) for fixing large OCD flaps and recently, successful long-term results have been reported for this technique (Sparks et al, 2011a). In the recent series of cases reported, cartilage was reattached when it had persisting perimeter continuity, the surface was not deeply fissured or irregular, and the cartilage was not protuberant or extensively mineralized. With this technique a 3-mm instrument portal was made directly over the affected trochlear to allow drilling of a 1.3-mm K-wire perpendicular to the articular surface. A PDS pinning kit

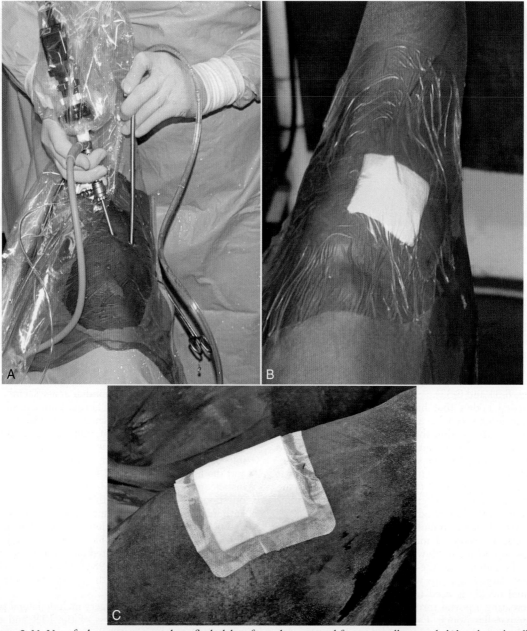

Figure 6-41 Use of a large egress cannula to flush debris from the proximal femoropatellar pouch **(A)** and sterile adhesive drape application after suturing **(B). C,** Use of Covaderm Plus® composite dressing after arthroscopic surgery of stifle.

(Orthosorb pins, DePuy Orthopaedics, Warsaw, Indiana) is used and the 40-mm × 1.3-mm diameter pins provided are cut in two to achieve a uniform length of 20 mm (Fig. 6-42). The length of the K-wire is set to terminate 1 mm short of the anticipated pin length, and multiple (10 to 15 per drill hole) passes in the same plane are used to allow smooth pin insertion. The precut PDS pin is then inserted into the cannula and pushed into place using the obturator. Approximately 1 to

2 mm of the pin are left protruding from the cartilage surface to allow for flattening of the pin head level with the articular surface to enhance stabilization. This technique is illustrated in Figures 6-43 and 6-44. The procedure is repeated at 10- to 15-mm intervals, as needed to achieve stable cartilage fixation, by changing the degree of joint flexion.

Postoperative Management

Horses generally receive perioperative antimicrobial drugs and phenylbutazone before surgery and for 5 successive days. This regimen is a precaution against any development of interfascial swelling. Most cases are simple to manage, and the horse can be discharged soon after surgery. Hand walking commences after 1 week to allow some clot organization within the defect. After this time, it is theorized that exercise will facilitate modulation of the tissue within the defect toward some form of fibrocartilage. On the basis of follow-up results, the horse can return to light training 3 to 4 months postoperatively, depending on the age of the animal.

Results

The results of arthroscopic surgery performed in the first 40 cases of OCD involving 24 horses were reported by McIlwraith & Martin (1985). In 1992, the results of arthroscopic surgery for the treatment of OCD in 250 femoropatellar joints in 161 horses were reported (Foland et al, 1992). There were 82 Thoroughbreds, 39 Quarter Horses, 16 Arabians, warmbloods, and 15 others of various breeds. There were 53 females and 108 males: 22 horses

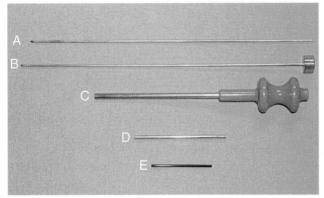

Figure 6-42 PDS Orthosorb® Fixation kit for reattachment of large OCD flap on lateral trochlear ridge of femur. *A*, K-wire for drilling, *B*, plunger for insertion of pin, C, cannula, *D*, protective sleeve of PDS pin, *E*, resorbable pin.

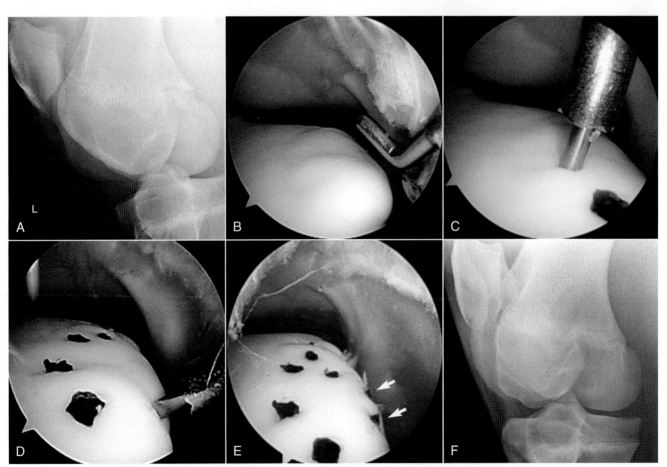

Figure 6-43 Radiograph **(A)** and arthroscopic views **(B-E)** of fixation of OCD flap of lateral trochlear ridge of femur with Orthosorb® PDS pins. Surgical technique for placing PDS pins, with arthroscope positioned normally, pin guide cannula *(arrow)* inserted perpendicular to the lateral trochlear ridge and immediately distal to the apex of the patella, and other instruments such as a probe used to hold the flap in place during reattachment. **F,** Postoperative view.

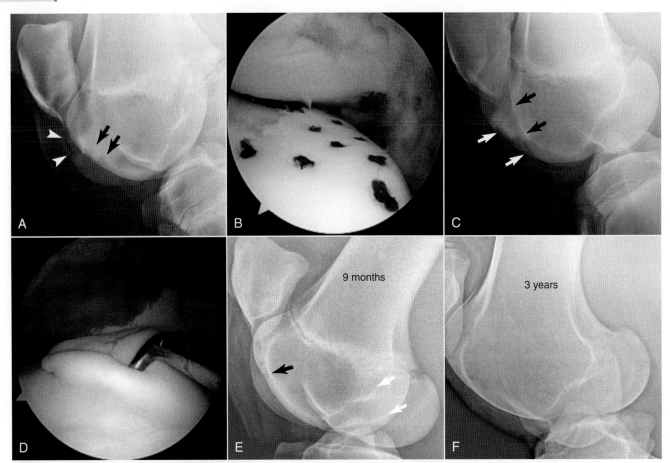

Figure 6-44 Preoperative and long-term radiographic appearance after PDS pinning of left stifle osteochondritis dissecans (OCD). **A,** Preoperative caudolateral to craniomedial oblique showing partially mineralized flap on lateral trochlear ridge (LTR) *(white arrows)* and lysis and irregularity suggesting a flap lesion on medial trochlear ridge (MTR) *(black arrows).* **B,** Intraoperative appearance after placing eight pins in LTR. **C,** Preoperative lateromedial radiograph showing extensive MTR OCD lesion *(white arrows)* and LTR lesion *(black arrows).* **D,** Arthroscopic image showing poor quality predominantly detached cartilage on MTR, which was debrided. **E,** Radiographic appearance 9 months after surgery showing fully restored subchondral plate on LTR and debrided site on MTR *(arrow).* **F,** Radiographs 3 years after surgery showing normal LTR and MTR. The horse had been successfully raced and had no symptoms related to the stifles (both left and right LTR repaired with PDS pins).

were younger than 1 year old at the time of surgery, 68 were yearlings, 36 were 2-year-olds, 21 were 3-year-olds, and 14 were either 4 years old or older; 91 had bilateral involvement and 70 had unilateral disease. It should be noted that OCD of the LTR of the femur has been recently reported in 4 ponies, and their clinical signs and pathologic features of the lesions are consistent with OCD of the LTR in horses (Voute et al, 2011).

Follow-up information was obtained on 134 horses, including 79 racehorses and 55 nonracehorses. Eighty-six (64%) of these 134 horses returned to their intended use, 9 (7%) were in training at the time of publication, 21 (16%) were unsuccessful, and 18 (13%) were unsuccessful due to other defined reasons. Horses with grade I lesions (<2 cm in length) had a significantly higher success rate (78%) than did horses with grade II (2 to 4 cm) or grade III (>4 cm) lesions (63% and 54% success rates, respectively). A significantly higher success rate was also noted for horses operated on as 3-year-olds compared with the remainder of the study population. A significantly lower success rate was noted for yearlings than for the remainder of the population. There was no significant difference as related to gender involved, racehorse versus nonracehorse, lesion location, unilateral versus bilateral involvement,

presence or absence of patellar or trochlear groove lesions, or presence or absence of loose bodies.

Although working soundness may reasonably be anticipated with this surgery in most cases, the nature of healing within the defects is less certain. On the basis of long-term follow-up radiographs obtained in horses that are sound, it seems irregular contours in the subchondral bone frequently persist. After debridement, defects presumably fill with fibrous tissue or fibrocartilage, but this supposition is based on minimal amounts of follow-up necropsy data (Pascoe et al, 1984) or second-look arthroscopy. Whatever the tissue that fills the defect, it seems to provide satisfactory stroma for articulation. No LTR lesion is necessarily too big to negate surgery, but more detailed follow-up evaluation of larger lesions in elite athletes would be appropriate and, as noted previously, the prognosis decreases with length of lesion (Foland et al, 1992). Limitations for healing have been described in the medial condyle of the femur (Convery et al, 1972), but the authors' clinical data support some form of functional filling of these defects on the trochlear ridges.

The healing potential of horses that have undergone operations at 2 to 3 years of age may be less than that of younger animals. Fortunately, these older horses typically have smaller

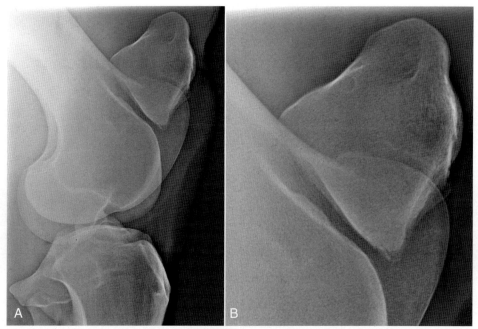

Figure 6-45 Lateromedial radiograph of the stifle **(A)** and lateromedial radiograph of the patella **(B),** showing fragmentation of the distal articular margin of the patella subsequent to medial patellar desmotomy.

defects, complete resurfacing of which may not be as critical for athletic function. Published data for 3-year-olds supports this conclusion (Foland et al, 1992). As presented previously, arthroscopic reattachment of OCD cartilage flaps has been demonstrated to salvage OCD cartilage by integration with the underlying bone (Nixon et al, 2004; Sparks et al, 2011b). Long-term results were presented for reattachment of OCD lesions with PDS pins in 40/44 joints from 27 horses by Sparks et al (2011a). Breeds included Thoroughbred (*n* = 18), Quarter Horse (*n* = 4), warmblood (*n* = 3), Standardbred (*n* = 1), and Arabian (*n* = 1). Mean age was 9.7 months and radiographic lesion length ranged from 1.5 cm to 6.3 cm. Reattachment alone was used in 32 of 44 affected joints, a combination of debridement and reattachment in 8 joints, and debridement alone in 4 joints. One horse was euthanized due to a tendon laceration. Of the remaining 26 horses, mean duration of follow-up was 15.6 months (range 2 months to 12 years). Radiographic resolution of OCD lesions treated with reattachment was significantly improved at 6 months (Fig. 6-45). Twenty horses had long-term performance data in which 19 were sound and had reached intended athletic potential. One horse remained lame, and an additional 6 were sound but remained unbroken or were convalescing at the time of publication. The overall success rate based on continued soundness in performing horses was 95% (19/20) (Sparks et al, 2011a). This was good evidence that with extensive OCD flaps, salvage by reattachment in the appropriate case could result in normal radiographic subchondral bone contour and long-term athletic performance.

A common question from clients regarding surgery for OCD of the stifles is: What is the likelihood of having more lesions develop or will the problem develop in other joints? Of the 161 horses operated on for femoropatellar OCD, 12 underwent concurrent surgery for other lesions, as well as femoropatellar arthroscopy (Foland et al, 1992). Five of these horses had OCD lesions in both metatarsophalangeal joints, 4 horses had OCD of the tarsocrural joint, 2 horses had subchondral cystic lesions of the medial femoral condyle, and 1 horse had OCD of a scapulohumeral joint. In other words, the likelihood of lesions developing elsewhere is low. Also, a

more recent work by Dik et al (1999) demonstrated that there is very low likelihood of additional lesion development in the femoropatellar joint after 11 months of age.

Fragmentation of the Distal Patella

This condition has been reported in the literature (McIlwraith, 1990) and its pathogenesis explored (Gibson et al, 1989). The condition is characterized by osteochondral fragmentation of the distal aspect of the patella. In the initial report of 15 horses, the problem was unilateral in 6 and bilateral in 9 horses and occurred in 8 Quarter Horses, 3 Thoroughbreds, 2 American Saddlebreds, 1 American Paint, and 1 warmblood/Thoroughbred cross. A previous medial patellar desmotomy had been performed on 12 of the 15 horses.

The condition manifests as hindlimb lameness and stiffness ranging from mild to severe. There is fibrous thickening in the stifle area in all cases associated with previous medial patellar desmotomy (the fibrosis is centered over the desmotomy site); synovial effusion is normally present and recognizable if the fibrosis is not too extensive. The radiographic changes include bony fragmentation, spurring (with or without an associated subchondral defect), subchondral roughening, and subchondral lysis of the distal aspect of the patella (see Fig. 6-45).

The treatment is arthroscopic surgery. In the initial series the lesions at arthroscopy varied from flaking, fissuring, undermining, or fragmentation of the articular cartilage to fragmentation or lysis of the bone, or both, at the distal aspect of the patella (Fig. 6-46). The subchondral bone was involved in all cases that had a previous medial patellar desmotomy. Of the 12 horses that had a previous medial patellar desmotomy, 8 horses became sound for their intended use, 1 horse was sold in training without problems, 1 horse was in early training without problems at the time of publication, 1 horse never improved, and 1 horse was in convalescence. Of the three cases that did not have a medial patellar desmotomy, 2 horses performed their intended use, but 1 horse was unsatisfactory. In these instances, there was no severe bone involvement. It is possible that such cases are equivalent to the chondromalacia syndrome described by Adams (1974).

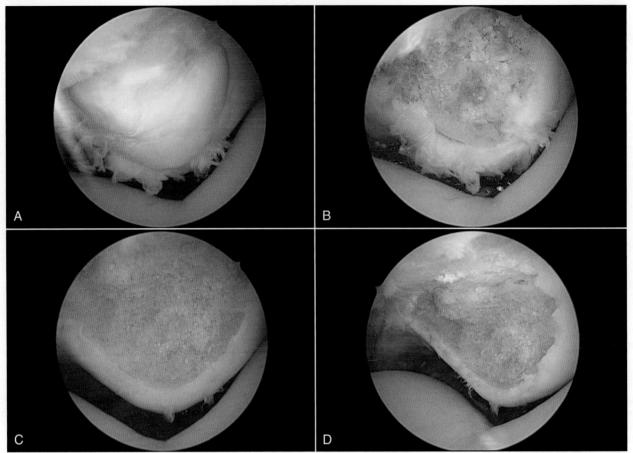

Figure 6-46 A, Arthroscopic appearance of the distal aspect of the patella demonstrating protuberant fragmentation covered by articular cartilage and with tufts of tissue extruded between the fragmentation and parent bone, lateral trochlear ridge to the left, and medial trochlear ridge to the right. **B,** Lesion appearance following removal of fragmentation demonstrating crumbling disorganized bone at the remaining distal aspect of the patella. **C,** Arthroscopic appearance of completion of debridement demonstrating organized bone on the patella with a well-defined osteochondral junction. **D,** Arthroscopic image at completion of debridement as in **C** (above) but with the lens angle rotated to view cranially and laterally demonstrating the debrided origin of the middle patellar ligament and the cranial margin of the fragmentation, lateral trochlear ridge to the left, and medial trochlear ridge to the right.

Preoperative Considerations

The history in these cases usually involves the development of hind limb lameness referable to the stifle, usually after medial patellar desmotomy. In most instances, the specific indication for the medial patellar desmotomy is unknown (performed by other veterinarians). Subsequent to desmotomy, a gonitis develops and persists. Femoropatellar effusion may be present in addition to pericapsular fibrosis. The lameness is typically obvious at the trot but is observable commonly at the walk. Radiographs of the femoropatellar joint reveal either a defect in the bone at the distal aspect of the patella or bony fragmentation (usually associated with an observable defect) of the distal aspect of the patella (see Fig. 6-46). On the basis of a lack of clinical improvement, as well as the presence of radiographic lesions in these cases, arthroscopic surgery is recommended.

Technique

An arthroscopic examination of the femoropatellar joint is performed as previously described. The lesion is identified on the distal patella and any other changes in the joint are noted. A distal lateral arthroscopic portal is made to allow an arthroscopic approach as illustrated in Figure 6-26. A probe is used initially to evaluate the lesion, which typically consists of elevated or fragmented articular cartilage with or without bone fragmentation. The defective tissue is removed by using rongeurs, a curette, a motorized abrader, or a combination of these. The joint is then lavaged in typical fashion.

Postoperative Management and Results

The overall prognosis is good. The incidence of these cases has now subsided, presumably due to recognition that medial patellar desmotomy can potentially lead to this complication (Gibson et al, 1989). In that study medial patellar desmotomy was performed in one stifle of 12 horses and a sham surgery performed in the opposite stifle. Lameness could be recognized by an observer unaware of the treatment groups at 1, 2, and 3 months after surgery, and at 3 months 8/12 showed radiographic lesions at the apex of the patella and 12/12 had arthroscopic fragmentation. Since that study the records of 78 horses with intermittent or permanent upward fixation of the patella were analyzed retrospectively (Dumoulin et al, 2007). Seventy-six horses were treated conservatively with corrective farriery, exercise, and dietary changes. Follow-up was available for 64 conservatively treated horses and was successful in 51.6% of patients, while 20.3% improved partially. In 18 cases with no response to conservative treatment and in 2 cases with permanent fixation, medial patellar desmotomy was performed. This corrected the fixation in 17/18 patients followed up. However, gait abnormalities were seen in 7 of those

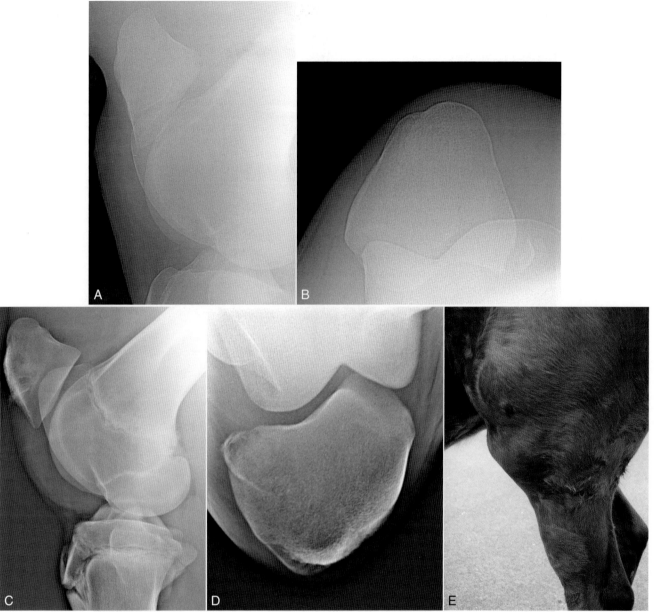

Figure 6-47 Lateral **(A)** and skyline **(B)** radiographic views of a femoropatellar joint with a fracture fragment off the medial aspect of the patella (arthroscopic views in Fig. 6-48). **C,** Lateromedial radiograph of displaced fragment protruding cranially from a defect in the patella—fragment sufficiently large and displaced to be visible on this radiographic view. **D,** Flexed cranioproximal-craniodistal oblique projection demonstrating same fracture off the medial pole of the patella. **E,** The affected femoropatellar joint demonstrates soft tissue swelling consistent with synovial fluid distention.

17 horses with the incidence being lower in horses that had been rested for at least 3 months (25%) compared with horses that had only rested for less than 1 month (66.6%), indicating that the longer convalescence is advantageous. More recently a controlled study evaluating the effects of medial patellar desmotomy combined with exercise restriction was done. The authors demonstrated that medial patellar desmotomy leads to patellar instability, and this can be demonstrated by radiographic changes. A 120-day rest period did not prevent the lesions caused by postsurgical patellar instability (Baccarin et al, 2009).

Patellar Fractures

Selected fracture fragments off the patella can be removed arthroscopically. Each case operated arthroscopically by the authors involved a traumatic incident and severe lameness referable to the stifle. Femoropatellar joint distension is frequently accompanied by general swelling of the stifle. Although conventional radiographs showed suspicious changes, accurate definition of the fracture required a skyline radiograph of the femoropatellar joint (Fig. 6-47). Fractures are typically medial but have also been seen on the lateral side.

Diagnostic arthroscopic examination reveals the distal articular part of the fracture in each case (Fig. 6-48), as well as damage elsewhere (seen occasionally). The fragments are removed by using a medial or lateral portal as appropriate. Instruments may include a banana blade, elevator, Ferris-Smith rongeurs, and motorized abrader. In occasional instances, a fracture of the medial patellar fibrocartilage without osseous involvement may be seen (see Fig. 6-48).

A retrospective study of five performance horses with patellar fractures treated with arthroscopic removal has been

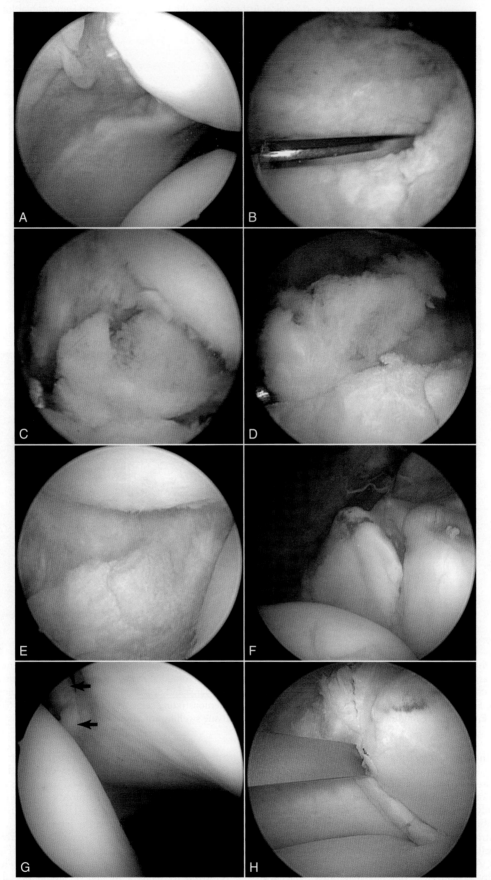

▶ **Figure 6-48** Arthroscopic views of fracture fragment of medial aspect of patella **(A)** with fracture fragment attached to medial patellar fibrocartilage **(B)** the medial patellar ligament fibrocartilage attachment being severed from the medial side of the fracture fragment **(F)**. **C,** After separation of fracture fragment. **D,** Fracture fragment totally free, which is needed before removal. **E,** After fragment removal and debridement of defect in medial aspect of patella. **F,** Arthroscopic view of distal margin of the patella of displaced fracture off distal medial pole of the patella as depicted in radiograph Figure 6-47C to D. **G,** Arthroscope moved forward beneath patella to reveal an intact proximal medial margin and proximal portion of the medial patellar fibrocartilage with fracture plane distally *(arrows)*. **H,** Sectioning of the medial margin of the fracture fragment from the medial patellar fibrocartilage with a menosectomy knife.

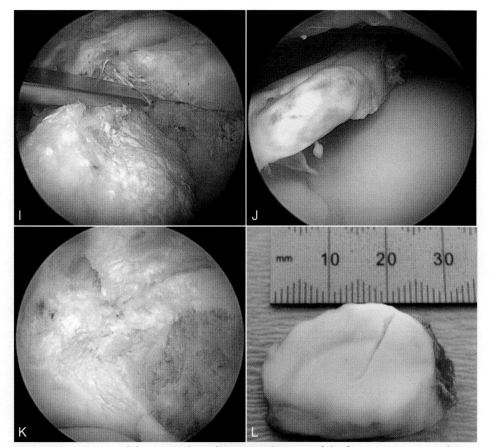

Figure 6-48, cont'd I, Continued dissection along the proximal margin of the fracture. **J,** Fragment following dissection lying adjacent to the medial trochlear ridge of the femur. **K,** Arthroscopic appearance of the fracture bed following fragment removal and demonstrating an intact medial patellar fibrocartilage. **L,** Fracture fragment following removal demonstrating distal (articular) surface.

reported (Marble & Sullins, 2000). Four of five horses had fractures of the medial aspect of the patella, and one horse had a fracture of the lateral aspect. Arthroscopy was performed in the femoropatellar joint using techniques described previously. There were no complications. Recovery periods ranged from 3 to 5 months. All horses recovered completely from surgery and performed at the same or a higher level of competition as before arthroscopy.

Recently, three cases of concurrent medial patellar fracture and lateral collateral ligament avulsion fracture have been reported. Both lesions were visible ultrasonographically and radiographically. Arthroscopic surgery to remove the patella fracture was attempted in one horse with severe desmitis of the lateral collateral ligament, and it remained lame afterwards (McLellan et al, 2012). The other two horses with less severe collateral ligament damage were managed conservatively and returned to athletic use despite the lack of surgical intervention to repair the patella fractures. The authors concluded that ultrasonographic findings pertaining to the collateral ligament may be prognostically important in such cases and this may be the limiting factor when such combined injuries occur.

Osteoarthritis and Osteophytosis of Femoropatellar Joint

Identification of osteoarthritis and accompanying osteophytosis of the femoropatellar joint involving the femoral trochlea or patella, or both, have been more recently identified based on referral for diagnostic arthroscopy. Cases may be referred on the basis of persistence of problems in the femoropatellar joint that are unresponsive to therapy and sometimes are accompanied by osteophytosis that is visible on the radiographs (Fig. 6-49). Diagnostic arthroscopy confirms the presence of varying levels of loss of articular cartilage on the trochlea and patella (see Fig. 6-49C-E). Treatment involves selective removal of osteophytes (see Fig. 6-49) and debridement of any elevated and separated articular cartilage. When there is extensive loss of articular cartilage, the prognosis is guarded.

ARTHROSCOPIC SURGERY OF THE MEDIAL FEMOROTIBIAL JOINT

Cystic Lesions of the Medial Condyle of the Femur

Cystic lesions of the femoral condyles remain one of the most common indications for stifle arthroscopy in the horse. In immature horses, many are simple cartilage apertures with deeper bone collapse and can be dealt with in a variety of definitive ways, including corticosteroid injection, debridement, and simple bone or cell grafting. Complicated cases with osteoarthritis can be more challenging, and widespread cartilage erosion and secondary meniscus failure generally signal the need for ancillary arthroscopic repair, using cell grafts and other biological repair systems to overcome the joint degenerative load. Despite the degree of complexity, arthroscopy remains the start point for diagnosis, staging, and subsequent choice of repair.

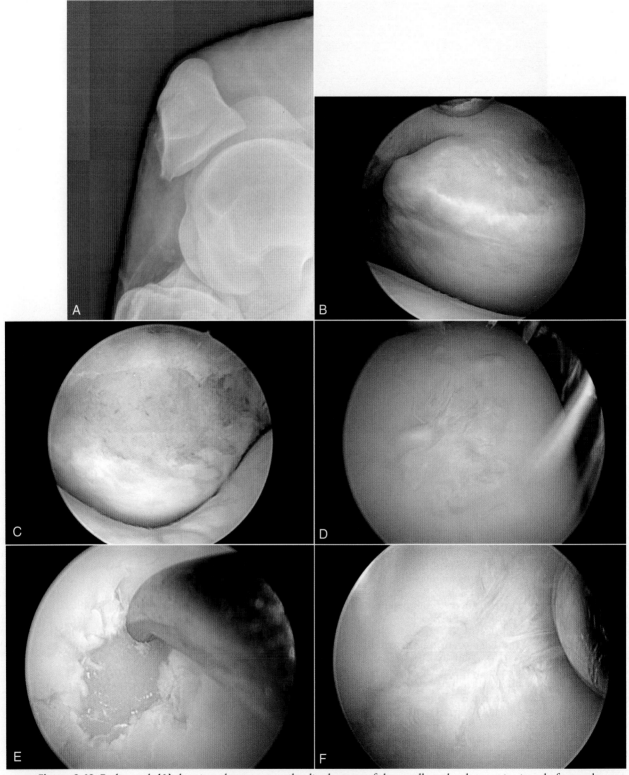

Figure 6-49 Radiograph **(A)** showing a large spur on the distal aspect of the patella and arthroscopic views before and after removal **(B** and **C). D** and **E,** Separation of articular cartilage on lateral trochlear ridge before and after debridement. **F,** Fibrillation and erosion on medial trochlear ridge and trochlear groove.

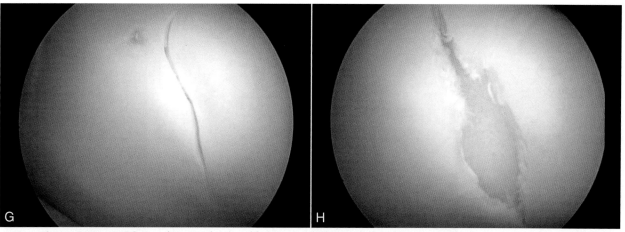

Figure 6-49, cont'd G and **H,** Crack in trochlear groove before and after debridement back to attaching cartilage.

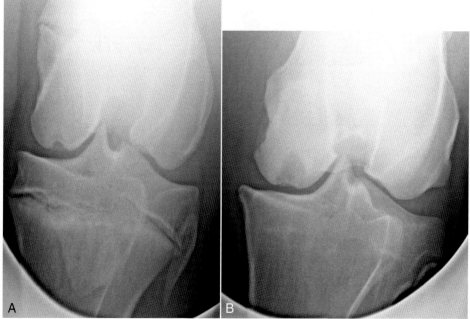

Figure 6-50 Radiographs of subchondral bone cysts as initially classified by White et al, 1988. **A,** Type I dome-shaped lesion. **B,** Type II circular lucent defect.

Preoperative Considerations

The typical clinical sign is lameness in one or both hindlimbs at a trot. In some horses, lameness is subtle and is noticeable only during riding. Historically, some of these horses can be in training for considerable periods of time, with clinical signs manifesting only after a certain amount of work has been done. Most horses swing the leg medially, and the lameness is accentuated when trotting in a circle with the affected leg inside. Medial femorotibial analgesia localizes the lesion, but a response can also be obtained with analgesia of the femoropatellar joint. There can be mild to moderate distention of the femorotibial joint, but it is more common to see femoropatellar effusion (Howard et al, 1995).

The lesion is apparent radiographically. Caudocranial, caudolateral-craniomedial oblique, and flexed lateral views are useful to ascertain the nature, location, and size of the lesion. There have been a number of radiographic classifications of subchondral cystic lesions (SCLs) of the medial femoral condyle (MFC). In the initial description of surgical treatment (White et al, 1988) there were two types: type I (dome-shaped

lesions) and type II (circular, lucent defects) (Fig. 6-50). Most recently, clinical lesions have been identified as four types with one having two subtypes (Wallis et al, 2008):
- Type 1: a dome-shaped lucent area opening to the surface
- Type 2: full cystic lesions with a and b subtypes depending on the opening at the joint surface
- Type 3: flattening or irregular contour of the subchondral bone
- Type 4: a SCL with no radiographic evidence of a cloaca in the subchondral bone plate (Fig. 6-51)

With the advent of digital radiography equipment and survey radiographs at yearling sales, more attention has been paid to minor subchondral defects and even flattening of the medial femoral condyle (Contino et al, 2012). Such lesions may be bilateral. A typical case may have a small type 3 lesion in one stifle opposite to one manifesting clinically and exhibiting a large cystic lesion or, more commonly, a type 3 defect being seen as an incidental finding on prepurchase radiographs of yearlings (Contino et al, 2012; Whitman et al, 2006).

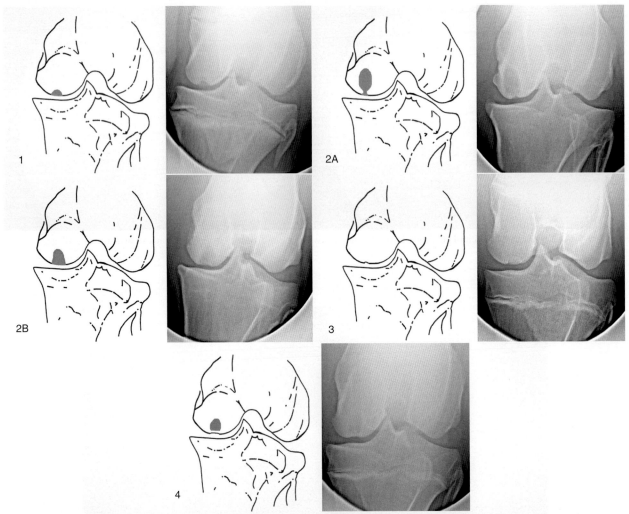

Figure 6-51 More recent classification of subchondral cystic lesions (SCLs) of the medial femoral condyle (MFC). Type 1 lesions are defined as being less than 10 mm in depth and are usually dome shaped. Type 2a lesions are >10 mm in depth and have a lollipop or mushroom shape with a narrow cloaca and a round cystic lucency. Type 2b lesions are greater than 10 mm in depth with a large dome shape extending down to a large articular surface defect. Type 3 lesions are defined as condylar flattening or small defects in the subchondral bone, usually noted in the contralateral limb to that of a clinically significant SCL. Type 4 lesions are classified as those that have a lucency in the condyle with or without an articular defect but no radiographic evidence of a cloaca in the subchondral bone plate. *(Reprinted with permission from Wallis et al, 2008.)*

The development of subchondral cystic lesions has been associated with both osteochondrosis and trauma. Whereas osteochondrosis was initially considered the exclusive pathogenesis, observations of cystic enlargement after surgery prompted further investigation into the pathogenesis of these lesions and to reasons why they may potentially expand. Work in the first author's (C.W.M.) laboratory (Ray et al, 1996) showed that it was possible to consistently produce (5/6 cases) subchondral cystic lesions by creating a 5-mm diameter, 3-mm deep defect in the subchondral bone at the central weight-bearing portion of the medial condyle of the femur. Other work then revealed that the fibrous tissue of subchondral cystic lesions (removed surgically) released nitric oxide, PGE_2, and neutral metalloprotases into culture media after in vitro culturing. It was also shown that conditioned media of the cultured tissue was capable of recruiting osteoclasts and increasing their activity (von Rechenberg et al, 2000). It was therefore believed that the inflamed fibrous tissue lining could play an active role in the pathologic processes of bone resorption occurring in the subchondral cystic lesions and may be partially responsible for the slow healing

rate and expansion of these lesions. Following these studies, the first author (C.W.M.) started injecting corticosteroids at the time of surgical debridement, which then progressed to direct injection of SCL (Wallis et al, 2008); this is presented in detail later.

Treatment Options

Although surgical debridement of cystic lesions has been the standard treatment for some time and is being described here, a number of other options have been used. Historically, cancellous bone grafting has been used (Kold & Hickman, 1984), but results with this technique, through arthrotomy at least, were not as good as simple debridement (White et al, 1988). A controlled study since then with cancellous bone grafting in experimentally created 12.7-mm diameter and 19-mm deep defects in the medial femoral condyle showed that healing was similar in grafted and ungrafted defects in the equine medial femoral condyle over a 6-month reevaluation period (Jackson et al, 2000). This suggested that surgical debridement alone rather than adjunctive bone grafting of cystic lesions could be the principal contributor.

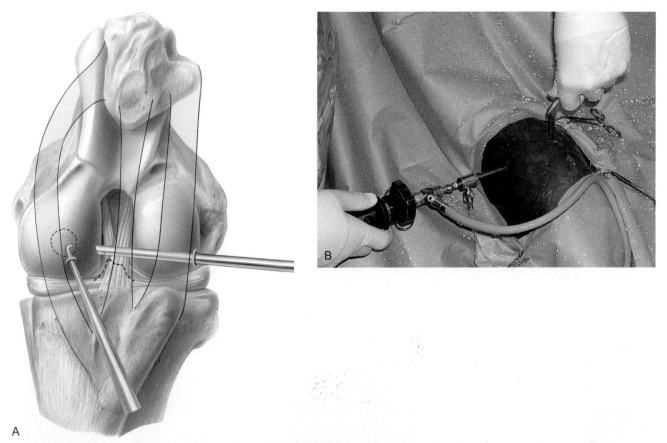

Figure 6-52 A, Diagram and external view **(B)** of arthroscope and instrument position during operations involving subchondral cystic lesions on the medial condyle of the femur.

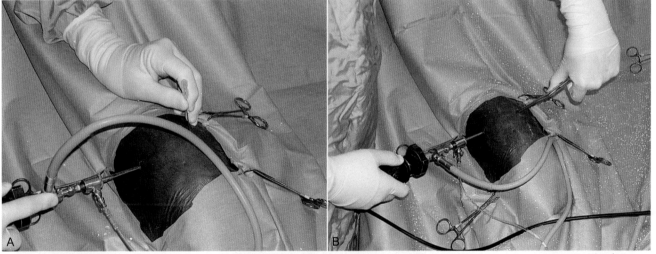

Figure 6-53 A, Using a spinal needle to determine the ideal instrument portal placement for operating on cystic lesions of the medial condyle of the femur. The arthroscope is placed through a lateral portal. **B,** Ferris-Smith rongeurs are placed in cranial instrument portal for operating on a cystic lesion of the medial condyle of the femur.

▶ *Arthroscopic Debridement of SCLs of Medial Condyle of Femur*

Debridement of SCLs was initially reported using arthrotomy (White et al, 1988), and an arthroscopic technique first described by Lewis (1987). Results for arthroscopic surgery for SCLs in the medial femoral condyle have since been reported (Howard et al, 1995; Sandler et al, 2002; Smith et al, 2005).

The authors use the technique developed by Lewis (1987), and this technique is illustrated in Figures 6-52 to 6-54. The procedure is performed with the horse under general anesthesia in dorsal recumbency. The leg is flexed such that the stifle and hock are approximately at 90-degree angles. Stabilizing the leg in this position is recommended. The medial femorotibial joint can be distended with irrigating solution, but for experienced surgeons, this is not necessary. The arthroscope is inserted through the

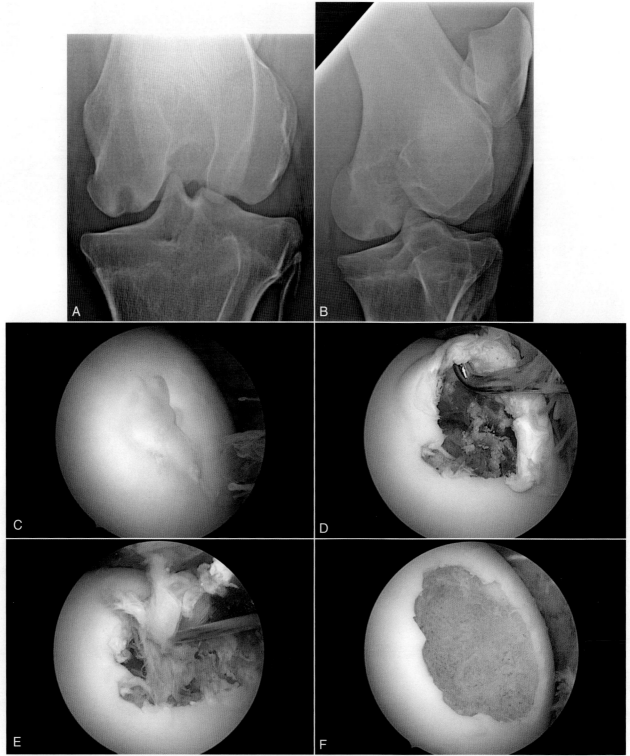

Figure 6-54 A, Caudocranial radiograph demonstrating subchondral cystic lesion (SCL) of medial femoral condyle (MFC). **B,** Caudolateral-craniomedial oblique projection illustrating a wide articular deficit. **C,** Arthroscopic appearance of same SCL illustrating irregular concavity with crevices in articular cartilage at the margin of the cystic opening. **D,** Elevation of the cartilage at the cyst opening with an arthroscopic probe revealing hemorrhagic, disorganized underlying tissue filling the cystic lumen. **E,** Fibromyxoid cyst lining being removed with arthroscopic rongeurs. **F,** Arthroscopic appearance at completion of evacuation and debridement.

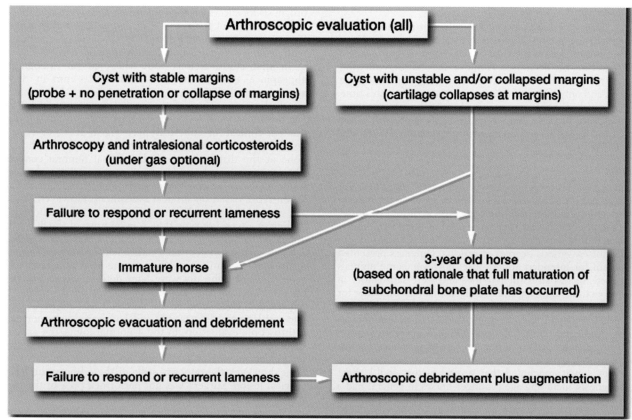

Figure 6-55 Algorithm of treatment decisions/pathways with subchondral cystic lesions of medial condyle of femur. This is an amalgamation of the three authors.

lateral portal between the lateral patellar ligament and the origin of the long digital extensor tendon, and examination of the medial femorotibial joint is performed as previously described.

The characteristic defect (dimple or slit) in the articular cartilage overlying the subchondral cystic lesion is visualized (see Fig. 6-54), and the location for the instrument portal is determined by placement of a needle (see Figs. 6-53A and 6-54B). This must be positioned so that the instruments contact the site of the lesion perpendicular to the articular surface, to enable effective surgical manipulations. The instrument portal is then made using an 8-mm incision through the skin and fascia and a stab through the joint capsule with a No. 11 blade (see Figs. 6-53B and 6-54C). The defective articular cartilage and subchondral bone are removed by using a curette and rongeurs (see Fig. 6-54). Sometimes a motorized resector is useful to assist in removing the fibromyxoid lining and other degenerate tissue.

The configurations of the cystic lesions at arthroscopy vary and can be multiloculated. Typically debridement of the subchondral tissue continues to normal bone. Because cancellous bone in young horses is quite soft anyway, this can be a difficult decision. Cartilage that is overhanging the hole is conservatively cut back to gain sufficient access to the SCL, but not more than that. Although drilling of the SCL has been abandoned because it appeared to be associated with enlargement of cysts (Howard et al, 1995), microfracture has been performed in the walls of the SCL and it is a subjective impression that it is quite useful.

Following debridement, the joint is lavaged liberally and application of suction can be useful. Care is taken during initial debridement of the contents of the cyst to remove defective tissue immediately from the joint and to minimize debris accumulation elsewhere. Inevitably some debris is released into the joint, and it generally accumulates in the intercondylar

area lateral to the medial condyle. A special effort is made during lavage and suctioning of the joint to remove all debris from this area. Finally, the skin portals are closed with simple interrupted sutures.

This technique of debridement is still practiced for certain indications as presented in the flow chart illustrated in Figure 6-55. Intralesional injection of triamcinolone acetonide (C.W.M. and A.J.N.) and methylprednisolone acetate (I.M.W.) into the fibrous tissue of SCLs is used as the primary procedure in cases with stable margins (see Fig. 6-55). Augmentation following debridement is being used increasingly when intralesional injection fails. This augmentation can take a number of forms, including cancellous bone grafting with or without chondrocytes or mesenchymal stem cells (MSCs) in fibrin glue or simple fibrin bone marrow–derived mesenchymal stem cells (BMSCs).

Treatment of shallow, crater-like femoral condyle lucencies, particularly those in the other stifle of a horse with a subchondral cyst, remains controversial. Arthroscopic examination of the lesser affected femorotibial (FT) joint seems prudent. A decision on debridement can be made after visual assessment and probing of the lesion to detect detached regions. Partially detached cartilage that is still smooth and hyaline in appearance may be salvaged by reattachment using PDS pins (Sparks et al, 2011b), as previously described for OCD flaps in the femoropatellar joint (Sparks et al, 2011a). Drilling the denser subchondral bone of the condyle takes more time, and the pins are inserted obliquely to the cartilage surface to minimize the potential for cyst formation (see Fig. 6-57). Resolution of the cartilage crater has been evident in three horses, which improves the potential for permanently avoiding later problems, including subchondral cyst formation.

Postoperative Management

Horses receive perioperative antimicrobial drugs and phenylbutazone. The patient is confined to a stall for 2 months. Hand walking commences at the time of suture removal, or 2 weeks later if grafting has been used. A minimum of 4 more months' pasture rest is recommended before training commences or resumes and only if the horse is sound at a trot after this time. In the series of cases reported by Lewis, the postoperative convalescence in cases that were ultimately successful varied from 4 to 18 months and averaged approximately 7½ months (Lewis, 1987).

Results

In the series reported by Lewis, complete soundness for intended use was achieved in 34 of the 67 cases on the basis of follow-up information from the owners. In addition, 14 horses were sound enough that they were used as intended, despite occasional mild lameness in the affected limb. Of the remaining 19 horses, various degrees of residual lameness presented a problem for intended athletic use; however, some animals were used for less stressful activities and were satisfactory in that respect. In summary, the overall satisfactory outcome for intended use was 72% (48 of the 67 cases). Of the 19 failures for intended use, 11 were from a group of 28 potential racehorses, producing a 39% failure rate. Eight were from a group of 39 horses intended for other use (cutting, reining, roping, and pleasure), representing a 21% failure rate in these types of horses. Lewis concluded that several factors could affect the prognosis, including age (younger horses in general had a better prognosis), unilateral versus bilateral lesions (cases of bilateral involvement were somewhat less successful), significant training or use before surgery (generally decreased the prognosis), previous administration of intraarticular medication (subjectively, the author thought prior corticosteroid injection was detrimental to the ultimate outcome), radiographic appearance (the broader opening of the cyst at the articular surface was associated with a less favorable prognosis), preexisting degenerative joint disease (poorer prognosis), and intended use (racehorses were the most difficult to return to intended use).

Howard et al (1995) described the results of arthroscopic surgery for SCL in the medial femoral condyle in 41 horses. There were 17 Quarter Horses, 15 Arabians, 8 Thoroughbreds, and 1 Holsteiner with 28 (68%) of the horses being 1 to 3 years old. For all horses, the owner's complaint was mild to moderate hindlimb lameness or an altered gait. Bilateral radiographic abnormalities of the medial femoral condyle were detected in 27 horses. Nineteen of the 27 horses had lesions identified bilaterally at arthroscopic surgery. In addition to the SCL, 13 joints in 11 horses had an OCD lesion on the articular surface of the medial femoral condyle that extended from the opening of the SCL. Surgical debridement performed by arthroscopy was the only treatment for 37 lesions in 23 horses. Debridement followed by drilling of the defect bed was performed in 23 lesions of 18 horses. Complete follow-up information was obtained for 39 horses: 22 (56%) horses had a successful result and 17 (44%) horses had an unsuccessful result.

Analyzing the Howard (1995) data by excluding horses with unsuccessful results because of factors not directly attributed to the SCL of the medial femoral condyle (censored analysis), 23 of 31 (74%) horses had a successful result and 8 of 31 (26%) horses had an unsuccessful result. Within this group of horses, the prognosis for a successful result after arthroscopic surgery was not associated with age, sex, size of lesion, unilateral or bilateral lesions, whether the lesion was drilled, the presence of OCD associated with the SCL, or whether the lesion enlarged after surgery. Compared with Thoroughbreds and Arabians, Quarter Horses had a poorer

prognosis for success. Follow-up radiographs were available for 14 horses. In 9 of these, the SCL had enlarged after surgery. Postoperative cystic enlargement was associated significantly with drilling of the lesion bed at the time of surgery.

In that study, lesions were classified on radiographic appearance as either type I lesions (≤10 mm in depth, appearing as shallow, saucer, or dome-shaped defects in the weight-bearing surface of the medial femoral condyle) (see Fig. 6-50A), type II lesions (>10 mm in depth and typically domed, conical, or spherical) (see Fig. 6-50B), or type III lesions (flattened or irregular contours of the subchondral bone at the distal aspect of the medial femoral condyle). Linear regression showed a significant association between lesion types as assessed from preoperative radiographs and lesion types based on surgical assessment. However, surgical assessment of lesions did not correspond to the radiographic finding of a type I or type II SCL in 6 joints; of the SCLs that appeared to be type I radiographically, 1 was a type II SCL, 1 had a cartilage defect only, and 2 had no surgical lesion at arthroscopic examination. Two lesions that appeared to be type II radiographically were later determined to be type I on the basis of arthroscopic findings. Of the 15 joints that appeared to have subchondral defect, 3 had a type I SCL, 6 had cartilaginous defects only, and 4 appeared to be normal at arthroscopic evaluation. In the 4 normal joints, the articular cartilage was firm and well attached to the subchondral bone on palpation with a probe and no surgical treatment was done; however, the opposite stifle of these horses did have a surgical lesion. Surgery was not performed on 2 of the joints with a subchondral defect.

A more recent paper published the results of arthroscopic debridement of SCL of the medial femoral condyle in Thoroughbred horses (Sandler et al, 2002). The depth and width of each lesion was measured radiographically as either type II or I, as previously described (Howard et al, 1995). Additionally, the amount of cartilage surface disrupted by the injury was measured arthroscopically at the time of surgery and the horses were divided into two groups: those with lesions that involved 15 mm or less cartilage surface and those with greater than 15 mm of disruption. During the period between 1989 and 2000, 150 clinically lame Thoroughbred horses with a total of 214 SCL underwent surgery. Eighty-six (58%) horses had unilateral lesions and 64 (42%) horses had bilateral lesions. A total of 96 (64%) of the operated horses raced, compared with 77% of their siblings; 48% of females raced, whereas 71% of males raced; 28% (42) of the horses that were operated on raced as 2-year-olds, 61% (79) as 3-year-olds, and 51% (55) as 4-year-olds. The number of starts and average earnings per start for the horses that had been operated on were less than their maternal siblings for their 2- and 3-year-old racing careers but were similar to their siblings for the 4-year-old racing year. Of the 49 horses with type I lesions, 34 (69.3%) horses started a race in their career, whereas 62 (61.3%) horses with type II lesions started. This indicated that radiographically assessed lesion depth was of little consequence in defining the prognosis. Additionally, there were 91 (60.6%) horses with less than or equal to 15 mm of surface debridement and 59 (39.3%) horses with greater than 15 mm of surface debridement. Of the 91 horses with 15 mm or less of surface disrupted, more than 70% started at least one race, whereas only about 30% of the 59 horses with greater than 15 mm of cartilage surface involvement started a race. Thus, the area of cartilage surface affected appeared to be a better predictor of success than lesion depth.

The age of the horse was considered to be an important prognostic factor in a retrospective study by Smith et al (2005) in which the medical records from six equine referral centers identified 85 horses that underwent arthroscopic debridement of SCLs. Twenty-five of 39 horses aged 0 to 3 years were debrided (64%, 95% CI 49% to 70%) returned to soundness compared with 16 of 46 horses aged older than 3 years (35%, 95% CI 21% to 49%). In addition, cartilage damage at sites other than the MFC negatively affected prognosis ($p = 0.05$). The presence of cartilage lesions or radiographic signs of OA negatively affecting prognosis is therefore consistent across a number of studies (Howard et al, 1995; Smith et al, 2005; Wallis et al, 2008), but age of horse seems to be less significant when SCLs are treated by direct intraarticular injection of corticosteroids without debridement (Wallis et al, 2008) (see next section).

There has been some relatively recent evidence of a potential clinical relationship between debridement of SCLs of the medial femoral condyle and development of a meniscal lesion. Six horses developed a meniscal lesion subsequent to SCL debridement (and two developed an SCL subsequent to a medial meniscal injury) (Hendrix et al, 2010). The authors of that study suggested that the sharp edge of a debrided SCL potentially caused trauma to the cranial pole of the medial meniscus or the cranial ligament of the medial meniscus, or both.

Arthroscopic Injection of Corticosteroids into the Fibrous Tissue of Subchondral Cystic Lesions

In the third edition of this text it was mentioned that one author (C.W.M.) has treated a number of cases with intralesional injection of corticosteroid (triamcinolone acetonide) under arthroscopic visualization (Fig. 6-56) with positive preliminary results. Since then the results of SCLs in the MFC treated with arthroscopic injection of corticosteroids into the lining of the cyst have been reported (Wallis et al, 2008). This more recent surgical technique has the rationale of injecting the cystic lining to reduce the production of local inflammatory mediators. These inflammatory mediators found in the fibrous tissue within the cysts recruit osteoclasts and have been demonstrated to cause active resorption of bone in vitro (von Rechenberg et al, 2000). On the basis of this research involving one of the authors (C.W.M.), the arthroscopic technique for corticosteroid injection was developed. Hypothesized advantages of the technique included a similar or increased chance of success as compared with debridement, shorter convalescence, lower risk of cystic enlargement, and minimal disruption of the articular surface. In addition, it was believed that if the procedure was unsuccessful, other surgical therapies could be offered, such as arthroscopic debridement with or without other reconstructive techniques.

The surgical technique involves a standard lateral arthroscopic approach to the medial femorotibial joint. The cranial pouch of the medial femorotibial joint is thoroughly explored, and in some instances loose tissue is removed from the MFC defect. A cranial instrument portal is created to provide direct vertical access to the area of the cyst. The probe is used to evaluate firmness of tissue, and then an 18-gauge spinal needle is placed into the depth of the cyst and 6 to 10 mg of triamcinolone acetonide injected. The total dose of TA used is usually 18 mg (3 mL). If no corticosteroid leaks from the cloaca, then an additional amount can be injected. Otherwise, the spinal needle is relocated and TA injected in another location (it is not uncommon to place the needle through cartilage peripheral to the cloaca to maximize deposition of TA in the lining).

Postoperative Care

The horse is stall rested for 2 weeks with sutures removed at 10 to 12 days. At 2 weeks hand walking is instituted for 5 minutes once or twice a day and walking increased by 5 minutes each week until 60 days postsurgery. At this time the horse is reevaluated at the walk and trot and, if there is no lameness, put back into training.

Results

Overall 35/52 (67%) cases (horses) were classified as successful, involving 73 joints of which 56 (77%) were classified as successful; an additional 5 horses, giving a total of 40/52 horses (77%), were considered sound on veterinary examination but for various reasons were not performing their intended use. There was no significant association between age group (age <3 years vs. >3 years) or cyst configuration on outcome. Forty-three/55 (78%) SCLs in horses aged 0 to 3 years and 13/18 (72%) SCLs in horses older than 3 years were classified successful. This equates to 27/39 (69%) 0 to 3 years and 8/13 (62%) age older than 3 years were classified as successful. Significantly more unilateral SCLs (28/31; 90%) were classified as successful with bilateral (28/42; 67%) cases being successful. Follow-up was available for 59 SCLs where preoperative radiographs were available for determination of lesion type. There was no significant association between lesion type and success. Radiographic findings of osteophytes were found on preoperative radiographs or listed in the radiograph report of 16/61 SCLs (26%). There was a significant association between absence of these osteophytes and success ($p = 0.04$). Ten/16 limbs (63%) with these radiographic signs were classified as successful as compared with 39/45 (87%) without any radiographic osteophytes being classified as successful.

There was a trend toward successful association ($p = 0.07$) between breed and success. Six/6 SCLs (100%) of Arabians, 1 (100%) Hanoverian, 18/20 (90%) of Thoroughbreds, 26/36 (72%) of American Quarter Horses, and 5/10 (50%) of American Paint Horses were classified as successful. Cartilage damage, not associated with the cloaca of the SCL, was found in 8/68 cases. Of these 8 SCLs, 5 were classified as successful (63%) compared with 46/60 (77%) without signs of cartilage damage being classified as successful, which is not statistically significant. However, there was a trend toward a significant difference ($p = 0.08$) in success based on the presence of other soft tissue damage within the joint, such as fraying of the medial cranial meniscotibial ligament (most common finding). Only 4/8 (50%) SCLs with other soft tissue damage of the joint were classified as successful compared with 47/60 (78%) SCLs without other soft tissue damage being successful. There was also a significant association between time to first reevaluation (and, therefore, return to exercise if the horse was sound) and success ($p = 0.02$). Eight/9 (89%) SCLs reevaluated at 30 days and 33/38 (87%) at 60 days were successful, whereas only 15/26 (58%) SCLs were successful when they were not first re-evaluated until 90 days postoperatively (Wallis et al, 2008).

Cancellous Bone Grafting and Mosaic Arthroplasty

Use of cancellous bone grafting was initially described by Kold and Hickman (1984) using arthrotomy. A case series was presented with results appearing inferior to another study in which debridement alone was performed (White et al, 1998). More recently, cancellous bone grafting for experimentally induced SCLs showed disappointing results owing to necrosis of the grafted bone, with secondary cyst formation and lesion enlargement by 6 months in 80% of grafted cases (Jackson et al, 2000). Long-term studies were not conducted, so the final morphological outcome of cancellous bone grafting is unknown.

Mosaic arthroplasty has been reported to restore articular surfaces of SCLs (Bodo et al, 2004). A case series of SCLs in four locations (medial femoral condyle 5 horses, lateral femoral condyle 1 horse, distal metacarpus 4 horses, and distal metatarsus 1 horse). Osteochondral autograft transplantation (mosaic athroplasty) was performed taking grafts from the abaxial border of the medial femoral trochlear of the unaffected limb. Graft implantation was achieved through a small

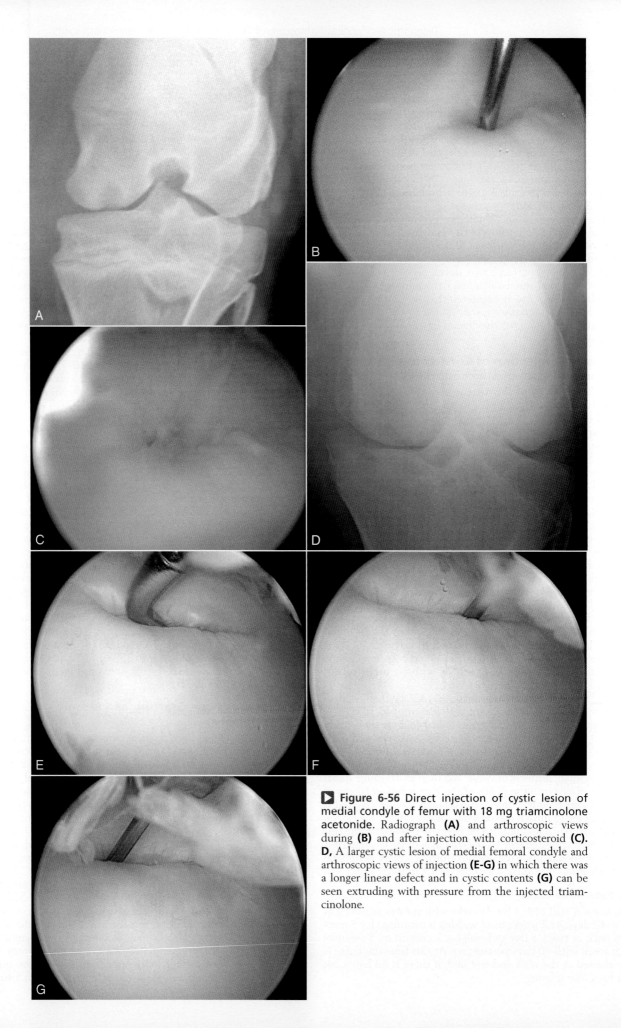

Figure 6-56 Direct injection of cystic lesion of medial condyle of femur with 18 mg triamcinolone acetonide. Radiograph **(A)** and arthroscopic views during **(B)** and after injection with corticosteroid **(C)**. **D,** A larger cystic lesion of medial femoral condyle and arthroscopic views of injection **(E-G)** in which there was a longer linear defect and in cystic contents **(G)** can be seen extruding with pressure from the injected triamcinolone.

arthrotomy or arthroscopy depending on SCL location. All horses improved postoperatively; 10 had successful outcomes with radiographic evidence of successful graft incorporation, and 7 returned to a previous or higher activity level. On follow-up arthroscopy in 5 horses there was successful reconstitution of a functional gliding surface. The authors of this study recognized limitations of this technique, including size and depth of cystic lesions, the time-consuming and invasive nature of harvesting grafts, and the risk of donor site morbidity with larger grafts. The technique is technically demanding, and inserting a graft at an angle and leaving exposed subchondral bone in the side wall of the recipient hole is an unacceptable technical error (Bodo et al, 2004). A study mapping donor and recipient site properties for osteochondral graft reconstruction of SCLs in the equine stifle joint showed that the material properties of the grafts from the trochlear groove and axial aspect of the LTR were the closest match for those found in the medial condyle, whereas the properties of the lateral condyle were most similar to those found in the trochlear groove and axial aspect of the MTR (Changoor et al, 2006).

Chondrocytes or Mesenchymal Stem Cells in Fibrin Glue

The potential for implantation of chondrocytes or mesenchymal stem cells in fibrin glue has been proposed (Fortier and Nixon, 2005), and such techniques for articular cartilage repair are presented in Chapter 16. Recently the use of chondrocytes cultured from articular cartilage of healthy horses younger than 1 year old at postmortem together with recombinant human IGF-1 was reported (Ortved et al, 2012). Arthroscopic cyst debridement followed by filling of the bone void with

autologous cancellous bone (45 horses) or tricalcium phosphate granules (4 horses) was performed (Fig. 6-57). A paired syringe containing a fibrinogen and chondrocyte mixture in one syringe and calcium activated bovine thrombin with IGF in the other was used to cover the surface.

A successful outcome was achieved in 36/49 (74%) horses, of which 33 horses had unilateral and 15 bilateral lesions; 1 horse had bilateral SCLs of the lateral femoral condyle. Median age of the horses was 3.3 years. Fifteen horses had preoperative radiographic and arthroscopic evidence of OA. Grafting resulted in success for 80% of horses older than 3 years old and 80% of horses with OA. The technique is illustrated below (see Fig. 6-59). The authors concluded that implantation of allogenic chondrocytes and IGF-1 into arthroscopically debrided SCLs of the equine femoral condyle leads to improved longterm clinical outcome (Ortved et al, 2012). This technique appeared particularly effective in horses that have had poorer prognoses with traditional therapies, including mature horses, horses with preexisting OA, and horses with upright hindlimb conformation. The authors also noted that simpler surgical methods, including debridement or intralesional corticosteroid injection, should still be considered for younger, nonarthritic horses. This technique certainly represents an option when either injection of an SCL or curettage alone has failed. Subchondral cyst cases since 2005 have also been grafted by one of the authors (A.J.N.) with autologous BMSCs secured in platelet-rich plasma (PRP) as a source of growth factor–rich fibrin, but there has been no published comparison of outcome compared with previous studies by Ortved (2012) using allograft chondrocytes implanted in fibrin. Experimental evidence (Wilke et al, 2007) suggests MSCs implanted in

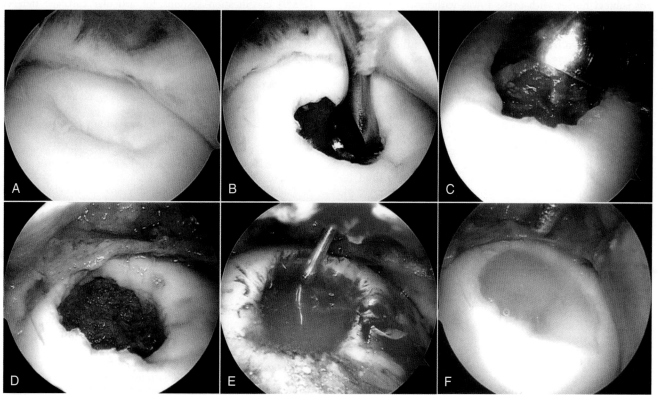

Figure 6-57 Surgical technique for cyst debridement and chondrocyte graft. **A,** Cyst in medial femoral condyle. **B,** Debridement of cyst with curette. **C,** Packing cancellous bone into depth of cyst under gas arthroscopy. **D,** Completing bone packing in cyst. **E,** Needle attached to paired syringes delivering chondrocytes and insulin-like growth factor-1 to surface of debrided cyst. **F,** Completed graft showing sealed cyst opening after returned to liquid distention. *(Reproduced with permission from Ortved KF, Nixon AJ, Mohammed HO, Fortier LA. Treatment of subchondral cystic lesions of the medial femoral condyle of mature horses with growth factor enhanced chondrocyte grafts: a retrospective study of 49 cases, Equine Vet J 2012;44:606–613.)*

cartilage lesions in the femoral trochlear using fibrin vehicle substantially improved the early repair but had less long-term superiority compared with fibrin alone.

Reattachment of the articular cartilage component of type I subchondral cystic lesions of the medial femoral condyle with polydiaxanone pins has been described in three horses in 2011 and provides a successful option for reconstitution of the articular surface (Sparks et al, 2011).

Management of Medial Femoral Condylar Cystic Lesions and Defects Detected on Sale Radiographs

Although not normally treated with arthroscopic surgery, the significance of lesions in the medial femoral condyle of Thoroughbred sale yearlings, as well as other breeds and disciplines, is an emerging issue. Survey radiographs at public auction have become standard procedure, and variable interpretation of radiographs has been a concern to both consigners and buyers. A review in Thoroughbreds divided radiographic lucencies of the medial femoral condyle into subchondral lucencies (SCL) along the distal aspect of the MFC that were shallow lesions, compared with MFC cysts, which were rounded lucencies within the condyle (Whitman et al, 2006). There were 25 horses with MFC cysts (6 bilateral, 3 left hind only, 16 right hindlimb only) and 27 horses with SCL (8 bilateral, 6 left, 13 right). No radiographic evidence of OA was seen in the affected medial femorotibial joints. Control horses (closest hip number with a radiographic report) had no MFC abnormalities and were chosen at the same sale. For control horses, 2 horses were withdrawn from sale, 7 did not attain their reserve, and 43 (83%) were sold for a median price of $95,000 (range $7,000 to $600,000). For subject horses with cysts, 1 was withdrawn, 9 did not meet reserve, and 15 (60%) were sold for a median price of $32,000 (range $6,200 to $100,000). For horses with SCL, 1 was withdrawn from the sale, 2 did not meet their reserve, and 24 (89%) were sold for a median price $34,000 (range $2,500 to $410,000). Control horses sold for more money than horses with MFC cysts or SCL ($P < 0.01$), and fewer horses with MFC cysts were sold compared with controls or SCL horses ($P < 0.05$).

The percentage of horses starting a race as a 2-year-old was 42% for control horses, 40% for horses with MFC cysts, and 41% for horses with SCL. The percentage of horses starting at least 1 race from ages 2 to 4 years was 90% for control horses, 88% for horses with MFC cysts, and 93% of horses with SCL. Neither the number of limbs affected nor the presence of radiographic abnormalities had an effect on racing records, and there were no statistical differences between horses with MFC cysts or SCL and control horses for any racing outcome measured. Nonsignificant P values for racing parameters between cases and controls analyzed included ability to start as a 2-year-old ($P = 1.0$), number of 2-year-old starts (starters only; $P = 0.57$), winning percentage of 2-year-old starts (starters only; $P = 0.23$), total starts 2 to 4 years of age ($P = 0.35$), win percentage from 2 to 4 years of age (starters only; $P = 0.2$), and lifetime earnings ($P = 0.44$). The authors note that a significant weakness in their study was that no follow-up lameness data were available and there was a lack of information about lameness caused by MFC lucencies or any treatments in the subjects. They also acknowledge that some horses with MFC cysts became lame and some of these horses required treatment.

More recently, studies have been done on cutting-bred Quarter Horse yearling survey radiographs. There was a high incidence of MFC lucencies, and outcome parameters did not indicate significant failure to compete or decreased earnings in both 3- and 4-year-olds (Barrett et al, unpublished data 2012; Contino et al, 2012).

Articular Cartilage Lesions on the Medial Condyle of the Femur

These lesions will be detected during diagnostic arthroscopy of the medial femorotibial joint. A typical signalment will be lameness with possible synovial effusion, positive response to hindlimb flexion tests and response to intraarticular analgesia of the stifle (Schneider et al, 1997). In a report of 15 cases there were subtle radiographic evidence of osteochondral lesions (Scott et al, 2004). Diagnostic arthroscopy of the medial femorotibial joint is performed as previously described. Of 12 joints in 11 horses that were affected with this condition and described by Schneider et al (1997), all horses had focal areas of damage to articular cartilage on the weight bearing surface of the medial femoral condyle. Cartilage was dimpled, wrinkled, and folded and was not firmly attached to the subchondral bone. Palpation of damaged cartilage with a blunt arthroscope probe consistently revealed an area of loose cartilage through which the probe could be easily inserted into the subchondral bone. Fibrillation and exposure of subchondral bone were also evident in some horses. The location of the lesions was at the same site as medial femoral SCL. Areas of separated cartilage should be debrided. In some instances of extensive damage, what can be done surgically is limited because extensive debridement will not produce a successful result. Since publication of this paper, diagnostic arthroscopy of the femorotibial articulations has increased greatly and the authors of this text have identified a wide range of pathologic changes. Figure 6-58 illustrates the range of lesions that are encountered ranging from small clefts, through larger multiple clefts into flaplike defects, and full-thickness erosion.

In the papers of Walmsley et al (2003) and Cohen et al (2009) classification systems for articular cartilage defects have been proposed.

Walmsley et al (2003) used the Outerbridge (1961) human grading system for articular cartilage lesions. Lesions in the articular cartilage of the medial femoral condyle (MFC) or lateral femoral condyle (LFC) were recorded as follows:

- Circumscribed areas of prominent fibrillation less than 1.5 cm in diameter (similar to those graded as Outerbridge grade 2)
- Superficial, mild fibrillation over larger area (similar to mild Outerbridge grade 3)
- Generalized fibrillation extending over larger areas, associated with apparent thinning of the articular cartilage (similar to Outerbridge grade 3)
- Full-thickness lesions of variable size in which the subchondral bone could be palpated with a probe (similar to Outerbridge grade 4)
- Shear lesions or chondral flaps characterized by the presence of torn flaps of articular cartilage
- Thickened, softened, enfolded, or fissured articular cartilage (similar to Outerbridge grade 1, but more severe and with fissuring)
- Small (about 3 mm), raised plaques of firm cartilage tissues sometimes containing shiny, yellowish tissue

In a more recent paper by Cohen et al (2009), articular cartilage lesions were reported using a modified Outerbridge scoring system:

- Grade 1 = superficial changes and softening of the cartilage
- Grade 2 = deep changes with no exposed bone
- Grade 3 = full-thickness lesions with exposed subchondral bone

Full-thickness lesions were then defined as focal (involving <25% of the articular surface) or diffuse (>25% of the articular surface). The worst grade documented at surgery was used to assign the overall chondral grade for the horse.

In the report by Schneider et al (1997) six of seven horses that were treated for focal cartilage lesions recovered

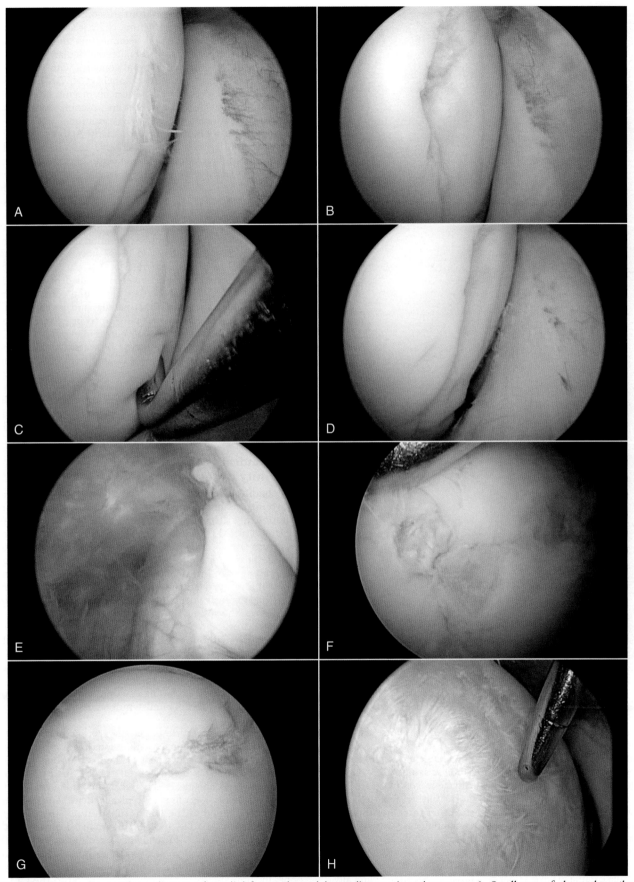

Figure 6-58 Articular cartilage disease of medial femoral condyle at diagnostic arthroscopy. **A,** Small area of elevated cartilage. **B,** After debridement of separated cartilage. **C,** Second area of separated cartilage on more caudal region of medial femoral condyle. **D,** After debridement of second area of separated cartilage. **E,** Very mild osteophytosis on medial intercondylar eminence indicating inflammation. **F,** Multiple areas of erosion before and **G,** after debridement. **H,** More diffuse erosion.

Continued

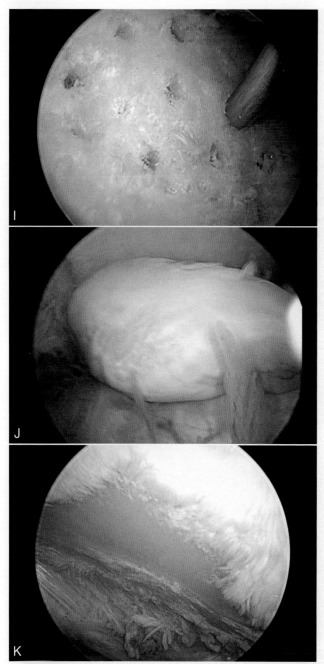

Figure 6-58, cont'd I, After debridement and microfracture of defect. **J,** Large osteophytosis of medial intercondylar eminence associated with **K,** more severe erosion on medial femoral condyle.

evidence of joint effusion after arthroscopically guided abrasion arthroplasty and microfracture. There is also a recent case report describing arthroscopic examination of a 4-year-old Thoroughbred gelding that had bilateral articular cartilage fissure defects of the medial femoral condyles with concurrent cranial cruciate ligament injury (Raheja et al, 2011). BMSCs were cultured and delivered with a fibrin glue arthroscopically into the defects 90 days after arthroscopic examination. Follow-up treatments included two additional injections of MSCs at 5 and 13 months intraarticularly. Arthroscopic evaluation 4 months after the initial MSC treatment revealed marked smoothing, reduction in the depth of cartilage defects, and moderate improvement in the cranial cruciate ligament. Approximately 15 months after treatment, the horse returned to racing. However, it is possible that this is the normal progress of these such lesions without any treatment.

In a review of long-term outcome in 44 horses with stifle lameness after arthroscopic exploration and debridement, chondral lesions were observed in 37 horses (84%); grades ranged from 0 to 3 with a median of 2 (Cohen et al, 2009). Full-thickness cartilage defects were identified in several different locations, including the medial femoral condyle, lateral femoral condyle, proximal tibia, patella, and proximal LTR. A microfracture technique was performed in 12 of 21 horses with either deep cartilage defects or areas of exposed bone. No significant association was observed between chondral grade and any of the authors' measures of long-term outcome, and no significant difference in long-term outcome was observed when comparing horses in which a microfracture technique was used with those without microfracture. However, higher meniscal grades of damage were negatively associated with return to previous level of function (meniscal tears are discussed in a later section).

Subchondral Cystic Lesions of the Proximal Extremity of the Tibia

This condition is relatively uncommon but typically presents at a young age. In one report of 12 cases, the mean age at presentation was 12.3 months, with a range of 6 to 24 months (Textor et al, 2001). Horses presented with severity of lameness from 0 to 3, but in all cases lameness was exacerbated by stifle flexion. Stifle joint effusion (with pouch undefined) was present in 6. Intraarticular analgesia was performed in 6 horses; it improved lameness in 4 and this was unchanged in 2 (these had extensive deep lesions of the lateral tibial condyle). In 6 horses the lesions were considered to be the result of osteochondrosis and were solitary lesions involving the lateral tibial condyle without other signs of joint disease (Fig. 6-59). In 5 out of 6 horses in which the lesions were considered to be the result of osteoarthritis (OA), there was a well-defined cystic lesion of the medial condyle of the tibia and signs of mild to marked OA, including osteophyte formation on the medial aspect of the tibia and femur, and subchondral bone sclerosis.

A technique for arthroscopic surgery has been reported (Textor et al, 2001). In horses with lesions involving the lateral tibial condyle, the lateral aspect of the femorotibial joint was arthroscoped using a medial portal, as described previously, with the arthroscope inserted between the middle and medial patellar ligaments. Lesions were typically identified cranial and immediately lateral to the lateral tuberosity of the intercondylar eminence (see Fig. 6-59). The cranial ligament of the lateral meniscus (CLLM) usually obscured the stoma, and the ligament was retracted cranially or bluntly divided with the probe to expose the stoma. Lesions were curetted to healthy bone. In some instances the stoma was caudal to the CLLM, making exposure relatively simple.

If the lesion was located in the proximomedial aspect of the tibia (medial to the intercondylar eminence), the medial

completely and resumed activities (racehorse, horse used in three-day eventing, jumper, dressage horse, trail riding horse, and pleasure horse). One racehorse that had intermittent lameness in the affected limb did not resume activities. Only one of the four horses with generalized damage to articular cartilage became clinically normal (show horse that was retired and used for pleasure riding). Two of the other three horses were Standardbred racehorses, and the remaining case was a Quarter Horse used for ranch work. These horses were unable to resume their previous activities as a result of persistent lameness. It was therefore concluded that horses with generalized cartilage damage have a poor prognosis for becoming clinically normal and performing well after treatment. In the report of Scott et al (2004), only two of six horses with generalized cartilage lesions were reported to be sound and without any

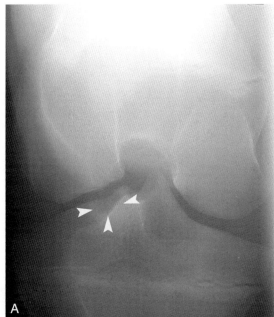

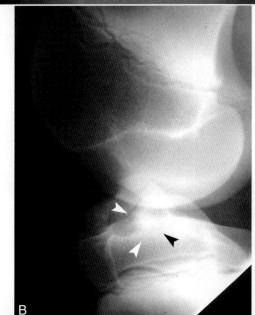

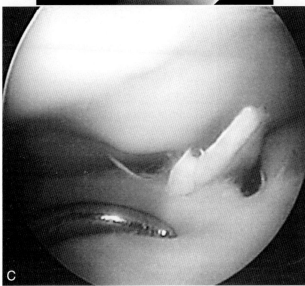

Figure 6-59 **A,** Preoperative radiograph of a yearling with a proximal tibial subchondral lucency *(arrows)* consistent with osteochondrosis of the lateral condyle of the proximal tibia. **B,** Lateral radiograph showing the subchondral cystic lesion of the proximal tibia *(arrows)*, involving the cranial one third of the tibial plateau, and accessible using cranial arthroscopic approaches. **C,** Cartilage flap and underlying subchondral defect associated with osteochondrosis of the proximal tibia. The cartilage defect is immediately caudal to the cranial ligament of the lateral meniscus, which is under the arthroscopic probe.

femorotibial joint was approached through a lateral portal and, again, lesions were identified by probing through the fibers of the cranial ligament of the medial meniscus in a manner similar to that described for lesions lateral to the intercondylar eminence. Proximal tibial cysts due to OA were often in the inaccessible central region of the medial condyle of the tibial plateau, and careful scrutiny of the lateromedial radiographs should be done before arthroscopic surgery to determine likely access compared with the need for extraarticular extirpation or transcystic lag screw. In the paper by Textor et al (2001), arthroscopic debridement was performed in 4 horses in which the lesions were considered to be the result of osteochondrosis and in 3 horses with osteoarthritis. Three horses in which SCLs were considered to be the result of osteochondrosis performed athletically after debridement. Two horses with moderate OA returned to work after arthroscopic debridement but at a lower level of athletic performance. One horse with SCL related to osteochondrosis responded to medical treatment and went on to race. More recent cases (4) have been debrided and grafted with tricalcium phosphate (Fig. 6-60). All four were in the lateral portion of the tibial plateau, and all had to be accessed through the cranial ligament of the lateral meniscus. Three of these were Thoroughbred weanlings; two went on to race and one developed OA and was destroyed.

Fracture of the Medial Tibial Intercondylar Eminence

Although these fractures were initially considered to be associated with avulsion of the insertion of the cranial cruciate ligament (Mueller et al, 1994; Prades et al, 1989), it is the authors' experience, as well as that of Walmsley (2002), that this is not usually the case. It is quite common to have these fractures with minimal damage to the cranial cruciate ligament (Figs. 6-61 to 6-62), even when they are quite large. The injury can of course be accompanied by damage to other structures. Lameness is obvious, and signs localize the problem to the medial femorotibial joint. The fracture can be diagnosed on radiographs. The usual treatment is removal of the fractured portion through a cranial instrument portal in the medial femorotibial joint (Mueller et al, 1994) (see Fig. 6-62). Some dissection from the cranial cruciate ligament and cranial ligament of the medial meniscus at the lateral and cranial margins, respectively, of the fracture may be necessary. Successful treatment of a medial intercondylar eminence fracture in a stallion using a cranial arthroscopic approach through the femoropatellar joint and into the medial compartment of the femorotibial joint has also been described (Grzybowski et al, 2008). One author has pointed out that if the fracture causes significant disruption to the surrounding tissues, lag screw fixation is preferred (Walmsley, 1997). In the case described, fixation was performed using a cranial arthroscopic portal with an extra instrument portal in line with the angle of the implant. The prognosis in these cases is related to absence or presence

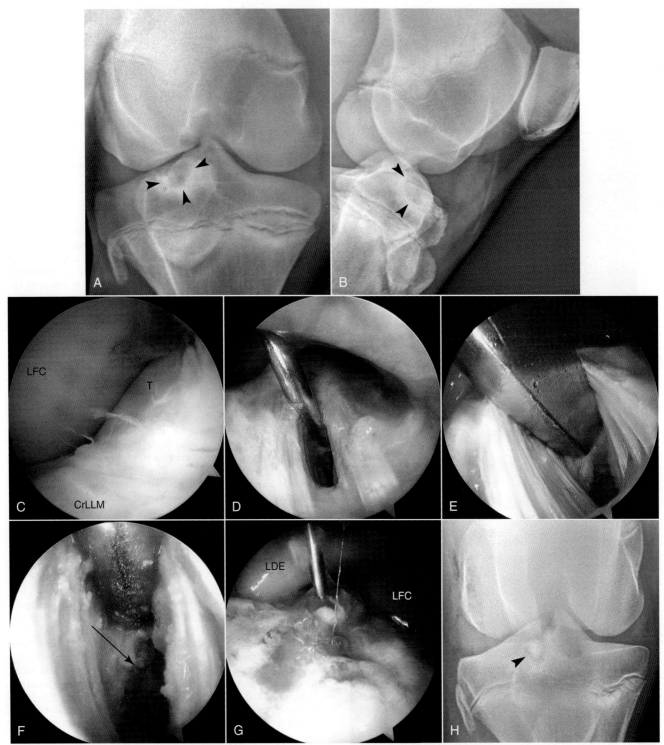

Figure 6-60 Arthroscopic debridement of subchocndral bone cyst in the lateral condyle of the tibia, followed by tricalcium phosphate (TCP) and stem cell packing. **A** and **B,** Preoperative radiographs showing subchondral cyst in lateral condyle of tibia *(arrowheads)*. **C,** Arthroscopic view showing normal lateral femoral condyle *(LFC)* and tibia *(T)*, with cranial ligament of lateral meniscus *(CrLLM)* showing minor fiber disruption but no landmarks to suggest underlying cyst. **D,** Intraoperative radiographs were used to target a needle into cyst, followed by minor separation of the cranial ligament. **E,** Separated cranial ligament showing debrided tibial cyst. **F,** Cyst lightly packed with TCP granules. **G,** Packed cyst and separated meniscal ligament sealed with cultured MSCs in a PRP vehicle under gas distension. *LDE,* Long digital extensor origin; *LFC,* lateral femoral condyle. **H,** Postoperative radiograph 3 days after surgery, showing TCP graft in place *(arrowhead)*.

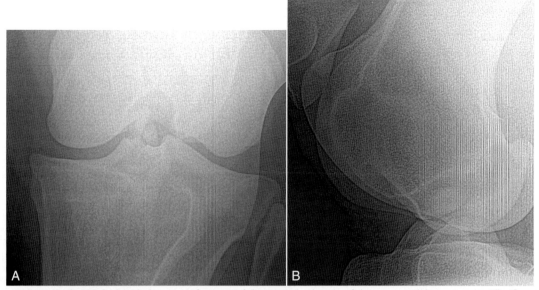

Figure 6-61 Radiographs **(A-B)** showing a fracture of the medial tubercle of the intercondylar eminence. The fracture fragment was removed surgically.

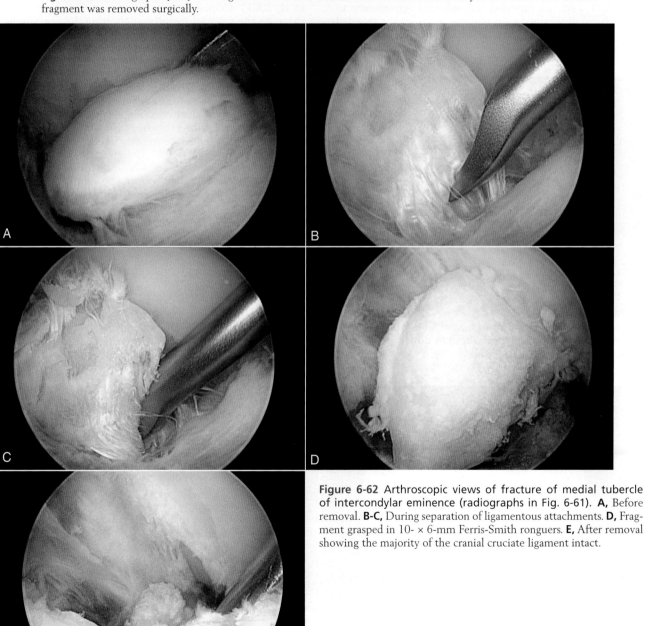

Figure 6-62 Arthroscopic views of fracture of medial tubercle of intercondylar eminence (radiographs in Fig. 6-61). **A,** Before removal. **B-C,** During separation of ligamentous attachments. **D,** Fragment grasped in 10- × 6-mm Ferris-Smith ronguers. **E,** After removal showing the majority of the cranial cruciate ligament intact.

of other injury in the joint. The authors have treated cases both with arthroscopic removal and by internal fixation.

Injuries to the Cruciate Ligaments

Cruciate ligament injury in the horse was initially described as a clinical entity by Sanders-Shamis et al (1988) and Prades et al (1989), but these papers did not involve arthroscopic evaluation. Complete rupture of the cranial cruciate ligament in the horse is catastrophic, and it is unusual to examine these cases arthroscopically (Fig. 6-63). Less severe injuries to cruciate ligaments can be diagnosed with arthroscopy. It has been pointed out that sometimes strains and partial ruptures may be diagnosed ultrasonographically if the examiner has considerable experience (Cauvin et al, 1996). However, decades later it is still widely acknowledged that only the insertion of the cranial cruciate can be imaged satisfactorily by ultrasound examination (Barrett et al, 2012), and arthroscopy is the preferred choice for a definitive diagnosis. Gradually improving access to wide-bore and open-field magnetic resonance imaging (MRI) units has provided the only real opportunity to gain preoperative information that may improve the targeted arthroscopic examination and potential biologic treatment of cruciate injuries.

Diagnostic arthroscopy of the cranial pouch of the medial femorotibial joint can be done through a lateral or cranial portal. The cranial portal will give better overall visualization of the cruciate ligaments in the intercondylar notch, but both approaches can be used. A typical partial-thickness tear will involve the body of the cranial cruciate ligament, rather than the insertion. This is consistent with experimental work that has shown that cranial cruciate ligaments fail in midbody (Rich & Glisson, 1994), at least in the ponies. However, avulsion at both the tibial and femoral insertions of the cranial cruciate ligament has been reported (Edwards & Nixon, 1996; Prades et al, 1989). Caudal cruciate ligament injury has been described in the literature (Moustafa et al, 1987) but is uncommon. Caudal cruciate injuries observed arthroscopically generally appear as longitudinal shredding of the femoral origin (Fig. 6-64), although radiographic lesions associated with the tibial insertion of the caudal cruciate can occasionally be seen (Fig. 6-65). A caudal cruciate ligament avulsion in the horse has been defined with imaging (Rose et al, 2001). Cranial cruciate injury can vary from hemorrhage on the synovial membrane covering the cruciate ligaments or mild fiber disruption to more severe fiber disruption (see Fig. 6-65). Moderate to severe injuries will have concomitant rupture of the median septum. In such cases, even though the arthroscope is in the medial femorotibial joint, it can pass through and visualize the lateral femorotibial joint. Anecdotal data of the authors dictate a reasonably good prognosis for mild to moderate tearing. Another author (Walmsley, 2002) has described the prognosis for severe injuries as poor (0/4), with moderate injuries having a 50% prognosis for returning to work (9/18). Cohen et al (2009) reported follow-up information on 3 of 4 horses with cruciate injuries. One horse had a complete tear and was euthanized shortly after surgery for persistent lameness. One horse with a partial tear became sound and returned to its previous level of performance, while the other horse with a partial tear improved but did not become completely sound. There are no published reports of successful cranial cruciate ligament reparative techniques, although partial tears respond satisfactorily to debridement of surface fraying. Injecting biologics such as cell or plasma derivatives into partially torn ACL has been described in man and experimental models, and one of the authors (A.J.N.) has treated several cases of partial cranial cruciate tear with minor debridement followed by MSCs in PRP or bone marrow aspirate concentrate (see Fig. 6-70). Follow-up data support this modality, but longer-term studies

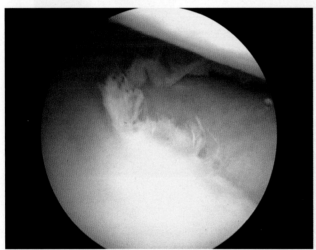

Figure 6-63 Arthroscopic view of medial femorotibial joint in which complete rupture has occurred in both cruciate ligaments. The caudal border of the meniscus is clearly visible.

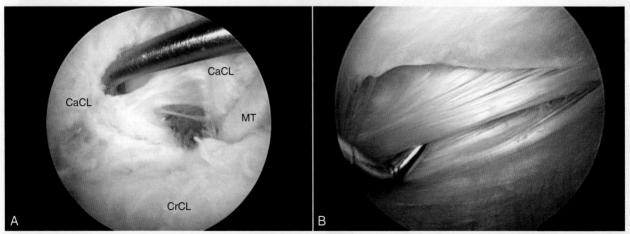

Figure 6-64 A, Tearing of the femoral origin of the caudal cruciate ligament. **B,** Linear tear in caudal cruciate ligament with probe inserted in tear. Probe is in shredded caudal cruciate fibers, exposing axial edge of medial condyle in background and leaving residual caudal cruciate fibers more caudal and cranial to tear. *CaCL,* Caudal cruciate ligament; *CrCL,* cranial cruciate ligament; *MT,* medial tubercle of intercondylar eminence.

and additional animals would be necessary before this treatment can be recommended.

Identification of caudal cruciate injury at the femoral origin has increased, and one of the authors (AJN) considers this syndrome may have been commonly overlooked in the past. Severe disruption across the fibers and even shredding down the fiber axis has been recognized as a singular cause of lameness (Fig. 6-66). Complete disruption at the femoral origin of the caudal cruciate has not been recorded, and most partially disrupted CaCL respond well to debridement and injection of biologics directly into the residual fiber bundles. Avulsion of the CaCL insertion onto the tibia is more devastating (see Fig. 6-68) because all of the fibers are generally involved. The bony fragment can be several centimeters long and retract back into the caudal compartment of the medial FT joint. This makes them accessible to surgical removal using arthroscopic means to access the caudal compartment. However, the dissection is quite deep, and the popliteal artery is immediately adjacent. Lag screw reaffixation has not been recorded.

▶ Meniscal and Meniscal Ligament Injuries

Arthroscopy has proved to be invaluable in the diagnosis of tears of the menisci and the meniscal ligaments. As has been previously pointed out, limited amounts of the meniscus are visible with arthroscopy and, the most complete examination is achieved by arthroscopic examination of both cranial and caudal aspects (cranial and caudal pouches of the medial or lateral femorotibial joints, respectively). It has been recognized that lesions are more commonly seen in the cranial pouch (Walmsley, 1995; Walmsley et al, 2003). Lesions also occur three times more commonly in the medial than in the lateral meniscus (Walmsley et al, 2003). Walmsley et al (2003) described a grading system according to the severity of the visible injury:

- Grade I, a tear in the cranial ligament extending into the meniscus but without significant separation of the tissues
- Grade II, a complete tear in the cranial horn (pole) of the meniscus and the cranial ligament where the limits are visible arthroscopically
- Grade III, a severe tear of the meniscus and ligament that extends beneath the femoral condyle so that the limits of the tear cannot be seen

It is less common to see tears of the meniscus in the caudal pouch of either the medial or lateral femorotibial joint. This probably reflects both the reduced frequency that surgeons examine the caudal pouches and the limited exposure of the contact areas of the meniscus that this affords.

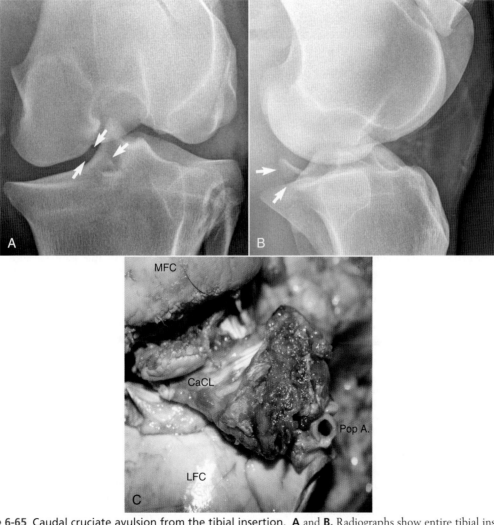

Figure 6-65 Caudal cruciate avulsion from the tibial insertion. A and **B,** Radiographs show entire tibial insertion, which has separated and rotated into the caudal compartment of the medial femorotibial joint. **C,** Necropsy showing caudal cruciate avulsion of bone bed, and adjacent popliteal artery. *CaCL,* Caudal cruciate ligament; *LFC,* lateral femoral condyle; *Pop A,* popliteal artery; *MFC,* medial femoral condyle. *(Images courtesy Dr. Greg Staller.)*

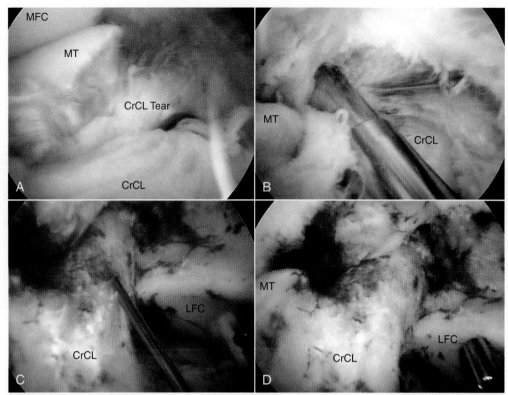

Figure 6-66 Partial tear of the cranial cruciate ligament. **A,** Arthroscopic image showing tear in medial aspect of cranial cruciate ligament *(CrCL)*. **B,** Synovectomy of tear and surface of CrCL. **C,** Debrided CrCL during injection of mesenchymal stem cells in a vehicle of bone marrow aspirate concentrate. **D,** Increased bulk of CrCL after stem cell. *LFC,* Lateral femoral condyle; *MFC,* medial femoral condyle; *MT,* medial tubercle of intercondylar eminence.

For tears in the cranial portion of the medial meniscus, the arthroscope is usually placed through the lateral portal. This provides good visualization and is out of the way of instrument entry through the cranial portal. Meniscal injuries seen in the horse can be categorized as vertical radial (transverse), vertical longitudinal, vertical flap, bucket handle, or as horizontal transverse (Fig. 6-67). True bucket handle tears, as seen in man, are an extensive vertical longitudinal tear with the thin separated border displaced to the axial side of the femoral condyle and are quite rare in the horse. For tears in the cranial horn or cranial ligament of the medial meniscus, a cranial instrument portal is made and the torn portion removed. This can be accomplished with a combination of Ferris-Smith rongeurs, biopsy suction forceps, or motorized equipment (Figs. 6-68 to 6-69). Sometimes the torn meniscal tissue will be hinged on the cranial ligament of the meniscus (also called meniscotibial ligament), which can be divided using arthroscopic (meniscectomy) scissors. Tears can also involve the cranial ligament (also called *meniscotibial ligament*) of the meniscus (see Fig. 6-68) or tears in the body of the meniscus itself (see Fig. 6-69). The aim is to leave a clean edge of healthy meniscal ligament or meniscus. One of the authors (A.J.N.) has used intraarticular suturing of the meniscus in six horses. The meniscal tear should be clean, vertical, and relatively fresh. Suturing can be achieved by using flexible needles (Fig. 6-70) (Nitinol, Arthrex Corporation, Florida) to tie mattress sutures through the tear, using an outside-to-inside technique. Alternatively, the Joystick™ cannula technique (Arthrex) allows utilization of a pair of flexible needles with a swedged-on fiberwire suture loop (Fig. 6-71) to form an inside-outside simple interrupted suture. All inside techniques such as the meniscal cinch™ (Arthrex) have also been used in the horse, but are designed for the transarticular repair of the caudal horn of man, and are difficult to get adequate purchase into the cranial horn of the

medial meniscus in horses. The joystick approach is inexpensive and has worked the best of the three systems in a limited case series. Transverse vertical tears can be more difficult to trim or suture because they orientated across the structure of the meniscus (Fig. 6-72). Additionally, they occur more commonly in the central (medial) to caudomedial portion of the meniscus and can be difficult to even visualize.

Tears of the lateral meniscus can be found on exploration of the lateral femorotibial joint using the portal that was developed over the medial femorotibial joint. Access can be a little more difficult in this joint because the long digital extensor tendon and popliteal tendon are both intraarticular. Avulsion fracture of the insertion of the cranial ligament of the lateral meniscus can cause meniscal instability. This site is predisposed, and in one author's opinion (A.J.N.), occurs as frequently as tears in the lateral meniscal body.

In the initial report of Walmsley (1995), there were five horses with a vertical tear in the cranial horn and cranial ligament of the medial meniscus and two horses with similar injuries in the lateral meniscus. All the lesions had similar characteristics, and the tear was about 1 cm from the junction of the axial border of the meniscus and the cranial ligament of the meniscus. In all but one case it was incomplete, with much of the torn tissue loosely attached to the axial part of the meniscus from where it was removed. The remaining meniscus abaxial to the tear was displaced cranially and abaxial, and its torn edges were debrided. In those cases, three horses returned to full competition, one horse was useable for hacking, two were convalescing, and one was still lame after 1 year. Walmsley (1995) pointed out that these lesions were quite different from the vertical meniscal tears, which occurred in the cranial horn of the meniscus at least 1 cm abaxial to the junction of the meniscus and its cranial ligament and involved separation of meniscal tissue on either side of the tear. The author

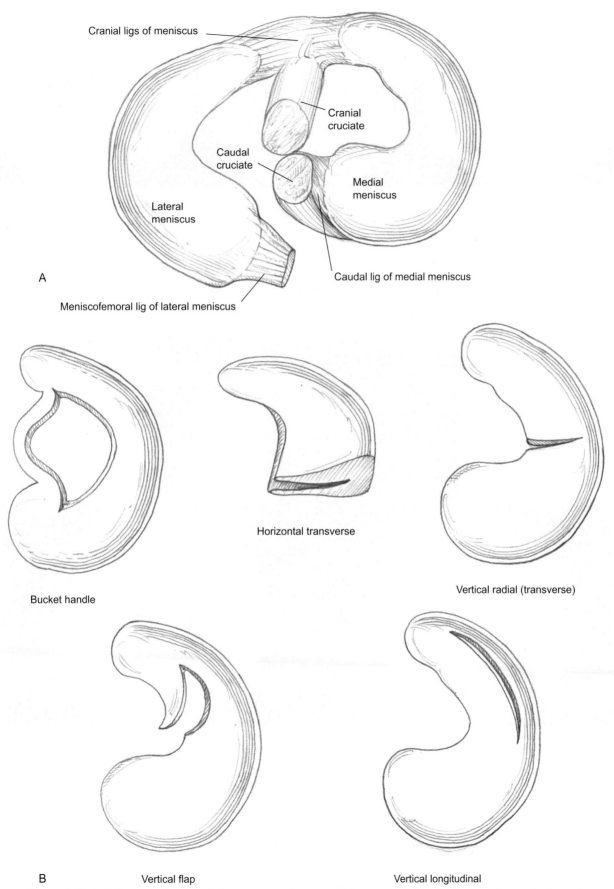

Left tibia

Cranial ligs of meniscus

Cranial cruciate

Caudal cruciate

Medial meniscus

Lateral meniscus

Caudal lig of medial meniscus

Meniscofemoral lig of lateral meniscus

A

Bucket handle

Horizontal transverse

Vertical radial (transverse)

B   Vertical flap

Vertical longitudinal

Figure 6-67 A, Schematic diagram of the menisci and associated ligaments. **B,** Types of meniscal tears: horizontal, vertical radial, vertical longitudinal, bucket handle, and flap.

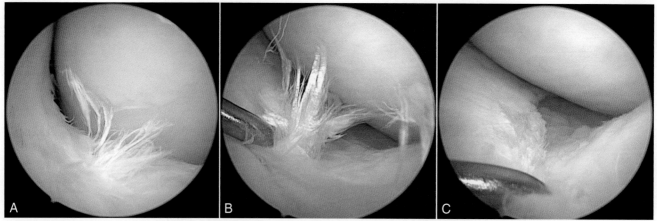

Figure 6-68 Tearing of the cranial ligament of the medial meniscus. **A,** Initial arthroscopic appearance. **B,** Tearing exposed further by eversion with an arthroscopic probe. **C,** Arthroscopic appearance at completion of debridement.

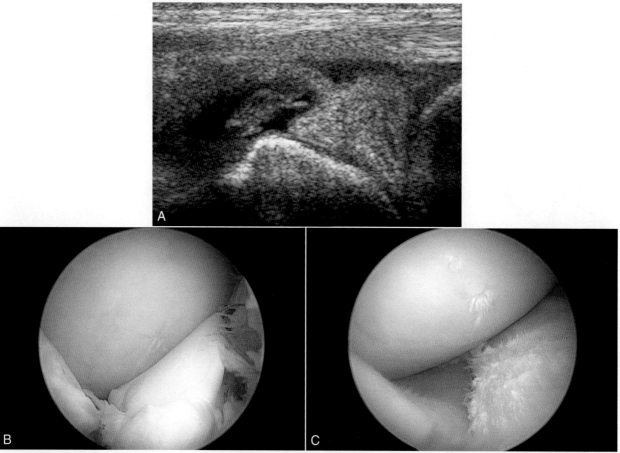

Figure 6-69 Tearing of the cranial horn of the medial meniscus. **A,** Transverse ultrasonographic image of the medial femorotibial joint (proximal to the left) demonstrating distension with irregular echogenic material proximal and cranial of the medial meniscus. **B,** Arthroscopic appearance from a craniolateral portal revealing extrusion of the torn cranial horn of the medial meniscus, hinged on the cranial meniscal ligament into the cranial compartment of the medial femorotibial joint. **C,** Arthroscopic image following removal of the torn tissue and debridement. The defect created exposes a larger portion of the medial articular surface of the tibia than is normally apparent.

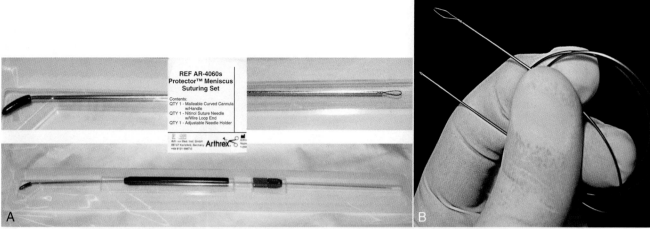

Figure 6-70 Simple disposable suture devices that work in the equine meniscus. **A,** The Protector™ (Arthrex) malleable curved cannula and nitinol needle, including a needle holder (purple) and the wire loop end suture retriever. The cannula is used to pass an inside-out strand of suture of the surgeon's choice, and the cannula and loop end of the needle are used to retrieve the free end in the joint to create a second inside-out strand. The ends are then tied in the subcutaneous perimeniscal tissue. **B,** The cheapest solution is just the nitinol® needle (Arthrex) used for meniscus repair using "outside-in" suture technique. The needle point is used to draw suture across the meniscus tear and into the joint, and the wire loop is used to retrieve the free end within the joint (introduced via 14-gauge needle) to return the suture to the outside for tying in a subcutaneous location.

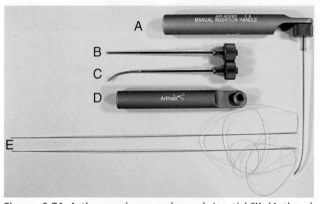

Figure 6-71 Arthroscopic cannula and Joystick™ (Arthrex) inside out meniscal suture and needles. *A,* Assembled handle and curved cannula to guide double armed needles. *B,* Straight and *C,* curved cannulae, with *D,* handle. *E,* Double-armed flexible needle with No. 2 fiberwire loaded.

was also uncertain as to whether fraying was symptomatic or associated with age and use. This paper served as the hallmark for making meniscal injuries a recognizable syndrome.

A later retrospective study described 80 cases of meniscal tears in horses (Walmsley et al, 2003). Inclusion criteria were as follows:
1. Lameness localized to the femorotibial joint with clinical confidence (in most cases with intraarticular analgesia)
2. Diagnostic arthroscopy identifying an abnormality in one or both menisci
3. The meniscal injury was considered to be the primary lesion in the joint

The medial meniscus was involved in 60 cases and the lateral in 20 cases. Forty-three tears were grade I, 20 were grade II, and 17 were grade III. Distention of either or both the femoropatellar and femorotibial joint was recorded in 31 horses, but in 14 of these, distention was recorded in only the femoropatellar joint. The relative likelihood of joint distention was nine times greater among horses with grade II and III injuries

(17/20, 13/17), respectively, as compared with horses with grade I injuries (4/43). The median lameness grade was 3 (on a scale of 5); the response to intraarticular analgesia was positive in 59/65 horses in which it was performed, and in 45/76 horses in which the information was recorded, the flexion test worsened the lameness. Radiographic abnormalities were seen in 38 horses and increased with severity of lesions. New bone formation on the medial intercondylar eminence of the tibia occurred in 23 cases, and OA of the femorotibial joint was evident in 18 cases. Mineralization of soft tissue structures was seen in 6 cases.

Walmsley et al (2003) used the Outerbridge (1961) human grading system to describe accompanying articular cartilage lesions in those cases. Arthroscopically diagnosed abnormalities of the femoral or tibial articular cartilage were recorded in 61 horses. These abnormalities were seen with 36 of 43 grade I tears, 13 of 20 grade II tears, and 12 of 17 grade III tears. Full-thickness cartilage defects and generalized fibrillation of the articular cartilage (Outerbridge grades 3 and 4) lesions were recorded in 31 horses, and these had a median age of 10 years old (range 3 to 22). Concurrent cranial cruciate ligament injury was seen in 12 cases. Twenty-five other horses showed fibrillation of the cranial ligament of the other meniscus, and 5 horses had disruption of the septum between medial femorotibial and lateral femorotibial joints.

Overall, 47% of affected horses returned to full use, including 63% of grade I tears, 56% of grade II tears, and 6% of grade III tears. Ten of 12 horses with concurrent cruciate injury were followed up and 6 horses returned to full use. Of the horses with radiographic abnormalities before surgery, significantly more (27/36; 75%) were lame at follow-up as compared with those that did not have a radiographic lesion before surgery (10/34 or 29%). In the series of cases by Walmsley et al (2003), grade I lesions were not debrided. Suturing was not considered practical in most cases, but one grade III lesion was sutured using the equivalent of the laparoscopic extracorporeal knotting technique (Soper & Hunter, 1992) with No. 3 polyglactin 910 (Vicryl).

In another publication (Cohen et al, 2009), when sonographic diagnosis was compared with arthroscopic findings of meniscal tears, an ultrasonographic diagnosis of meniscal tear

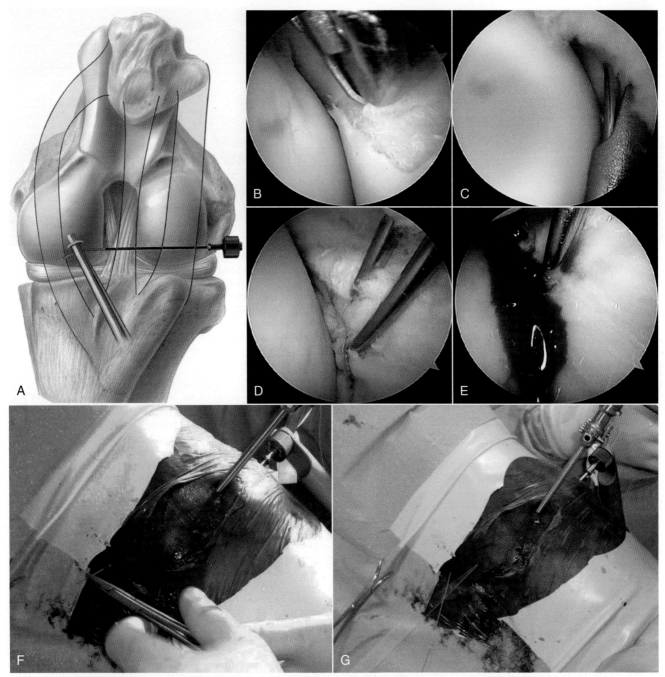

Figure 6-72 Inside-out suture repair of vertical flap in cranial horn of medial meniscus in a 15-year-old warm-blood mare. **A,** Schematic showing "joystick" cannula being introduced from lateral portal and threaded across to medial femorotibial (FT) joint. **B,** Arthroscopic image showing meniscal tear **(C)** Curved cannula being used to guide flexible needle from inside edge of meniscus to outside. A second needle penetrates on the other side of tear. **D,** Suture has been placed, and both arms of the suture have been exteriorized and tied in perimeniscal perimeter. **E,** Injection of mesenchymal stem cells in PRP vehicle under gas arthroscopy, in and around meniscal tear. **F,** Exterior view showing first needle exiting the skin over craniomedial aspect of the medial FT joint. **G,** Both sutures have been exteriorized. One suture arm is tunneled subcutaneously and tied to the other arm to complete a single interrupted loop.

was confirmed at surgery in 11 horses, whereas a false-positive ultrasonographic diagnosis of a meniscal tear was made in 4 horses. Conversely, ultrasound correctly identified 5 horses as having a normal appearance to the meniscus but failed to diagnose meniscal lesions that were later identified at surgery in 3 horses. Meniscal tears were present in 30 horses (68%), with 24 horses having tears in the medial meniscus and 7 having tears in the lateral meniscus (Cohen et al, 2009). Lesions involving the cruciate ligaments were present in 4 horses (9%), and only 1 of these lesions was a complete tear. With regard to success rate with meniscal tears, for grade I lesions 8/11 (73%) improved with 6/11 (55%) becoming sound and 4/11 (36%) returning to previous use. With grade II lesions 6/7 (86%) improved, 4/7 (57%) became sound, and 2/7 (29%) returned to previous use. With grade III lesions 0/4 improved, became sound, or returned to previous use.

In a more recent study of 33 horses with soft tissue injury of the femorotibial joint treated with intraarticular autologous BMSCs 4 weeks after surgery (Ferris et al 2013), a higher percentage of horses were able to go back to work after meniscal injury when treated with surgery plus BMSCs compared with the previous reports of surgery alone. Twenty-four horses had the presence of meniscal damage recorded; 9 with grade I, 7 with grade II, and 8 with grade III scores. Fibrillated areas of meniscal damage were mechanically debrided; none of the horses had their menisci sutured. Of the 9 horses given a meniscal score of one, 5 (56%) returned to their previous level of work and 4 (44%) returned to same work for an overall return to work of 9/9 (100%). Of the 7 horses with a meniscal score of two, 2 (29%) returned to their previous level of work and 2 (29%) returned to less work for a total returning to work of 4/9 (57%). Of the 8 horses with a grade III meniscal score, 2 were able to return to their previous function (25%) and 3 (37%) returned to less work, for a total of 5/8 (63%) working. These 62% of horses with a grade III meniscal tear were able to return to some level of function following treatment with BMSCs and surgical debridement, which compares favorably with a 0% success rate reported by Cohen et al (2009) and a 6% (1/17) success reported by Walmsley et al (2003).

The question of whether arthroscopic partial menisectomy results in knee OA has been addressed in humans. A systematic review of patients following arthroscopic, partial menisectomy with a minimum of 8 years follow-up showed that radiographic signs of OA are significant at 8 and 16 years follow-up, but clinical symptoms of knee arthritis are not significant (Petty and Lubowitz, 2011). It appears from clinical results in horses that grade III tears of the meniscus result in long-term problems but that these can be improved by intraarticular MSC therapy. A clinical study with BMSCs mentioned earlier (Ferris et al, 2013) was initiated after review of the study in goats where meniscal regrowth and decreased OA was reported following intraarticular administration of BMSCs (Murphy et al, 2003). Changes that occur following a grade III cranial horn tear have been investigated in an in vitro equine cadaveric study, in which creation and resection of grade III cranial horn tears were evaluated at full extension (Fowlie et al, 2011a). The study showed that resection of grade III cranial horn tears in the medial meniscus resulted in a central focal region of increased pressure on the medial tibial condyle at a 160-degree stifle angle, and this increased pressure was related to smaller joint contact area at 160 degrees. An earlier study by the same group had shown that axial compression and cranial displacement of the cranial horn of the medial meniscus occurs at a 160-degree stifle angle based on three-dimensional MRI (Fowlie et al, 2011b). The authors also noted that there were limitations in extrapolating these findings to clinical cases because in clinical cases the torn segment of tissue is often severely fibrillated and displaced and hence provides minimal mechanical support, whereas in the simulated grade III tear the meniscus remained in place as the load was applied. Additionally, the load applied was only equivalent to that experienced at a walking gait.

Meniscal tears, particularly the longitudinal tears described by Walmsley et al (2003) as grade III, can progress into the midportion and even the caudal horn of the meniscus. Any meniscal tear where the abaxial and caudal terminations cannot be discerned needs to be explored further by examination through the caudal joint pouch of the femorotibial joint. Discrete tears of the caudal horn of the medial meniscus can also occur (Fig. 6-73). The authors now always examine the caudal portion of the medial femorotibial joint, even if a tear in the cranial horn appears contained. The medial meniscus is most commonly affected; the caudal horn of the lateral meniscus is rarely affected. Vertical longitudinal tears of the

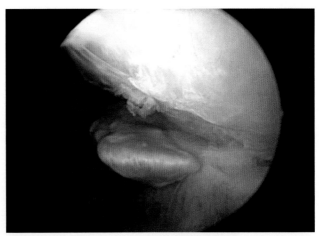

Figure 6-73 Chronic tear of caudal horn of medial meniscus as visualized with the arthroscope placed in the caudal pouch of the medial femorotibial joint.

medial meniscus have also been seen (see Fig. 6-80). Mineralization of the meniscus is a late-stage development (see Fig. 6-81) and frequently signals chronic meniscal tearing. Surgical aims in mineralized cases should be to trim all protruding portions that impinge on the caudal surface of the femoral condyle, debride free or fibrillated soft portions of the meniscus, and suture any longitudinal tears that are not disintegrated. Manipulation of instruments in the caudal compartment is not easy, particularly since the depth of the damaged meniscus from the skin surface is often 6 to 8 cm. Trimming of caudal horn meniscal tissue is best accomplished with a motorized resector, particularly the large-format tooth synovial resectors such as the orbit incisor or Synovator. Removal of mineralization may require an arthroburr. A single report of mineralization of the caudal meniscal horn in association with a vertical longitudinal tear of the medial meniscus has been reported (Janicek and Wilson, 2007). The authors suspected that the caudal meniscotibial ligament was disrupted on the basis of caudal displacement of the caudal meniscal horn. However, caudal horn laxity is a common feature with advanced meniscal disease and OA, particularly as the articular cartilage thins and the meniscus body loses its shape and resiliency. Either MRI or the cranial approach to the caudal compartment of the medial FT joint would be needed to confirm caudal meniscal ligament disruption. (This is an uncommon finding based on the authors' experience because unless the cranial approach to the caudal compartment of the medial FT joint is used, the caudal ligament of the medial meniscus is not seen.) Mineralized meniscus was removed arthroscopically; suturing of the meniscal tear was not attempted because of poor accessibility. On the basis of owner follow-up, there was no lameness observed at a walk 12 months after surgery.

In common with other species, macerated tears of the menisci carry a poor prognosis for return to working soundness because the loss of fibrocartilagenous meniscal tissue is usually marked. These injuries frequently also extend into the central inaccessible body of the meniscus, so removal of torn tissue is often incomplete.

Meniscal Cysts

Meniscal cysts have been recently described in the horse (Sparks et al, 2011c). Meniscal cysts have been described in the human orthopedic literature, but the term is often used interchangeably with a ganglion cyst. Most reports published in the human literature recognize meniscal cysts as always appearing with an adjacent meniscal tear (Scott, 2012). Sparks et al (2011c) reported clinical symptoms, treatment,

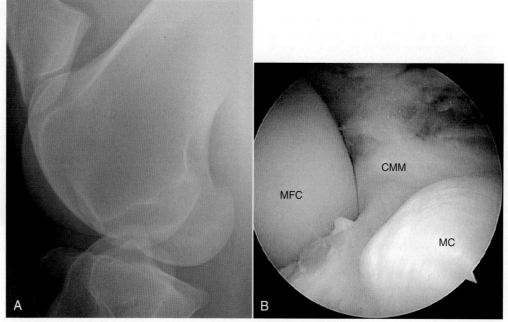

Figure 6-74 Meniscal cyst. **A,** Radiograph showing minimal changes other than mild mineralized density in the cranial region of the femorotibial joint. **B,** Arthroscopic view of a meniscal cyst near the junction of the cranial ligament and cranial horn of the medial meniscus, visualized using a routine, lateral arthroscopic approach to the cranial compartment of the right medial femorotibial joint. *CMM,* Cranial ligament of medial meniscus; *MC,* meniscal cyst; *MFC,* medial femoral condyle. *(From Sparks HD, Nixon AJ, Boening KJ, Pool RR. Arthroscopic treatment of meniscal cysts in the horse. Equine Vet J 43:669-675, 2011.)*

and outcome of seven cases treated with arthroscopic cyst excision and meniscal debridement in horses. Five horses had lameness attributable to femorotibial joint pathology, while the remaining two horses had meniscal cysts found incidentally during diagnostic arthroscopy for the treatment of OCD of the LTR of the femur. All lesions were identified along the medial meniscus at or near the junction of the cranial ligament with the cranial horn of the medial meniscus. They appeared arthroscopically as circular soft tissue structures having a broad attachment with smooth glistening synovial tissue covering their exterior surface (Fig. 6-74).

Five of six horses with long-term follow-up were sound, and a seventh horse was improved 11 months after surgery. The authors concluded that meniscal cysts, while uncommon, can be associated with progressive lameness in the horse and that surgical excision of the cysts resulted in resolution or improvement of symptoms, without evidence of recurrence on follow-up examination.

Other Indications for Arthroscopic Surgery in Caudal Pouches of the Femorotibial Joints

The use of arthroscopic surgery to define and treat lesions of the caudal aspect of the femoral condyles in foals through examination of the caudal pouches has been described (Hance et al, 1993). The etiology of this syndrome remains controversial, with sepsis being a prominent finding in many cases in the original publication. However, nonseptic causes have also been described, and the authors of this text consider some caudal femoral condyle lesions in foals and weanlings may be extensive OCD-like lesions of the medial femoral condyle (Fig. 6-75). The lateral femoral condyle is rarely involved. Treatment by arthroscopic access to the caudal pouch of the medial FT joint uses the more proximal caudomedial approach as originally described by Hance et al (1993). This allows instrument entry to debride the cartilage or mineralized cartilage flaps (see Fig. 6-75). The dissection can be extensive and challenging. Despite the extensive loss of joint surface, most cases

are weanlings and some can race after arthroscopic debridement. The prognosis is poor without surgery.

The authors have also used this approach to examine and remove cartilage and mineralized fragments in the caudal aspect of the medial femorotibial joint of mature horses (Fig. 6-76). Acute trauma can result in cartilage debris and small bony fragments (see Fig. 6-76). The caudal compartment of the medial femorotibial joint is quite voluminous. Free fragments swirl in this cavity and can be difficult to reach. Pre-placing a 7.5-cm spinal needle before developing the instrument portal is vital in reaching the fragments and avoiding instruments and the arthroscope interfering with each other as they penetrate deeper to retrieve free pieces.

Cartilage or osteochondral fragments that arise on the condylar surface often settle in the cranial or caudal pouch of the medial FT joint. In chronic cases, continued growth is common, resulting in fragments up to 3 cm across. Surgical removal uses the caudomedial approach close to the saphenous vein (Watts and Nixon, 2006). Retrieval of large fragments often leaves an aperture in the joint capsule that precludes joint distension (see Fig. 6-75), so any exploration and debridement, or cell grafting, of the cranial or caudal femoral condyle needs to be done before fragment removal.

The caudal portion of the caudal cruciate ligament may also be viewed deep (axially) in the caudal compartment of the medial femorotibial joint. However, in the experience of the authors, disruption at the insertion of this cruciate (evident radiographically) may not be visible during arthroscopy unless it is a large avulsion fracture that markedly retracts (see Fig. 6-65). Moreover, the popliteal artery is 1 cm caudal to this ligament and exposure of the caudal cruciate by motorized resection of the covering joint capsule would be hazardous.

Standing Diagnostic Arthroscopy of the Stifle
Contributed by David D. Frisbie

A technique for standing arthroscopic evaluation of the equine stifle was developed by the author to obtain diagnoses

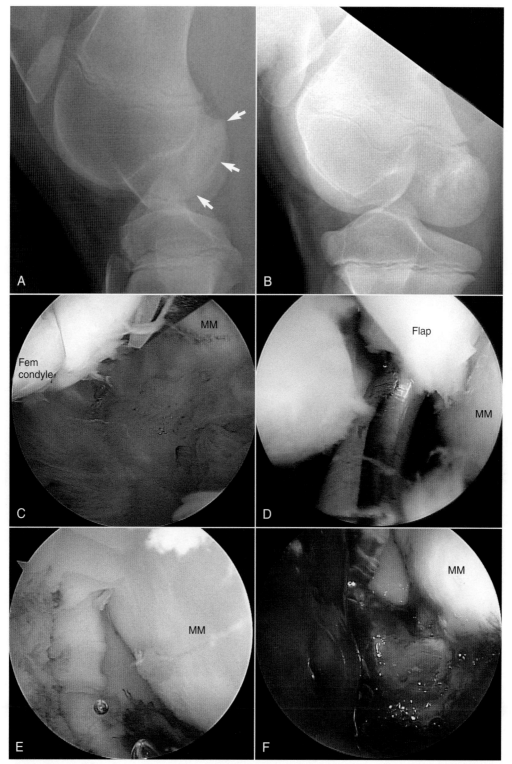

Figure 6-75 Thoroughbred weanling with caudal femoral condyle osteochondritis dissecans (OCD) affecting the medial condyle. A and **B,** Lateral and oblique radiographs show extensive OCD flap extending from proximal extremity of condyle to region articulating with medial meniscus *(arrows).* **C,** Arthroscopic view in caudal pouch of medial femorotibial joint showing caudal condyle, OCD flap *(flap)* and medial meniscus *(MM).* **D,** Flap was elevated and removed in pieces. **E,** Debrided medial condyle, showing thick cartilage, and exposed gap articulating with medial meniscus *(MM).* **F,** Debrided bone was grafted with bone marrow aspirate concentrate *(BMAC)* under gas arthroscopy.

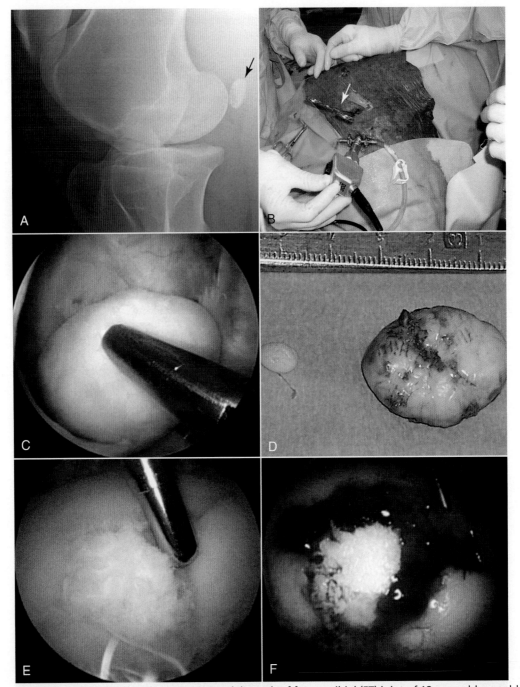

Figure 6-76 Osteochondral free fragment in caudal pouch of femorotibial (FT) joint of 12-year-old warmblood jumper. **A,** Oblique radiograph showing chronic fracture fragment in caudal pouch *(arrow)*. **B,** Surgical view showing caudomedial approach to caudal pouch of medial FT joint, with Ochsner forcep *(arrow)* inserted to retrieve fragment. **C,** Arthroscopic view of ochsner retrieving free fragment. **D,** Removed fragments. **E,** Cranial aspect of medial femoral condyle, showing partially healed defect of origin for the osteochondral fragment in the central weight-bearing region. **F,** Debrided regions during mesenchymal stem cells graft.

in a group of athletic horses that had clinical evidence of stifle disease based on diagnostic analgesia, equivocal changes on radiographic and ultrasonographic examinations, but owners were reluctant to elect for conventional arthroscopy. Use of an 18-gauge (1.3-mm) needle arthroscope in the standing sedated horse allows shortened postprocedure rehabilitation and can help identify presence or absence of a significant lesion. It is not a treatment modality. The goal is to distinguish between horses in which training can, with appropriate management, reasonably be expected to continue and those in which arthroscopic surgery under general anesthesia is indicated. The reader should

also be cautioned that considerable conventional arthroscopic surgical experience (particularly in the stifle joints) is necessary before this technique is considered.

A recently published study detailed the proof of principle work describing needle arthroscopy, including its ability to provide diagnostically useful information in the joint structures (Frisbie et al, 2013). In cases that the author has then followed up with routine 4-mm arthroscopy under general anesthesia to address a specific lesion, there were no further lesions that were not identified with the needle arthroscope. Thus, at this point it is apparent that similar diagnoses can

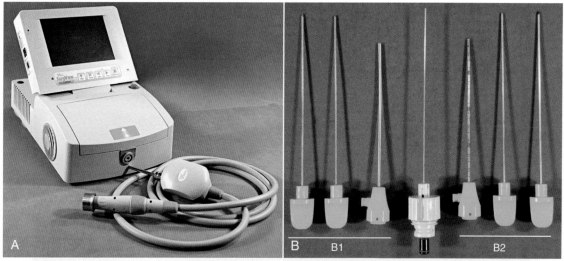

Figure 6-77 A, Integrated fiberoptic xenon light source, 6-4" high-resolution LCD monitor and light cable/480-line, high-resolution camera. **B,** 18-gauge flexible arthroscope, *(B1)* sharp and blunt obturator and stiff cannula, and *(B2)* sharp and blunt obturator and standard cannula. *(From Frisbie DD, Barrett MF, McIlwraith CW, Ullmer J. Diagnostic stifle joint arthroscopy using a needle arthroscope in standing horses.* Vet Surg *43:12-18, 2014.)*

be made using this technique as described previously using a standard 4-mm arthroscope.

Equipment

The 18-gauge needle arthroscope (1.3-mm diameter) (BioVision Technologies, Golden, Colorado) is a compact and portable unit that consists of a light source and imaging processor in one console and a camera attached to a cable, which connects with the base console (Fig. 6-77). The standard 100-mm long arthroscope and cannula/obturator (2-mm outer diameter, OD) systems are disposable and come in a 10-degree and special-order 30-degree configurations. A separate, stiffer cannula/obturator (2.5-mm OD) with a 30-degree scope lens system is available from the manufacturer and was used in all clinical cases (see Fig. 6-77). Fluid distention of the joints is necessary and may be achieved through either the use of a 60-mL syringe, a fluid pressure bag on a 1-L fluid bag, or an automated pressure-sensitive arthroscopic fluid pump system. The fluid used to distend the joint during surgery should have 200 mL of 2% lidocaine/mepivacaine added per liter of fluid.

Patient Preparation

Patients are typically given 2 g of phenylbutazone before surgery and then 2 g daily for 3 additional postoperative days. The first 10 to 15 patients to undergo the procedure received a single perioperative IV dose of ceftiofur (2.5 mg/kg). Gentamicin (6.6 mg/kg) systemic antibiotics have not been used on subsequent cases. Throughout the procedures horses are administered light to moderate sedation; they are also typically restrained with a nose twitch and in some cases using stocks. Horses are routinely sedated with 10 mg of detomidine intramuscular (IM) at the time of initial site preparation. The joints to undergo the procedures are blocked separately using approximately 20 to 30 mL of local anesthetic, optimally at least 20 minutes before the onset of the procedure. Next, depending on the amount of organic debris and hair length, the stifle area is clipped with a No. 40 clipper blade and prepared in an aseptic manner as for routine arthroscopic surgery. In some horses that have very short coats, the hair is not clipped. Just before local skin and tissue anesthesia, the horses are typically given 3 mg of detomidine and 5 mg of butorphanol IV. Approximately 5 to 10 mL 2% mepivacaine hydrochloride is used to block the skin and deeper tissues at each of the entry portals (described in the next section). An

additional aseptic preparation of the portal sites follows with final positioning of the limb. The team typically consists of a surgeon and assistant wearing sterile gloves, as well as an assistant to position and help balance the hindlimb.

The preferred limb positioning is flexed similar to standard arthroscopy described earlier in this chapter. In refractory horses the stifle joints can be entered in a weight-bearing position, but the surgeon needs to be aware that this changes the shape and position of soft tissue structures, most notably the appearance of the menisci (Fig. 6-78). If the limb is entered in a weight-bearing position (minority of the cases), the limb is flexed manually for a short period to visualize the more distal extent of the condyle.

The author has used several positioning devices, including a custom bracket fixed to a set of stocks at the Orthopaedic Research Center, Colorado State University (Fig. 6-79). More recently a customized stand was made to hold the limb in flexion with more versatility (see Fig. 6-79). Using this technique the distal limb is bandaged with a quilt and bandage and then placed in a Kimzey leg save splint (Kimzey, Inc., Woodland, California). A custom base (BioVision Technologies, Golden, Colorado) has been manufactured to accept the Kimzey splint and allow for variable flexion of the limb on the basis of how high the base was from the ground (see Fig. 6-79). A modified Kimzey splint is being designed to obviate the need for the custom base and allow various degrees of flexion.

At the end of the procedure, either 125 mg of amikacin or 600 mg of ceftiofur are administered into the joint undergoing needle arthroscopy. The small size of the skin incisions means that no suture or other methods of closure is necessary; however, the author has used tissue glue in cases where bleeding was an issue. Horses are normally stall confined and observed twice daily for 3 days, and then the level of work appropriate to the arthroscopic findings is in the proof of principle study. Horses were ready for normal activity after 3 to 5 days.

Portal Placement

It is imperative that the workup include diagnostic anesthesia of the stifle joints, just as in any presurgical routine. In some cases this will limit the number of compartments to be examined using the needle arthroscope. In the author's practice, the medial femorotibial joint is followed by the lateral femorotibial joints.

A stab incision just big enough to introduce the sharp tip of the trocar can be made using a No. 15 or 11 blade. However,

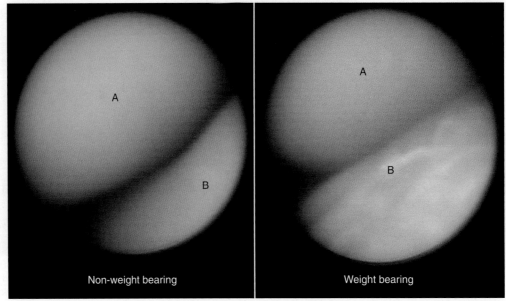

Figure 6-78 Comparison of the cranial aspect of the medial femorotibial joint in a non–weight-bearing (left image) and weight-bearing (right image) position in the same horse. The configuration of the medial meniscus changes considerably when the joint is being loaded. *A*, Medial femoral condyle; *B*, medial meniscus.

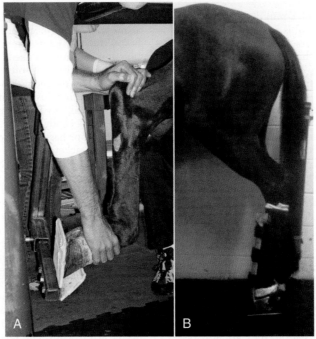

Figure 6-79 A, Stationary limb-positioning stand. **B,** Mobile limb-positioning device.

the author has more recently used the sharp trocar to introduce the stiff arthroscopic cannula through the skin and soft tissues before advancement of the cannula into the joint using the blunt obturator. Distention of the joint is not necessary before cannula placement; this is aided by the previously administered 20 to 30 mL of local anesthetic. Additionally, the caudal aspect of the medial femorotibial joint is usually done after the cranial compartment, thus providing some caudal distention. The author believes this aids entrance.

The cranial compartment of the medial femorotibial (MFT) joint is assessed from a standard approach lateral to the lateral patellar ligament and then a cranial approach between the lateral and medial patellar ligaments (McIlwraith et al, 2005) in either flexed or extended limb positions (Fig. 6-80).

The lateral approach optimizes visualization of the cranial ligament and axial portion of the medial meniscus easier. The cranial approach allows easier visualization of the intercondylar area (cruciate ligaments) and the medial collateral ligament (Fig. 6-81) (Barrett et al, 2012). The caudal approach to the MFT uses the description of Trumble et al (1994) and can be used in both flexed and weight-bearing positions (McIlwraith et al, 2005) (see Fig. 6-80). The author's approach of choice to the cranial compartment lateral femorotibial (LFT) joint is that first described by Moustafa et al (1987) using the previous lateral portal (lateral to the lateral patellar ligament) to the cranial MFT joint, although the portal for the cranial MFT joint can also be used (McIlwraith et al, 2005) to help visualize more lateral structures. The caudal pouch of the LFT joint is

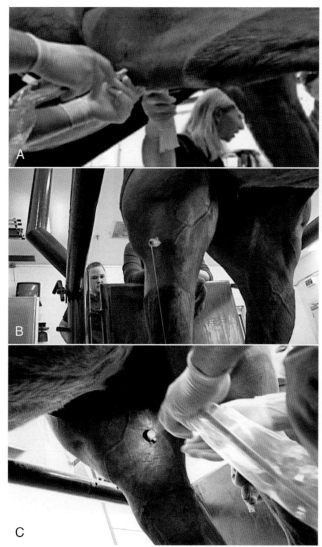

Figure 6-80 A, Simultaneous diagnostic arthroscopy and ultrasonographic examination in a standing horse with the operated limb flexed. **B,** Synovial fluid draining from a stiff (2.5-mm) cannula inserted in the cranial compartment of the medial femorotibial (MFT) joint from a lateral portal in a standing horse. **C,** Cannula placement in the caudal compartment of the MFT joint in a standing horse. *(From Frisbie DD, Barrett MF, McIlwraith CW, Ullmer J. Diagnostic stifle joint arthroscopy using a needle arthroscope in standing horses.* Vet Surg *43:12-18, 2014.)*

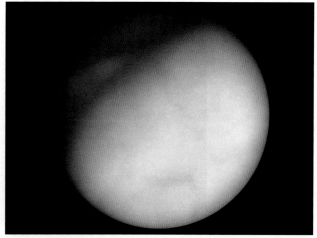

Figure 6-81 View of a normal cranial cruciate ligament just caudal to the attachment at the medial tibial eminence as it courses through the intercondylar notch area.

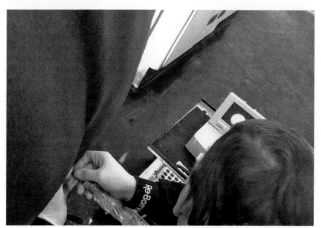

Figure 6-82 Correct hand placement on the cannula, which is used to manipulate the scope in the joint. No torque is being placed on the scope or camera.

entered using an approach that is 2.5 cm proximal to the tibial plateau and 3 cm caudal to the lateral collateral ligament; the author has only performed this in the flexed position. The femoropatellar joint is entered through a standard craniolateral approach with the limb extended (McIlwraith et al, 2005).

A combination of these approaches allows a complete examination of the stifle. It should be noted that all movements of the cannula around the joint should be made by placing pressure on the cannula itself, and not on the scope or camera, because these are prone to breakage (Fig. 6-82). Because this weak point is outside the joint, no morbidity to the patient would be encountered if breakage were to occur. The author has not experienced this and typically uses a single scope for four to five procedures or until visible damage to the scope is observed.

The procedure permits simultaneous arthroscopic and ultrasonographic examinations (Barrett et al, 2012) (see Fig. 6-80).

A broad range of lesions have been identified using the needle scope as described. These include full-thickness cartilage erosion of articular cartilage (Fig. 6-83), horizontal articular

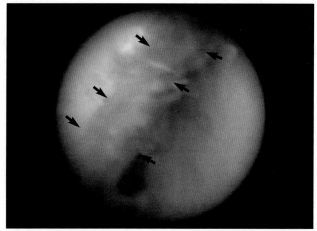

Figure 6-83 Full-thickness erosion on the medial condyle (outlined by *black arrows*) just adjacent to the medial tibial eminence (right side of picture).

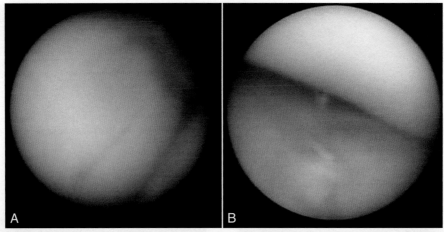

Figure 6-84 Full-thickness lacerations in the medial condyle **(A)** adjacent to a medial meniscal lesion **(B).**

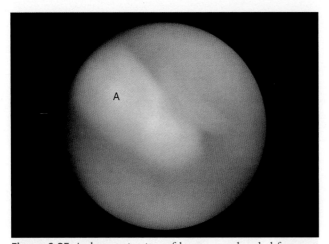

Figure 6-85 Arthroscopic view of loose osteochondral fragment *(A)* in the intercondylar area.

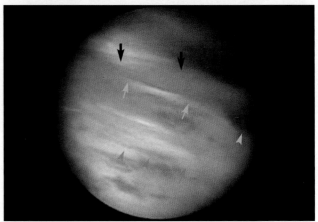

Figure 6-86 Image of the cranial compartment of the medial femorotibial, weight-bearing position. The *black arrows* delineate the margin of the proximal articular margin of the medial condyle and reflection of synovial membrane. The *green arrows* delineate the proximal boarder of the medial meniscus. The *orange arrows* delineate the horizontal tear in the medial meniscus, which was noted to become larger as the horse became more non-weight bearing.

cartilage lacerations and an axial lesion of the medial meniscus (Fig. 6-84), and a loose body identified in the intercondylar area (undetected on radiographs and ultrasound) (Fig. 6-85). Other syndromes include a horizontal meniscal lesion (in a weight-bearing stifle) (Fig. 6-86) and tearing of the cranial ligament of the lateral meniscus (Fig. 6-87). It is important to note that the smaller-diameter arthroscope means a smaller field of view and the surgeon must scan the joint to ensure that a complete exploratory examination is performed. If this is done, there should be no limitations to the technique in accurately diagnosing stifle lesions without the need for general anesthesia.

In some cases blood contamination limits the visualization of intraarticular structures. Increasing the intraarticular pressure can improve this issue. A second method of clearing blood from the joint is by passive egress of fluid through the arthroscopic cannula (typically by partial removal of the arthroscope).

A rational choice can then be made for medical therapy and return to exercise or arthroscopic treatment using standard arthroscopic equipment and surgical triangulation to address the specific lesions.

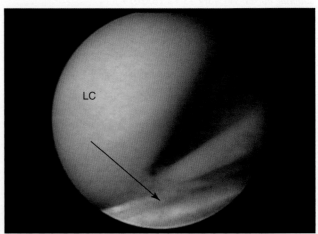

Figure 6-87 Lateral condyle *(LC)* and longitudinal tear in the cranial ligament of the lateral meniscus *(arrow).*

REFERENCES

Adams OR: *Lameness in Horses*, ed 3, Philadelphia, 1974, Lea & Febiger.

Baccarin RYA, Martins EAN, Hagen SFC, Silva LCLC: Patellar instability following experimental medial patellar desmotomy in horses, *Vet Comp Orthop Traumatol* 22:27–31, 2009.

Barrett MF, Frisbie DD, McIlwraith CW, Werpy NM: The arthroscopic and ultrasonographic boundaries of the equine femorotibial joints, *Equine Vet J* 44:57–63, 2012.

Bodo G, Hangody L, Modis L, Hurtig M: Autologous osteochondral grafting (mosaic arthroplasty) for treatment of subchondral cystic lesions in the equine stifle and fetlock joints, *Vet Surg* 33:588–596, 2004.

Boening KJ: Die Arthroskopie des Kniegelenks beim Pferd uber einen 'Centralen' Zugang, *Teil 1: Methodik Pferdheilkund* 11:247–257, 1995.

Bourzac C, Alexander K, Rossier Y, Laverty S: Comparison of radiography and ultrasonography for the diagnosis of osteochondritis dissecans in the equine femoropatellar joint, *Equine Vet J* 41:686–692, 2009.

Cauvin ER, Munroe GA, Boyd JS, Paterson C: Ultrasonographic examination of the femorotibial articulation in horses: imaging of the cranial and caudal aspects, *Equine Vet J* 28:285–296, 1996.

Changoor A, Hurtig MB, Runciman RJ, Quesnel AJ, Dickey JP, Lowerison M: Mapping of donor and recipient site properties for osteochondral graft reconstruction of subchondral cystic lesions in the equine stifle, *Equine Vet J* 38:330–336, 2006.

Cohen JM, Richardson DW, McKnight AL, Ross MW, Boston RC: Long-term outcome in 44 horses with stifle lameness after arthroscopic exploration and debridement, *Vet Surg* 38:543–551, 2009.

Contino EK, Park RD, McIlwraith CW: Prevalence of radiographic changes in yearling and 2-year-old Quarter Horses intended for cutting, *Equine Vet J* 44:185–195, 2012.

Convery ER, Akeson WH, Keown GH: The repair of large osteochondral defects; an experimental study in horses, *Clin Orthop Rel Res* 82:853–862, 1972.

Desjardins MR, Hurtig MB: Diagnosis of equine stifle disorders: 3 cases, *Can Vet J* 33:543–550, 1991.

Dik KJ, Enzerink E, van Weeren PR: Radiographic development of osteochondral abnormalities in the hock and stifle of Dutch Warmblood foals, from age 1 to 11 months, *Equine Vet J* 31(Suppl 1):9–15, 1999.

Dumoulin M, Pille F, Desmet P, DeWulf J, Steenhaut M, Gasthuys F, Martens A: Upward fixation of the patella in the horse. A retrospective study, *Vet Comp Orthop Traumatol* 20:119–125, 2007.

Edwards RB, Nixon AJ: Avulsion of the cranial cruciate ligament in a horse, *Equine Vet J* 18:334–336, 1996.

Ferris DJ, Frisbie DD, Kisiday JD, McIlwraith CW, Hague BA, Major MD, Schneider RK, Zubrod CJ, Kawcak CE, Goodrich LR: Clinical follow-up of thirty-three horses treated for stifle injury with bone marrow derived mesenchymal stem cells intra-articularly, *Vet Surg*, 2013, In Press.

Foland JW, McIlwraith CW, Trotter GW: Arthroscopic surgery for osteochondritis dissecans of the femoropatellar joint, *Equine Vet J* 24:419–423, 1992.

Fortier LA, Nixon AJ: New surgical treatments for osteochondritis dissecans and subchondral bone cysts, *Vet Clin North Am Equine Pract* 21:673–690, 2005.

Fowlie J, Arnoczky S, Lavagnino M, Maerz T, Stick J: Resection of Grade III cranial horn tears of the equine medial meniscus alter the contact forces on medial tibial condyle at full extension: an in-vitro cadaveric study, *Vet Surg* 40:957–965, 2011a.

Fowlie JG, Arnoczky SP, Stick JA, Pease AP: Meniscal translocation and deformation throughout the range of motion of the equine stifle joint: an in vitro cadaveric study, *Equine Vet J* 43:259–264, 2011b.

Frisbie DD, Barrett MF, McIlwraith CW, Ullmer J: Diagnostic arthroscopy of the stifle joint using a needle arthroscope in standing horses: a novel procedure, *Vet Surg*, 2013, In Press.

Gibson KT, McIlwraith CW, Park RD, Norrdin RW: Production of patellar lesions by medial patellar desmotomy in normal horses, *Vet Surg* 18:466–471, 1989.

Grzybowski M, Brehm W, Werren C, Tessier C: Successful treatment of a medial intercondylar eminence fracture in a stallion by arthroscopic removal, *Vet Rec* 162:756–758, 2008.

Guhl JF: Arthroscopic treatment of osteochondritis dissecans, *Clin Orthop* 167:65–74, 1984.

Hance SR, Schneider RK, Embertson RM, Bramlage LR, Wicks JR: Lesions of the caudal aspect of the femoral condyles in foals: 20 cases (1980-1990), *J Am Vet Med Assoc* 202:637–646, 1993.

Hendrix SM, Baxter GM, McIlwraith CW, Hendrickson DA, Goodrich LR, Frisbie DD, Trotter GW: Concurrent or sequential development of medial meniscal and subchondral cystic lesions within the medial femorotibial joint in horses (1996-2006), *Equine Vet J* 42:5–9, 2010.

Howard RD, McIlwraith CW, Trotter GW: Arthroscopic surgery for subchondral cystic lesions of the medial femoral condyle in horses: 41 cases (1988-1991), *J Am Vet Med Assoc* 206:842–850, 1995.

Jackson WA, Stick JA, Arnoczky SP, Nickels FA: The effect of compacted cancellous bone grafting on the healing of subchondral bone defects on the medial femoral condyle in horses, *Vet Surg* 29:8–16, 2000.

Janicek JC, Wilson DA: Vet Med Today What is your diagnosis? *J Am Vet Med Assoc* 230:1149–1150, 2007.

Kold SE, Hickman J: Results of treatment of subchondral bone cysts in the medial condyle of the equine femur with an autogenous cancellous bone graft, *Equine Vet J* 16:414, 1984.

Lewis RD. A retrospective study of diagnostic and surgical arthroscopy of the equine femorotibial joint. Proceedings 23rd Annual Meeting AAEP, 1987.

McIlwraith CW: Experience in diagnostic and surgical arthroscopy in the horse, *Equine Vet J* 16:11–19, 1984.

McIlwraith CW: Osteochondral fragmentation of the distal aspect of the patella in horse, *Equine Vet J* 22:157–163, 1990.

McIlwraith CW: *Diagnostic and Surgical Arthroscopy in the Horse*, ed 2, Philadelphia, 1990, Lea & Febiger.

McIlwraith CW. Osteochondritis dissecans of the femoropatellar joint. Proceedings 39th Annual Meeting AAEP, 1993:73–77.

McIlwraith CW, Martin GS: Arthroscopy and arthroscopic surgery in horse, *Compend Cont Educ* 6:S43–S53, 1984.

McIlwraith CW, Martin CS: Arthroscopic surgery for the treatment of osteochondritis dissecans in the equine femoropatellar joint, *Vet Surg* 14:105–116, 1985.

McIlwraith CW, Nixon AJ, Wright IM, Boening KJ: *Diagnostic and Surgical Arthroscopy in the Horse*, ed 3, Elsevier-Mosby Limited, 2005.

McIntosh SC, McIlwraith CW: Natural history of femoropatellar osteochondrosis in three crops of Thoroughbreds Equine, *Vet J* 16(Suppl):54–61, 1993.

McLellan J, Plevin S, Taylor E: Concurrent patella fracture and lateral collateral ligament avulsion as a result of trauma in three horses, *J Am Vet Med Assoc* 240:1218–1222, 2012.

McNally TP, Slone DE, Lynch TM, Hughs FE: Use of a suprapatellar pouch portal and laparoscopic cannula for removal of debris or loose fragments following arthroscopy of the femoropatellar joint on 168 horses (245 joints), *Vet Surg* 40:886–890, 2011.

Marble GP, Sullins KE: Arthroscopic removal of patellar fracture fragments in horses: 5 cases (1989-1998), *J Am Vet Med Assoc* 216:1799–1801, 2000.

Martin GS, McIlwraith CW: Arthroscopic anatomy of the equine femoropatellar joint and approaches for treatment of osteochondritis dissecans, *Vet Surg* 14:99–104, 1985.

Moustafa MAI, Boero JJ, Baker GJ: Arthroscopic examination of the femorotibial joints of horses, *Vet Surg* 16:352–357, 1987.

Mueller POE, Allen D, Watson E, Hay C: Arthroscopic removal of a fragment from an intercondylar eminence fracture of the tibia in a 2-year-old horse, *J Am Vet Med Assoc* 204:1793–1795, 1994.

Murphy JM, Fink DJ, Hunziker EB, et al.: Stem cell therapy in a caprine model of osteoarthritis, *Arthritis Rheum* 48:3464–3474, 2003.

Muurlink T, Walmsley J, Young D, Whitton C: A cranial intercondylar arthroscopic approach to the caudal medial femorotibial joint of the horse, *Equine Vet J* 41:5–10, 2009.

Nickels FA, Sande R: Radiographic and arthroscopic findings in the equine stifle, *J Am Vet Med Assoc* 181:918–924, 1982.

Nixon AJ, Fortier LA, Goodrich LR, Ducharme NG: Arthroscopic reattachment of select OCD lesions using resorbable polydioxanone pins, *Equine Vet J* 36:376–383, 2004.

Ortved KF, Nixon AJ, Mohammed HO, Fortier LA: Treatment of subchondral cystic lesions in the medial femoral condyle of mature horses with growth factor enhanced chondrocyte grafts: a retrospective study of 49 cases, *Equine Vet J* 44:606–613, 2012.

Outerbridge RE, Outerbridge HK: The etiology of chondromalacia of the patella, *J Bone Joint Surg (Br)* 43B:752–757, 1961.

Pascoe JR, Wheat JD, Jones KL: A lateral approach to the equine femoropatellar joint, *Vet Surg* 9:141–144, 1980.

Pascoe JR, Pool RR, Wheat JD, O'Brien TR: Osteochondral defects of the lateral trochlear ridge of the distal femur of the horse. Clinical, radiographic, and pathologic examination of results of surgical treatment, *Vet Surg* 13:99–110, 1984.

Peroni JF, Stick JA: Evaluation of a cranial arthroscopic approach to the stifle joint for the treatment of femorotibial joint disease in horses: 23 cases (1998-1999), *J Am Vet Med Assoc* 220:1046–1052, 2002.

Petty CA, Lubowitz JH: Does arthroscopic partial meniscectomy result in knee osteoarthritis? A systematic review with a minimum of 8 years follow-up, *Arthroscopy* 27:419–424, 2011.

Prades M, Grant VD, Turner TA: Injuries of the cranial cruciate ligament and associated structures: summary of clinical, radiographic, arthroscopic and pathological findings from 10 horses, *Equine Vet J* 21:354–357, 1989.

Raheja LF, Galuppo LD, Bowers-Lepore J, Dowd JP, Tablin F, Yellowley CE: Treatment of bilateral medial femoral condyle articular cartilage fissures in a horse using bone marrow-derived multipotent mesenchymal stromal cells, *J Equine Vet Sci* 31:147–154, 2011.

Ray CS, Baxter GM, McIlwraith CW, Trotter GW, Powers BE, Park RD, Steyn PF: Development of subchondral cystic lesions after articular cartilage and subchondral bone damage in young horses, *Equine Vet J* 28:225–232, 1996.

Rich RF, Glisson RR: In vitro mechanical properties and failure mode of equine (pony) cranial cruciate ligament, *Vet Surg* 23:257–265, 1994.

Rose PL, Graham JP, Moore I, Riley CB: Imaging diagnosis – caudal cruciate avulsion in a horse, *Vet Radiol Ultrasound* 42:414–416, 2001.

Sanders-Shamis M, Bukowiecki CF, Biller DS: Cruciate and collateral ligament failure in the equine stifle: 7 cases (1975-1985), *J Am Vet Med Assoc* 193:573–576, 1988.

Sandler EA, Bramlage LR, Embertson RM, Ruggles AJ, Frisbie DD. Correlation of lesion size with racing performance in Thoroughbreds after arthroscopic surgical treatment of subchondral cystic lesions of the medial femoral condyle: 150 cases (1989-2000). Proceedings 48th AAEP 255–256, 2002.

Schneider RK, Jenson P, Moore RM: Evaluation of cartilage lesions on the medial femoral condyle as a cause of lameness in horses: 11 cases (1988–1994), *J Am Vet Med Assoc* 20:1649–1652, 1997.

Scott GSP, Crawford WH, Colahan BT: Arthroscopic findings in horses with subtle radiographic evidence of the medial femoral condyle, *J Am Vet Med Assoc* 224:107–112, 2004.

Scott WN: *Insall & Scott Surgery of the Knee*, ed 5, Philadelphia, PA, 2012, Elsevier/Churchill Livingstone.

Smith MA, Walmsley JP, Phillips TJ, Pinchbeck GL, Booth TM, Greet TR, Richardson DW, Ross MW, Schramme MC, Singer ER, Smith RK, Clegg PD: Effect of age at presentation on outcome following arthroscopic debridement of subchondral cystic lesions in the medial femoral condyle: 85 horses (1993-2003), *Equine Vet J* 37:175–180, 2005.

Soper NJ, Hunter JG: Suturing and knot tying in laparoscopy, *Surg Clin N Am* 72:1139–1152, 1992.

Sparks HD, Nixon AJ, Boening KJ, Pool RR: Arthroscopic treatment of meniscal cysts in the horse, *Equine Vet J* 43:669–675, 2011c.

Sparks HD, Nixon AJ, Bogenrief DS: Reattachment of the articular cartilage component of type 1 subchondral cystic lesions of the medial femoral condyle with polydioxanone pins in 3 horses, *J Am Vet Med Assoc* 238:636–640, 2011b.

Sparks HD, Nixon AJ, Fortier LA, Mohammed HO: Arthroscopic reattachment of osteochondritis dissecans cartilage flaps of the femoropatellar joint: long-term results, *Equine Vet J* 43:650–659, 2011a.

Steinheimer DN, McIlwraith CW, Park RD, Steyn PF: Comparison of radiographic subchondral bone changes with arthroscopic findings in the equine femoropatellar and femorotibial joints. A retrospective study of 72 horses, *Vet Radiol* 36:478–484, 1995.

Textor JA, Nixon AJ, Lumsden J, Ducharme NG: Subchondral cystic lesions of the proximal extremity in horses: 12 cases (1983–2000), *J Am Vet Med Assoc* 218:408–413, 2001.

Trotter CW, McIlwraith CW, Norrdin RW: A comparison of two surgical approaches to the equine femoropatellar joint for the treatment of osteochondritis dissecans, *Vet Surg* 12:33–40, 1983.

Trumble TN, Stick JA, Arnoczky SP, Rosenstein D: Consideration of anatomic and radiographic features of the caudal pouches of the femorotibial joints of horses for the purpose of arthroscopy, *Am J Vet Res* 55:1682–1689, 1994.

Vinardell T, Florent D, Morisset S: Arthroscopic surgical approach and intra-articular anatomy of the equine suprapatellar pouch, *Vet Surg* 37:350–356, 2008.

von Rechenberg B, Guenther H, McIlwraith CW, et al.: Fibrous tissue of subchondral cystic lesions in horses produce local mediators and neutral metalloproteinases and cause bone resorption in horses, *Vet Surg* 29:420–429, 2000.

Voute LC, Henson FMD, Platt D, Jeffcott LB: Osteochondrosis lesions of the lateral trochlear ridge of the distal femur in four horses, *Vet Rec* 168:265–269, 2011.

Wallis TW, Goodrich LR, McIlwraith CW, Frisbie DD, Hendrickson DA, Trotter GW, Baxter GM, Kawcak CE: Arthroscopic injection of corticosteroids into the fibrous tissue of subchondral cystic lesions of the medial femoral condyle in horses: a retrospective study of 52 cases (2001-2006), *Equine Vet J* 40:461–467, 2008.

Walmsley JP: Vertical tears of the cranial horn of the meniscus and its cranial ligament in the equine femorotibial joint: 7 cases and their treatment by arthroscopic surgery, *Equine Vet J* 27:20–25, 1995.

Walmsley JP: Fracture of the intercondylar eminence of the tibia treated by arthroscopic internal fixation, *Equine Vet J* 29:148–150, 1997.

Walmsley JP: Arthroscopic surgery of the femorotibial joint, *Clin Techn Equine Prac* 1:226–233, 2002.

Walmsley JP, Philips TJ, Townsend HGG: Meniscal tears in horses: an evaluation of clinical signs and arthroscopic treatment of 80 cases, *Equine Vet J* 35:402–406, 2003.

Watts AE, Nixon AJ: Comparison of arthroscopic approaches and accessible anatomic structures during arthroscopy of the caudal pouches of equine femorotibial joints, *Vet Surg* 35:219–226, 2006.

White NA, McIlwraith CW, Allen D: Curettage of subchondral bone cysts in medial femoral condyles of the horse, *Equine Vet J Suppl* 6:120–124, 1988.

Whitman JL, Moorehead JP, Prichard MA, Hance SA, Keuler NS, Santschai EM: Radiographic lucencies in the medial femoral condyle of Thoroughbred sale yearlings a preliminary investigation of the effect on race records, *Proccedings AAEP* 52:416–419, 2006.

Wilke MM, Nydam D, Nixon AJ: Enhanced early chondrogenesis in articular defects following arthroscopic mesenchymal stem cell implantation in an equine model, *J Orthop Res* 25:913–925, 2007.

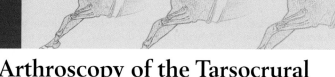

CHAPTER 7

Diagnostic and Surgical Arthroscopy of the Tarsocrural (Tibiotarsal) Joint

The tarsocrural (tibiotarsal) joint has proven highly amenable to both diagnostic and surgical arthroscopy. The most common indication is osteochondritis dissecans (OCD). However, as in the other joints, new discoveries have produced further indications for diagnostic arthroscopy, as well as an increase in the spectrum of surgical conditions in the tarsocrural joint. For instance, before the use of arthroscopy, surgical intervention was not considered appropriate for a tarsocrural joint manifesting effusion or lameness, or both, unless it had a radiographic lesion. Now veterinarians know that not all cases of tarsocrural OCD, for instance, manifest radiographically. Although this finding further confirms the limitations of radiographs, it does, however, allow for defining and treating cases of "idiopathic synovitis" that would otherwise have remained undefined. In addition, as in other joints, OCD can be treated conveniently with arthroscopic surgery and the same advantages exist.

DIAGNOSTIC ARTHROSCOPY OF THE TARSOCRURAL JOINT

Two approaches for diagnostic arthroscopy in the tarsocrural joint are described: dorsal and plantar. The dorsal approach involves a dorsomedial arthroscopic portal except for fractures of the lateral malleolus of the tibia when a dorsolateral arthroscopic portal is used. The plantar approach involves a plantarolateral or plantaromedial arthroscopic portal.

In all situations, the patient is in dorsal recumbency. This positioning not only allows convenient access to either side of the joint, which is important for triangulation, but also the degree of flexion of the joint is easily controlled. The use of dorsal recumbency also minimizes the risk of losing loose fragments. The leg may be suspended or hangs free with the former preferred.

The tarsocrural joints are clipped circumferentially (some of the authors also shave at portal sites). The draping system includes an adhesive barrier and impermeable drapes (Fig. 7-1). The joint is distended before making the skin incisions. The skin incisions for the arthroscopic and instrument approaches are located to the sides of the group of extensor tendons on the dorsal aspect of the joint (the long digital extensor, the peroneus tertius, and the cranialis tibialis tendons). These structures are collectively referred to in the remainder of the text as the *extensor tendons*. As a general principle, all portals are made close to (≈1 cm from) the extensor tendons to maximum visualization.

Arthroscopic Examination Using a Dorsomedial Approach

The dorsomedial approach is used most commonly. If the arthroscopic portal is made close to the cranialis tibialis and peroneus tertius tendons, a large portion of the dorsal aspect of the joint can be seen. The approach provides excellent visualization of the dorsal compartment of the joint, including the trochlear ridges and trochlear groove of the talus. Flexing and extending the joint, which brings different areas of the trochlear ridges into view, can increase the area of visualization. The corresponding area of the distal tibia from the medial malleolus to the distal intermediate ridge is also visible. Most adult horses also have an opening that allows visualization of the proximal intertarsal (talocentral) joint distally. Inspection of the synovial lining of the dorsal aspect of the tarsocrural joint can also be performed.

The joint is distended using a needle placed through the dorsomedial pouch with the leg in extension (see Fig. 7-1). The skin portal is made slightly dorsal to the center of the distended dorsomedial outpouching and just below the palpable distal end of the medial malleolus, and the arthroscopic sleeve and conical obturator are inserted (Fig. 7-2). If the arthroscope is placed more medially, it is difficult to pass the arthroscopic sheath over the trochlear ridges of the talus across the joint. The skin portal is made sufficiently large (8 to 10 mm) to ensure that the saphenous vein is not directly beneath the incision and to avoid its penetration. In many horses, the arthroscope portal can be made between the saphenous vein and the extensor tendons, and this location provides optimal visualization of the deeper region of the intermediate ridge. A No. 11 blade is then used to continue the portal through the fibrous capsule. The sleeve and conical obturator are then inserted until contact with the medial side of the talus is made (see Fig. 7-2). The joint is then flexed, enabling the arthroscopic sleeve and obturator to pass across the joint, over the top of the trochlear ridges, and beneath the extensor tendons (this maneuver is impossible in an extended joint).

The arthroscopic portal can also be made with the joint flexed, eliminating the need to flex the joint during placement of the sheath; however, the landmarks (as well as location of the saphenous vein) are more easily identified with the limb in extension.

Examination commences on the lateral side of the joint, looking at the proximal aspect of the lateral trochlear ridge and its articulation with the tibia. This view includes the lateral malleolus (Fig. 7-3). The arthroscope is then rotated to visualize the central lateral trochlear ridge, and further distad, the distal part of the lateral trochlear ridge comes into the visual field (see Fig. 7-3). In this fashion, the trochlear ridge can be visualized by using minimal movement of the arthroscope. The view of the arthroscope is then returned to the junction of the trochlear ridge and the tibia, and the arthroscope is withdrawn slightly with the lens still oriented in a plantar direction to visualize the distal intermediate (sagittal) ridge of the tibia and the proximal portion of the trochlear groove of the talus (see Fig. 7-3). The remainder of the trochlear groove is visible further distally. In addition, the talocentral (proximal intertarsal) joint can be visualized. This communication is not usually patent in very young foals. A synovial fossa may be observed in the trochlear groove of the talus, a normal finding, or, less frequently, on the medial trochlear ridge of the talus (see Fig. 7-3).

Further withdrawal of the arthroscope accompanied by rotation, so that the view is proximal and plantar, enables visualization of the proximal aspect of the medial trochlear ridge and its articulation with the distal tibia (see Fig. 7-3). If the tip of the arthroscope is moved more medially, examination of the medial malleolus is possible. The more distal aspects of the medial trochlear ridge can be examined by rotating the lens plantar and then distal and flexing the hock or by moving the arthroscope distad. A synovial fossa may also be seen rarely on the medial trochlear ridge of the talus. Retraction of the arthroscope allows examination of the medial side of the talus and the dorsomedial pouch (see Fig. 7-3).

With this approach, imposition of soft tissue sometimes makes examination of the lateral trochlear ridge and other areas of the lateral part of the joint challenging. It requires the end of the arthroscope to be close to the lateral trochlear ridge of the talus along with the use of the instrument to retract soft tissue. However, with practice, this becomes reasonably easy.

▶ Arthroscopic Examination Using Plantar Lateral or Plantar Medial Approaches

These approaches are used less commonly. They allow excellent visualization of the portions of the lateral and medial trochlear ridges that are not visualized using the previously described dorsal approaches. Each trochlear ridge is best evaluated by using an arthroscopic approach through the same side (Fig. 7-4). The principal uses of the plantar approaches are allowing examination of defects in the proximal portion of the trochlear ridges, the removal of fragments, and the treatment of sepsis and osteomyelitis. This approach can be useful to access fractures of the lateral malleolus of the tibia. Virtually all of the synovial lining of the plantar joint pouch can be inspected through these approaches. Additionally, the plantar aspect of the distal tibia and the deep digital flexor tendon (DDFT) within its tendon sheath can be seen, but these observations have not proven to be of major clinical relevance. The approach to the plantar pouch was reported by Zamos et al (1994). Joint distention is critical and can be performed dorsally or by placing a needle in the center of the plantar pouch, which usually allows adequate distention. The skin portal is made in the center of the plantar outpouching with the tarsus

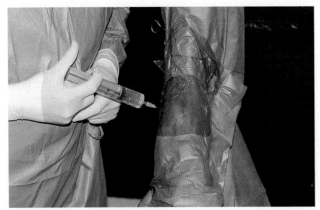

Figure 7-1 Tarsus draped for surgery and tarsocrural joint being distended.

flexed at 90 degrees. The arthroscopic sheath is placed in the joint using the blunt obturator. The surgeon should be careful to avoid damaging the trochlear ridges of the talus. Viewing commences with the hock flexed (see Fig. 7-4).

Introduction of the arthroscope through a plantaromedial or plantarolateral portal puts the arthroscope immediately dorsal to the tarsal synovial sheath surrounding the DDFT and plantar to the trochlear ridges of the talus. This permits evaluation of the plantar aspects of the medial and lateral trochlear ridges of the talus, as well as the trochlear groove, distal tibia (plantar aspect of intermediate ridge), and articular portion of the tendon sheath containing the DDFT (see Fig. 7-4). Through a plantarolateral arthroscopic portal, the plantarolateral cul-de-sac of the tarsocrural joint, synovial membrane, and lateral malleolus can also be observed if the arthroscope is directed dorsad. Withdrawing the arthroscope slightly allows observation of the plantar talocalcaneal ligament connecting the lateral trochlear ridge of the talus to the coracoid process of the calcaneus and the joint space of the proximal region of the talocalcaneal articulation.

If a plantaromedial arthroscopic portal is used, directing the arthroscope dorsally allows observation of the dorsomedial cul-de-sac, but the medial malleolus cannot be seen. However, using a medial portal, the lateral malleolus can be observed when the arthroscope is advanced across the joint.

By extending the joint to approximately 120 degrees, the medial and lateral dorsal cul-de-sacs of the joint can be observed more easily. On the other hand, with more flexion, an enhanced examination of the proximal areas of the medial and lateral trochlear ridges is possible.

Diagnostic Arthroscopy of the Tarsocrural Joint

The most common indication for arthroscopy in the tarsocrural joint is for the surgical treatment of OCD. In some instances, however, OCD is radiographically silent, and surgical treatment in these cases begins as a purely diagnostic examination. For this reason, diagnostic arthroscopy in the tarsocrural joint may be indicated if idiopathic effusion (bog spavin) is noted in the young horse, even when the radiographic signs are negative. In addition, arthroscopy is an excellent means by which to evaluate the joint in cases of persistent synovitis, suspected soft tissue lesions, osteoarthritis, or sepsis. The general aspects of such diagnostic examinations were discussed in Chapter 3. Septic osteomyelitis lesions in the young horse can be evaluated and treated (curettage and lavage) arthroscopically, and this is discussed in more detail in Chapter 14. Arthroscopy also permits identification of soft tissue lesions such as tears of the collateral ligaments, within or communicating with the tarsocrural joint. As in other locations, arthroscopy is the imaging modality of choice for surface lesions in the tarsocrural joint.

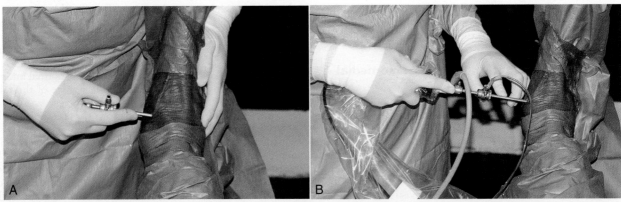

Figure 7-2 A, Insertion of the arthroscopic sleeve for a dorsomedial approach to the tarsocrural joint. **B,** Arthroscope positioned for beginning of examination.

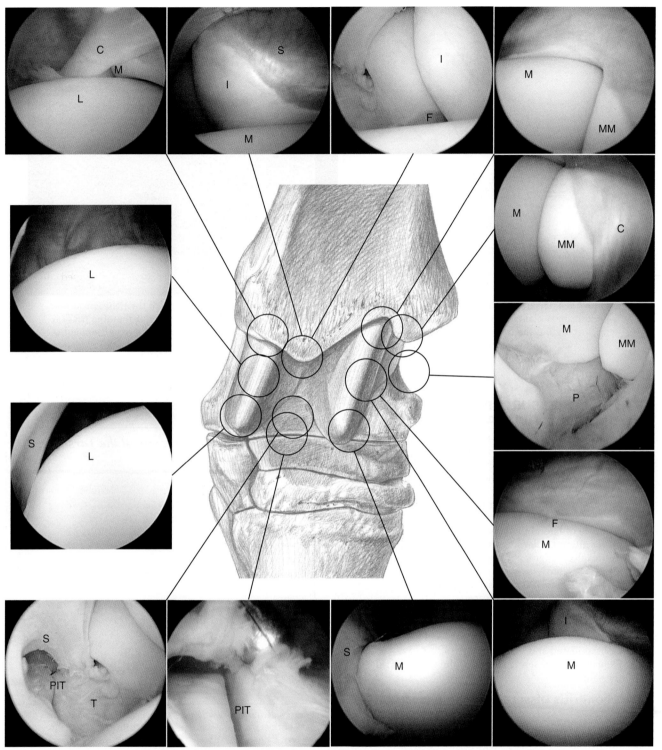

Figure 7-3 Composite of arthroscopic images obtained from tarsocrural joint using dorsomedial arthroscopic approach. *C,* Short lateral collateral ligament; *F,* synovial fossa; *L,* lateral trochlear ridge of talus; *LDE,* long digital extensor tendon; *LM,* lateral malleolus of tibia; *M,* medial trochlear ridge of talus; *MM,* medial malleolus of tibia; *PIT,* proximal intertarsal joint; *PT,* peroneus tertius; *TC,* tibialis cranialis; *S,* synovial membrane; *T,* trochlear groove of talus.

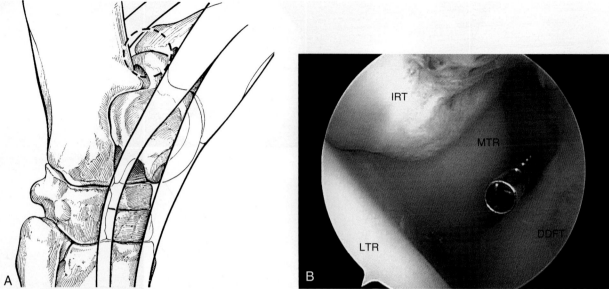

Figure 7-4 Diagram of arthroscopic field **(A)** and arthroscopic view **(B)** of the plantar pouches of the right tarsocrural joint, using a plantarolateral entry. With the horse in dorsal recumbency, the intermediate ridge of the tibia *(IRT)* is uppermost and the lateral trochlear ridge *(LTR)* and medial trochlear ridge *(MTR)* are visible. An egress cannula has been inserted in the plantaromedial cul-de-sac of the joint and used to caudally retract the deep digital flexor tendon *(DDFT)* within the tarsal sheath.

ARTHROSCOPIC SURGERY OF THE TARSOCRURAL (TIBIOTARSAL) JOINT

Arthroscopic surgery has proven to be an excellent tool in the tarsocrural joint and is indicated for the following conditions:

1. OCD of the distal intermediate ridge of the tibia
2. OCD of the lateral and medial trochlear ridges of the talus
3. Cystic lesions of the proximal trochlea of the talus
4. OCD of the medial malleolus of the tibia
5. Removal of lateral malleolar fragments
6. Other intraarticular fractures of the tarsocrural joints
7. Retrieval of fragments from the talocentral (proximal intertarsal joint)
8. Tears/avulsions of the collateral ligaments
9. Tears/avulsion of the joint capsule
10. Treatment of some forms of proliferative synovitis
11. Traumatic lesions and osteoarthritis, including diagnostic arthroscopy in cases of lameness and hemarthrosis
12. Contaminated and infected joints
13. Debridement of septic lesions of the trochlear ridges of the talus

Osteochondritis Dissecans of the Tarsocrural Joint

In the authors' experience, OCD of the dorsal aspect of the distal intermediate (sagittal) ridge of the tibia is the most common indication for arthroscopic surgery in the equine tarsocrural (tibiotarsal) joint. A review of a series of cases of OCD of 318 tarsocrural joints treated by arthroscopic surgery (McIlwraith et al, 1991) provides an indication of the location of these lesions (Box 7-1).

Lesions were seen most frequently on the intermediate ridge of the distal tibia, followed by the lateral trochlear ridge of the talus and the medial malleolus, respectively. Lesions were also seen at multiple sites in 22 joints. Loose bodies were present in 8 joints; 5 of them had separated from intermediate ridge lesions and 3 fragments had separated from lateral trochlear ridge lesions. The breed distribution in the 203 affected horses is given in Box 7-2.

Box • 7-1

Osteochondritis Dissecans of the Tarsocrural Joint

Location	Number of Joints
Intermediate ridge of the distal tibia	244
Lateral trochlear ridge of the talus	37
Medial malleolus of the tibia	12
Intermediate ridge of the tibia plus the lateral trochlear ridge (both)	11
Intermediate ridge plus medial malleolus of the tibia (both)	4
Intermediate ridge plus medial trochlear ridge of talus	3
Lateral trochlear ridge of the talus and the medial malleolus of the tibia (both)	3
Medial trochlear ridge of the talus	3
Lateral and medial trochlear ridges of the talus (both)	1
Total	318

From McIlwraith CW, Foerner JJ, Davis DM. Osteochondritis dissecans of the tarsocrural joint: results of treatment with arthroscopic surgery. *Equine Vet J* 1991;23:155–162.

Horses with OCD of the intermediate ridge of the tibia usually have joint effusion or lameness, or both. Commonly, the clinical situation is joint effusion in the young horse of yearling age; lameness is often not evident. Careful examination, however, often reveals subtle gait abnormality, such as decreased flexion in the tarsus owing to increased synovial fluid pressure.

In the 1991 retrospective study of 303 joints in which synovial effusion was recorded, it was the presenting clinical sign in 261 (86.1%). In racehorses, effusion was present in 166 joints (81%) and absent in 39 joints. In nonracehorses, effusion was

Box • 7-2

Osteochondritis Dissecans of the Tarsocrural Joint by Type of Horse

Racehorses	Number of Joints
Standardbred	106
Thoroughbred	30
Quarter Horse	18
Total	154
Nonracehorses	
Arabian	20
Quarter Horse	18
Warmblood	13
Appaloosa	4
American Saddlebred	4
Thoroughbred	4
Draught breeds	3
American Paint	2
Morgan	1
National Show Horse	1
Lipizzaner	1
Total	71

From McIlwraith CW, Foerner JJ, Davis DM. Osteochondritis dissecans of the tarsocrural joint: results of treatment with arthroscopic surgery. *Equine Vet J* 1991;23:155–162.

Box • 7-3

Horses Presenting with Synovial Effusion

Type	Age (Yr)	Number	Percentage
Racehorse	1	34	22.1
	2	68	44.2
	3	36	23.4
	4	8	5.2
	5	4	2.6
	6	1	0.6
	7	2	1.3
	9	1	0.6
Nonracehorse	1	33	46.5
	2	18	25.3
	3	6	8.5
	4	6	8.5
	5	1	1.4
	7	1	1.4
	8	1	1.4
	9	1	1.4
	10	1	1.4
	13	2	2.8
	14	1	1.4

From McIlwraith CW, Foerner JJ, Davis DM. Osteochondritis dissecans of the tarsocrural joint: results of treatment with arthroscopic surgery. *Equine Vet J* 1991;23:155–162.

present in 95 joints (96.9%) and absent in 3 joints. The degree of lameness was not recorded consistently but usually was designated as mild. The exception was when a severe lesion was present on the lateral trochlear ridge of the talus (lesions involving the entire visible portion when viewed arthroscopically in the flexed position). Racehorses presented most often at 2 years old, having trained or raced, whereas nonracehorses presented most often as yearlings before training (Box 7-3) (McIlwraith et al, 1991).

Whether or not to treat these cases surgically has been a historic debate (McIlwraith, 1983). However, with arthroscopic surgery, the authors recommend surgery in all instances if an athletic career is planned. The authors also believe that arthroscopic surgery is appropriate in young horses that may show only tarsocrural effusion. The prognosis after arthroscopic surgery in terms of athletic soundness is excellent. It is also reasonably good for the resolution of synovial effusion, and with competent surgeons and anesthetists the risks are small.

It is worth noting that in a longitudinal radiographic study in Dutch Warmblood foals that were radiographed at age 1 month and subsequently at intervals of 4 weeks, resolution of radiographic lesions commonly occurred (Dik et al, 1999). At 1 month old, the appearance of the intermediate ridge of distal tibia was frequently abnormal. Abnormal appearances of the distal aspect of the lateral trochlear ridge of the talus were less common. Initial abnormalities of the intermediate tibial ridge showed a marked tendency for regression. Progression was less common. Normal appearances rarely turned into abnormal. Abnormalities of the distal aspect of the lateral trochlear ridge of the talus showed a strong tendency toward resolution. Progression of lesions never occurred, and normal appearances seldom turned into abnormal. For both predilection sites in the hock, normal and abnormal appearances were permanent beyond age 5 months (Dik et al, 1999). On the basis of this information, in warmbloods, at least, it would seem that making a surgical decision in the hock before 5 months would be premature.

For arthroscopic surgery, the patients are placed in dorsal recumbency. This position not only facilitates the triangulation process but also minimizes the chances of losing a fragment. Fragments can break off during manipulation of the primary lesion; if the animal is in lateral recumbency, these fragments can easily settle into a position of the joint that cannot be easily visualized with the arthroscope or reached with the instrument. In dorsal recumbency, the leg can be suspended or tied, in which case it is raised or lowered or the cord is shortened or lengthened to achieve different degrees of flexion, or it can be free. Tying the limb has an advantage in that the surgeon is assured that the limb remains in a fixed position. Having an assistant hold the limb results in position changes, which can change the position of the instrument portal and make the operation more difficult.

Arthroscopic Surgery for Osteochondritis Dissecans of the Distal Intermediate Ridge of the Tibia

The presence of OCD is confirmed radiographically (see Figs. 7-7A to 7-9A). The radiographic manifestations range from subtle irregularity of the intermediate ridge up to large defects containing fragments (Hoppe, 1984). Some cases of OCD on the intermediate ridge and in other locations do not manifest radiographically or the lesions are subtle (see Fig. 7-10).

The arthroscopic portal is always through the dorsomedial pouch (McIlwraith et al, 1991). The use of this medial approach is important because the medial trochlear ridge of the talus projects further dorsad than the lateral trochlear ridge and any instrument passage over the medial trochlear ridge would not be able to reach the intermediate ridge of the tibia. After insertion of the arthroscope, a complete examination of the joint is made. The triangulation technique for arthroscopic surgery for a distal intermediate ridge (DIR) OCD is illustrated in Figure 7-5.

To create the instrument portal, the surgeon turns off the ingress fluids and passes a percutaneous needle through the distal dorsal aspect of the distended dorsolateral joint pouch lateral to the extensor tendons to confirm correct positioning of the instrument portal (Fig. 7-6A). A skin incision is then

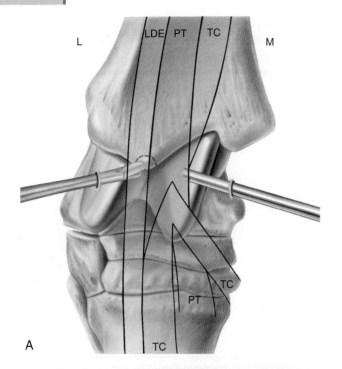

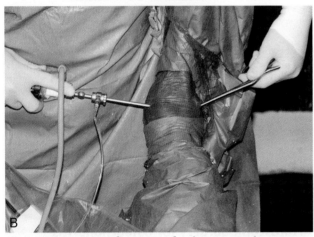

Figure 7-5 Diagram of position of arthroscope and instrument during operations involving an osteochondritis dissecans lesion of the dorsal aspect of the intermediate ridge of the tibia **(A)** and external view **(B)**. *L*, Lateral trochlear ridge of talus; *LDE*, long digital extensor tendon; *M*, medial trochlear ridge of talus; *PT*, peroneus tertius; *TC*, tibialis cranialis.

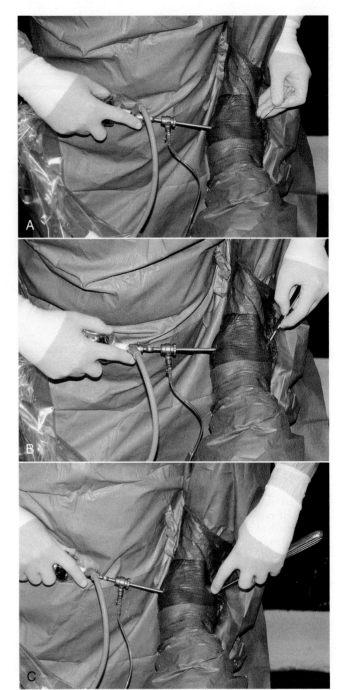

Figure 7-6 A, Spinal needle through the distended dorsolateral joint pouch confirms correct positioning of the instrument portal. **B,** A skin incision is made at the proposed site of the instrument portal and the portal is completed with a stab through the joint capsule. **C,** Instrument is inserted.

made and the instrument portal is completed with a stab through the joint capsule (see Fig. 7-6B). If the ingress of fluids is not stopped while establishing this instrument portal, rapid subcutaneous extravasation of fluid may occur around the area of the instrument portal. Similarly, the skin incisions should be sufficiently generous to maintain a clean entry for instruments and exit for fluids.

A probe or egress cannula is inserted to provide initial evaluation of the lesion (see Fig. 7-6C). Minimal correlation exists between the radiographic appearance of an OCD lesion and the degree of attachment of the fragment as found arthroscopically. Some of the fragments are attached by a single strand of fibrous tissue and fall away when touched by the probe or egress cannula. Other lesions that have an identical radiographic appearance are firmly attached by fibrous tissue. Figure 7-7 illustrates a typical sequence in the removal of a small OCD lesion off the distal intermediate ridge, and

medium and larger DIT fragments are illustrated in Figures 7-8 and 7-9, respectively. The fragment is elevated until it is almost completely loose (see Figs. 7-7C to 7-9C). Elevation is usually achieved by inserting a periosteal elevator. If the fragment is firm and difficult to separate, an osteotome or light tapping of the elevator may be used. Repeated attempts at trying to elevate a firmly attached fragment by using the periosteal elevator can cause small fragments to break off and become loose bodies. The use of a blunt osteotome or Milk's tooth elevator rather than a sharp osteotome can minimize the risk of creating new fragments or fracture lines. Once the

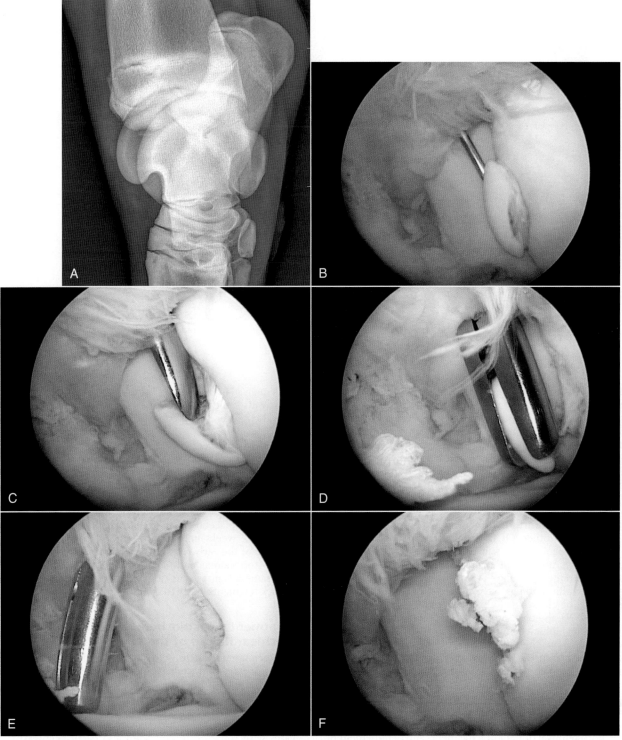

Figure 7-7 Dorsomedial to plantarolateral oblique radiograph **(A)** and arthroscopic views of small osteochondritis dissecans (OCD) of distal intermediate ridge of tibia. **B,** Arthroscopic view of OCD fragment with spinal needle placed to evaluate ideal arthroscopic portal. **C,** Elevation of OCD fragment. **D,** Removal of fragment with Ferris-Smith rongeurs. **E,** Defect prior to debridement of osteochondrotic tissue. **F,** Elevation of defective osteochondrotic tissue from defect.

Continued

fragment is elevated, an appropriately sized pair of grasping forceps is introduced and the fragment is grasped (see Figs. 7-7 to 7-9). The grasping forceps are then rotated to break down any remaining soft tissue attachments and withdrawn. As discussed in Chapter 4, the forceps should enclose the fragment. In many instances in the tarsocrural joint, however, due to the large size of fragments this is not always possible. As the

fragment is pulled through the joint capsule, fluid flow is again stopped to minimize the development of subcutaneous fluid extravasation. Larger fragments may necessitate enlargement of the skin incision; otherwise, the surgeon runs the risk of losing the fragment subcutaneously.

The defect from which the fragment was removed is then evaluated (see Figs. 7-7 to 7-9) and any additional fragments

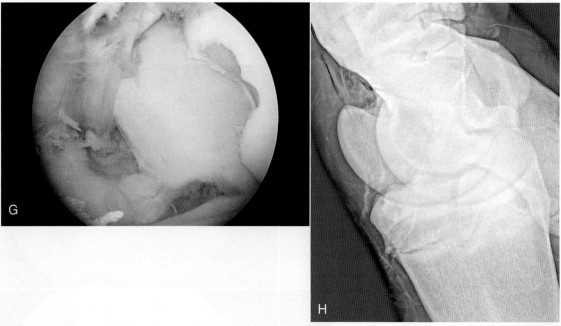

Figure 7-7, cont'd G, Defect after completion of debridement. **H,** Postoperative radiograph demonstrating removal of fragment.

are removed. Light curettage elevates any tags of tissue within the defect or at the edge of the defect, which are removed with forceps or rongeurs. The surgeon must pay particular attention to the most plantar portion of the defect, where fragments may remain but cannot be visualized. Reduced flexion, rotation of the arthroscope, and careful probing of the defect along the edge facing the trochlear groove can reveal additional fragments that need to be loosened and removed. The joint is then lavaged copiously. Postoperative radiographs are obtained to check for any remaining or dislodged fragments that were not detected during the arthroscopic examination.

As with all other OCD lesions, the radiographic and arthroscopic manifestations in OCD of the distal intermediate ridge vary. Any number of fragments or fragments of any size can be removed. Figure 7-10 illustrates a case in which the radiographic findings were negative, but an OCD fragment could be elevated. Note also that in the case illustrated in Figure 7-10, the opposite tarsocrural joint had an effusion but no radiographic changes were evident. An osteochondral fragment of about the same size as that illustrated was found and removed from the intermediate ridge in the other joint. Fragments may also dislodge from the primary lesion and be located elsewhere in the joint (Fig. 7-11). Loose fragments can move into the plantar pouch of the tarsocrural joint or descend through the communicating foramen into the talocentral joint and can be retrieved from these positions. In such cases, both removal of the loose fragments and debridement of the primary lesion are necessary.

The stab incisions are closed with one or two sutures, and a bandage—consisting of a sterile pad, adhesive gauze (Kling®), and Elasticon®—is used over the hock immediately after the operation. Maintenance of hock bandages until the sutures are removed is particularly important because these incisions are prone to dehiscence and subsequent sepsis.

The patients can be discharged from the clinic on the first postoperative day. Therefore the protocol depends on the severity of the case. Animals should be hand walked for 4 weeks and then allowed small paddock or controlled light exercise for an additional 4 weeks. Some clinicians consider the use of hyaluronan (HA) or polysulfated glycosaminoglycan

(Adequan®) useful 30 days postoperatively. A study published shortly after the third edition of this text reported on the use of oral HA after arthroscopic surgery for tarsocrural OCD and provided interesting evidence of benefit (Bergin et al, 2006). Oral HA (Conquer®) was given after arthroscopic surgery for tarsocrural OCD in 24 yearlings at a dose of 100 mg orally for 30 days and results compared with 24 other yearlings treated with an oral placebo for 30 days. A blinded examiner scored the effusion at 30 days from grade 0 to 5. The mean 30-day effusion score in the treated group was 0.67 compared with 2.05 in the placebo group ($P < 0.0001$). Training can resume in 8 to 12 weeks unless some other clinical problem arises. Because of the early return to exercise, trainers are more willing to stop training and remedy the problem while it is fresh. The same advantages as discussed with regard to carpal and fetlock fragments apply to operations involving the tarsocrural joint.

Treatment of Osteochondritis Dissecans of the Trochlear Ridges of the Talus

The technique for arthroscopic surgery of lesions on the lateral trochlear ridge of the talus is illustrated in Figure 7-12. Typical cases of OCD of the lateral trochlear ridge are illustrated in Figures 7-13 to 7-15. Lesions may range from small fragments (see Fig. 7-13) to large cartilaginous flaps (see Fig. 7-14) or multiple osteochondral fragmentation (see Fig. 7-15). Chronic cases with rounded, loose bodies also occur (Fig. 7-16). The presenting clinical signs associated with OCD of the lateral trochlear ridge of the talus may be the same as with lesions on the intermediate ridge of the tibia or they may be more severe. The severity of the clinical signs is usually related to the amount of lateral trochlear ridge that is affected.

For cases of OCD or fragmentation of the trochlear ridges, a triangulation approach using a medial arthroscope and lateral instrument portals is used (see Fig. 7-12). As discussed in the section concerning diagnostic arthroscopy, when a dorsomedial arthroscopic approach is made, the medial trochlear ridge on the near side is visualized easily, but the lateral trochlear ridge may be difficult to visualize because of the closer apposition of the extensor tendon bundle and associated joint

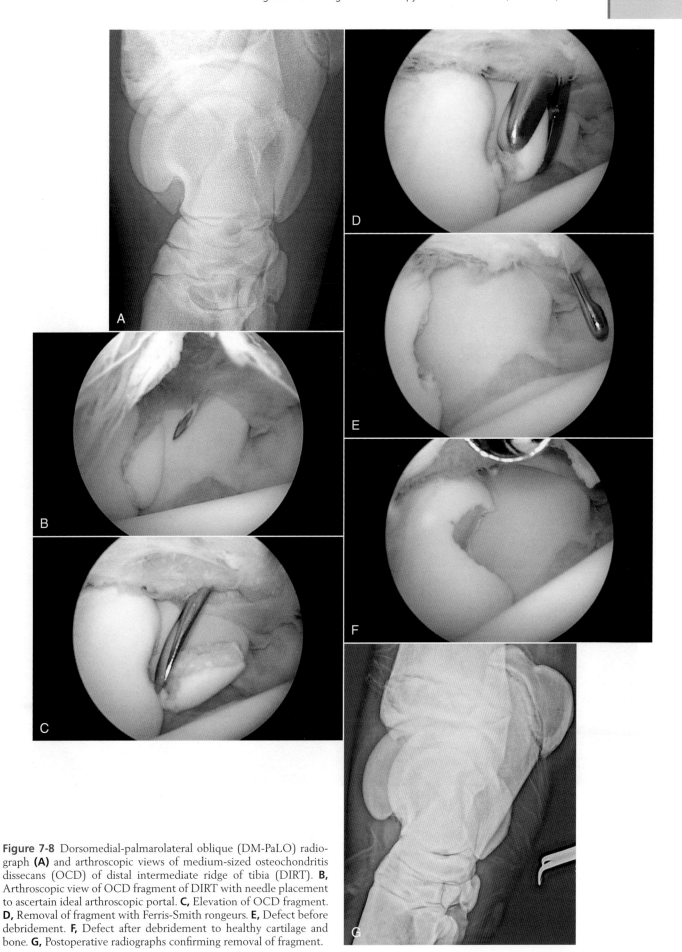

Figure 7-8 Dorsomedial-palmarolateral oblique (DM-PaLO) radiograph **(A)** and arthroscopic views of medium-sized osteochondritis dissecans (OCD) of distal intermediate ridge of tibia (DIRT). **B,** Arthroscopic view of OCD fragment of DIRT with needle placement to ascertain ideal arthroscopic portal. **C,** Elevation of OCD fragment. **D,** Removal of fragment with Ferris-Smith rongeurs. **E,** Defect before debridement. **F,** Defect after debridement to healthy cartilage and bone. **G,** Postoperative radiographs confirming removal of fragment.

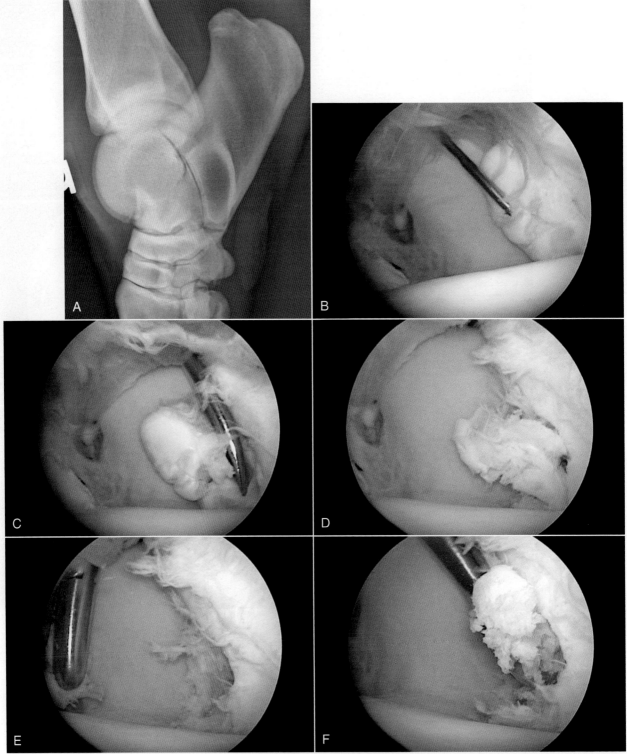

Figure 7-9 Dorsomedial to plantarolateral oblique radiographic view **(A)** of larger fragment off distal intermediate ridge of tibia (DIRT) and arthroscopic views **(B)** of the osteochondritis dissecans (OCD) lesion with multiple fragments. **C,** Elevation of largest fragment. **D,** Second fragment remaining after removal of larger fragment. **E,** After removal of fragment showing residual osteochondrotic tissue in defect. **F,** Debridement of defective osteochondrotic tissue with a curette.

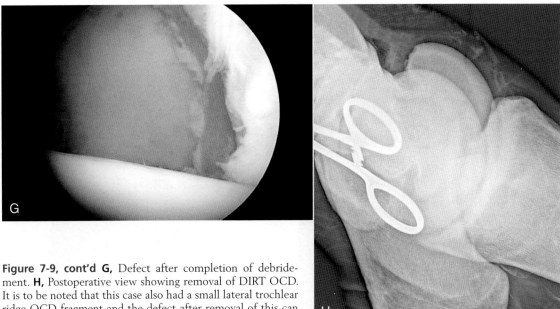

Figure 7-9, cont'd G, Defect after completion of debridement. H, Postoperative view showing removal of DIRT OCD. It is to be noted that this case also had a small lateral trochlear ridge OCD fragment and the defect after removal of this can also be seen.

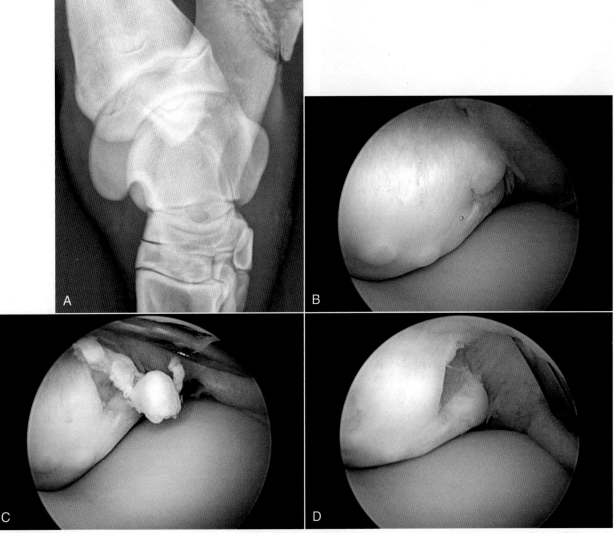

Figure 7-10 An osteochondritis dissecans (OCD) lesion present on the distal intermediate ridge of the tibia (DIRT) found at diagnostic arthroscopy. A, Radiograph showing absence of visible lesion. B, Arthroscopic view showing nondisplaced fragment. C, After elevation of fragment. D, Defect after removal of fragment.

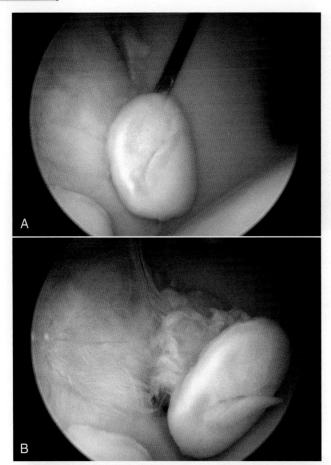

Figure 7-11 Arthroscopic views **(A** and **B)** of loose fragment (with old defect in distal intermediate ridge present).

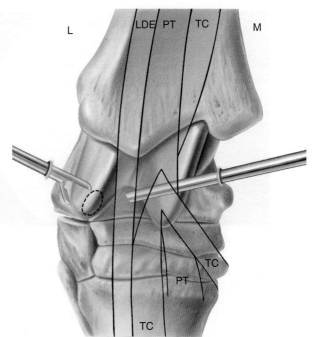

Figure 7-12 Diagram of position of arthroscope and instrument during operations involving an osteochondritis dissecans lesion of the lateral trochlear ridge of the talus using arthroscopic and instrument approaches from opposite sides of the joint. *LDE*, Long digital extensor tendon; *PT*, peroneus tertius; *TC*, tibialis cranialis.

capsule on this side. In all instances, use of a needle to ascertain the optimal site for the instrument portal is recommended. It should be recognized that the technique for lateral trochlear ridge debridement is more difficult than that used for intermediate ridge lesions. In the report on arthroscopic surgery for the treatment of OCD in 318 tarsocrural joints (McIlwraith et al, 1991), one of the two surgeons was still doing arthrotomy for lateral trochlear ridge lesions. Therefore, in that published report, the relative percentage of lateral trochlear lesions is smaller than a large population would provide because only the first author's (C.W.M.) lateral trochlear ridge cases were included. Although arthroscopic surgery for lateral trochlear ridge lesions is more challenging than for distal intermediate ridge problems, all lateral trochlear ridge lesions can be effectively managed using arthroscopic techniques.

The principles of fragment removal are the same as described for OCD of the intermediate ridge. Debridement to healthy subchondral bone is important in the more involved trochlear ridge lesions. Any osteochondral flap or fragment on the trochlear ridge is elevated and removed and the lesion is debrided (see Figs. 7-14 and 7-15). Loose bodies are removed, and degenerative changes of articular cartilage on the talus may be seen in such cases (see Fig. 7-16). Fragments embedded in the synovial membrane are removed if they are visible.

OCD lesions on the medial trochlear ridge of the talus are rare but do occur occasionally. They are typically on the trochlear ridge immediately distal to the tibia when the leg is straight (Fig. 7-17). There were three cases in the initial series published by McIlwraith et al (1991). All cases presented as typical undermining of the cartilage in this location (see Fig. 7-17). The arthroscopic approach is illustrated in Figure 7-18.

Bone spurs and fragments (so-called dewdrop lesions) have been identified distal to the medial trochlear ridge of the talus. These spurs and fragments are typically embedded in joint capsule or are extraarticular and are generally considered normal radiographic variations that are of no clinical significance (Shelley & Dyson, 1984) (Fig. 7-19). Surgical intervention is only occasionally indicated (see Fig. 7-19). Most articular lesions (depressions) on the medial trochlear ridge of the talus are incidental findings at arthroscopy.

Osteochondritis Dissecans of the Medial Malleolus of the Tibia

Fragmentation of the medial malleolus is the third most common location, and the clinical, radiographic, surgical, and histologic findings are consistent with OCD. The axial intraarticular portion of the medial malleolus is affected. Such lesions must be distinguished from fractures of the medial malleolus that typically involve the entire malleolus, extending proximally well beyond the joint capsule boundaries. The clinical manifestations of OCD in the medial malleolus are similar to those of the disease affecting other locations in the tarsocrural joint. Effusion or lameness, or both, are apparent, and in the authors' experience, the more common situation is the development of effusion or lameness, or both, when animals are being trained or beginning with race training or racing. Dorsoplantar or dorsolateral-plantaromedial (DLPMO) radiographs usually confirm the presence of a lesion (Fig. 7-20), but sometimes a radiographically silent lesion is detected only during arthroscopy.

A dorsomedial arthroscopic portal is used (Fig. 7-21). The hock is extended. A needle is then used to decide on the optimal position for the instrument portal, but because of the positioning of the fragment it needs to also be in the dorsomedial pouch. The instrument portal is axial and usually slightly distal to the level of the arthroscopic portal (see Fig. 7-21). The fragment is then elevated away using an elevator or osteotome, depending on the degree of attachment remaining before fragmentation is removed and the defect debrided (Figs. 7-22 and 7-23).

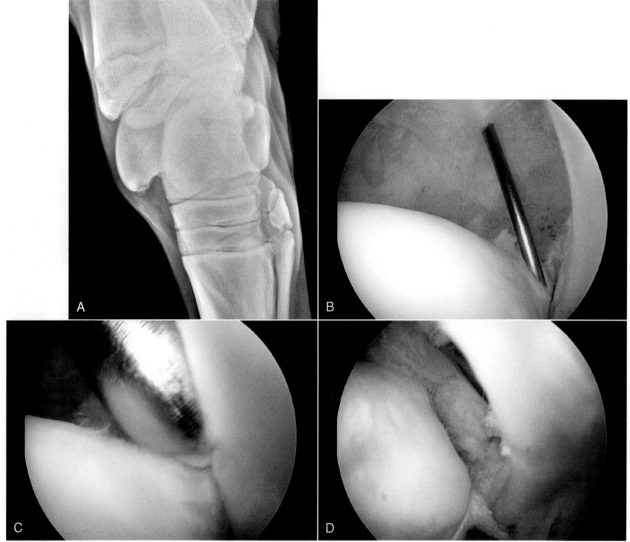

Figure 7-13 Small osteochondritis dissecans (OCD) lesion of the lateral trochlear ridge (LTR) of the talus. **A,** Radiograph showing small fragment. Arthroscopic views before **(B)** with fragments in forceps **(C)** and after debridement **(D).**

Lesions can extend plantarly along the axial margin of the medial malleolus. This may not be immediately apparent, following removal of dorsal fragments, and requires rotation of the arthroscope and sometimes movement of the limb to identify and remove.

Results of Arthroscopic Surgery for Treatment of Osteochondritis Dissecans of the Tarsocrural Joint

The results of arthroscopic surgery for the treatment of OCD in 318 tarsocrural joints in 225 horses have been reported (McIlwraith et al, 1991). The overall functional ability and cosmetic appearance of the limbs were excellent. Postsurgical follow-up information was obtained for 183 horses, of which 140 (76.5%) horses raced successfully or performed their intended use following surgery. Of the remaining 43 horses, only 11 horses were still considered to have a tarsocrural joint problem. Nineteen horses developed other problems precluding successful performance, 8 horses were considered poor racehorses without any lameness problems, 3 horses were euthanized because of septic arthritis (all associated with the horse getting the bandage off within 24 hours of surgery), and 2 horses died from other causes. There was no significant effect of age, sex, or limb involvement on the outcome. The success

rate relative to three size groups for intermediate ridge lesions was 27/33 (81.8%) for lesions 1 to 9 mm in width, 86/116 (74.1%) for lesions 10 to 19 mm in width, and 41/47 (87.2%) for lesions 20 mm or more in width (no significant difference).

When success rate was considered relative to the findings of additional lesions at arthroscopy, 16/19 (84.1%) with articular cartilage fibrillation, 5/10 (50%) with articular cartilage erosion or wear lines (Fig. 7-24), 3/5 (60%) with loose fragments, 0/2 with proliferative synovitis, and 0/1 with joint capsule mineralization were successful. There was a significantly poorer outcome in racehorses with articular cartilage degeneration or erosion ($P < 0.05$). Figure 7-25 indicates the natural healing that can occur in chronic cases.

The synovial effusion resolved in 117/131 racehorse joints (89.3%) and in 64/86 nonracehorse joints (74.4%). The outcome for synovial fluid effusion was significantly inferior for lesions of the lateral trochlear ridge of the talus and medial malleolus of the tibia compared with distal intermediate ridge lesions. There was no significant relationship between resolution of effusion and successful performance outcome.

In 1994, Beard et al compared the results of 64 Thoroughbreds and 45 Standardbred horses treated for OCD of the tarsocrural joint with arthroscopic surgery before 2 years of age to those of other foals from the dams of the surgically treated

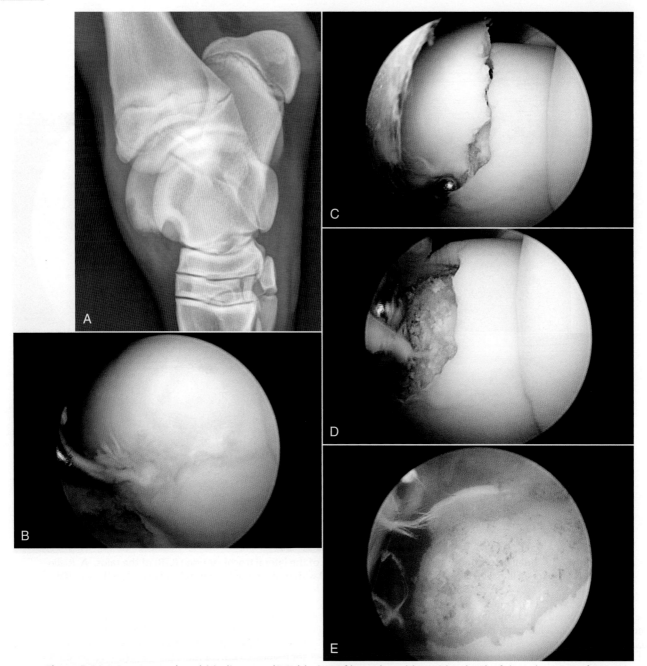

Figure 7-14 Larger osteochondritis dissecans (OCD) lesion of lateral trochlear ridge (LTR) of the talus. **A,** Radiograph showing fragmentation at distal aspect and defect extending 3 cm up LTR. **B,** Arthroscopic view of OCD flap delineated by cleft that probe is in. **C,** Use of probe to separate OCD flap and define limits. **D,** After removal of flap evaluating defective tissue underneath. **E,** After debridement of osteochondrotic tissue down to healthy, bleeding bone and smooth edges of cartilage, which is still attached to the bone.

horses. For the Standardbreds, 22% of those who had surgery raced as 2-year-olds and 43% raced as 3-year-olds, compared with 42% and 50% of the siblings that raced as 2-year-olds and 3-year-olds, respectively. For the Thoroughbreds, 43% of those that had surgery raced as 2-year-olds and 78% raced as 3-year-olds compared with 48% and 72% of the siblings that raced as 2-year-olds and 3-year-olds, respectively. The median number of starts for surgically treated horses was lower than the median number of starts for siblings for all groups except 3-year-old Thoroughbreds. Median earnings were lower for affected horses than for siblings for both breeds and both age groups. There was a tendency for horses with multiple lesions

to be less likely to start a race than horses with only a single lesion; however, the difference was significant only for 2-year-old Standardbreds. Affected Standardbreds and Thoroughbreds were less likely to race as 2-year-olds than were their siblings. It is noted that this study was quite different from the first follow-up study (McIlwraith et al, 1991); the selection criteria and control groups were different and racing performance was not analyzed by year in the earlier report. In another study, horses treated for OCD of the distal intermediate ridge of the tibia performed as well as matched controls (Laws et al, 1993).

In a recent study the presence and degree of tarsocrural joint effusion and lameness and the results of a hindlimb

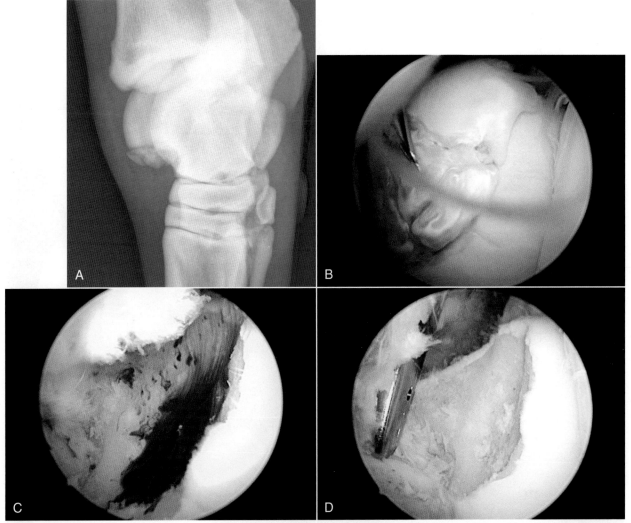

Figure 7-15 Large fragmented osteochondritis dissecans (OCD) lesion of lateral trochlear ridge (LTR) of the talus. Radiographic **(A)** and arthroscopic views: **B,** initial appearance of the lesion with probe distal to largest fragment and proximal to more distal multiple fragments, **C,** after removal of fragments with flap remaining proximally and hemorrhage from defect on talus, and **D,** appearance of defect after debridement of pathologic tissue.

flexion test were scored subjectively in 79 horses before, and 6 weeks to 20 months after, arthroscopic surgery to remove OCD fragments (Brink et al, 2009). The group consisted of 30 Standardbreds, 46 Warmblood riding horses, and 1 each of Andalusian, Friesian, and American Paint horses. The age distribution was 25 yearlings, 35 two- and 3-year-olds, and 19 between 4 and 9 years of age. The scores of all three variables improved significantly after surgery. The score reductions for the right and left hindlimbs, respectively, were 82% and 95% for lameness, 48% and 41% for joint effusion, and 89% and 84% for reaction to flexion ($P < 0.01$). The oldest horses reacted more favorably to the arthroscopic surgery as measured by the reaction to the flexion tests, but age was not significantly related to changes in lameness or joint effusion. There was no significant correlation between the time of follow-up examination and the effect of surgery on lameness and reaction to flexion, but an increased time to follow-up was associated with decreased joint effusion.

Subchondral Cystic Lesions of the Tarsocrural Joint

Subchondral cystic lesions (SCLs) are uncommon compared with the femorotibial joint but have been identified in

multiple locations, including the medial and lateral malleoli and distal intermediate ridge of the tibia, as well as lateral and medial trochlear ridges and the intertrochlear groove of the talus (Garcia-Lopez and Kirker-Head, 2004; , Janicek et al, 2010; Montgomery and Juzwiak, 2009) (Fig. 7-26). In a series of four cases of the lateral trochlear ridge of the talus, all cases could be identified with digital radiographs alone with the flexed lateromedial view giving the best demonstration of the lesion (Montgomery and Juzwiak, 2009). Other authors have reported lack of radiographic demonstration in a series of cases but increased radiopharmaceutical uptake on scintigraphy in the distal tibia or talus of all horses with further characterization by computed tomography (Garcia-Lopez and Kirker-Head, 2004). The case illustrated in Figure 7-26 showed an increased uptake of technetium on a bone scan and diagnostic arthroscopy detected a hole and cystic lesion in the trochlear groove (using a plantar approach). A medial plantar arthroscope approach and a lateral plantar instrument entry allowed debridement of that trochlear groove cystic lesion. Some lesions can be quite deep, despite minor radiographic abnormalities (see Fig. 7-26). Flexion of the joint after insertion of the arthroscope was used to expose the cyst entry. Needle insertion then guided the instrument portal. Arthroscope

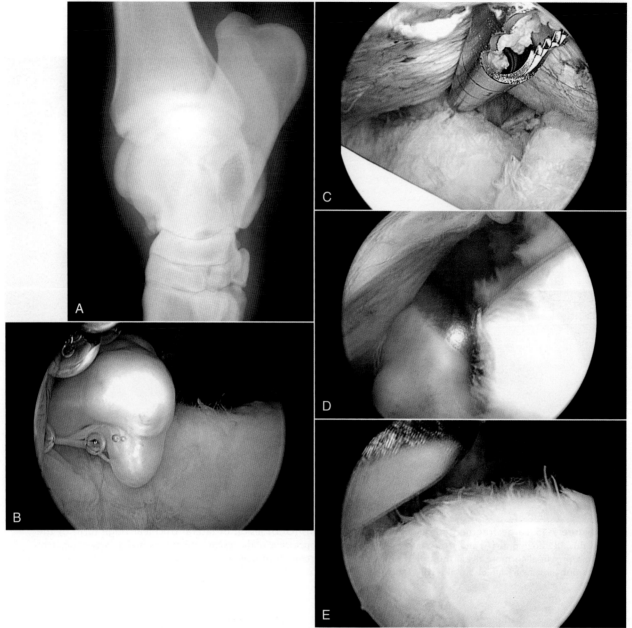

Figure 7-16 Radiograph **(A)** and arthroscopic view **(B)** of loose body that was presumed to have developed after separation from a chronic OCD of the lateral trochlear ridge (LTR) of talus. **C,** Arthroscopic view of LTR after removal of fibrous tissue over defect. **D,** Removal of loose body with Ferris-Smith rongeurs. **E,** Distal aspect of medial trochlear ridge after removal of loose body and articular cartilage fibrillation and focal zone of erosion on medial trochlear ridge of talus.

and instrument portals will vary with other locations. As with treatment options for SCLs of the femorotibial joint, treatment options have increased with SCLs in the tarsocrural joint. A series of four cases on the lateral trochlear ridge of the talus were treated successfully with intralesional injection of triamcinolone acetonide, simulating the protocol of Wallis et al (2008) on the medial femoral condyle (Montgomery and Juzwiak, 2009). All lesions were on the proximal lateral trochlear ridge and so were approached through the plantar pouch. This treatment protocol was successful in all four cases, but it was noted that there was an OCD elsewhere within the joint in all four cases and these were treated as well. A case of a severe SCL on the proximal medial trochlear ridge of the talus was treated with osteochondral mosaicplasty in one report (Janicek et al, 2010).

▶ Fractures of the Lateral Malleolus

These fragments are encountered less commonly than OCD fragments and appear to be traumatic in origin. The important point to note with fragments of the lateral malleolus is that a relatively small portion of the lateral malleolus is actually intraarticular; most of it is enclosed within the collateral ligaments. A case example of a fracture associated with direct trauma is provided in Figure 7-27. Figure 7-28 illustrates a fracture of the lateral malleolus that was a consequence to a rough recovery from anesthesia.

Horses are operated in dorsal recumbency with the affected limb suspended and protracted caudally with a tarsal angle of approximately 130 degrees. The ability to vary limb position can be useful. An Esmarch and tourniquet applied to the proximal crus aids visibility and reduces surgery time

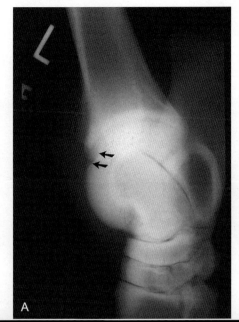

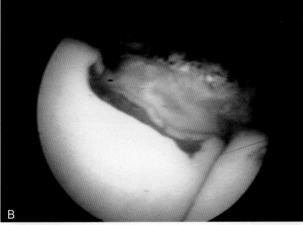

Figure 7-17 Radiograph **(A)** and arthroscopic view **(B)** of osteochondritis dissecans of medial trochlear ridge of talus (after debridement).

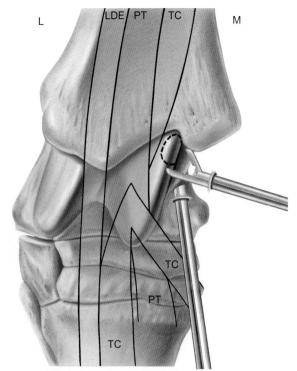

Figure 7-18 Diagram of position of arthroscope and instrument during operations involving an osteochondritis dissecans lesion of the medial trochlear ridge using arthroscopic and instrument approaches from the same side of the joint. *LDE*, Long digital extensor tendon; *PT*, peroneus tertius; *TC*, tibialis cranialis.

(Smith & Wright, 2011). Surgery is most readily performed with the surgeon standing at the medial aspect of the limb. Both dorsolateral arthroscope and instrument portals are used with arthroscope portal axial to the instrument portal. Both have almost vertical orientation (i.e., perpendicular to the long axis of the tibia).

Fractures vary in size, degree of comminution, and amount of displacement. The principal fracture fragment most frequently rotates, hinged on the short collateral ligament. Small fragments can be scattered throughout dorsal and plantar compartments and in the former commonly will descend through the dorsal communication to lie adjacent to the central tarsal bone. As a general rule, displaced fragments in the dorsal compartment are removed first.

Fractures disrupt varying amounts of the origins of the short lateral collateral ligaments. Fragment removal always requires dissection from the short collateral ligament. Both straight and curved fixed blade knives and scissors are used. Frequent clearing of the dissection plane with a motorized synovial resector aids this process. Sometimes it is necessary to push large fragments that run the full dorsoplantar width of the lateral malleolus into the plantar pouch in order to visualize and divide the entire ligament attachments. Dissection at

this point usually requires creation of a plantarolateral instrument portal. Large fragments frequently expose the long lateral collateral ligament and, on occasions, the tendon of insertion of the lateral digital extensor and its synovial sheath. Large fragments usually require 6- × 10-mm arthroscopic rongeurs for removal. Debridement of osseous and soft tissue defects follow in line with general surgical principles.

Since the last edition there have been two reports of results of arthroscopic treatment of the lateral malleolus of the tibia (O'Neill & Bladon, 2010; Smith & Wright, 2011). The first case series retrospectively reviewed 13 horses over a 10-year period that underwent arthroscopic removal of fractures of the lateral malleolus. Of the 13 horses presented, 12 were Thoroughbreds, 9 of which were United Kingdom National Hunt racehorses and 3 were flat racehorses. The other horse in the study was used for general purpose riding. All cases presented with an acute unilateral fracture. Eleven/13 had greater than 6 months' postoperative follow-up and all were sound. Of the 12 Thoroughbreds, 10 raced again, a total of 104 times (median 5 times) and the median time from surgery to return to racing was 241 days (180 to 366 days). It was concluded that horses with fractures of the lateral malleolus have an excellent prognosis for return to full athletic activity following arthroscopic debridement and that arthroscopic fragment removal is an appropriate treatment for fractures of the lateral malleolus (O'Neill & Bladon, 2010). In a second retrospective study there were 25 Thoroughbreds and 1 sport horse (Smith & Wright, 2011). The horses were used for a variety of purposes: racing (*n* = 17), intended for racing (*n* = 4), intended for eventing (*n* = 1), intended for dressage (*n* = 1), general purpose (*n* = 2), and breeding (*n* = 1). Fractures were successfully removed arthroscopically in all cases following dissection from the short lateral collateral ligament. Significant

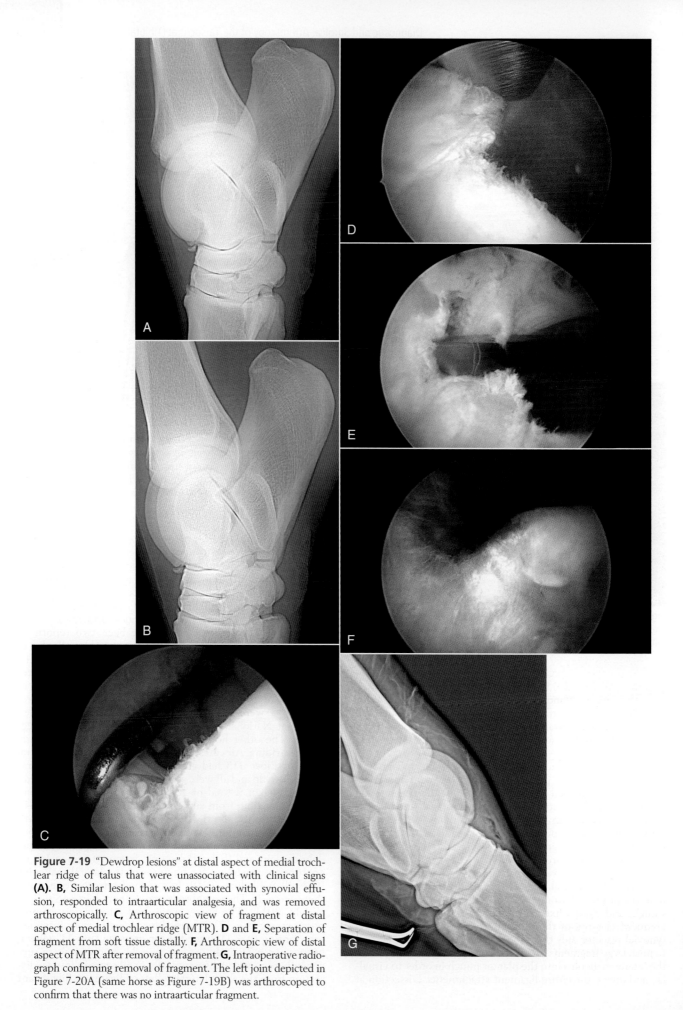

Figure 7-19 "Dewdrop lesions" at distal aspect of medial trochlear ridge of talus that were unassociated with clinical signs **(A)**. **B,** Similar lesion that was associated with synovial effusion, responded to intraarticular analgesia, and was removed arthroscopically. **C,** Arthroscopic view of fragment at distal aspect of medial trochlear ridge (MTR). **D** and **E,** Separation of fragment from soft tissue distally. **F,** Arthroscopic view of distal aspect of MTR after removal of fragment. **G,** Intraoperative radiograph confirming removal of fragment. The left joint depicted in Figure 7-20A (same horse as Figure 7-19B) was arthroscoped to confirm that there was no intraarticular fragment.

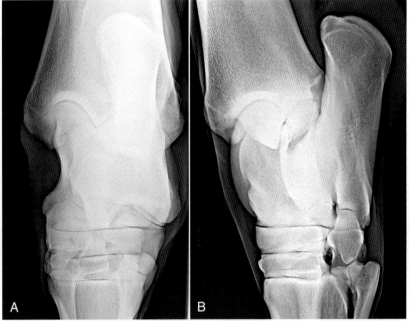

Figure 7-20 Dorsoplantar **(A)** and dorsolateral-plantaromedial oblique (DLPLMO) **(B)** radiographs of osteochondritis dissecans of medial malleolus. In **A** there is a clearly defined fragment. In **B** bony lucency is the manifestation.

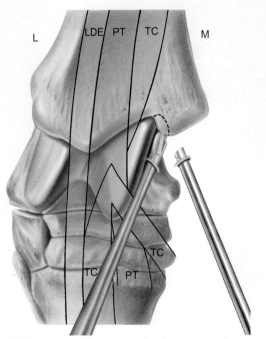

Figure 7-21 Diagram of position of arthroscope and instrument during operations involving a lesion of the medial malleolus. *LDE,* Long digital extensor tendon; *PT,* peroneus tertius; *TC,* tibialis cranialis.

postoperative complications occurred in only 1 horse. All other horses recovered well from surgery and of 22 horses with long-term follow-up, 18 returned to their previous use. The authors concluded that arthroscopic removal of fractures of the lateral malleolus of the tibia is technically demanding but can be performed with minimal complications, with low patient morbidity and short periods of hospitalization. The majority of horses are able to successfully return to work following the procedure.

Other Intraarticular Fractures of the Tarsocrural Joint

These fractures are relatively uncommon. Figures 7-29 to 7-31 show some examples of cases that may be encountered. Fractures can occur through the medial malleolus of the tibia and will show different manifestations than medial malleolus OCD. There will be an obvious linear fracture line and usually the fragment is displaced distally. The fragments are removed arthroscopically, and prognosis will be related to whether the long medial collateral ligament can be left intact. Fragments may occur off the proximal plantar aspect of the medial trochlear ridge (see Figs. 7-29 and 7-30) and are operated on using an approach through the plantar pouch. Larger displaced fracture fragments may also occur off the medial trochlear ridge of the talus (see Fig. 7-30). Figure 7-31 illustrates a case in a 4-month-old colt and an image of a direct penetrating injury to the tarsocrural joint with a fragment and defect on the lateral trochlear ridge of the talus. This was removed arthroscopically and was accompanied by severe synovitis.

Occasionally, fractures amenable to lag screw fixation will occur in the talus; these are usually in a sagittal plane (Fig. 7-32). Small linear fractures have been repaired with one screw. The cases illustrated in Figure 7-32 required three cortical screws. In a retrospective study of 11 racehorses (8 Standardbreds and 3 Thoroughbreds) that had incomplete sagittal fractures of the talus that were treated conservatively, follow-up information was available for 8 horses, of which 7 raced after injury. Performance in 3 horses was improved, in 1 it was unchanged, and in 3 horses performance declined (Davidson et al, 2005). The need for lag screw fixation of these incomplete fractures is therefore considered questionable.

A single case has been published of loose fragmentation in the plantar pouch of the tarsocrural joint that was hypothesized to originate from small fragments detaching from the epiphyseal growth cartilage by trauma and continuing to grow within in the synovial fluid. The authors suggested that trauma during the animal's first days of life could have released cartilaginous tissue from the tibial articular growth plate growth

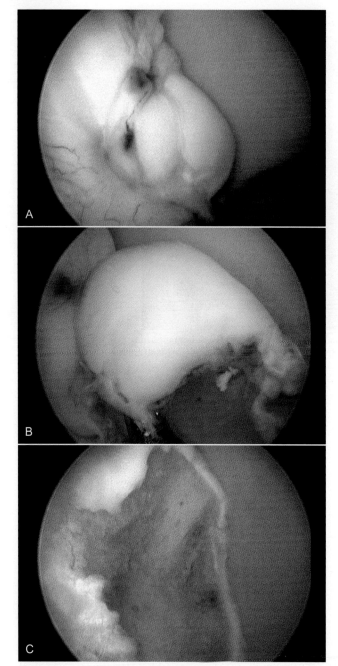

Figure 7-22 Arthroscopic views of medial malleolus OCD before **(A)** and following **(B)** elevation of the fragment. **C,** After removal and debridement.

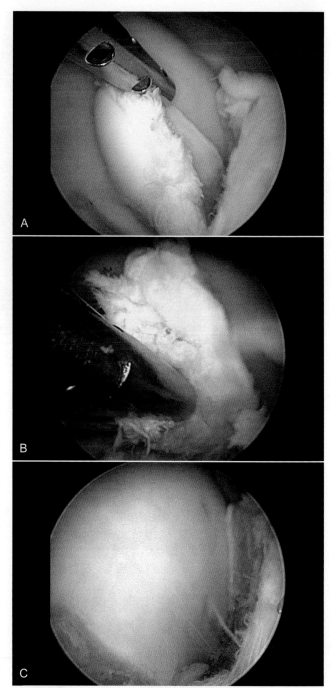

Figure 7-23 Large fragment of the medial malleolus (radiographs shown in Fig. 7-28). **A,** Loose fragment palpated with egress cannula. **B,** Fragment being removed with Ferris-Smith rongeurs. **C,** View after removal and debridement.

cartilage complex (this was based on the presence of radiolucency at the caudolateral aspect of the tibia) (Carstanjen et al, 2005).

Retrieval of Fragments from the Talocentral (Proximal Intertarsal) Joint

Fragments will occasionally be seen in the dorsal talocentral joint. They are often under the plica or a fibrous membrane that incompletely separates the tarsocrural and talocentral joints. Most fragments originate from other locations in the dorsal tarsocrural joint and migrate to this dependant cul-de-sac. The dorsomedial arthroscopic portal is the same for all other surgery and allows visualization sinto the talocentral joint (Fig. 7-33). A needle is used to decide on optimal placement

of the instrument portal. In some cases, a medial instrument portal will be satisfactory, whereas in most the authors have used a lateral instrument portal to retrieve the fragment from under the joint capsule or plica. Exchange of arthroscope and instrument portals may be useful and in several cases, a third incision, medial and distal, in the dorsomedial joint pouch has been required. Resection of the perimeter of the opening between the tarsocrural and talocentral joints is often necessary to identify and retrieve loose fragments from the dorsomedial recess of the joint and a second instrument portal is sometimes useful (see Fig. 7-33).

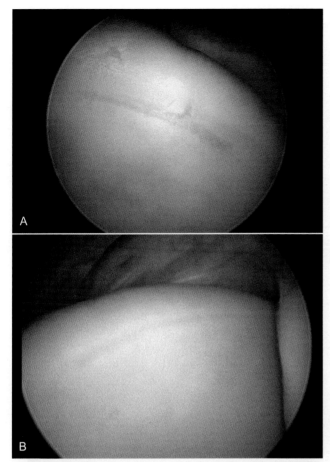

Figure 7-24 Wear lines on medial trochlear ridge of talus. A, Secondary to large medial malleolus osteochondritis dissecans. **B,** Associated with chronic osteochondritis dissecans and loose body.

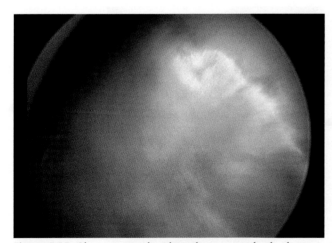

Figure 7-25 Chronic osteochondritis dissecans with a healing primary lesion.

Tears and Avulsions of the Collateral Ligaments of the Tarsocrural Joint

Barker et al (2013) described 20 horses with tears of the collateral ligaments. All involved the short collateral ligaments, and in 4 horses the long collateral ligaments were also affected. Lesions were identified ultrasonographically before surgery in 18 of 20 cases (Fig. 7-34). At arthroscopy most horses had concurrent tearing of the joint capsule. The morphology of the collateral ligament tears varied; some were full and some partial thickness. Invariably torn fibers were extruded into the joint lumen. Medial collateral ligaments were torn in 9, lateral collateral ligaments in 6, and both medial and lateral ligaments in 5 horses. Collateral ligament disruption was frequently accompanied by additional (remote) capsular disruption (17 horses) or disruption of the dorsal plica (5 horses), or both, and tears into the extensor bundle (4 horses). Disruption of the collateral ligaments and adjacent capsule was seen as the sole lesion in only 1 animal. In all cases treatment consisted of removal of torn tissue principally with motorized synovial resector (see Fig. 7-34). Fourteen horses returned to previous level of performance, 4 remained lame, and 2 were lost to follow-up.

Tearing of the Joint Capsule

Tearing of the tarsocrural joint capsule has been identified as a sole lesion and in conjunction with tearing of the collateral ligaments in horses with lameness localizing to the tarsocrural joint. This was identified in 25 out of 30 horses with soft tissue injuries of the tarsocrural joint (Barker et al, 2013). In most instances this was identifiable ultrasonographically before surgery. At arthroscopy torn capsular tissue was extruded into the synovial environment (Fig. 7-35). When extensive there was expansion of the joint outside its normal confines, and when the capsule was avulsed from its osseous attachment, areas of bone that cannot normally be seen arthroscopically were exposed (Fig. 7-36). Treatment consisted of removal of torn, extruded tissue with a goal of creating an inert scar. Three horses that failed to return to work had extensive tearing affecting dorsal and plantar compartments of the joint capsule.

Treatment of Proliferative Synovitis

Occasionally, severe proliferative synovitis occurs in the tarsocrural joint, and debridement of some of the tissue (partial synovectomy) can offer some relief. The authors have used both hand instrumentation and motorized instrumentation (the latter is usually better) for debridement in these cases.

Treatment of Septic Arthritis and Septic Osteomyelitis

The use of arthroscopy in the treatment of septic osteomyelitic lesions of the talus was mentioned previously. Arthroscopy has also been used to remove fibrin from patients with septic arthritis and is considered to emulate the successful results achieved with arthrotomy (Bertone et al, 1987). The management of sepsis in synovial structures is discussed in Chapter 14.

Aftercare

Careful maintenance of a bandage postoperatively is critical (Fig. 7-37). As discussed with regard to OCD in the intermediate ridge, routine aftercare involves 1 month of stall rest with hand walking and then some limited exercise before training commences at 2 to 4 months, depending on the amount of disease. In cases of osteoarthritis or septic arthritis, the period of convalescence may vary. In cases of proliferative synovitis, antiinflammatory therapy is often indicated. Intraarticular corticosteroid administration has also been used.

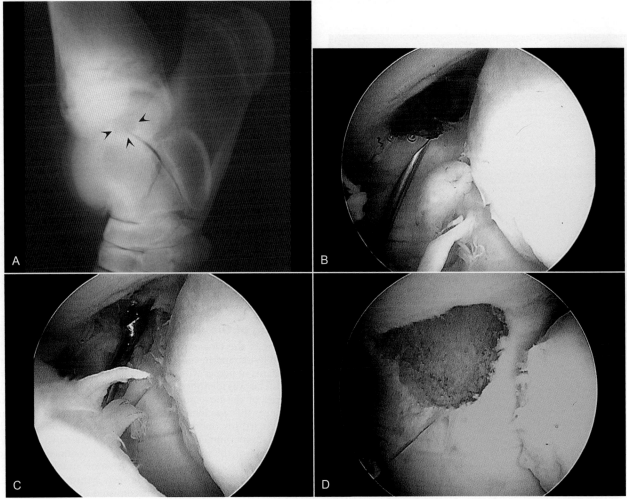

Figure 7-26 A, Lateral to medial radiograph of a yearling Arabian with a subchondral cystic lesion of the proximal region of the trochlear groove of the talus *(arrowheads).* **B,** Arthroscopic image showing the opening to the subchondral cyst in the trochlear groove, viewed using a plantaromedial arthroscope portal and needle inserted using a plantarolateral portal. The plantar aspect of the intermediate ridge of the tibia is articulating with the trochlear groove. **C,** A curette has been introduced through the plantarolateral portal, allowing debridement of the cyst content. **D,** The appearance of the cyst after arthroscopic debridement.

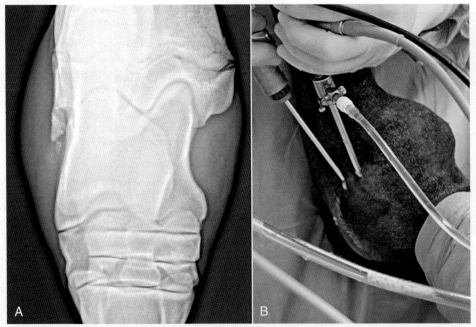

Figure 7-27 A, Dorsoplantar radiograph showing large and smaller intraarticular fractures of the lateral malleolus of the tibia. **B,** External view of position of arthroscope and instrument to remove fragmentation of the lateral malleolus of tibia.

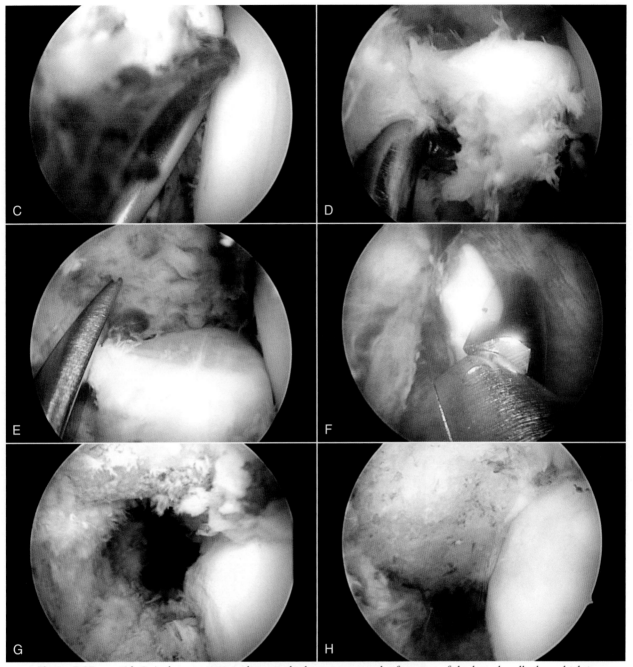

Figure 7-27, cont'd C, Arthroscopic view showing the large intraarticular fragment of the lateral malleolus, which is adjacent to the lateral trochlear ridge (LTR) and partially embedded in the short collateral ligaments. **D,** A probe placed between the fracture fragment and the short lateral collateral ligament after dissection of the large fracture fragment from ligamentous attachments. **E,** Complete separation of the large fracture fragment. **F,** Removal of second, smaller fragment with Ferris-Smith ronguers. **G,** Defect created by removal of fragments with parent lateral malleolus above *(arrow)* and cavity leading into lateral plantar pouch of tarsocrural joint. **H,** Defect in parent bone after debridement.

Continued

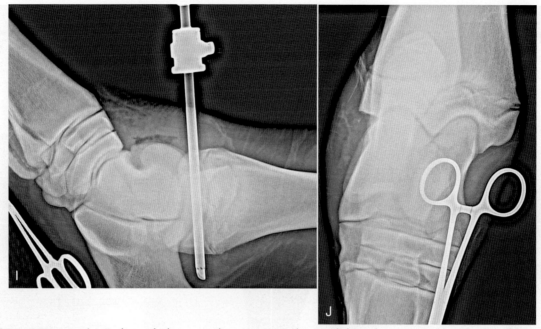

Figure 7-27, cont'd I, Radiograph showing arthroscopic cannula passed through gap created by removal of fracture fragments into lateral plantar pouch. **J,** Postoperative radiograph showing the lateral malleolus after fracture fragment removal.

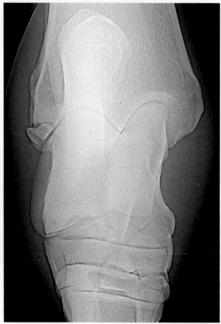

Figure 7-28 Dorsoplantar radiograph showing a fracture of the lateral malleolus that was a consequence to a rough recovery from anesthesia.

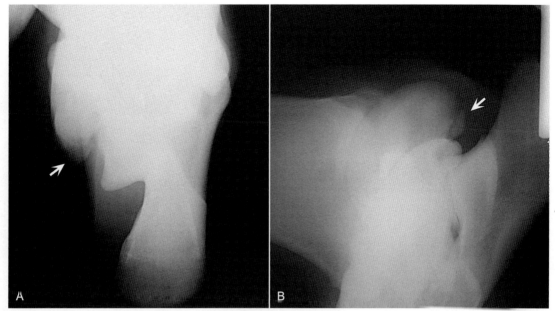

Figure 7-29 A, A skyline radiograph of the tarsus showing a fracture of the proximal plantar aspect of the medial trochlear ridge *(arrow)* in a 2-year-old Percheron-cross filly. The fracture resulted from a kick 2 months before radiography. **B,** An oblique flexed lateral radiograph projects the proximoplantar extent of the medial trochlear ridge and the fracture *(arrow)*.

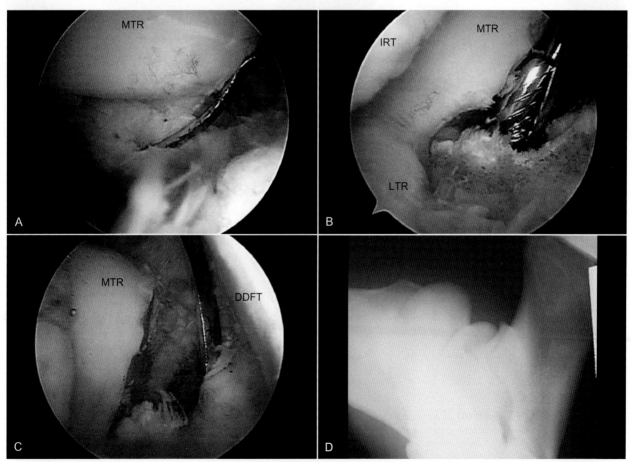

Figure 7-30 A, Arthroscopic view of the fracture of the proximal plantar aspect of the medial trochlear ridge *(MTR)* (case in Fig. 7-29). The MTR with an elevator in the fracture plane. **B,** The major portion of the fracture has been removed, and the fracture bed is being smoothed with a motorized burr. The MTR and lateral trochlear ridge *(LTR)* are evident, and the caudal aspect of the intermediate ridge *(IRT)* of the tibia is evident articulating in the trochlear groove. **C,** The arthroscopic view after removal of diagnostic fracture fragment showing the proximal extent of the medial trochlear ridge and the adjacent tarsal sheath containing the deep digital flexor tendon *(DDFT)*. **D,** Postoperative radiograph showing the residual trochlear ridge after removal of the fracture fragment.

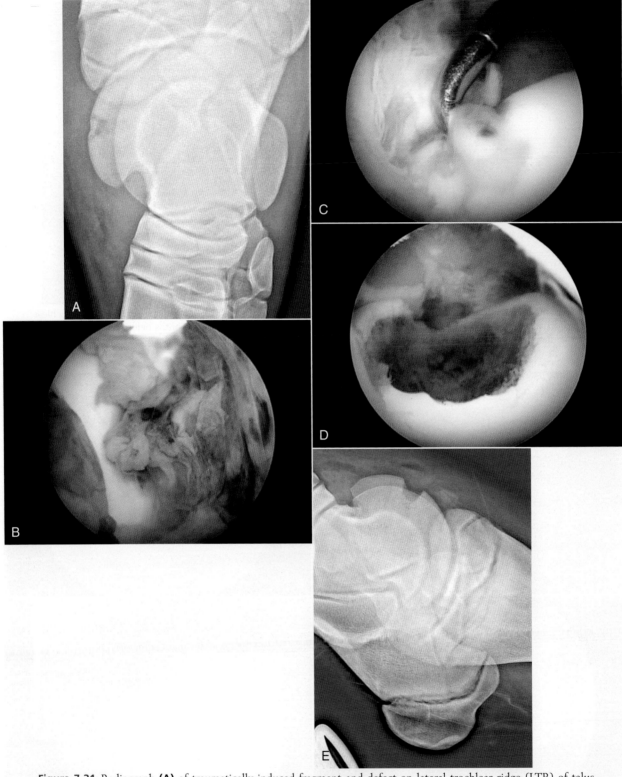

Figure 7-31 Radiograph **(A)** of traumatically induced fragment and defect on lateral trochlear ridge (LTR) of talus associated with direct trauma. Arthroscopic views of fibrinous synovitis **(B)** and the fragment and defect before removal **(C). D,** The defect after debridement and postoperative radiograph **(E).**

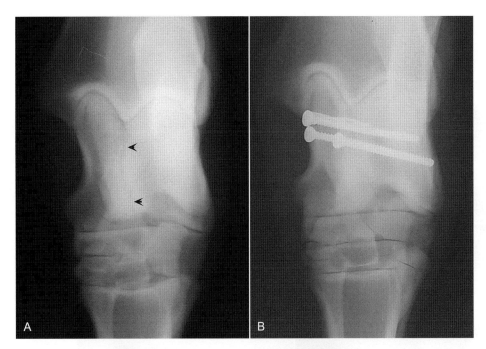

Figure 7-32 A, Preoperative dorso-plantar radiograph showing a sagittal fracture of the talus *(arrowheads).* The fracture propagated from the central proximal region of the trochlear groove to obliquely split the medial trochlear ridge distally. **B,** Arthroscopic guidance was used to allow lag screw repair using three cortical screws. Notice also a broken drill bit, which occurred during extension of the tarsocrural joint for an intraoperative radiograph. Motion of the soft tissue medially, particularly the medial collateral ligament, was thought to create the shear required to break the drill.

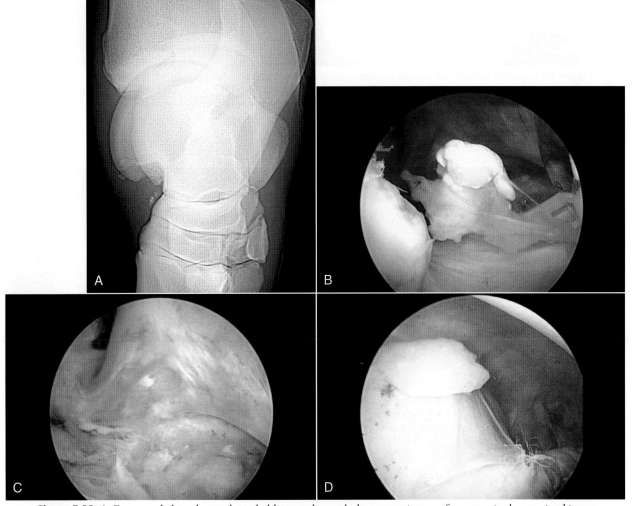

Figure 7-33 A, Dorsomedial to plantarolateral oblique radiograph demonstrating two fragments in the proximal intertarsal (centrodistal) joint. There was also a small fragment associated with the distal aspect of the lateral trochlear ridge (LTR) of the talus. Arthroscopic views of one fragment loosely attached in centrodistal joint **(B).** View into joint after removal of fragment **(C).** Visualization of a second loose fragment that had floated up from the joint and is overlying the distal intermediate ridge of tibia **(D).**

Continued

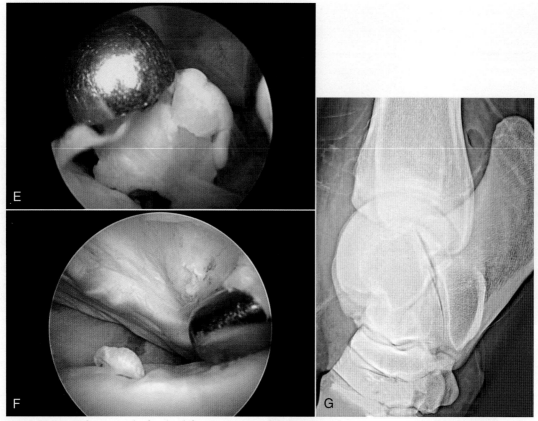

Figure 7-33, cont'd Removal of a third fragment using the dorsolateral instrument portal **(E)**. Removal of a small fragment in the medial aspect of the joint at the distal aspect of the MRT of the talus that required creating a second instrument portal dorsomedially **(F)**. Intraoperative radiograph showing removal of fragments **(G)**.

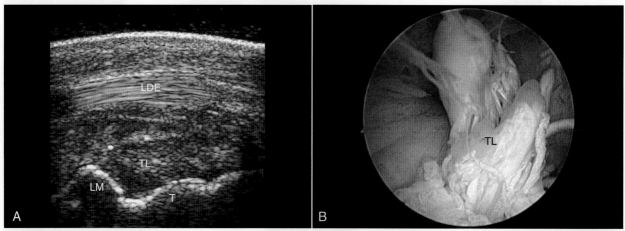

Figure 7-34 Tearing of the short lateral collateral ligaments. **A,** Longitudinally oriented ultrasonograph. **B-E,** Arthroscopic images of the lesion identified in **(A)**, visualized from a dorsomedial arthroscopic portal. **B,** Torn short collateral ligament imaged on its lateral malleolar origin and recoiled proximally.

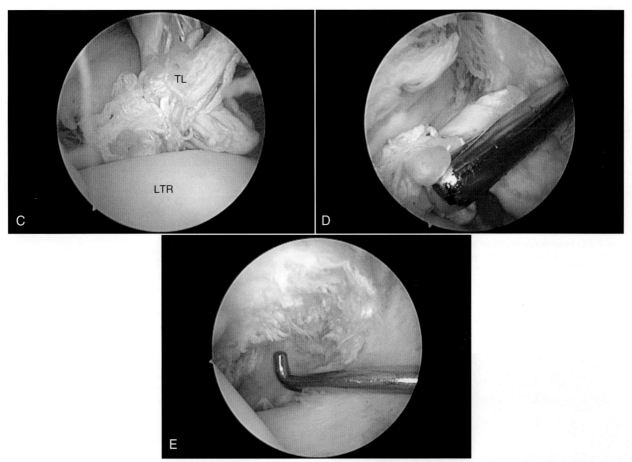

Figure 7-34, cont'd C, Slightly further distal view than **B. D,** Removal of the torn ligament with a motorized synovial resector. Note suction used to pull the torn tissue into the blades. **E,** Appearance following removal of the torn ligament with a probe passing distal to the debrided lateral malleolar origin toward the plantar compartment of the joint. *LDE,* Lateral digital extensor tendon; *LM,* lateral malleolus; *LTR,* lateral trochlear ridge of talus; *T,* talus; *TL,* short lateral collateral ligament.

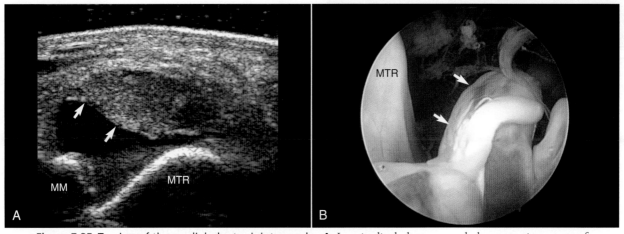

Figure 7-35 Tearing of the medial plantar joint capsule. A, Longitudinal ultrasonograph demonstrating a mass of organized tissue protruding from the medial joint capsule into the distended joint. **B,** Arthroscopic appearance of the tear. *MM,* Medial malleolus of tibia; *MTR,* medial trochlea ridge of tallus; white arrows indicate torn joint capsule in both images.

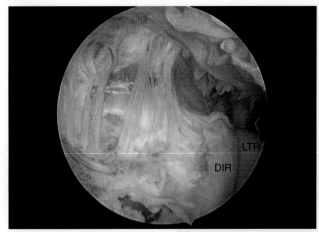

Figure 7-36 Tearing/avulsion of the dorsal joint capsule from distal tibia exposing areas of bone that are normally covered by the capsular reflection. *DIR*, Distal intermediate ridge of tibia; *LTR*, lateral trochlear ridge of talus.

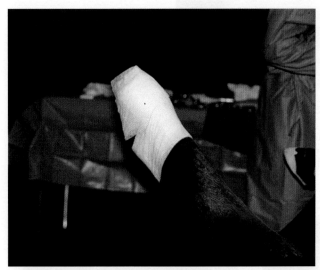

Figure 7-37 Placement of nonadhesive pad followed by Kling® gauze over tarsus after arthroscopic surgery. After two layers of Kling®, a final layer of Elastikon® is then applied.

REFERENCES

Barker WJH, Smith MRW, Minshall GJ, Wright IM: Soft tissue injuries of the tarsocrural joint: a retrospective analysis of 30 cases evaluated arthroscopically, *Equine Vet J* 45:435–441, 2013.

Beard WL, Bramlage LR, Schneider RK, Embertson RM: Post-operative racing performance in Standardbreds and Thoroughbreds with osteochondrosis of the tarsocrural joint: 109 cases (1984-1990), *J Am Vet Med Assoc* 204:1655–1659, 1994.

Bergin BJ, Pierce SW, Bramlage LR, Stromberg A: Oral hyaluronan gel reduces postoperative tarsocrural effusion in the yearling Thoroughbred, *Equine Vet J* 38:375–378, 2006.

Bertone AL, McIlwraith CW, Jones RL, et al.: Comparison of various treatments for experimentally induced equine infectious arthritis, *Am J Vet Res* 48:519–529, 1987.

Brink P, Dovik NI, Tverdal A: Lameness and effusion of the tarsocrural joints after arthroscopy of osteochondritis dessicans in horses, *Vet Rec* 165:709–712, 2009.

Carstanjen B, Couturier L, Cauvin E: Ectopic cartilage formation of unknown origin in the plantar pouch of the tarsocrural joint in a yearling, *Vet Rec* 157:630–632, 2005.

Davidson EJ, Ross MW, Parente EJ: Incomplete sagittal fracture of the talus in 11 racehorses: outcome, *Equine Vet J* 37:457–461, 2005.

Dik KJ, Emerink E, van Weeran PR: Radiographic development of osteochondral abnormalitis in the hock and stifle of Dutch Warmblood foals from age 1 to 11 months, *Equine Vet J* 31(Suppl 1):9–15, 1999.

Garcia-Lopez JM, Kirker-Head CA: Occult subchondral osseous cyst-like lesions of the equine tarsocrural joint, *Vet Surg* 33:557–564, 2004.

Hoppe F: Radiological investigations of osteochondrosis dissecans in Standardbred Trotters and Swedish Warmblood horses, *Equine Vet J* 16:425–429, 1984.

Janicek JC, Cook JL, Wilson DA, Ketzner KM: Multiple osteochondral autografts for treatment of a medial trochlear ridge subchondral cystic lesion in the equine tarsus, *Vet Surg* 39:95–100, 2010.

Laws EG, Richardson DW, Ross MW, et al.: Racing performance in Standardbreds following conservative and surgical treatment for tarsocrural osteochondrosis, *Equine Vet J* 25:199–202, 1993.

McIlwraith CW: Surgery of the hock, stifle and shoulder, *Vet Clin North Am Large Anim Pract* 5:333–362, 1983.

McIlwraith CW, Foerner JJ, Davis DM: Osteochondritis dissecans of the tarsocrural joint: results of treatment with arthroscopic surgery, *Equine Vet J* 23:155–162, 1991.

Montgomery LJ, Juzwiak JS: Subchondral cyst-like lesions in the talus in four horses, *Equine Vet Educ* 21:629–647, 2009.

O'Neill HD, Bladon BM: Arthroscopic removal of fractures of the lateral malleolus of the tibia in the tarsocrural joint: a retrospective study of 13 cases, *Equine Vet J* 42:558–562, 2010.

Shelley J, Dyson S: Interpreting radiographs. 5. Radiology of the equine hock, *Equine Vet J* 16:488–495, 1984.

Smith RMW, Wright IM: Arthroscopic treatment of fractures of the lateral malleolus of the tibia: 26 cases, *Equine Vet J* 43:280–287, 2011.

Wallis TW, Goodrich LR, McIlwraith CW, Frisbie DD, Hendrickson DA, Trotter GW, Baxter GM, Kawcak CE: Arthroscopic injection of corticosteroids into the fibrous tissue of subchondral cystic lesions of the medial femoral condyle in horses: a retrospective study of 52 cases (2001-2006), *Equine Vet J* 40:461–467, 2008.

Zamos DT, Honnas CM, Hoffman AG: Arthroscopic approach and intra-articular anatomy of the plantar pouch of the equine tarsocrural joint, *Vet Surg* 23:161–166, 1994.

CHAPTER 8

Diagnostic and Surgical Arthroscopy of the Scapulohumeral (Shoulder) Joint

Arthroscopic surgery of the shoulder is not a common procedure in horses, and two of the authors' (C.W.M. and A.J.N.) experience over 25 years includes only 180 cases, with all but 30 of those cases involving osteochondrosis. (It is to be noted in this discussion that *osteochondrosis* is a collective term for osteochondritis dissecans [OCD] and subchondral cystic lesions [SCLs] because both commonly occur together in the shoulder and will be collectively abbreviated as OC from now on.) The need for diagnostic arthroscopy for lameness originating from the shoulder in mature horses has become increasingly common, while presentation of younger horses for treatment of shoulder OCD has seemingly declined. The reduced numbers of weanlings and yearlings with shoulder OCD may be real, although the recent literature suggests a rather poor prognosis for athletic performance with or without surgical debridement of shoulder OCD (Jenner et al, 2008). This, combined with the difficulty in performing shoulder arthroscopy and the rare instance where conservative therapy resulted in successful athletic function, may have tempered the demand for surgical intervention for shoulder OCD.

Two techniques for performing arthroscopic surgery of the shoulder have been described: a craniolateral approach, in which the arthroscope is inserted cranial to the infraspinatus tendon, and a lateral approach, in which the arthroscope penetrates the shoulder joint immediately caudal to the infraspinatus tendon (Bertone & McIlwraith, 1987b; Nixon, 1987). The choice of surgical approach is largely defined by the location of the lesion and the previous experience of the operator. Two reports of outcome following treatment for OCD of the shoulder indicate the outlook varies from good (9 of 11 horses returning to soundness) (Bertone & McIlwraith, 1987a) to poor with 30% of horses returning to soundness (Jenner et al, 2008). Clearly, patient selection, early intervention, choice of approach, and operator experience all factor in outcome after arthroscopic debridement of shoulder OCD.

Conservative (nonsurgical) treatment of OC of the shoulder been reported to have minimal success, particularly in the limited numbers of horses able to enter athletic activities (Jenner et al, 2008; Meagher et al, 1975; Nyack et al, 1981; Rose et al, 1986). However, early recognition of lesions can lead to a successful outcome, particularly with lesions limited to the glenoid. Rapid onset of osteoarthritis and a general delay in definitive diagnosis often limit the response to surgery. Early surgical reports describe several animals that responded well to treatment by arthrotomy (DeBowes et al, 1982; Mason & Maclean, 1977; Nixon et al, 1984; Schmidt et al, 1975); however, extensive soft tissue dissection is necessary during arthrotomy and the craniomedial aspect of the joint may not be visualized (Nixon et al, 1984). Other complications include loss of lateral joint stability (Schmidt et al, 1975) and seroma formation (Nixon et al, 1984). These complications are not only avoided with arthroscopy but also the minimally invasive nature of arthroscopy provides many of the intraoperative and postoperative advantages seen in other joints. Other than part of a broader approach for distal scapula fracture repair and open repair of shoulder luxation, there is no place for shoulder arthrotomy in the horse. Arthroscopy for intraarticular disease is the preferred method for OCD and other conditions strictly involving the shoulder joint. On the other hand, arthroscopy of the shoulder is more technically complex, and in adult horses it can be a particular challenge, even for experienced arthroscopists.

SURGICAL ANATOMY OF THE SHOULDER

The shoulder is a relatively tightly articulated diarthrodial joint and consists of the rounded articular surface of the humeral head and the depressed concavity of the glenoid surface of the scapula. Collateral and stabilizing support for the shoulder is derived from periarticular tendons and ligaments. Lateral support is provided by the supraspinatus and infraspinatus tendons of insertion, while medial support is formed by the subscapularis tendon of insertion and a plical fold, referred to as the *medial glenohumeral ligament*. The primary cranial stabilizer is the biceps tendon of origin. Similarly, caudal support is derived from the tendons of origin of the teres minor and deltoideus muscles. Access for the arthroscope and instrument entry is limited to the lateral aspects by the close association of the scapula with the thorax. Finally, the accessible portions of the shoulder are functionally divided into cranial and caudal regions by the infraspinatus tendon of insertion.

▶ DIAGNOSTIC ARTHROSCOPY OF THE SHOULDER JOINT

Insertion of the Arthroscope

The horse is positioned in lateral recumbency, with the affected limb uppermost and supported in a slightly adducted position. The leg is draped so that traction can be applied to the limb during surgery. After aseptic preparation and draping of a wide sterile field, the appropriate landmark for insertion of a spinal needle immediately cranial to the infraspinatus tendon and proximal to the notch dividing the greater tubercle of the humerus into cranial and caudal components is identified (Fig. 8-1). If the joint is predistended (one of the authors A.J.N. does this), an 18-gauge, 3-inch spinal needle is inserted at this location at an angle approximately 25 degrees caudal and distal to penetrate the shoulder joint cranial cul-de-sac (Fig. 8-2). The needle is advanced until the tip contacts articular cartilage, and about 60 mL of a balanced electrolyte solution are then injected to distend the joint (Fig. 8-3).

The spinal needle is removed, and if the craniolateral approach to the shoulder is selected, a 5-mm vertical skin incision is made in the same location (if it is not made before placement of the spinal needle). For the lateral approach, the skin incision for the arthroscope portal is made 1 cm caudal to the palpable caudal border of the infraspinatus tendon. The proximal aspect of the greater tubercle is also palpable, and the incision for the lateral approach is made 1 cm proximal to this landmark. The arthroscope cannula and conical obturator are then inserted through the joint capsule in the same direction as the 18-gauge spinal needle under the infraspinatus tendon toward the caudal aspect of the joint (Fig. 8-4). Entry into the joint is confirmed by removing the obturator and observing a flow of fluid from the cannula. The arthroscope is then placed within the cannula, and the diagnostic arthroscopic evaluation can commence from this position (Fig. 8-5).

Normal Arthroscopic Anatomy—Craniolateral Approach

Systematic examination of the joint using the craniolateral approach begins with the tip of the arthroscope in the caudal aspect of the joint. In this position, the caudal humeral head

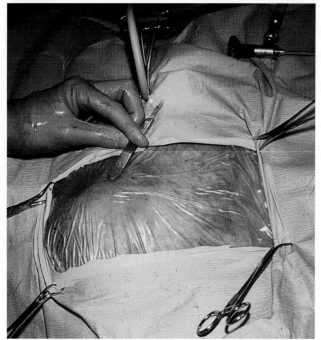

Figure 8-1 Identifying the infraspinatus tendon using a scalpel. The site for the arthroscopic portal is proximal to the cranial aspect of the greater tubercle of the humerus (cranial to and above the distal end of the scalpel).

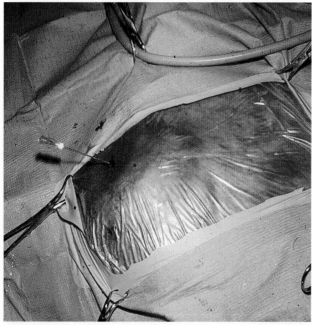

Figure 8-2 Shoulder joint arthrocentesis cranial to infraspinatus tendon. An 18-gauge spinal needle is inserted through the indentation and angled approximately 25 degrees caudally and distally.

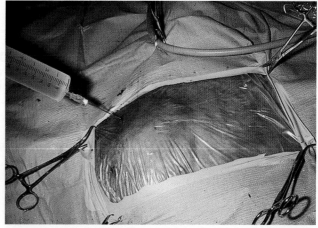

Figure 8-3 Distention after incision. Injection of sterile, balanced electrolyte solution to distend the shoulder.

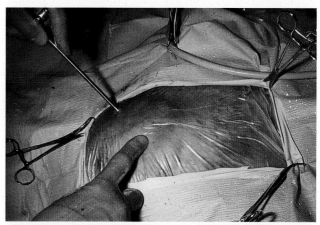

Figure 8-4 Insertion of the arthroscopic sheath and obturator.

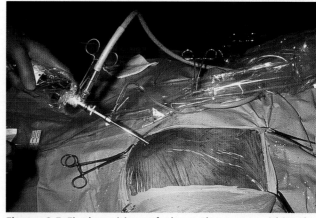

Figure 8-5 Final position of the arthroscope within the sheath, with the tip in the caudal aspect of the shoulder joint.

(ventrally), glenoid (medially), and synovial membrane (laterally) can be visualized (Fig. 8-6). The arthroscope and cannula are then withdrawn along the lateral aspect of the joint to allow visualization of the lateral rim of the glenoid medially, the humeral head ventrally, and the synovial surface of the infraspinatus tendon laterally. The synovial membrane adjacent to the infraspinatus tendon is arranged in longitudinal bands and is relatively devoid of villi (Fig. 8-7). At this stage, elevation

of the limb to a position parallel to the floor (as opposed to the adducted position) brings the lateral aspect of the humeral head, lateral reflection of the joint capsule on the humeral head, and the lateral cul-de-sac of the shoulder joint into view (Fig. 8-8). Returning the limb to an adducted position exposes more of the medial surface of the humeral head. The tip of the arthroscope is then moved craniomedially to visualize the cranial rim of the glenoid, the synovial membrane underlying

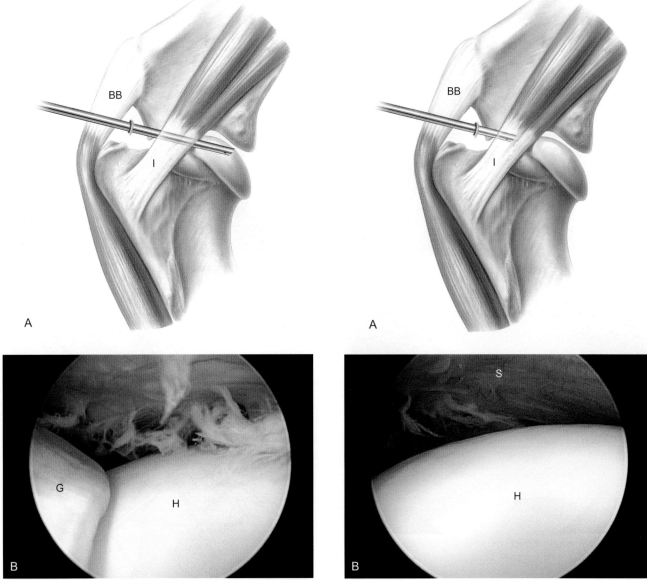

Figure 8-6 Caudal aspect of the scapulohumeral joint. **A,** Diagram of arthroscope position. **B,** Arthroscopic view: *(BB)* tendon of origin of biceps brachii; *(G),* caudal rim of glenoid; *(H),* caudal humeral head; *(I)* tendon of insertion of infraspinatus.

Figure 8-7 Lateral aspect of the humeral head *(H)* and longitudinal bands of the infraspinatus tendon visible beneath the villous synovial membrane *(S)*. *(BB)* Tendon of origin of biceps brachii and *(I)* tendon of insertion of infraspinatus covered by synovial membrane *(S)*. **A,** Diagram of arthroscope position. **B,** Arthroscopic view.

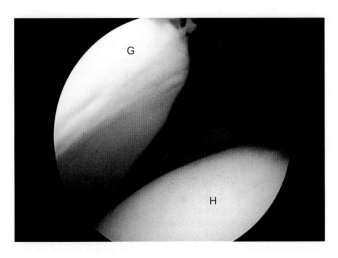

Figure 8-8 Separation of humeral head and glenoid to allow deeper evaluation of the articular surfaces. Lateral aspect of the scapulohumeral joint with the arthroscope between the glenoid and humeral head (separation achieved with fluid distention): *(G)* lateral glenoid, *(H)* humeral head.

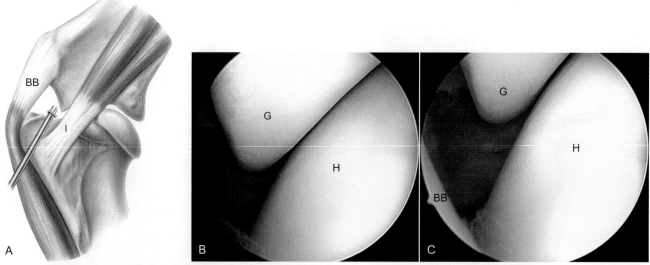

Figure 8-9 Cranial aspect of the scapulohumeral joint. **A,** Diagram of arthroscope position. **B** and **C,** Arthroscopic views: (G), cranial rim of the glenoid; (H), cranial aspect of the humerus. (BB) indentation produced by biceps brachii.

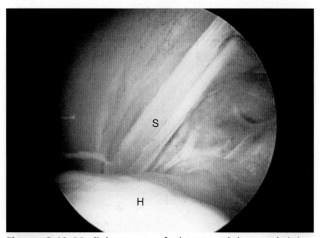

Figure 8-10 Medial aspect of the scapulohumeral joint. Arthroscopic view: H, humeral head; S, medial synovial membrane with the normal plica (glenohumeral ligament).

the biceps tendon, and the cranial aspect of the humerus (Fig. 8-9). With the joint maximally distended so that the glenoid and humeral head are separated, the tip of the arthroscope is inserted over the humeral head and under the glenoid toward the medial side of the joint. The articular surface of the glenoid or caudomedial humeral head, or both, can be closely examined by rotating the viewing angle of the scope 180 degrees. Traction on the limb at this stage also facilitates the procedure. The medial aspect of the glenoid and humeral head are inspected, as well as the medial surface of the synovial membrane, which contains a normal plica, devoid of villi, that has been referred to as the *medial glenohumeral ligament* despite the fact that it is not truly a ligament (Fig. 8-10). In mature horses, complete examination of the medial and caudomedial aspects of the shoulder joint become more difficult. Additional traction can aid exposure, but access can be limited unless erosion and malformation of the humeral head are extensive.

Normal Arthroscopic Anatomy—Lateral Approach

An alternative approach for arthroscopic examination of the shoulder joint uses a direct lateral approach (Nixon, 1987) and is favored when the target lesion is on the caudal, medial, or caudomedial surface of the humeral head or glenoid cavity. In

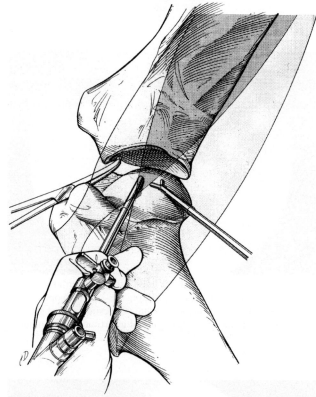

Figure 8-11 Lateral approach to the shoulder joint. The arthroscope entry is placed 1 cm caudal to the infraspinatus tendon, and instrument portal 4 to 5 cm caudal to the arthroscope. *(From Nixon AJ. Diagnostic and surgical arthroscopy of the equine shoulder joint. Vet Surg 1987;16:44–52 with permission.)*

this technique, the arthroscope penetrates the joint 1 to 2 cm caudal to the infraspinatus tendon, entering between the infraspinatus and teres minor muscles (Fig. 8-11). This approach allows examination of the cranial, lateral, and caudal portions of the humeral head and the glenoid cavity, as well as portions of the medial aspect depending on the age of the horse and extent of disease. In most situations it allows good visualization of the caudomedial aspect of the humeral head (Fig. 8-12), which can be difficult to examine using the craniolateral approach. Additionally, it also leaves the portal cranial to the

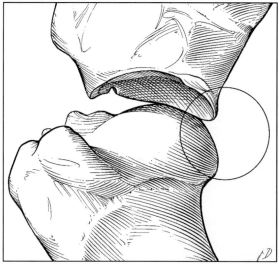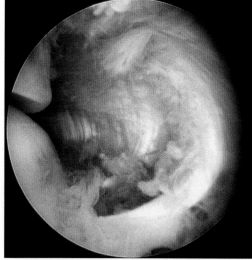

Figure 8-12 Caudal aspect of the scapulohumeral joint. Arthroscopic view of the caudal aspect of the shoulder joint using the lateral arthroscope entry portal. *(Modified from Nixon AJ. Diagnostic and surgical arthroscopy of the equine shoulder joint. Vet Surg 1987;16:44–52 with permission.)*

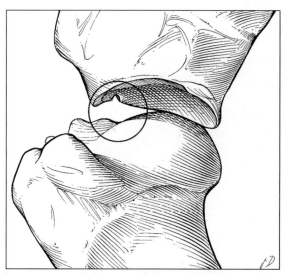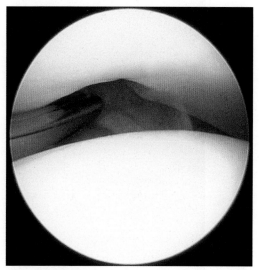

Figure 8-13 Medial aspect of the scapulohumeral joint showing glenoid notch. Arthroscopic view of the medial aspect of the joint with curved forceps providing joint distraction. *(Modified from Nixon AJ. Diagnostic and surgical arthroscopy of the equine shoulder joint. Vet Surg 1987;16:44–52 with permission.)*

infraspinatus tendon available for the egress cannula. In adult horses the cranial portal can also provide access for the surgeon to insert a curved, blunt-tipped forceps across the nonarticular portion of the shoulder joint to engage the glenoid notch and distract the humeral head from the glenoid by rotation of the forceps. This allows the arthroscope to be advanced safely to the medial aspect of the joint (Fig. 8-13). A third portal, 2 to 4 cm caudal to the arthroscope entry portal, is used as an instrument portal for arthroscopic surgery by triangulation. This method of internal distraction precludes the need for external traction; however, because it risks iatrogenic damage to the cranial aspect of the humeral head, it is generally used only in heavily muscled mature horses. For surgical debridement of most OCD lesions, the younger age of the horse and the chronicity of the disease provide sufficient laxity that fluid distention and axial traction are adequate to allow access to most regions of the articulation.

Specific Indications and Technique

The primary indication for diagnostic arthroscopy of the shoulder joint is the evaluation and treatment of OC. Diagnostic arthroscopy is also indicated when lameness is localized to the shoulder by response to intraarticular anesthesia but radiographic signs are equivocal (Doyle and White, 2000). This paper also described the value of nuclear scintigraphic evaluation in 6 of the 15 horses and described radiographic findings suggesting shoulder disease including glenoid sclerosis, focal glenoid lysis, small glenoid cysts, and alterations in the contour of the humeral head. Arthroscopic evaluation confirmed shoulder disease in all 15 horses with a variety of cartilage lesions, including glenoid cysts, humeral head cysts, and fibrillation of the humeral and glenoid surfaces. One horse had a nondisplaced fracture of the humeral head, and one of the authors (C.W.M.) has encountered a similar case. As in other joints with OCD, the arthroscopic findings do not always correlate with the radiographic changes and the diagnostic examination is a critical part of the arthroscopic procedure. Arthroscopy is also appropriate in cases of septic arthritis, both for evaluating the articular cartilage and for treatment.

Using a probe during diagnostic arthroscopy of the shoulder joint is critical. An instrument portal is necessary for probe placement, and creation of this portal is described in the next section. The optimal site to insert the probe is ascertained using an 18-gauge, 3-inch spinal needle.

In addition to defining intraarticular disease entities, shoulder arthroscopy in human patients has been extensively used

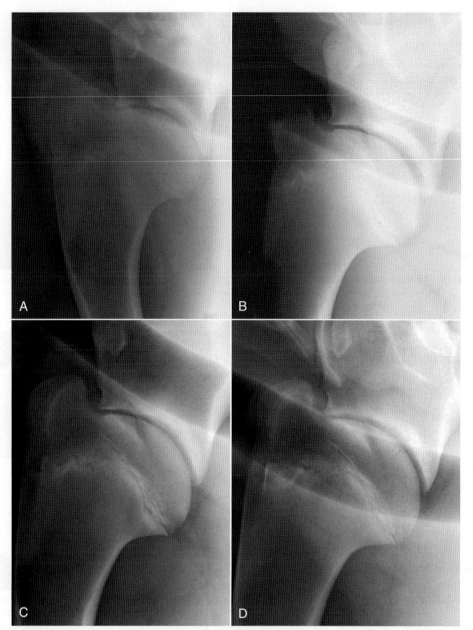

Figure 8-14 Radiographic improvement with conservative management of glenoid osteochondrosis. Radiographs taken December 31, 2010, **A,** obvious osteochondrosis lesion of the glenoid. Follow-up radiographs February 1, 2011 **(B)**, March 15, 2011 **(C)**, and April 14, 2011 **(D)** showing resolution of the defect in the glenoid with some subchondral sclerosis appearing along with the healing process. *(Courtesy Dr. L.R. Bramlage.)*

for rotator cuff repair to stabilize shoulders and loose body removal (Johnson, 1986), and in assessing cases of supraspinatus tendinitis and labrum impingement (Cofield, 1983), and ruptured biceps tendon. The value of arthroscopic evaluation and debridement of arthritis in young and middle-aged patients has also been described, both for staging the disease and allowing definitive treatment (Bhatia et al, 2012). Some of these indications have not been recognized in the horse as yet; the horse does not have a rotator cuff or glenoid labrum.

Arthroscopic Surgery of the Shoulder Joint for Treatment of Osteochondrosis

As mentioned previously, nonsurgical treatment of OC in the equine shoulder has rarely allowed horses to regain athletic capability. It is uncommon but not impossible for a radiographically obvious lesion to resolve without OA with conservative management (Fig. 8-14). More often a delay in definitive

arthroscopic repair simply results in expansion of the lesion, OA, and a reduced response when surgery is finally instituted. Historically, three different arthrotomy approaches have been used to treat cases of OC in the equine shoulder. Complications including loss of lateral support (Schmidt et al, 1975), limited access (DeBowes et al, 1982), and seroma formation (Nixon et al, 1984) have been seen, but probably of more importance is the fact that complete visualization of the articulation is not possible with an arthrotomy incision (Nixon et al, 1984). Extensive traction is also critical to the performance of the procedure.

Arthroscopy provides advantages over arthrotomy by avoiding these limitations and complications, as well as providing better visualization and earlier rehabilitation as a benefit of the minimally invasive approach. It should be stressed, however, that adequate arthroscopic visualization and surgical manipulation in the equine shoulder joint are more difficult than in other joints described previously in this text.

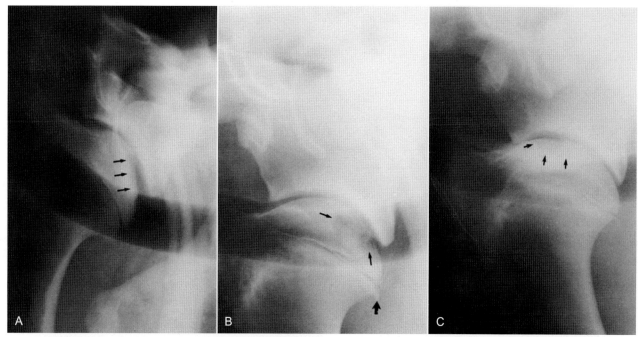

Figure 8-15 Osteochondritis dissecans involving only the humeral head. **A–C,** Radiographs from three cases involving osteochondritis dissecans lesions *(arrows)* of the humeral head. **B,** The larger *arrow* indicates an enthesophyte. **C,** The lesion is in an unusually cranial position.

The material presented is based on the experience of the authors, both in evaluating the approaches in cadavers and involvement in 119 clinical cases, including a previously published series of cases of OC with follow-up (Bertone & McIlwraith, 1987a; Nixon, 1986).

Preoperative Considerations

Most shoulder OCD cases show clinical signs before 1 year of age. The age at presentation does depend somewhat on the observation skills of the owners. In some cases, a recent history of lameness may be described. Contracted appearance to the hoof on the lame limb often correlates with the duration of shoulder OCD. Preoperative clinical signs include lameness with a shortened cranial phase of stride. Some horses have palpable distension of the joint capsule cranial to the infraspinatus tendon, and others show resentment to firm digital pressure caudal to the infraspinatus tendon. Extension and flexion of the shoulder joint is also resented in some cases. Intraarticular anesthesia of the shoulder joint improves or eliminates the lameness in most cases. However, when the articular cartilage over subchondral bone defects is still intact, intraarticular local anesthesia may not generate a response. Intraarticular anesthesia is performed by using the same landmark as previously described for placing the spinal needle during arthroscopy. The absence of these localizing clinical signs, however, does not rule out the presence of OC in the shoulder. In many instances, the shoulder is evaluated after the elimination of problems in the lower limb with the use of nerve blocks.

The diagnosis of OC is confirmed radiographically. Standing radiographs may be taken, and these images help to provide a provisional diagnosis in most cases. Radiographs obtained with the horse under general anesthesia are sometimes necessary to provide images of sufficient quality to rule out the presence of lesions in the joint. Good-quality digital radiographs now make the need for plain radiographs under general anesthesia much less likely. Radiographic signs of OCD in the humeral head include malformation of the epiphysis with flattening and/or undulation of the bone caudally, uneven bone density throughout the epiphysis, and an irregular joint space (Fig. 8-15). Lipping and osteophyte development on the caudal

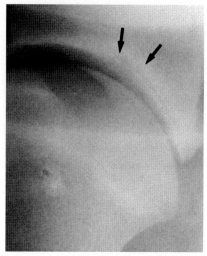

Figure 8-16 Osteochondritis dissecans of the glenoid *(arrows).*

portion of the humeral head, particularly at the physeal junction, may be seen. Occasionally, osteophyte development is evident without other radiographic signs of OCD.

Radiographic abnormalities in the scapula that are considered to relate to OC include subchondral cystic lesions, focal decreased subchondral bone density typical of OCD, osteochondral fragmentation, and abnormal flattening of the glenoid cavity (Figs. 8-16 and 8-17). In most instances, the glenoid cavity develops an abnormal shape with osteophyte development on the caudal border. More chronic shoulder OCD cases have osteophyte formation on both caudal and cranial glenoid rims. Conversely, as in the humeral head, changes may be limited to osteophyte formation on the caudal aspect of the glenoid. In such instances, however, pathologic changes are frequently found on the articular cartilage within the glenoid (Bertone & McIlwraith, 1987a).

Arthrography of the shoulder joint has been described as a technique to diagnose OCD, but more importantly, to evaluate which cases can still be helped by surgery compared with

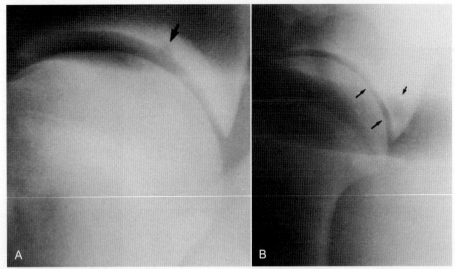

Figure 8-17 Cystic lesions of the shoulder. A, Cystic lesion *(arrow)* of the glenoid. **B,** Cystic lesion of the glenoid and an osteochondritis dissecans lesion of the humerus *(arrows)*.

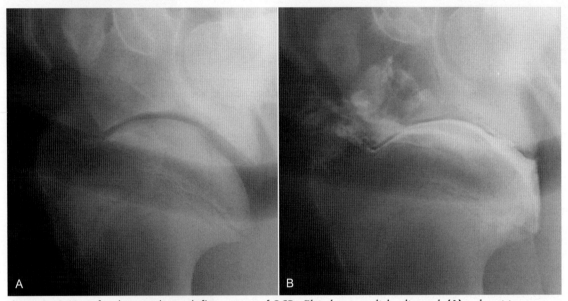

Figure 8-18 Use of arthrography to define extent of OCD. Plain lateromedial radiograph **(A)** and positive contrast arthrogram **(B)** of the shoulder showing underrun cartilage flaps of the humeral head and opposing region of the glenoid cavity. The prognosis with surgery remains poor.

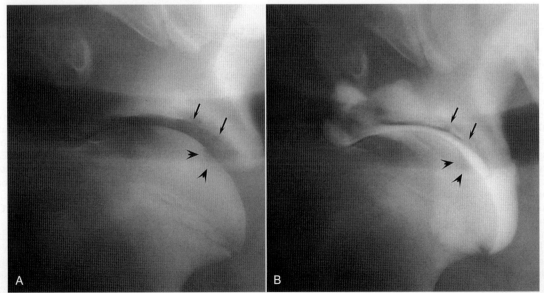

Figure 8-19 Arthrography defines cartilage dissection from underlying bone and assists with prognosis. Plain lateromedial radiograph **(A)** and positive contrast arthrogram **(B)** of the shoulder from a yearling Thoroughbred with lucency of both articular surfaces of the shoulder, but with intact humeral head cartilage. The outlook with surgery is relatively good.

those that are eroded to the extent that they are beyond salvage (Nixon & Spencer, 1990). A critical determinant is the extent of eroded cartilage on opposing surfaces of the humeral head and glenoid cavity (Fig. 8-18). Preoperative confirmation that one cartilage surface remains intact, despite radiographic evidence of subchondral lucency, improves an otherwise poor prognosis and can lead to surgery and generally a better outlook (Fig. 8-19).

▶ Arthroscopic Technique

A thorough exploration of the scapulohumeral joint, as previously described, is performed as the first step. This exploration involves probing all visible lesions and normal-appearing articular cartilage. The normal instrument entry for triangulation during arthroscopic surgery in the shoulder is illustrated in Figure 8-20. The instrument portal is selected to permit access to the caudal humeral head and central articular surface of the glenoid. To determine the location, an 18-gauge spinal needle is inserted about 6 cm caudal to the infraspinatus tendon and 4 cm distal to the arthroscopic portal (Fig. 8-21). This location usually places the needle directly over the caudal humeral head. The needle is inserted through the

deltoid muscle mass and into the distended joint with the limb perpendicular to the body and resting in slight adduction; it must penetrate 6 to 8 cm of muscle mass to reach the joint. The tip of the needle is visualized. At this time, the surgeon must ascertain that the direction of the portal is such that instruments can pass into the space between the glenoid and the humeral head. The entry should be placed more distal if the lesion is confined to the glenoid cavity so that instruments can penetrate to the depths of the glenoid erosions.

When the needle position is judged to be satisfactory, an 8-mm skin incision is made at that location and a stab incision is continued into the muscle mass with the use of a No. 11 or 15 blade (Fig. 8-22). A conical obturator is inserted along the same path to ensure the presence of a workable portal. It is important that fluid pressure be at a minimum at this time. When the portal is unobstructed, intramuscular and subcutaneous accumulation of fluid is minimal, although it usually becomes a problem later during surgery, regardless of the portal size. The shoulder is one of the few sites where screw-in self-sealing cannulae are useful to prevent massive subcutaneous fluid accumulation. Because they limit the size of instrument entry, they must have at least a 7-mm internal diameter to be useful (described in Chapter 2). A blunt probe is initially passed through the instrument portal to evaluate the lesions in the joint, to palpate the articular cartilage peripheral to the defects, and to explore the extent of the undermined cartilage in OCD lesions, as well as the openings of subchondral cystic lesions. The presence of all lesions and their degree is ascertained before any surgical manipulations are performed (Figs. 8-23 to 8-32).

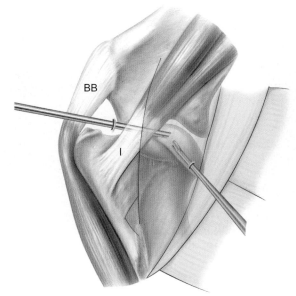

BB

I

Figure 8-20 Usual triangulation position for craniolateral approach to arthroscopic surgery in the shoulder joint. The arthroscope is inserted cranial to the infraspinatus tendon. The instrument portal is caudal and distal to the arthroscopic portal.

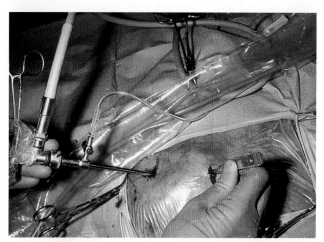

Figure 8-22 An instrument portal being made with a No. 15 scalpel blade.

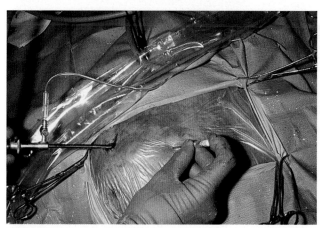

Figure 8-21 A spinal needle is used to ascertain the position of the instrument portal.

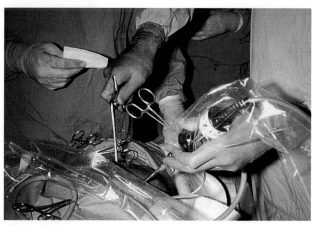

Figure 8-23 Use of the Ferris-Smith rongeurs to remove flap.

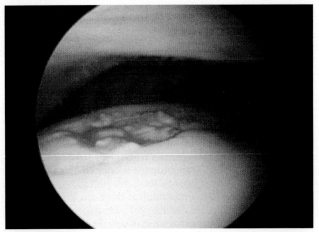

Figure 8-24 Humeral head OCD. Localized osteochondritis dissecans lesion on the medial aspect of the humeral head.

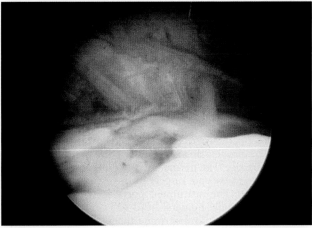

Figure 8-25 Extensive humeral head OCD. More widespread osteochondritis dissecans lesions on the humeral head.

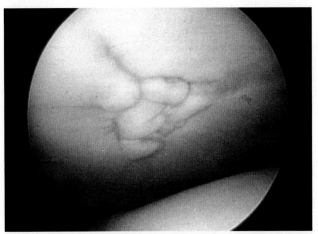

Figure 8-26 Subchondral cyst of glenoid. Arthroscopic view of surface defect associated with subchondral cystic lesion in the glenoid.

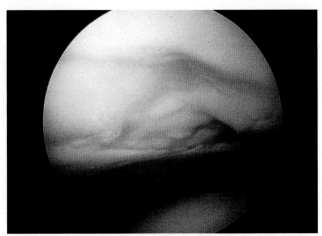

Figure 8-27 OCD of the glenoid. Osteochondritis dissecans lesion of the glenoid.

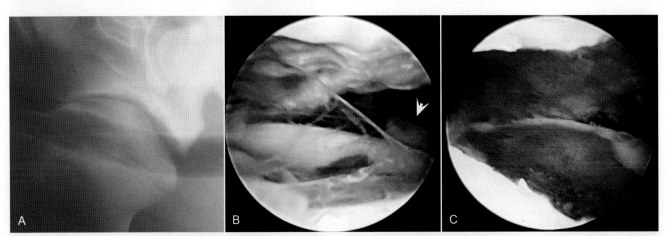

Figure 8-28 Osteochondritis dissecans lesions affecting extensive portions of both articular surfaces of the shoulder have a poor prognosis for return to athletic capabilities. **A,** Preoperative radiograph showing involvement of more than 50% of the articular surface of the glenoid cavity and humeral head. The caudal humeral head is irregularly flattened, and there is divergence of the caudal joint space and extensive remodeling of the caudal glenoid angle. **B,** Arthroscopic view before debridement reveals many of the cartilage flaps have detached and formed free bodies in the caudal joint pouch *(arrow)*. **C,** Following debridement and free body removal.

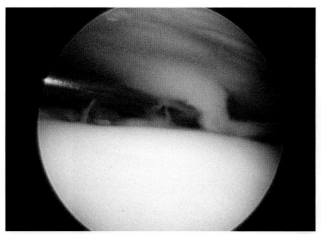

Figure 8-29 Defining lesion with probe. Probe is placed in extensively undermined cartilage on the glenoid. Note also a smaller lesion on the humeral head.

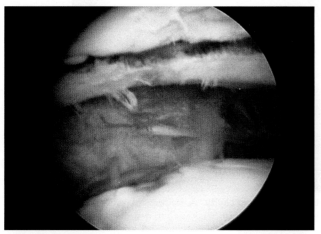

Figure 8-30 Glenoid fragmentation. Fragmentation of the lateral aspect of the glenoid in association with osteochondritis dissecans of the glenoid and humeral head.

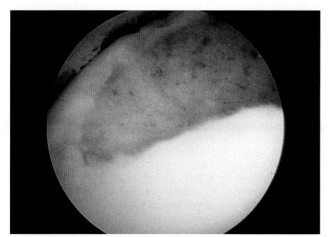

Figure 8-31 Focal humeral head OCD. After debridement of a relatively localized lesion on the humeral head.

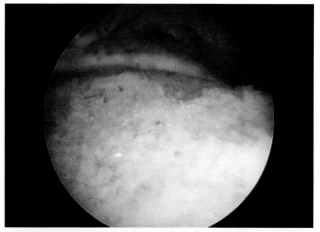

Figure 8-32 Humeral head OCD. After debridement of an extensive lesion of the humeral head.

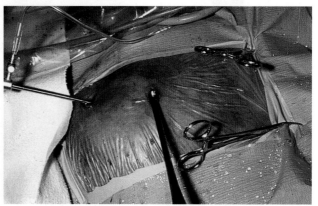

Figure 8-33 Cartilage fragment removal. Piece of cartilage being removed from joint with Ferris-Smith rongeurs.

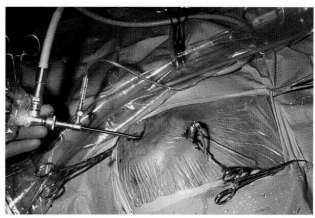

Figure 8-34 Final joint lavage. Use of 4.5-mm egress cannula in shoulder joint (note that it is inserted all the way to be in the joint).

This caudolateral instrument portal is used for debriding most lesions. Laterally located defects are easier to operate than medially placed lesions. Therefore, procedures involving lesions on the medial side of the joint are performed first while maximal joint distention is maintained and separation of the glenoid and humeral head is achieved. Adjunctive traction is also sometimes necessary at this stage. Surgical intervention on laterally placed lesions is still possible later, when joint distention has decreased.

Humeral head defects (see Figs. 8-24 and 8-25) are debrided initially with a hand curette or periosteal elevator; large pieces of cartilage are removed using Ferris-Smith rongeurs (Fig. 8-33). Small debris can be flushed from the joint using a large-bore (≈4.5-mm) egress cannula (Fig. 8-34). A motorized resector can be used for debriding large lesions.

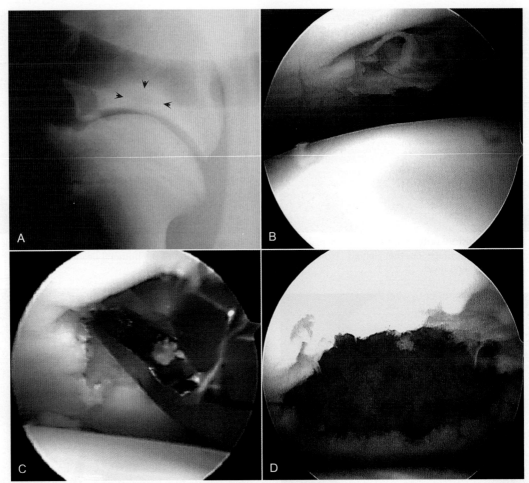

Figure 8-35 Angled rongeurs can be useful to debride cysts of the glenoid cavity. **A,** Radiograph showing 15-mm deep lysis of the glenoid *(arrows)*. **B,** Surface opening of lesion. **C,** Angled rongeur being used to debride the depths of the defect. **D,** Completed debridement of glenoid lesion.

The resector works well in the debridement of easily accessible humeral head lesions. When the defect is deeper within the subchondral bone, however, the resector or burr, or both, may not reach and a right-angled curette is used. Angled motorized resectors (see Chapter 2) can be helpful to accommodate the curvature of the humeral head. Similarly, small angled rongeurs (patellar forceps) can be helpful to enter deep OCD lesions and retrieve cartilage flaps or debride subchondral bone (Fig. 8-35). At the completion of subchondral bone debridement, the edges of the defect are debrided with a hand curette and Ferris-Smith rongeurs. When intact articular cartilage overlies a subchondral defect (a common manifestation with OCD in the shoulder), all cartilage superficial to the defect is removed and the defect beneath is debrided. Figures 8-31 and 8-32 depict defects on the humeral head after debridement.

Similarly, articular cartilage fissures, areas of erosion, cyst-like lesions, and detached articular cartilage in the glenoid (see Figs. 8-26 to 8-30) are debrided and removed by using Ferris-Smith rongeurs, patellar forceps, curettes (both straight and angled), and occasionally the motorized resector or burr. The concave shape of the glenoid sometimes makes accessibility with the straight resector blade difficult. An angled resector and the right-angled curette are particularly useful for debriding extensive lesions and deep lesions. Osteochondral fragments are rare in the shoulder, but detached OCD flaps frequently mineralize and grow and are then often lodged in the caudal cul-de-sac of the shoulder joint.

In some cases, an additional cranial incision or exchange of the arthroscope and instrument portals is necessary to gain instrument access to the cranial aspect of the joint (Figs. 8-36 and 8-37). Alternatively, using the lateral arthroscope entry technique, the arthroscope remains caudal to the infraspinatus tendon, leaving the existing portal cranial to the infraspinatus tendon free for rongeurs or curettes, which replace any egress cannula that may have been placed during the initial phase of surgery. Instrument entry through the cranial portal allows removal of free osteochondral fragments from the cranial cul-de-sac of the joint or access to lesions of the humeral head that extend more cranial than normal (Fig. 8-38).

At the completion of the procedure, the joint is lavaged by using a large-bore (4.5-mm) egress cannula through the instrument portal (see Fig. 8-34). Suction is usually applied at some stage to ensure removal of debris. As discussed in Chapter 3, the use of a motorized pump is important in cases involving extensive lesions. With an open large-bore egress cannula in position, fluid flow is usually set at maximal to lavage the joint effectively.

As recorded previously (Bertone & McIlwraith, 1987a), the lesions found at arthroscopy are usually more extensive than they appeared radiographically. In most instances, the cartilaginous changes extend beyond the limits of the subchondral bone abnormalities observed on the radiographs, particularly in the glenoid of the scapula. In some horses in which radiographically the lesion appears limited to the glenoid or humeral head, additional lesions are found arthroscopically on the opposing articular surface. The most common arthroscopic abnormalities

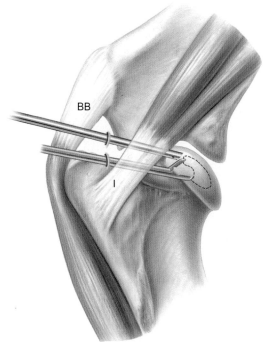

Figure 8-36 Craniolateral approach. Positioning of the arthroscope and the instrument for surgery on lesions of the cranial and lateral aspect of the humeral head.

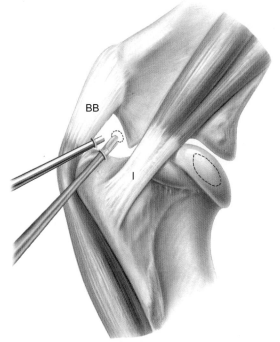

Figure 8-37 Craniolateral approach. Retrieval of a free osteochondral fragment from the cranial cul-de-sac with a Ferris-Smith rongeur introduced through a cranial instrument portal.

of the humeral head are cartilage discoloration with undermining and erosion down to subchondral bone on the caudal aspect of the articular surface (see Figs. 8-24 and 8-25). In some instances, a lesion is not visible initially and probing is required to ascertain the area of undermined cartilage. The most common arthroscopic abnormality in the glenoid is cracked undermined articular cartilage with fissure formation and fibrillation

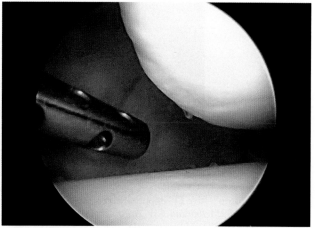

Figure 8-38 Lateral approach. Access to the cranial cul-de-sac using a lateral arthroscope entry 2 cm caudal to the infraspinatus tendon and instruments placed through the portal cranial to the infraspinatus tendon.

(see Figs. 8-26 to 8-30). An additional common finding is friable, defective subchondral bone, and these lesions may extend quite deeply. In most horses, the center of the glenoid cavity is most severely affected. Occasionally, however, lesions extend laterally to the glenoid rim, and the bone of the glenoid rim may also be fragmented (see Fig. 8-30). In other instances, the medial portion of the glenoid is affected. Although a diffuse OCD lesion is the most common finding, a focal subchondral cystic lesion may also be noted. In these cases, cartilage folds and crevices are confined to the immediate area around the opening of the cyst (see Fig. 8-26).

Postoperative Management

Antibiotics are administered perioperatively and for 2 days postoperatively. Phenylbutazone is administered on the day of the operation and for the successive 3 to 5 days. Horses are confined to a stall for 10 days, at which time hand walking commences. The authors usually start with hand walking for 5 minutes per day, with incremental increases of 5 minutes each week to 30 minutes per day. Horses are then turned out for periods of 4 to 12 months before forced exercise begins.

Problems and Complications

It should be reiterated that adequate arthroscopic visualization and surgical manipulation are more difficult in the equine shoulder joint than in most other joints in which arthroscopic surgery is commonly performed. A definite learning curve associated with the technique is noted, and speed and success improve with experience in a series of clinical cases. However, most people experience one or more of the following difficulties and complications.

Arthroscopic Placement in the Joint

Difficulty can be experienced with this step. Accurate placement of the spinal needle, predistention of the joint, and practice alleviate this problem.

Difficulty in Establishing Triangulation

Visualizing the spinal needle is difficult in certain cases due to the depths of the joint from the skin surface, but the severity of this problem decreases with surgical practice. Changes in limb position and difference in the size of the patient can confuse the operator. For most instances in which access to the joint was not achieved initially, the needle was placed too cranial or too proximal, or both. Maintaining the limb in an unsupported, adducted (resting) position facilitates joint entry by widening the lateral aspect of the joint.

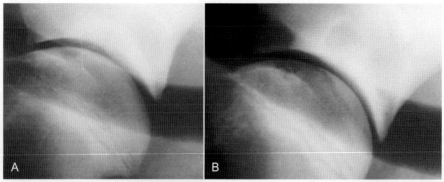

Figure 8-39 Glenoid cyst formation postoperatively. **A,** Preoperative view of a case of glenoid osteochondrosis. **B,** Postoperative (11 months) radiograph reveals cystic lesion of the scapula that developed after surgery. *(From Bertone AL, McIlwraith CW. Arthroscopic surgery for the treatment of osteochondrosis in the equine shoulder joint. Vet Surg 1987;16:303–311, with permission.)*

Extravasation of Fluids

Extravasation occurs in all shoulder arthroscopy cases to some degree. During surgery the amount of fluid in the periarticular tissue increases, causing increased extraarticular pressure. This increase in turn produces technical difficulty, such as collapse of the joint space and decreased ability to see and manipulate instruments. An efficient surgical procedure is critical in operations involving the shoulder. A clear, unobstructed instrument portal, careful control of fluid ingress, and judicious use of self-sealing cannulae also improve surgical procedures in this region.

Difficulty in Reaching Potential Lesions

In some instances, even with the lateral approach to the shoulder, the surgeon may visualize lesions and not be able to reach them with the instruments. These lesions are usually located on the caudomedial surface of the humeral head of adult horses and become even more difficult to access in well-muscled patients. In one series (Bertone & McIlwraith, 1987a), the problem of inadequate instrument length was encountered in three horses. Debridement of these areas can be performed in young horses without difficulty, where traction on the limb opens the joint space and facilitates curettage of the medial surfaces. However, the ideal instrument for reaching medial lesions in larger horses has not been found. Long rongeurs and long right-angled spoon curettes are helpful, but instruments with long shafts and with some curvature can be difficult to find. It is important to advise owners that complete debridement may not be achieved when the horse weighs 500 kg or more. Large accumulations of subcutaneous fluid also contribute to inadequate instrument length, and periodic application of pressure massage to drive fluid out the skin portals often improves access to remote regions of the humeral head.

Damage to Instruments

The instrument portal passes through 6 to 8 cm of muscle before entry into the joint. Manipulation of the instruments is restricted by this muscle mass. The instrument portal can be enlarged, but, in certain instances, the probe or trocar has been bent when removed.

One possible solution to the difficulty sometimes experienced in maintaining separation of the glenoid and humeral head (this distance becomes critical when fluid extravasation inhibits distention) is placing the patient in dorsal recumbency. By suspending the leg and lowering the table slightly, "gravity traction" may provide a less energy-consuming alternative. The authors have not tried this technique, but reports of its utility from other surgeons suggest it is a real option. The possibility of damaging the brachial plexus is one potential hazard. Transient paresthesia in the upper extremities after shoulder arthroscopy involving traction was reported in human patients, and brachial plexus strain versus joint accessibility with different shoulder positions has been described (Klein et al, 1987).

Results

There are two case series describing surgery and postoperative outcome in horses following arthroscopic debridement of OCD lesions. The initial series of 11 horses reported surgical outcome (Bertone & McIlwraith, 1987a). A more recent series described the outcome after conservative and surgical therapy in 32 horses (Jenner, 2008).

In the case series by Bertone & McIlwraith (1987a), leakage of lavage fluid resulted in subcutaneous and intramuscular swelling in all horses, which generally resolved within 7 days. None of the horses were more lame postoperatively, and all improved clinically from within 2 weeks of surgery until the time of follow-up evaluation. Nine of the 11 horses achieved soundness and 8 horses remained sound. Seven horses were completely sound at a jog within 4 months. Five horses were athletically sound and were being shown, ridden, or raced after 5 to 20 months. A sixth horse was sound when beginning race training. A seventh horse was pasture sound and was to begin race training at the time of the report. An eighth horse showed well in halter for 12 months, but shoulder lameness returned. This horse was donated, and a necropsy was performed. The ninth and tenth horses were not completely sound at 11 months. The eleventh horse improved but remained lame and could not be used for athletic performance.

Follow-up radiographic assessment revealed improvement in contour of the humeral head and joint space and more even density of the humeral epiphysis and the glenoid of the scapula in six horses. One of these horses showed marked improvement in subchondral bone density and surface contour of the glenoid cavity. In two of the remaining five horses, the caudal border of the glenoid cavity had remodeled to appear more like the contralateral joint. In the fourth of the six horses, radiographs obtained 1 year later showed a subchondral cystic lesion in the scapula (1.5 cm in diameter) that had not been present previously (Fig. 8-39). However, this horse was athletically sound. The contour of the glenoid articular surface and its caudal border was smoother postoperatively, and the subchondral osteosclerosis was reduced in thickness. In the fifth horse in this group, an osteophyte on the humeral head had enlarged, but improvement was noted in joint contour of both the humeral head and glenoid cavity (Fig. 8-40). Radiographs obtained from one of the two horses that improved but were still lame showed no improvement in the glenoid lesion radiographically. In the horse where euthanasia was chosen when it deteriorated clinically, the humeral epiphysis was severely distorted with a defect in the articular surface contour, a subchondral cystic lesion, and a small intraarticular fracture of the cranial margin of the glenoid cavity.

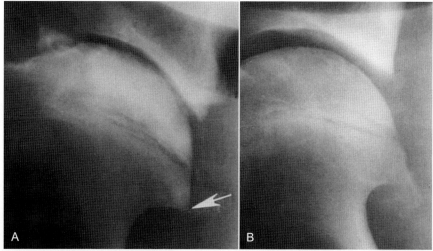

Figure 8-40 Humeral head recontouring postoperatively. Preoperative **(A)** and follow-up **(B)** radiographs of a case of humeral head osteochondrosis reveal remodeling of the humeral head and glenoid cavity with improvement in joint contour after 11 months. The osteophyte on the humerus *(arrow)* is larger. *(From Bertone AL, McIlwraith CW. Arthroscopic surgery for the treatment of osteochondrosis in the equine shoulder joint. Vet Surg 16:303–311, 1987, with permission.)*

In summary, all 11 horses improved clinically. Soundness was achieved in 9 horses, and 5 of 11 horses have been used athletically. Two horses did not become sound. One of these horses was young but had extensive lesions of the glenoid cavity and humeral head; a large osteophyte also developed. The other horse was 4 years of age at the time of surgical intervention and did show some clinical but no radiographic improvement. One horse developed severe degenerative changes in the joint after being sound for 8 months. It seems that considerable healing response can be obtained if surgical treatment occurs in a timely fashion.

Hand curettage was satisfactory for treating most lesions, but the motorized resectors and burr provided the most efficient debridement of articular cartilage and subchondral bone in both the scapula and humerus, and it avoided the potential difficulties associated with hand curettage. Osteochondrotic lesions of the humeral head were the easiest to debride, especially in horses that were yearlings or younger, because they had less muscle mass and more flexible periarticular structures. However, the lesions were accessible even in older horses when the joint was distracted. Traction is extremely important for access to extensive scapular lesions, but arthroscopic surgery in the treatment of these lesions is recommended only for surgeons with considerable experience with this technique.

Euthanasia was the eventual outcome after surgery for four horses in the Bertone and McIlwraith (1987a) study. The quality of the repaired tissue varied. From necropsy findings in three cases in which glenoid lesions were debrided, it seemed these lesions did not heal as well as similar lesions of the humeral head. The defects were filled with mixtures of fibrous tissue and fibrocartilage. In addition, cystic lesions in the bone also developed.

The development of cystic lesions in the subchondral bone of the glenoid subsequent to surgery is an interesting finding. This may be a sequel to untreated OCD or to debridement in which the articular cartilage is removed down to subchondral bone. Subchondral bone cystic lesions can form in normal joints if full-thickness articular cartilage defects are created surgically in weight-bearing areas (Kold et al, 1986). These lesions can develop within 6 months, and some authors state that intraarticular synovial fluid pressure may exceed subchondral bone pressure in weight-bearing areas, contributing to expansion of the cystic cavity in the bone (Landells, 1953).

The radiographic evidence of remodeling of the glenoid cavity and humeral head in six horses younger than 1 year of age may help explain the clinical improvement in severe cases that would otherwise have carried a less favorable prognosis. Since this published series, the authors have performed

surgery on horses with extensive involvement of the glenoid and humeral head and have achieved considerable levels of improvement. In general, extensive and opposing lesions of the glenoid and humeral head leave inadequate cartilage to avoid further joint deterioration and collapse, and careful case selection to avoid operating on these types of lesions usually needs high detail preoperative radiographs or even arthrography. Additionally, older horses may have a poor prognosis because cartilage remodeling decreases with advancing age. A more recent survey of 70 cases of one author (C.W.M.) reveals an overall success rate for return to athletic activity of 45%.

A more recent published series of shoulder OC cases treated surgically or conservatively has been published (Jenner et al, 2008). These horses were all younger than 2 years of age and included 16 of 32 with bilaterally affected shoulders. Nineteen of the 32 horses were operated and the remainder were continued to be treated conservatively. The overall outcome with or without surgery was considered poor. Only 4 of the 26 potential racehorses started a race (15.4%). However, 4 of the 6 nonracehorses (67%) did become sound for their intended use. There was no significant effect of unilateral or bilateral limb involvement, of the type of treatment used, or in the severity of the preoperative radiographic lesions. Conversely, the authors did identify a high positive correlation between severe lesions on the humerus and concurrent severe lesions on the glenoid.

ARTHROSCOPIC SURGERY FOR OTHER CLINICAL ENTITIES IN THE SHOULDER
Osteoarthritis

The authors have been involved in 10 cases in which the horse was considered to have degenerative articular cartilage lesions of the humeral head that differed from the typical cases of OCD. In each instance, the horse was mature and involved in athletic activity when the problem developed. The lesions manifested arthroscopically as areas of fibrillation and deeper bone involvement and were treated with debridement. Some shoulder cases in mature horses have cystic and wider lucent lesions on the humeral head, which generally result in radiographic evidence of early arthritis, including osteophytes on the glenoid perimeter (Fig. 8-41).

Arthroscopic assessment of early OA and OA related to cystic lesions of the glenoid have become a significant reason for arthroscopic exploration and staging. Many cases are mature horses that developed a lameness that is localized to the shoulder joint by intraarticular anesthesia. Many of these cases have

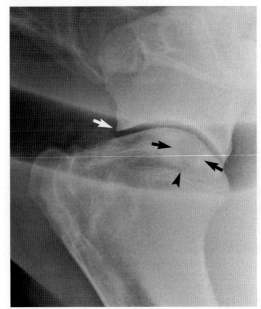

Figure 8-41 Humeral head subchondral bone cyst with osteoarthritis. Radiograph of a shoulder joint from a mature event horse with a subchondral lucency in the humeral head *(black arrows)* and secondary osteophyte development *(white arrow)* indicating early osteoarthritis.

subtle radiographic changes, similar to those described in the literature (Doyle and White, 2000). Scintigraphic evaluation is commonly required to assist in localizing the principal region of lameness within the shoulder (Fig. 8-42). With the availability of more sensitive digital radiographs, more discrete lesions can occasionally be seen. In mature horses the majority of the lesions involve shallow cystic defects in the center of the glenoid cavity and mild to moderate osteophyte formation on the cranial and caudal regions of the scapula (see Fig. 8-42). Exploratory arthroscopy is generally indicated if the radiographic extent of osteoarthritis is not severe. In a series of 15 horses with unilateral shoulder disease examined by arthroscopy (Doyle and White, 2000), 12 of the 15 affected horses had a narrow upright foot shape as a result of the chronic lameness. Nine of the 10 responded positively to intraarticular anesthesia, and scintigraphic evaluation was useful to detect the lesions in 4 of 6 horses where it was performed. Radiographic changes were subtle and included glenoid sclerosis, focal glenoid lysis, small glenoid cysts, and alterations in the humeral head contour. At surgery, arthroscopic evaluation identified clefts in the glenoid cartilage, glenoid cysts, a humeral head cyst, fibrillation of the humeral head cartilage, cartilage fragmentation, or a nondisplaced fracture of the humeral head. The outcome after surgery was apparently quite good, with 12 of the 15 horses returning to their previous level of performance. This case series indicates the value of arthroscopy to confirm the lesion, and the outcome data would suggest that debridement of the affected lesions is quite effective in returning horses to function.

The choice of arthroscopic approach in mature horses with shoulder disease varies depending on the radiographic and scintigraphic evidence of lesion location within the shoulder. The most versatile entry for complete examination is the lateral approach, which allows more thorough assessment of the entire humeral head. The arthroscope is inserted 1 to 2 cm caudal to the infraspinatus tendon as described previously. Some form of traction is vital for adequate separation of the humeral head and glenoid cavity (Fig. 8-43). Examination of the humeral head and glenoid surfaces is then performed. Particular attention to cartilage on the medial aspects of the humeral head and the central portions of the glenoid cavity should be done while the joint distension and traction

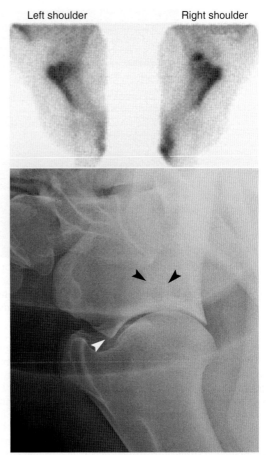

Left shoulder   Right shoulder

Figure 8-42 Glenoid cavity subchondral bone cyst with osteoarthritis. Scintigraphic appearance of central glenoid lesion in an 8-year-old warmblood jumping horse (top). Radiographs from the same horse (lower) showing radiographic evidence of a small glenoid cyst in the center of the glenoid *(black arrowheads)* in the same position as that identified on nuclear scintigraphy. Osteophytes *(white arrowhead)* indicate secondary osteoarthritis has developed.

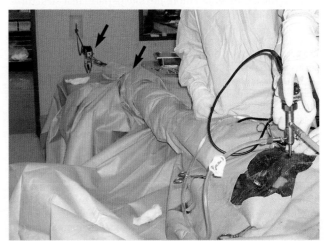

Figure 8-43 Axial traction of the shoulder joint in mature horses can be provided by traction devices *(arrows)* attached to the wall. Adequate stabilization of the horse on the surgery table is required to avoid pulling the horse onto the edge of the table.

provides adequate separation. In large horses, the arthroscope may be inserted to its fullest extent during this exploration. Similarly, instruments need to be long to gain access to lesions located deeper within the joint (Fig. 8-44). An instrument portal is then developed 3 to 4 cm caudal to the arthroscope

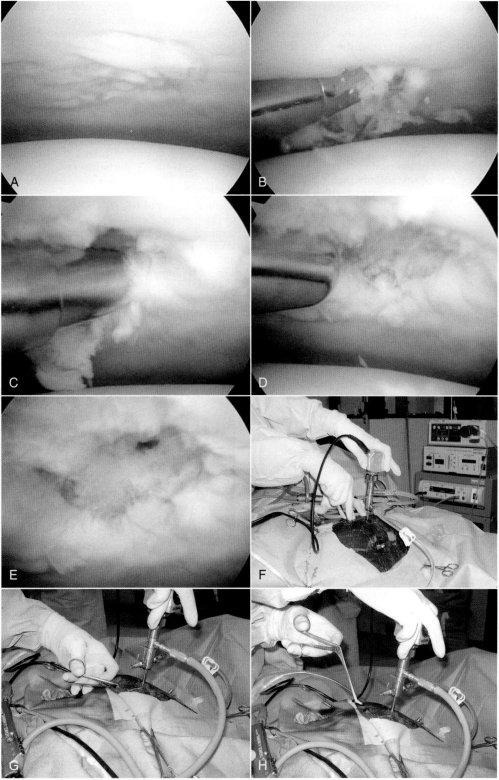

Figure 8-44 Glenoid cavity subchondral bone cyst and osteoarthritis. **A,** Surgical exploration of a shoulder joint in an adult event horse showing cartilage fibrillation and cracking overlying a subchondral cystic defect in the center of the glenoid cavity. **B,** Probing of this defect and debridement remove the necrotic bone. **C,** A curved rotatable shaver allows debridement and evacuation of necrotic tissue. **D,** Residual yellow or brown regions indicate necrotic bone, which must be debrided to its fullest extent. **E,** Final debridement of cartilage and bone show opening into deeper cystic structure, which is debrided with curved spinal needles, 90-degree 2-0 or 3-0 spoon curettes, and small ethmoid or patellar forceps. The defect was then filled with bone marrow aspirate concentrate. **F,** In large mature horses, the arthroscope and long spoon curettes are inserted almost their complete length. **G** and **H,** Many curved small forceps are also working at their maximal depth.

entry and 1 to 2 cm more distal, based on previous spinal needle insertion that appropriately targets the lesion. This incision should be well developed with the use of the blunt obturator or by insertion of a self-sealing cannula (see Chapter 2). Debridement of lesions on the glenoid cavity requires long instruments and cystic lesions in this region can be a particular challenge. Use of a 90-degree angled curette, small curved mosquito hemostat, and pointed up-biting patella forceps or ethmoid forceps are useful (Fig. 8-45). Motorized equipment with curvature on the distal extremity assists in debridement of glenoid lesions. The cartilage defects are then debrided to leave vertical walls to assist in healing. In middle-aged horses the use of biologics to improve the quality of cartilage repair has also been used by one of the authors (A.J.N.). While a cultured mesenchymal stem cell graft secured with a clottable

biologic such as platelet rich plasma is preferable, these are not always available within the time constraints of the diagnosis to surgery interval. In this circumstance use of a bone marrow aspirate concentrate (BMAC) has been useful. Bone marrow can be harvested from the proximal humerus (Fig. 8-46) and either used by direct injection to clot in the cartilage defect or centrifuged to provide BMAC. Injection into the depths of the glenoid region has required the use of a flexible Teflon catheter to provide access into the depths of debrided subchondral cysts in the glenoid. Resolution of radiographic lesions generally occurs, and the authors' experience is similar to that of Doyle and White (2000), with the majority of these horses returning to athletic performance.

Articular Fracture

Some fractures of the glenoid and portions of the perimeter of the humeral head can lead to severe lameness and require removal of fragments to improve the outcome. Fragmentation of the cranial or caudal glenoid rim can be removed arthroscopically, while larger fractures generally require fixation and compression by lag screw insertion. Extensive craniocaudally oriented fractures of the glenoid cavity, which extend proximally to involve the neck of the scapula, may require both arthroscopic debridement and small fragment removal, followed by screw compression. These types of fracture can appear normal on lateromedial radiographs, largely because of the minimal craniocaudal displacement of the fracture.

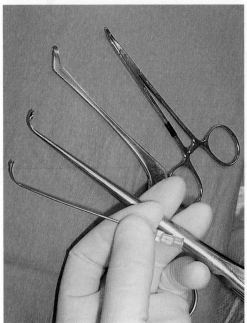

Figure 8-45 Customized instruments for identification, debridement, and packing of glenoid cysts. From top to bottom, curved hemostat, up-biting patellar forcep, ultra bent 2-0 spoon curette, and 90-degree angled spinal needle.

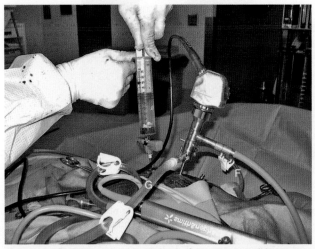

Figure 8-46 Bone marrow aspirate from proximal humerus. Harvest of bone marrow from the proximal humerus for development of bone marrow aspirate concentrate or direct use for packing of the debrided cyst.

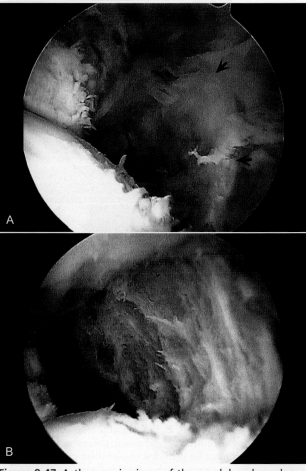

Figure 8-47 Arthroscopic views of the caudal and caudomedial portions of the shoulder of a chronic septic joint viewed using the lateral approach to the shoulder. A, Synovial proliferation and fibrinous deposits are evident *(arrows)*. **B,** After synovectomy the fibrous joint capsule is partially exposed.

Septic Arthritis/Osteomyelitis

Foals and weanlings are predisposed to septic physitis and osteomyelitis, which can seed a joint and necessitate further debridement. Routine arthroscopy of the shoulder for fibrinectomy and removal of inspissated debris are required for resolution in advanced cases. Lateral or cranial arthroscopic approaches provide visualization of the joint surfaces sufficient to allow debridement of synovial membrane and cartilage. The large caudal and cranial cul-de-sacs need particularly aggressive lavage and manual fibrin removal to reduce the bacterial load (Fig. 8-47). Debridement of deeper lesions involving cartilage and subchondral bone may occasionally be necessary. Placing ingress drains for antibiotic delivery can also improve the outcome. Additional detail is provided in Chapter 14.

REFERENCES

Bertone AL, McIlwraith CW: Arthroscopic surgery for the treatment of osteochondrosis in the equine shoulder joint, *Vet Surg* 16(4):303–311, 1987a.

Bertone AL, McIlwraith CW: Arthroscopic surgical approaches and intraarticular anatomy of the equine shoulder joint, *Vet Surg* 16:312–317, 1987b.

Bhatia S, Su A, Lin EC, Chalmers B, Ellman M, Cole BJ, Verma NN: Surgical treatment options for the young and active middle aged patient with glenohumeral arthritis, *Adv Orthop.* 843–846, 2012.

Cofield RH: Arthroscopy of the shoulder, *Mayo Clin Proc* 58:501–508, 1983.

DeBowes RM, Wagner PC, Grant BD: Surgical approach to the equine scapulohumeral joint through a longitudinal infraspinatus tenotomy, *Vet Surg* 11:125–128, 1982.

Doyle PS, White NA: Diagnostic findings and prognosis following arthroscopic treatment of subtle osteochondral lesions in the shoulder joint of horses: 15 cases (1996-1999), *J Am Vet Med Assoc* 217:1878–1882, 2000.

Jenner F, Ross MW, Martin BB, Richardson DW: Scapulohumeral osteochondrosis. A retrospective study of 32 horses, *Vet Comp Orthop Trauamatol* 21:406–412, 2008.

Johnson LL: *Arthroscopic surgery principles and practice*, ed 3, St. Louis, 1986, Mosby.

Klein AH, France JC, Mutschler TA, Fu FH: Measurement of brachial plexus strain in arthroscopy of the shoulder, *Arthroscopy* 3:45–52, 1987.

Kold SE, Hickman J, Melsen F: An experimental study of the healing process of equine chondral and osteochondral defects, *Equine Vet J* 18:18–24, 1986.

Landells JW: The bone cysts of osteoarthritis, *J Bone Joint Surg Br*, 35-B:643–649, 1953.

Mason TA, Maclean AA: Osteochondrosis dissecans of the head of the humerus in two foals, *Equine Vet J* 9(4):189–191, 1977.

Meagher DM, Pool RR, O'Brien TR: Osteochondritis of the shoulder joint in the horse, *Proc Am Assoc Equine Prac* 19:247–256, 1975.

Nixon AJ: Diagnostic and operative arthroscopy of the equine shoulder joint, *Vet Surg* 15:129, 1986.

Nixon AJ: Diagnostic and surgical arthroscopy of the equine shoulder joint, *Vet Surg* 16:44–52, 1987.

Nixon AJ, Spencer CP: Arthrography of the equine shoulder joint, *Equine Vet J* 22(2):107–113A, 1990.

Nixon AJ, Stashak TS, et al.: A muscle separating approach to the equine shoulder joint for the treatment of osteochondritis dissecans, *Vet Surg* 13:247–256, 1984.

Nyack B, Morgan JP, et al.: Osteochondrosis of the shoulder joint of the horse, *Cornell Vet* 71:149–163, 1981.

Rose JA, Sande RD, Rose EM: Results of conservative management of osteochondrosis in the horse, *Proc 31st Annual Conv AAEP*, 1986.

Schmidt GR, Dueland R, Vaughan JT: Osteochondrosis dissecans of the equine shoulder joint, *Vet Med/Small An Clin* 70:542–547, 1975.

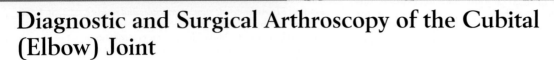

CHAPTER 9

Diagnostic and Surgical Arthroscopy of the Cubital (Elbow) Joint

INTRODUCTION

Although the elbow is not frequently a cause of lameness in the horse, it does occasionally develop intraarticular fragmentation, osteochondrosis and osteochondritis dissecans (OCD), osteoarthritis (OA), and secondary septic arthritis from adjacent physeal sepsis or direct penetrating injury. Other than OCD, there are no reports in the literature of case series involving any of these conditions in the elbow, although there are several case reports to provide clinical and radiographic perspective. The degree of lameness is largely dictated by the extent of derangement of the articular surface, except in the case of septic arthritis where the lameness is generally more profound. These surgical diseases are uncommon in the elbow joint of horses but arise with sufficient frequency to warrant techniques for arthroscopic surgery of the various pouches of the elbow joint. Subchondral cystic lesions of the medial humeral condyle or medial portion of the proximal radius have been described in two case series, one involving six horses (Bertone et al, 1986) and a second describing seven horses (Hopen et al, 1992). These studies indicate that some lesions can be conservatively treated, including cystic lesions of the proximal portion of the radius. Other lesions, including OCD of the humeral condyles, may be more appropriately treated by surgical debridement.

Because the elbow is so complex, one arthroscopic approach does not allow access to all relevant regions. However, a series of arthroscopic techniques provide access to the cranial portions of the humeral condyles using a craniolateral approach, to the caudal portions of the humeral condyles using a caudomedial approach, and to the proximal regions of both condyles and to the anconeal process of the ulna using a caudoproximal approach via the olecranon pouch. This chapter describes all three approaches. The relevant anatomy and choices for arthroscopic surgical approach to the equine elbow have been recently reviewed (Nixon, 2012). The complexity of periarticular neurovascular structures and inherent risks of elbow arthroscopy are well known in humans (Baker & Jones 1999; Lynch et al, 1986; Thomas et al, 1987), and similar risks are present with approaches to the elbow in the horse (Nixon, 1990). Overall, arthroscopic access to the cranial regions of the elbow in man and horses is relatively simple, while the caudal compartments are more challenging, with increased risk to adjacent neurovascular structures (Baker & Jones, 1999; Nixon, 1990; Poehling & Ekman, 1994).

ANATOMY

The elbow joint of the horse is a complex articulation of the humerus, radius, and ulna. All three bones are intimately connected by substantial collateral ligaments. As a result, distraction of the humeroradial articulation and humeroulnar articulation results in little separation of the articular surfaces and therefore limited access to regions predisposed to disease, particularly the proximal surface of the radius. For the humeral condyles, this can be overcome to some extent by the large range of motion of the elbow, allowing articular surfaces to be exposed by flexion or extension. The tight articulation essentially divides the elbow to a cranial joint pouch, a limited caudal joint pouch, and a large proximocaudal joint pouch surrounding the anconeal process.

Approaches to the cranial portion of the elbow joint place small terminal branches of the radial nerve at risk as they arborize and terminate in the antebrachial extensor muscle bellies. The arthroscope entry avoids these branches; however, instrument access cranially, through the muscle bellies, may affect several small branches of the radial nerve. No clinical repercussions, including extensor muscle dysfunction, have been recognized, although transient extensor paresis has been seen in one case where intraarticular Marcaine® (bupivacaine) leaked out of the instrument portal at the commencement of surgery. Recovery of function took several hours, and there was no long-term impact.

The caudomedial approach to the elbow joint penetrates between the muscle bellies of the flexor carpi radialis and flexor carpi ulnaris, and inadvertent entry caudal to the flexor carpi ulnaris places the arthroscope close to the ulnar nerve coursing over the caudomedial aspect of the humerus and continuing down the medial aspect of the ulna. Similarly, inadvertent entry to the elbow joint cranial to the flexor carpi radialis muscle belly places the median nerve at risk. During the caudomedial approach to the elbow, the instrument entry often penetrates through the flexor carpi ulnaris muscle belly, but also without repercussion. The caudal extremity of this approach may also affect portions of the ulnar nerve. The approach to the olecranon pouch of the elbow penetrates the distal terminal portions of the triceps musculature or tendon of insertion; however, no significant neurovascular structures are at risk using this approach.

ARTHROSCOPIC APPROACHES TO THE ELBOW JOINT

Positioning

Positioning for arthroscopy of the elbow is dictated by the site of surgical disease. Only dorsal recumbency will allow simultaneous access to all three pouches of the elbow joint. However, this can increase the degree of difficulty in arthroscopic access to the caudoproximal olecranon pouch. Additionally, in adults the surgeon has to reach across the horse from the opposite side of the surgery table to access the caudomedial portal. This can be taxing and may limit access to lesions on the humeral condyles. Conversely, in foals it is quite easy and dorsal recumbency works well for access to all three portals in these younger animals (Fig. 9-1). For access to specific disease conditions involving the cranial, caudal, or caudoproximal region of the elbow, lateral recumbency is preferred. The cranial pouch and caudoproximal pouch of the elbow can be accessed with the affected limb uppermost (Fig. 9-2), whereas access to the caudomedial pouch requires the affected limb to be placed down on the surgery table. Repositioning the horse from affected limb down to affected limb uppermost during the surgical procedure is another possibility, although this delays the surgical process, is manpower demanding, and risks breaks in sterile procedures.

Craniolateral Approach to the Elbow

The horse is positioned in lateral recumbency so that the limb can be manipulated into extension and flexion of the elbow joint (see Fig. 9-2). After preparation and draping, the

292

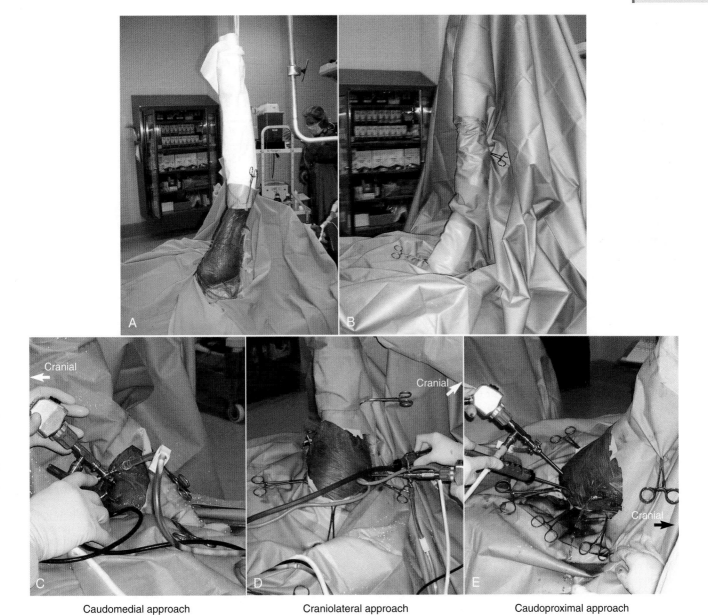

Caudomedial approach   Craniolateral approach   Caudoproximal approach

Figure 9-1 Positioning of foal in dorsal recumbency allows access to all compartments of the elbow joint using all three of the described approaches. **A,** Suspending the limb allows circumferential draping. **B,** Impervious drapes allow access for all three approaches after cutting appropriate windows. **C,** Caudomedial approach while reaching across the foal's sternum to the medial antebrachium. Note the distal to proximal entry angle of the arthroscope. A probe has been introduced through the portal several centimeters proximal and caudal to the arthroscope. **D,** An egress remains in the caudomedial portal, and the craniolateral approach has been performed with the operator standing alongside the affected limb. **E,** Caudoproximal arthroscope and instrument entry completes the examination routine. An egress remains in the craniolateral approach, and both arthroscope and shaver are introduced cranial to the olecranon process.

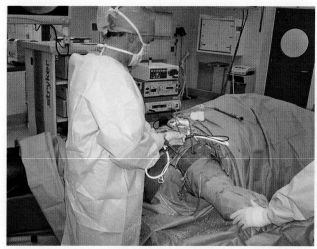

Figure 9-2 Lateral positioning is preferred in adults for the craniolateral and caudoproximal approaches. Illustration shows the craniolateral arthroscope and large bore (stifle) cannula being used to flush debris from the cranial compartment of the elbow after fracture removal.

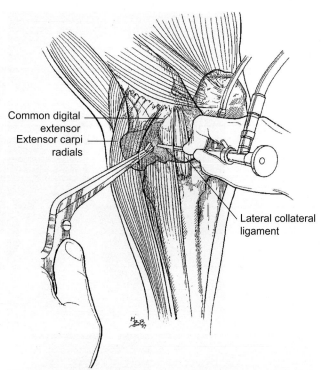

Figure 9-3 Arthroscopic technique for access to the cranial pouch of the elbow joint. Arthroscope entry is made in the triangle formed by the craniolateral curvature of the lateral condyle of the humerus, the proximal perimeter of the craniolateral surface of the radius, and the caudal border of the muscle belly of the common digital extensor tendon. Instrument entry can be made between the muscle bellies of the common digital extensor and extensor carpi radialis muscles (*From Nixon AJ. Arthroscopic approaches and intraarticular anatomy of the equine elbow.* Vet Surg 1990;19:93–101.)

elbow joint is distended through the cranial pouch with 40 to 60 mL of lactated Ringer solution. Addition of long-acting local anesthetic to the initial distending medium should be avoided to limit possible anesthesia of the radial nerve arborization to the antebrachial extensor muscles. The cranial perimeter of the humeroradial articulation is palpated cranial to the lateral collateral ligament, and a 5-mm stab incision made approximately 2 to 3 cm cranial to this palpable collateral ligament border. The muscle belly of the common digital extensor forms a cranial limit to the triangular target area for access of the arthroscope. If the entry is made too close to the cranial palpable border of the lateral humeral condyle, manipulation within the cranial pouch of the elbow becomes more difficult. The arthroscope sleeve is inserted across the cranial pouch of the elbow joint, and the obturator exchanged for the forward oblique-viewing arthroscope (Fig. 9-3). The cranial articular surfaces and cranial joint pouch of the elbow can then be examined (Fig. 9-4). The arthroscope is inserted as deeply as possible to examine the craniomedial margins of the radius and humerus. A 70-degree arthroscope may be useful in this region; however, it is not essential. Withdrawal of the arthroscope identifies the medial followed by the lateral condyles of the humerus, with a large synovial fossa interposed between the two (see Fig. 9-4). Further withdrawal of the arthroscope reveals the lateral portion of the humeroradial articulation and the lateral collateral ligament. The cranial joint pouch of the elbow is voluminous and easily examined.

An instrument portal can be made cranial to the arthroscope entry, after placing a 7.5-cm × 18-gauge spinal needle. This portal usually penetrates between the antebrachial extensor muscle bellies, generally where a shallow division can be palpated between the extensor carpi radialis and common digital extensor muscles. The midcranial region should be avoided to minimize potential damage to the transverse cubital artery. For lesions involving the craniolateral extremity of the radius or lateral humeral condyle, the arthroscope and instrument entry portal can be exchanged to provide instrument access to the lateral portions of the articular perimeter. Following completion of the procedure, fluid is expressed from the joint and the skin incisions are closed with interrupted sutures.

Caudomedial Approach to the Elbow Joint

The horse is positioned in lateral recumbency with the affected limb down, for access to the medial portion of the elbow joint.

Dorsal positioning can be used if access to the other elbow joint pouches is expected, as previously described. After preparation and draping, the site for arthroscope entry is identified by systematically palpating from cranial to caudal to identify the medial collateral ligament, the depression between the caudal aspect of the radius and the muscle belly of the flexor carpi radialis, and, finally, the division formed by the approximation of flexor carpi radialis and flexor carpi ulnaris muscle bellies. A needle is inserted to identify the humeroradial articulation, and a point 2 to 3 cm distal to this articular level and between the muscle bellies of the flexor carpi radialis and flexor carpi ulnaris is identified. The palpable division between these muscle bellies is identified more easily at the midradius level, and the separation tracked proximally to the point 2 to 3 cm distal to the level of the humeroradial articulation. The palpable landmarks for arthroscope entry tend to be obscured over the elbow by the overlying superficial pectoral muscles and antebrachial fascia. Insertion of the arthroscope proximal to the level of the humeroradial articulation places the ulnar neurovascular structures at risk, particularly if a second entry for instruments is then made caudal to the flexor carpi ulnaris muscle belly.

After insertion of the needle to the caudomedial aspect of the joint, the elbow is distended with 60 mL of lactated Ringer's solution and a 5-mm skin incision made for entry of the arthroscope sleeve and obturator (Fig. 9-5). The arthroscope sleeve with obturator in place is advanced proximally in an oblique direction to enter the caudomedial aspect of the elbow joint pouch. When cartilage or bone is encountered and joint fluid is returned through the egress outlets on the arthroscope sleeve, the conical obturator is replaced by the arthroscope. In many instances the arthroscope sleeve can be inserted to its limit, as it penetrates into the caudal cul-de-sac

In the figure labels:
Common digital extensor
Extensor carpi radialis
Lateral collateral ligament

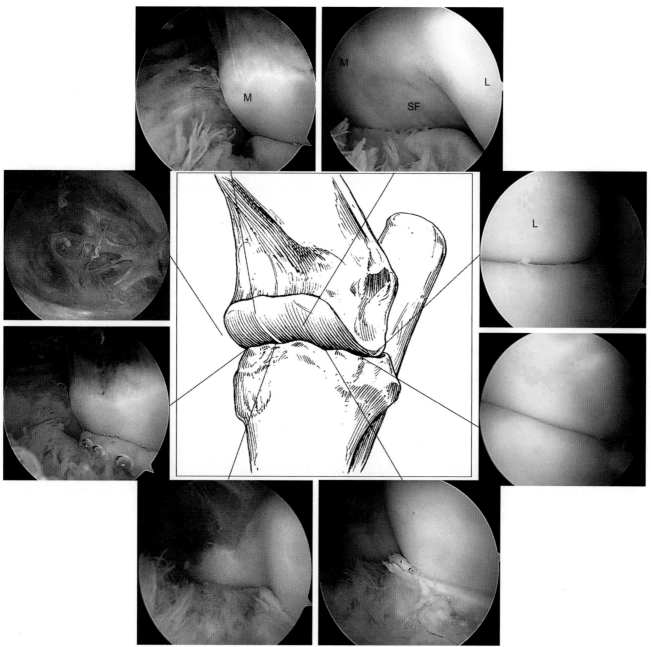

Figure 9-4 Composite illustration showing the visible regions of the cranial pouch of the elbow joint. The cranial portions of the lateral *(L)* and medial *(M)* condyles of the humerus are readily examined, including the voluminous cul-de-sacs of the cranial joint pouch. The humeral surface is interrupted at the junction of lateral and medial condyles by the synovial fossa *(SF)*. The proximal aspect of the radius is also visible, although none of the capitular fovea of the radius can be accessed.

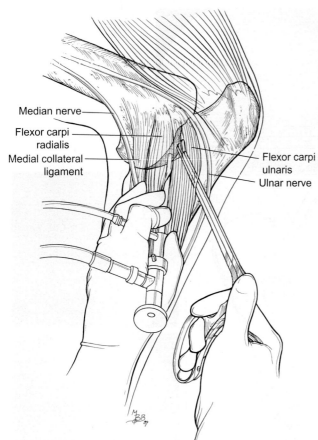

Median nerve

Flexor carpi radialis

Medial collateral ligament

Flexor carpi ulnaris

Ulnar nerve

Figure 9-5 Arthroscopic technique for access to the caudo-medial pouch of the elbow joint. The arthroscope portal is made between the muscle bellies of the flexor carpi radialis and flexor carpi ulnaris muscles, 2 to 3 cm distal to the level of the humeroradial articulation. The arthroscope then penetrates the caudomedial joint pouch of the elbow obliquely, allowing better visualization of the caudal surfaces of the humeral condyles. Instrument entry is made 2 to 3 cm proximal and caudal to the arthroscope entry, depending on the path defined by needle insertion. *(From Nixon AJ. Arthroscopic approaches and intraarticular anatomy of the equine elbow. Vet Surg 1990;19:93–101.)*

of the elbow and farther into the caudoproximal cul-de-sac surrounding the anconeal process. A standard forward oblique arthroscope is inserted, and the caudal regions of the elbow are examined. The medial humeral condyle is readily visible (Fig. 9-6). The caudal perimeter of the humeroradial articulation is a convenient landmark to commence examination of the joint (see Fig. 9-6). The articular surfaces of the humeral condyles, particularly the medial condyle, are readily evaluated. Flexion of the elbow improves the exposure of the caudal portions of the humeral condyles. Portions of the weight-bearing articular surface of the radius can be seen, but the arthroscope cannot be advanced between the radius and humerus (see Fig. 9-6). Distraction of the medial aspect of the humeroradial joint by abduction of the limb is made easier by positioning the horse in lateral rather than dorsal recumbency. Manipulating the tip of the arthroscope caudally exposes the trochlear notch of the ulna and the opposing articular surface of the humeral condyles (see Fig. 9-6). Further caudally, the intrusion of the medial epicondyle of the humerus and the proximal regions of the trochlear notch of the ulna are evident (see Fig. 9-6). The large tendon of origin of the humeral head of the deep digital flexor tendon is also visible. The space between the trochlear notch of the ulna and this mobile tendon provides access to

the caudoproximal cul-de-sac of the elbow. However, for ease of surgical manipulation, the caudoproximal approach to this cul-de-sac using a lateral access technique is recommended (described below).

Instrument entry portals are made through the muscle belly of the flexor carpi ulnaris, caudal to the arthroscope portal. The most suitable path for instrument entry is selected after inserting a 7.5-cm-long spinal needle. This provides ready access to the medial condyle and medial aspects of the lateral condyle. The central regions of the capitular fovea of the radius cannot be accessed surgically.

Caudoproximal Approach to the Elbow Joint

The voluminous caudoproximal pouch of the elbow joint can be accessed arthroscopically using approaches similar to those described for arthrocentesis of the elbow (Stashak, 1987). This approach is best done with the horse in lateral recumbency with the limb free to be manipulated through flexion and extension. Dorsal recumbency can suffice when approaches to all compartments are anticipated. However, manipulation of instruments can be limited. The joint is distended with 60 to 80 mL of lactated Ringer solution using a 7.5-cm spinal needle inserted over the lateral epicondyle to enter the lateral portion of the caudoproximal cul-de-sac of the joint. Needle entry is approximately level with the point of the elbow and caudal to the palpable lateral epicondyle of the humerus. The spinal needle is angled distally and cranially to target the anconeal process of the ulna. Following removal of the needle, the skin incision for arthroscope entry is made in a similar location and the arthroscope sleeve and conical obturator inserted, angling distally and cranially to contact the articular surface of the anconeal process (Fig. 9-7). The obturator is then exchanged for the arthroscope, allowing examination of the voluminous caudoproximal joint pouch (Fig. 9-8). The anconeal process and proximal portions of the humeral condyles are readily visible (see Fig. 9-8). Flexion of the elbow exposes the entire caudal one half of the humeral condyles for surgical procedures. The arthroscope can be manipulated distally along the medial aspect of the ulna junction with the medial surface of the humerus to insert along the ulna into the caudomedial pouch of the elbow. Visualization of the medial condyle and radius is not as clear as that obtained with the direct caudomedial approach. Instrument entry for access to lesions is then made by preplacing a 7.5-cm spinal needle to give direct access to lesions on the anconeal process or humeral condyles. This entry usually perforates terminal portions of the triceps musculature and occasionally the tendon of insertion on the olecranon. Hand instruments and motorized burrs can be inserted for surgical debridement.

▶ ARTHROSCOPIC SURGERY OF THE ELBOW JOINT

Fractures of the Craniolateral Portion of the Humerus

The craniolateral portion of the distal humerus, particularly the lateral portion of the humeral condyle, is exposed to external impact injury, which can dislodge intraarticular osteochondral fragments (Fig. 9-9). In some cases, an open wound with joint penetration also results in a septic elbow joint, which complicates treatment. Removal of these fragments is generally simple using the craniolateral arthroscopic access. After examination of the remainder of the cranial aspect of the elbow joint, the arthroscope and instrument portals are reversed, placing the arthroscope through an instrument portal approximately between the muscle bellies of the extensor carpi radialis and common digital extensor. This leaves the more lateral portal for rongeur entry for fracture removal.

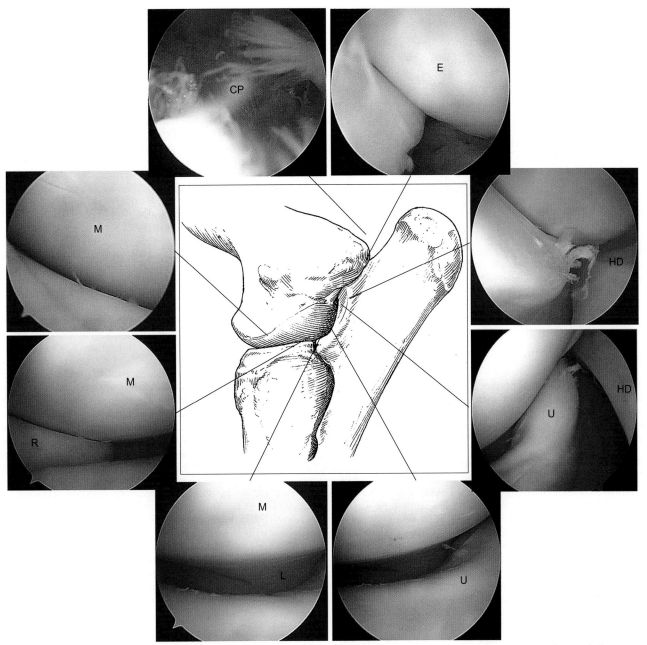

Figure 9-6 Composite of arthroscopic views of the caudomedial portions of the elbow joint. The medial humeral condyle *(M)* is easily examined over its caudal one-half, the medial aspect of the lateral humeral condyle *(L)* can be assessed, and the proximal portion *(R)* of the radius (capitular fovea) can be viewed but not accessed by instruments. Repositioning the arthroscope more proximal exposes the trochlear notch of the ulna *(U)*. The tendinous origin of the humeral head of the deep digital flexor muscle *(HD)* is always evident, and advancing the arthroscope beside this tendon and the medial humeral epicondyle *(E)* frequently allows entry to the spacious caudoproximal joint pouch of the elbow *(CP)*.

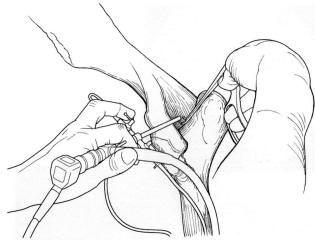

Figure 9-7 Arthroscopic technique for access to the caudo-proximal (olecranon) pouch of the elbow joint. The arthroscope portal is made over the lateral side of the elbow, between the lateral epicondyle of the humerus and the prominence of the proximal aspect of the olecranon. The arthroscope is angled cranially and distally to enter the elbow joint pouch over the anconeal process.

Debridement of the subchondral bed is routine, and debris can be flushed from the joint with a large egress cannula. The extent of articular involvement usually defines the expected outcome, although the predisposed area for impact fracture is generally 2 to 4 cm in length.

Fracture of the Cranial Aspect of the Radius

The cranial and craniolateral portion of the proximal radius is exposed to joint trauma in much the same way as the lateral portion of the humeral condyle. Fractures tend to be chronic by the time a diagnosis is established, which can also result in early OA. Radiographs generally define the fracture (Fig. 9-10). Some fractures also result in concurrent impact trauma to the humeral condyles, and others can result in erosion of the cartilage surface over the humeral condyle as a result of intrusion of the fracture of the radius into the joint space. Removal of osteochondral fragments from the cranial aspect of the radius uses similar approaches to those involving the cranial and craniolateral aspect of the humerus. The craniolateral arthroscopic access is the usual start point; instrument entry through the antebrachial musculature is then accomplished to allow probing and separation of the fracture fragment. Retrieval can then be accomplished easily using rongeurs. Most fractures are relatively chronic and further debridement of bony callus and secondary osteophytes is done using motorized equipment (see Fig. 9-10). At the end of the procedure, debris is flushed from the joint and intraoperative radiographs are obtained to ensure complete removal of the fracture fragment. The few cases in which fracture has involved the small, intraarticular portion of the radius have recovered from the presenting lameness within several months of surgical removal. Follow-up treatment of the joint with biological therapy, such as platelet rich plasma or cultured stem cells, may also be appropriate depending on the extent of cartilage erosion.

Fracture of the Caudal Aspect of the Radius

Although the caudal aspect of the radius is more protected from external impact trauma, arthroscopic removal of a fracture from the caudomedial perimeter of the radius has been described (Bobkiewicz and Hodgson, 2012). The caudomedial

approach was used, and the caudal and medial perimeter of the radius, including a chronic intraarticular fragment, identified (Fig. 9-11). An instrument portal proximal and slightly cranial to the arthroscope entry allowed fragment removal and fracture bed debridement. The horse recovered function.

Osteochondrosis and Osteochondritis Dissecans of the Elbow

Osteochondrosis of the elbow usually takes the form of either OCD flap lesions of the humeral condyles or subchondral cystic lesions of the proximal radius. To date, there are no arthroscopic techniques that will provide access to the head of the radius (capitula fovea of the radius). Conservative therapy of subchondral cystic lesions of the proximal radius is generally accepted as the treatment of choice for these subchondral cysts (Hopen et al, 1992) (Fig. 9-12), but surgical treatment has also been successful (Bertone et al, 1986). OCD lesions of the humeral condyles can involve the caudal one half of either the medial or lateral condyle (Hopen et al, 1992). The flap lesions present as lysis on radiographs, similar to OCD lesions in most other sites in the body (Fig. 9-13). Access to lesions of the medial humeral condyle is easily provided using the caudomedial arthroscopic approach (Fig. 9-14). This approach also provides visualization but difficult triangulation to lesions of the lateral condyle. Use of the caudoproximal approach with the elbow fully flexed provides better access to the caudal one third to caudal one half of the lateral condyle. Differences in available exposed surfaces with elbow flexion are due to fibrosis of the joint, which limits range of motion. Triangulation is also easily accomplished using instrument entry through the triceps muscle or the myotendinous junction. The caudal surfaces of the medial and lateral condyle are a rare site for OCD in the horse, and experience is limited to lesion debridement in four horses by one author (A.J.N.). The outcome in all four of these horses was favorable, with all going on to athletic work. Preoperative planning to decide the most appropriate arthroscopic approach to the humeral condyles requires a flexed lateral radiograph. If the lesion is evident at the level of the anconeal process with the elbow flexed, the caudoproximal approach is simpler and safer, and provides more extensive room to manipulate surgical instruments. Similar controversy surrounds the need for surgery and best approaches for treatment of elbow OCD in humans (Krijnen et al, 2003; Pill et al, 2003), although the results of debridement support surgical treatment.

Fragmentation of the Anconeal Process

The anconeal process can develop fragmentation as a manifestation of osteochondrosis, trauma, or the end result of a septic process (Hardy et al, 1986). Access to the anconeal process using the caudoproximal approach is relatively simple (Fig. 9-15). Fragment removal can be accomplished using triangulation techniques as described previously. OCD fragments are rare in this location, and many of these fragments should be considered trauma induced. Similarly, complex fractures of the olecranon occasionally result in a free portion of bone that is too small to be repaired by internal fixation. The open lateral approach to the anconeal process during plate application to the olecranon is not particularly simple, and arthroscopy can be used to assess or remove the free fragment either during the plating procedure (see Fig. 9-15) or later. Fragmentation of the anconeal process or epicondyle junction of the humeral condyles can also develop, potentially precipitating OA (Fig. 9-16). Removal of fragments and debridement of the bony callus overgrowth have returned two horses to competitive riding. More chronic joint disease results in the need for more extensive debridement of new bone formation (Fig. 9-17).

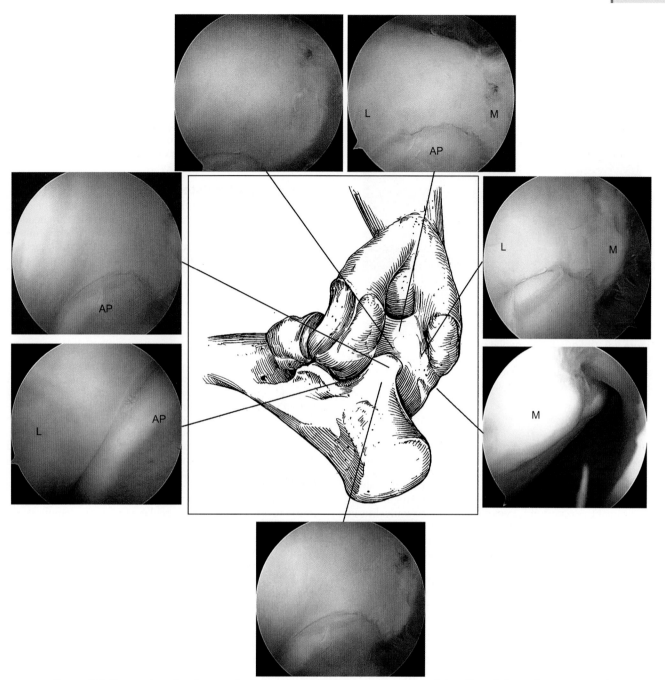

Figure 9-8 Composite of arthroscopic views of the caudoproximal aspect of the elbow joint, using a proximal caudolateral entry to place the arthroscope in the voluminous cul-de-sac over the anconeal process. The caudal portions of the medial *(M)* and lateral *(L)* humeral condyles are easily examined, and the anconeal process of the ulna can be viewed *(AP)*. Instrument access from either side of the arthroscope allows manipulation in many areas in the caudal joint pouch.

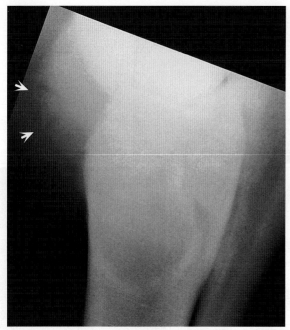

Figure 9-9 Oblique lateromedial radiograph showing a fracture of the cranial portion of the lateral humeral condyle *(arrows)*. The intraarticular fracture was easily removed using a craniolateral arthroscopic approach to the elbow.

Septic Arthritis

The elbow joint is a complex articulation and is occasionally involved in hematogenous septic processes in foals. The lateral aspect of the joint also has minimal soft tissue cover and is a common site for door latches or kicks from other animals to penetrate the joint through or adjacent to the lateral collateral ligament. A report of 5 cases of traumatic osteomyelitis of the proximolateral portion of the radius also indicates some of these traumatic episodes involve the proximal radius without septic arthritis of the elbow (Swinebroad et al, 2003). Lavage and flushing of all compartments of the elbow joint represents minimal therapy for septic arthritis (see Chapter 14). Recalcitrant cases need arthroscopic exploration, using debridement of inspissated and fibrinous material, and partial synovectomy of proliferative regions (Fig. 9-18). Arthroscopic exploration also allows evaluation of the cartilage surfaces of the humerus and ulna, and debridement of any areas that have developed separation from the subchondral bone. The access to the cranial pouch of the elbow joint is relatively simple using the craniolateral approach and, similarly, access to the proximal caudal joint pouch can be provided using the caudoproximal approach. Both can be accomplished with the patient in lateral recumbency. The necessity to enter the smaller joint pouch associated with the caudomedial arthroscopic approach is questionable. Most areas of the joint can be adequately lavaged and inspissated material removed from the more voluminous cranial and caudoproximal pouches. Drains can be instilled or antibiotic repository devices placed in either or both of the cranial or caudoproximal pouches (see Fig. 9-18). Use of resorbable calcium phosphate beads (Norian™, Synthes) has been shown to elute antibiotics over several weeks, and the beads are resorbed from the joint within 4 to 8 weeks (Watts et al, 2011). The outcome for synovial sepsis is described in Chapter 14, and is generally dictated by the extent of osteomyelitis in the subchondral bone.

Arthroscopy for Osteoarthritis

Arthroscopic exploration and debridement of areas of cartilage degeneration in OA is occasionally warranted, depending on the extent of osteophytosis in the elbow. The prominent regions for osteophyte formation include the cranial aspect of the radius, and the proximal joint capsule attachments on the cranial aspect of the humerus and over the anconeal process of the ulna. The therapeutic benefits of lavage and chondroplasty for arthritis are questionable (see review in Chapter 16); however, in the early stages, symptomatic relief may be provided for several years.

Postoperative Care

The skin incisions are sutured with monofilament nonresorbable material or covered with adhesive steristrips. Protection to avoid contamination from the environment is provided by self-adhesive wound coverings (Tegaderm™; 3M Healthcare, St. Paul, Minnesota) followed by sterile plastic adhesive incise drapes, such as Ioban iodine impregnated incise drapes (Fig. 9-19). The distal limb can be bandaged routinely to avoid edema and gravitational fluid accumulation.

COMPLICATIONS

Despite the complexity of the elbow articulation and the proximity to important neurovascular structures, complications with elbow arthroscopy are uncommon. The primary complication during arthroscopic procedures around the elbow is subcutaneous fluid accumulation, which can be extensive using the approaches described. Distention for visualization should be used in moderation, and the cranial and caudoproximal pouches of the joint are voluminous and easily examined with moderate distention.

Necropsy examination of horses used in the development of arthroscopic approaches to the elbow showed minor areas of muscle hemorrhage associated with instrument entry during triangulation (Nixon, 1990). The primary concern in elbow arthroscopy is surgical planning to provide access to the lesions without the necessity for repositioning the horse. The use of dorsal recumbency can result in difficulty in orientation and manipulation but should be taken into consideration when all three compartments of the joint need to be examined.

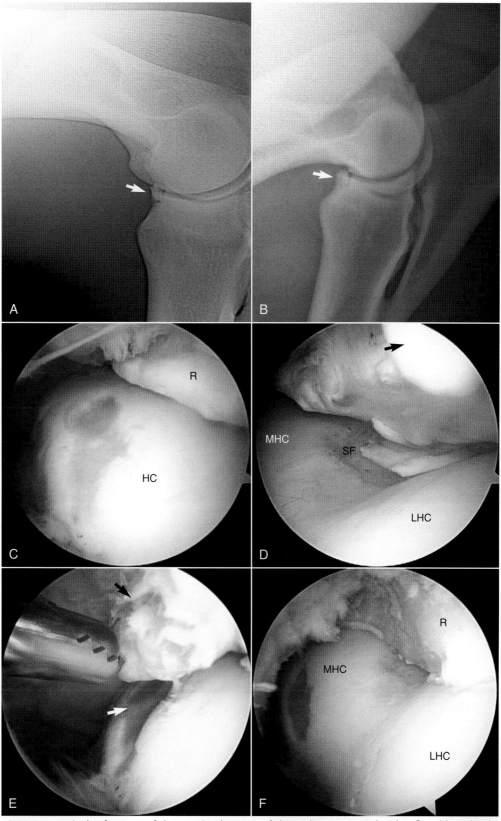

Figure 9-10 **Intraarticular fracture of the proximal aspect of the radius.** **A,** Lateral and **B,** flexed lateral radiographs showing fracture fragmentation of the cranial aspect of the radius *(arrows)*. **C,** Intraarticular image with arthroscope in craniolateral entry and shaver introduced through cranial portal between extensor carpi radialis and common digital extensor muscle bellies. Horse is in dorsal recumbency. The medial humeral condyle *(HC)* has a large impact cartilage injury. *R,* Radius. **D,** The synovial fossa *(SF)* has a detached cartilage flap laying in the recess between the lateral humeral condyle *(LHC)* and medial humeral condyle *(MHC)*. The fracture fragment is identified by *arrow.* **E,** A shaver is used to debride the fracture edges and fibrous attachment *(black arrow)*. The MHC impact injury is visible *(white arrow)*. **F,** Complete removal of fracture fragments with debrided radius *(R)* and debrided MHC lesion. *(Radiographs courtesy Dr. Ryland Edwards.)*

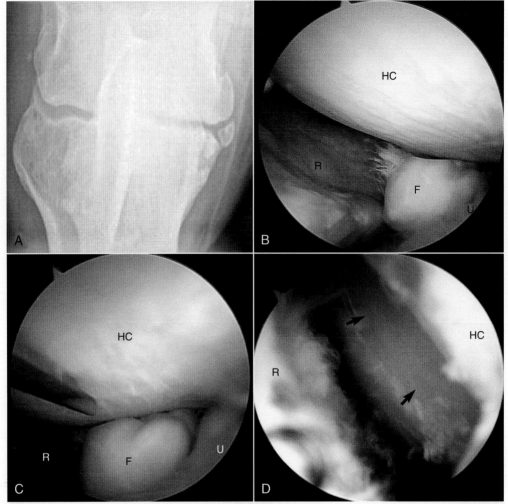

Figure 9-11 Intraarticular fracture of the caudomedial aspect of the radius. **A,** Craniocaudal radiograph shows chronic fracture fragment. **B,** Intraarticular view using caudomedial approach to the elbow. *F,* Osteochondral fracture; *HC,* humeral condyle; *R,* radius; *U,* ulna. **C,** An instrument entry was made proximal and slightly cranial to the arthroscope entry on the basis of spinal needle insertion. **D,** Additional damage to the medial HC *(arrows)* was debrided. *(Courtesy Dr. Bobkiewicz.)*

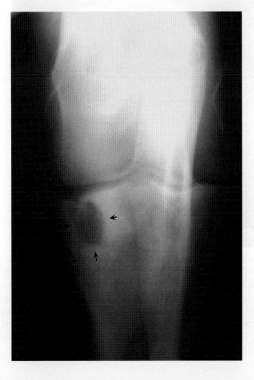

Figure 9-12 Subchondral cystic lesion of the medial portion of the capitular fovea of the proximal radius *(arrows).* Arthroscopic techniques may allow visualization of the articular stoma but not cyst debridement.

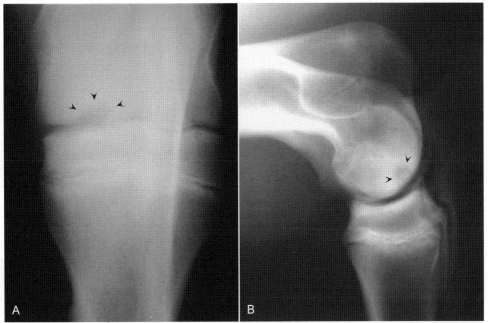

Figure 9-13 Osteochondritis dissecans (OCD) of the medial humeral condyle. A and **B,** Osteochondritis dissecans of the medial humeral condyle can be accessed using either the caudomedial approach or the caudoproximal approach, depending on the position of the lesion with the elbow fully flexed. The caudoproximal approach allows easier triangulation.

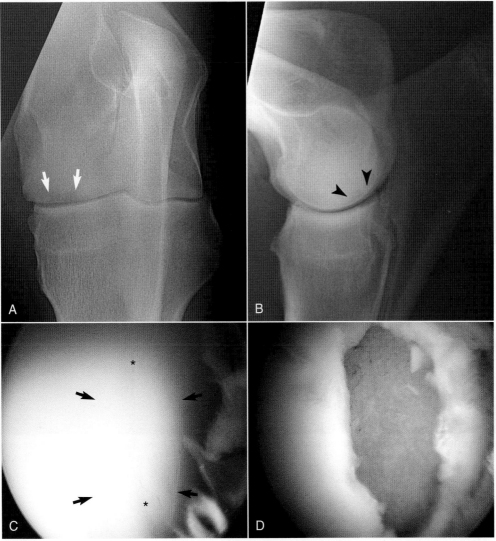

Figure 9-14 Debridement of osteochondritis dissecans (OCD) flap lesion of the medial humeral condyle. A and **B,** Radiographs show shallow OCD lesion in the central weight-bearing region of the medial condyle *(arrows).* **C,** Intraarticular view using the caudomedial approach to the elbow, showing edges of cartilage lesion *(arrows)* and additional linear crack *(asterisks).* **D,** Debridement of the OCD lesion leaves normal subchondral bone intact. *(Courtesy Dr. Bladon.)*

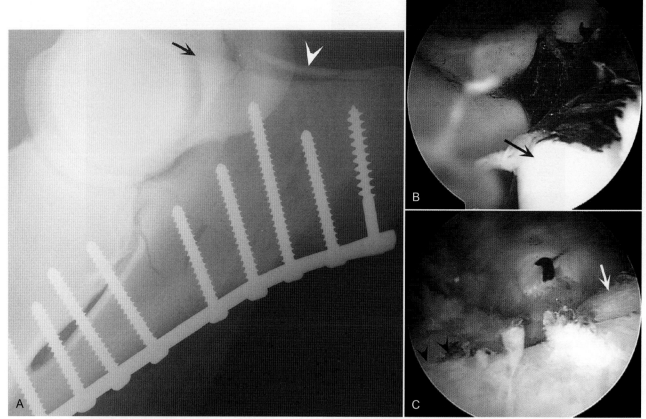

Figure 9-15 Intraarticular fracture of the anconeal process of the ulna. A, Radiograph after plate fixation of midshaft ulnar fracture, with a residual fracture of the anconeal process *(black arrow)* and a moderately displaced fracture of the cranial cortex of the olecranon *(white arrowhead).* **B,** Caudoproximal arthroscopic approach to the elbow joint exposes the anconeal process *(arrow)* and reveals blood clots overlying the intraarticular portion of the fracture. **C,** After removal of blood clots, the nondisplaced fracture of the anconeal process is visible and relatively immobile *(black arrowheads)*, while the free intraarticular portion of the cortex of the olecranon *(white arrow)* is trimmed back to the joint capsule. *(Photographs courtesy Dr. Lisa Fortier, Cornell University.)*

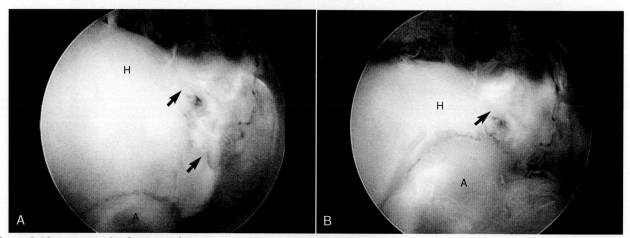

Figure 9-16 Intraarticular fracture of the medial epicondyle of the humerus. Arthroscopic view of fragmentation of the epicondyle junction of the humeral condyles *(arrows)* showing the lesion with the joint more flexed **(A)** and extended **(B).** The full extent of the epicondyle lesion is only obvious with flexion. *A,* Anconeal process; *H,* humerus.

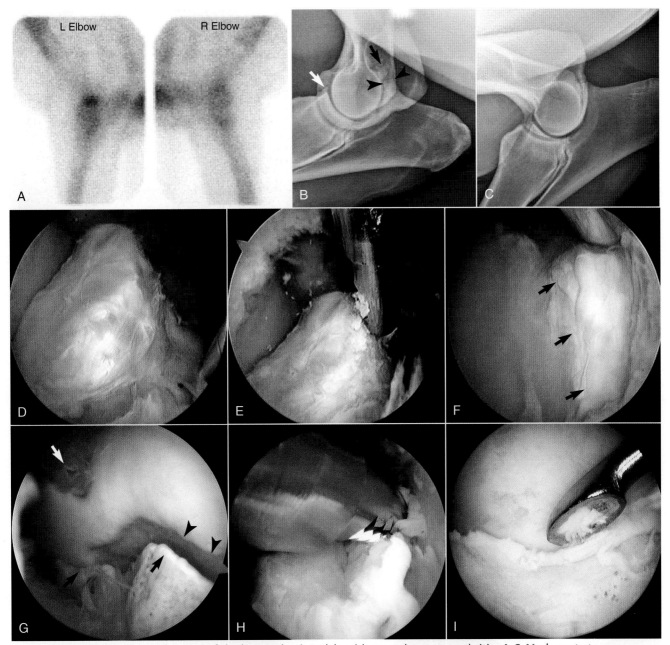

Figure 9-17 Chronic fracture of the humeral epicondyle with secondary osteoarthritis. A-C, Nuclear scintigram and radiographs of an 8-year-old event horse showing chronic fragmentation of the epicondyle *(black arrow)* of the left elbow, with secondary changes on the anconeal process *(arrowheads)*. A large osteophyte has developed on the cranial aspect of the radius *(white arrow)*. **D** and **E,** Intraarticular examination shows the chronic proliferative bone on the anconeal process before and after debridement. **F,** The medial epicondyle bone fragment *(arrows)* has also encroached on the elbow action and is being removed with a motorized abrader. **G,** In the cranial compartment of the elbow joint, the cartilage surface of the humerus has a traumatic cartilage lesion *(white arrow)* and the lateral humeral condyle has a lesion *(black arrowheads)* extending into the synovial fossa. The multiple large osteophytes from the radius protrude into the joint surface of the humerus. **H** and **I,** Motorized resector and curette being used to debride the radial osteophytes.

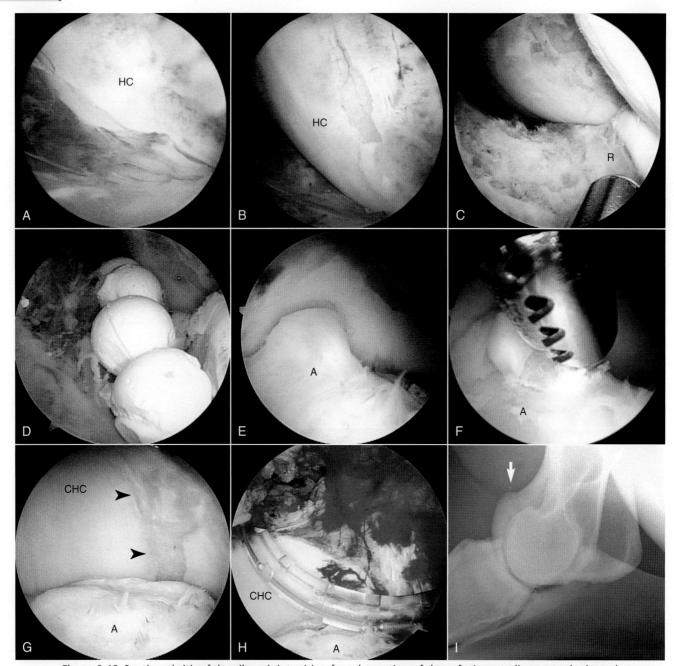

Figure 9-18 Septic arthritis of the elbow joint arising from laceration of the soft tissues adjacent to the lateral collateral ligament. **A,** Chronic proliferative synovial tissue, clots, and inspissated material in the cranial compartment accessed using the craniolateral approach with the horse in lateral recumbency. **B,** Cartilage erosion peeling from the humeral condyle. **C,** Inspissated material and synovial proliferation being removed with motorized shaver. **D,** Resorbable bone cement beads (Norian®) laden with antibiotics are delivered into the cranial compartment. **E,** Caudal compartment viewed using the caudoproximal approach. Inspissated material covers the anconeal process *(A)* of the ulna and the articular margin of the humerus. **F,** Purulent material is removed using the motorized shaver and "whisker" technique. **G,** Secondary full-thickness cartilage erosion *(arrows)* in the caudal region of the humeral condyle *(CHC)* is exposed with elbow flexion. **H,** After debridement and minimal synovectomy, an ingress drain (Davol ⅛ inch) is placed for delivery of antibiotics pending bacterial isolation and sensitivity. **I,** Radiographs 4 weeks after surgery show many of the beads have resorbed from the cranial compartment, with two small fragments remaining *(arrow)*. *HC*, Humeral condyle; *R*, radius.

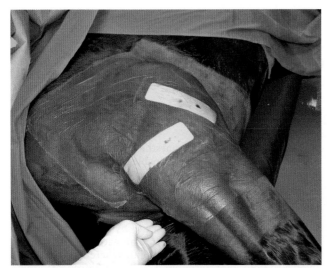

Figure 9-19 Adherent bandages following elbow arthroscopy. Postoperative bandaging for the elbow uses transparent adhesive dressings (Tegaderm™, 3M Healthcare, St. Paul, Minnesota) directly over the incisions (craniolateral and caudoproximal approaches), covered by Ioban sterile adhesive plastic drape.

REFERENCES

Baker Jr CL, Jones GL: Arthroscopy of the elbow, *Am J Sports Med* 27:251–264, 1999.

Bertone AL, McIlwraith CW, Powers BE, et al.: Subchondral osseous cystic lesions of the elbow of horses: conservative versus surgical treatment, *J Am Vet Med Assoc* 189:540–546, 1986.

Bobkiewicz J, Hodgson S: Arthroscopically-assisted removal of an osteochondral fragment from the equine elbow using a caudomedial approach, *Equine Vet Educ* 24:172–175, 2012.

Hardy J, Marcoux M, Eisenberg H: Osteochondrosis-like lesion of the anconeal process in two horses, *J Am Vet Med Assoc* 189:802–803, 1986.

Hopen LA, Colahan PT, Turner TA, Nixon AJ: Nonsurgical treatment of cubital subchondral cyst-like lesions in horses: seven cases (1983–1987), *J Am Vet Med Assoc* 200:527–530, 1992.

Krijnen MR, Lim L, Willems WJ: Arthroscopic treatment of osteochondritis dissecans of the capitellum: report of 5 female athletes, *Arthroscopy* 19:210–214, 2003.

Lynch GJ, Meyers JF, Whipple TL, Caspari RB: Neurovascular anatomy and elbow arthroscopy: inherent risks, *Arthroscopy* 2:190–197, 1986.

Nixon AJ: Arthroscopic approaches and intraarticular anatomy of the equine elbow, *Vet Surg* 19:93–101, 1990.

Nixon AJ: Elbow arthroscopy, indications, approaches, and syndromes, *Eq Vet Educ* 24:176–181, 2012.

Pill SG, Ganley TJ, Flynn JM, Gregg JR: Osteochondritis dissecans of the capitellum: arthroscopic-assisted treatment of large, full-thickness defects in young patients, *Arthroscopy* 19:222–225, 2003.

Poehling GG, Ekman EF: Arthroscopy of the elbow, *J Bone Joint Surg* 76A:1265–1271, 1994.

Stashak TS: Diagnosis of lameness. In Stashak TS, editor: *Adams' lameness in horses*, Philadelphia, 1987, Lea & Febiger, pp 150–153.

Swinebroad EL, Dabareiner RM, Swor TM, Carter GK, Watkins JP, Walker M, Schmitz DG, Honnas CM: Osteomyelitis secondary to trauma involving the proximal end of the radius in horses: 5 cases (1987-2001), *J Am Vet Med Assoc* 223:486–491, 2003.

Thomas MA, Fast A, Shapiro D: Radial nerve damage as a complication of elbow arthroscopy, *Clin Orthop* 130–131, 1987.

Watts AE, Nixon AJ, Papich MG, Sparks HD, Schwark WS: In vitro elution of amikacin and ticarcillin from a resorbable, self-setting, fiber reinforced calcium phosphate cement, *Vet Surg* 40:563–570, 2011.

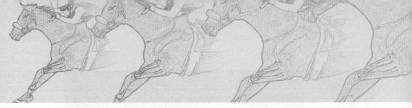

CHAPTER 10

Diagnostic and Surgical Arthroscopy of the Coxofemoral (Hip) Joint

iseases of the coxofemoral joint are being recognized more commonly, and the need for arthroscopic evaluation of the joint is growing. Nevertheless, reports of diagnostic arthroscopy and instances of surgical correction of problems in the hip are still relatively rare. This may be in part due to the inherent challenges of isolating problems to the coxofemoral joint, particularly in horses with chronic lameness. Moreover, the difficulties associated with surgical therapy often diminish enthusiasm for arthroscopic exploration. However, an increased awareness of hip joint diseases and the use of imaging modalities such as nuclear scintigraphy and standing digital radiography, coupled with increased use of intraarticular anesthesia, have increased the likelihood of establishing a definitive diagnosis of lameness associated with the coxofemoral joint. A logical extension of improved diagnostic capabilities is the use of arthroscopic examination with a view to surgical correction of some diseases. Arthrotomy of the hip joint is difficult, results in limited exposure of relevant structures, is debilitating for the horse and surgeon, and is accompanied by high wound-healing complication rates: Given this, it is rarely warranted for any surgical disease of the hip, other than repair of separation of the proximal femoral capital physis, or assisted reduction and stabilization of hip luxation. However, arthroscopy for diagnostic purposes is feasible, particularly in foals (Honnas et al, 1993), and with practice most adults can be examined with regular-length arthroscopes, and larger horses can be assessed using longer arthroscope and sleeve combinations (see Chapter 2).

Diagnostic arthroscopy has been used to evaluate tearing of the ligament of the head of the femur (round ligament), osteoarthritis (OA), fracture of the acetabulum, and osteochondrosis (OC) in the hip (Nixon, 1994). In humans, diagnostic arthroscopy of the hip is a useful technique to establish a diagnosis, as well as aid in treatment; it actually altered the preoperative diagnosis in 53% of 328 patients (Baber et al, 1999). Given the preoperative use of computed tomography (CT) and magnetic resonance imaging (MRI) in humans, these results represent a marked increase in diagnostic usefulness of arthroscopy. In humans the most common problem at diagnostic arthroscopy is labral tears (60%) followed by cartilage damage, OA, dysplasia, synovitis, loose bodies, and avascular necrosis (Byrd and Jones, 2010). In foals, arthroscopic surgery is particularly valuable in the treatment of sepsis involving the coxofemoral joint, in the evaluation and debridement of round ligament tears, and in the treatment of osteochondrosis (Nixon, 1994).

PREOPERATIVE ASSESSMENT

The clinical signs associated with clinical hip lameness in horses vary, depending on whether the derangement is a result of developmental disease in foals and weanlings, trauma to the hip resulting in tearing of the ligament of the head of the femur, degenerative OA, or fracture of various portions of the acetabulum (Miller & Todhunter, 1987; Nixon et al, 1988; Rose et al, 1981). Under the best of circumstances, the diagnosis of hip disease is often protracted, leading to OA as a common sequela. When the lameness is marked, muscle atrophy of the affected hind limb is evident in the gluteal and quadriceps musculature, facilitating an earlier diagnosis. More obscure upper hindlimb lameness may take more diligence in the work-up. Diagnostic manipulative tests are useful; however, the definitive diagnosis

often requires intraarticular anesthesia. Rectal examination is also recommended, although palpable enlargements have been recorded in only 50% of acetabular fractures (Rutkowski & Richardson, 1989), and many other conditions including OC and OA are not detected using rectal examination.

Ultrasonographic examination for hip disease is useful for fracture, luxation, and advanced OA (Brenner and Whitcomb, 2009). It has a vital role in eliminating pelvic fracture and moving the focus to the hip joint. Where a fracture does involve the hip joint, ultrasound examination can determine involvement of the periphery of the acetabulum compared with mid-acetabulum, provide a measure of fracture displacement, and reveal any sign of additional subluxation. Ultrasonographic examination and standing radiography provide complementary information in the assessment of hip disease in the horse (Gebruek et al, 2009).

With the availability of large-bore CT, there is a possibility for examination of the hip and pelvis in growing horses (Trump et al, 2011). The capabilities of obtaining a CT on an adult horse are less, depending on the bore size and configuration of the CT equipment.

Nuclear scintigraphy has improved the diagnostic specificity for chronic hindlimb lameness but still lacks the conclusive nature of intraarticular anesthesia. Blocking the hip can be difficult until some familiarity with the surface anatomic landmarks is gained. Later confirmation and staging of the degree of the hip joint involvement can be provided by radiographs. Good-quality radiographs require general anesthesia, and ventrodorsal and oblique ventrodorsal views are necessary for evaluation of the acetabulum and femoral heads. Moderate and severe degenerative OA, OC, osteochondritis dissecans (OCD), and luxation or subluxation of the hip are apparent on hip radiographs. The increased sensitivity of computed and digital radiographs has allowed reasonable-quality standing hip joint radiography (Barrett et al, 2006) (Fig. 10-1). Less obvious hip diseases, such as tearing of the ligament of the head of the femur and mild OA, may not be evident on routine radiographs. These lesions may need to be identified through direct visualization during arthroscopic examination.

▶ DIAGNOSTIC ARTHROSCOPY OF THE HIP JOINT

Arthroscopy is indicated for the diagnosis of hip joint disease, particularly in cases in which radiographs provide little additional information after a positive intraarticular anesthetic response has been obtained and as a therapeutic tool for other conditions. Arthroscopic examination of the hip joint in horses has been described in a limited case series (Honnas et al, 1993; Nixon, 1994). Arthroscopic visualization was useful in determining the extent of cartilage damage associated with fractures of the acetabular rim, in several cases where radiographically visible small fractures were identified associated with the periphery of the acetabular rim, in assessing the degree of tearing of the ligament of the head of the femur, and in cases where cartilage defects were evident during examination of horses with hip joint lameness but no radiographic lesions (Nixon, 1994). Intraarticular debridement of torn and partially torn ligaments of the head of the femur, debridement of OCD of the

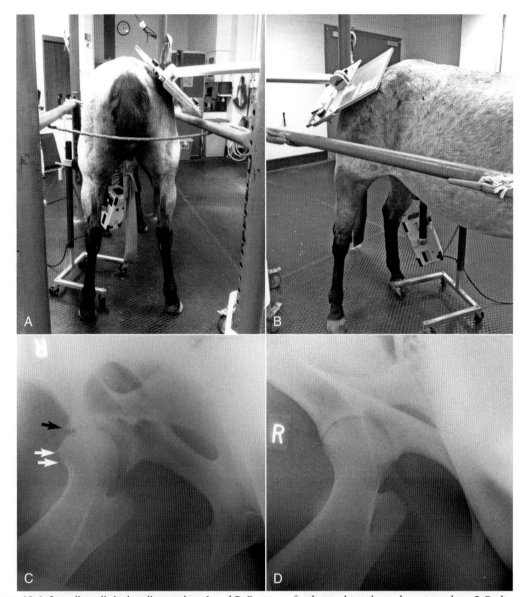

Figure 10-1 Standing digital radiography. A and **B,** Position of radiographic tube and receiver plate. **C,** Radiographs showing subluxation and early osteoarthritis of the right hip. Osteophytes are evident on the cranial region of the acetabulum *(black arrow)* and on the femoral head and neck *(white arrows)*. Arthroscopic assessment of the hip joint, particularly the ligament of the head of the femur, is warranted. **D,** Normal hip joint radiographs taken in the standing position. Images obtained with MinXray portable generator at 80KvP and 2 sec exposure. Canon CR system.

acetabulum, and cystic lesions of the femoral head have been described (Nixon, 1994). Similarly, arthroscopic lavage and synovectomy with debris removal is a useful method for improving the response in foals with infectious arthritis of the hip.

Surgical Technique

Arthroscopic examination of the hip joint is readily accomplished in foals and can be performed with some difficulty in horses up to 500 kg. Hip arthroscopy in horses heavier than 500 kg is possible but is facilitated by a longer arthroscope (see later). Regardless of equipment, in larger horses, examination of the articular structures is less complete; the procedure is more technically demanding and is associated with more surgical trauma to the articular and periarticular structures than encountered during hip arthroscopy in foals. However, hip joint laxity associated with persistent effusion provides a largely unrecognized advantage in arthroscopic examination of adult horses with chronic hip disease. With appropriate axial traction on the affected hindlimb, the femoral head can

be distracted from the acetabulum sufficiently to allow examination of large portions of the femoral head and acetabulum.

The horse is anesthetized and positioned in lateral recumbency with the affected limb uppermost. The entire lateral region of the hip and gluteal muscle is draped for surgery with the affected limb supported in the neutral position but free to be mobilized during surgery. An arthroscope entry portal is made at the site that has been previously described for intraarticular anesthesia (Stashak, 1987; Nixon, 1994). A skin incision is made between the cranial and caudal portions of the greater trochanter, entering approximately 2 cm proximal to the palpable level of the trochanter (intertrochanteric fossa) (Fig. 10-2). This provides arthroscopic access to both the cranial and caudal recesses of the hip joint. The joint is initially distended with 60 to 80 mL of lactated Ringer solution administered through a 15- to 20-cm spinal needle or the stylette from a 15-cm intravenous catheter. The arthroscope sleeve and conical obturator of a standard arthroscope are adequate to penetrate the joint of horses less than 400 kg. Larger horses can also be examined

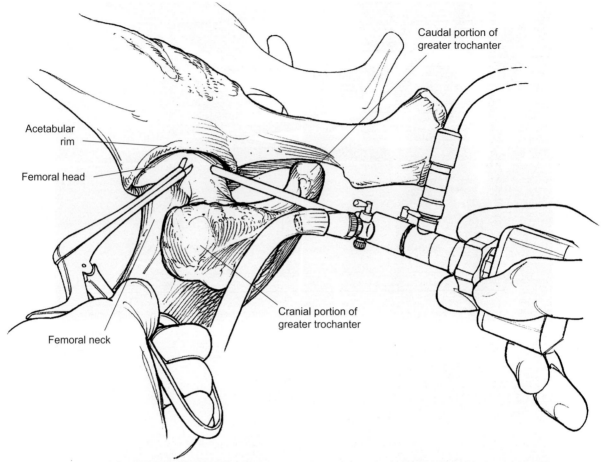

Caudal portion of
greater trochanter

Acetabular
rim

Femoral head

Cranial portion of
greater trochanter

Femoral neck

Figure 10-2 Arthroscopic technique for examination of the equine coxofemoral joint. The arthroscope skin portal is made 2 cm proximal to the greater trochanter, between the cranial and caudal portions of the trochanter.

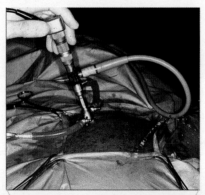

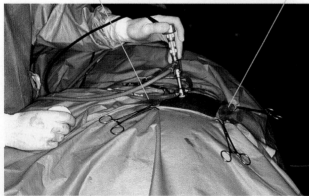

Figure 10-3 The horse is positioned in lateral recumbency and the arthroscope inserted to its full extent. Inset shows a 15-cm spinal needle used as an egress needle.

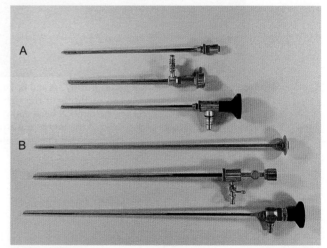

Figure 10-4 Arthroscopes suitable for hip arthroscopy. The normal 13- to 15-cm, 4-mm arthroscope **(A)** is suitable for hip arthroscopy in most horses. Larger horses may require a longer arthroscope **(B)**.

using a standard arthroscope sleeve and 4-mm forward oblique viewing arthroscope (Fig. 10-3). However, a longer arthroscope (25-cm arthroscope, Karl Storz Endoscopy, Goleta, CA) is useful for more complete examination in heavier adult horses (Fig. 10-4). The arthroscope sleeve and conical obturator are inserted through the skin and angled 20 degrees ventral and 20 degrees cranially, to follow the dorsal (proximal) contour of the femoral neck (see Fig. 10-2). The lateral portion of the hip joint is penetrated, the obturator removed, and the arthroscope inserted.

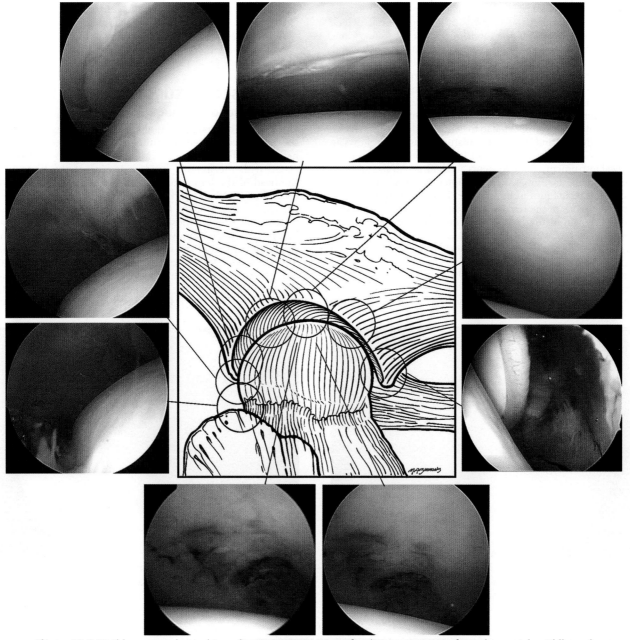

Figure 10-5 Visible regions during hip arthroscopy. Composite of arthroscopic images from the cranial, middle, and caudal aspects of the hip joint.

The standard 25-degree or 30-degree forward oblique viewing arthroscopes are satisfactory for examination of most regions of the hip joint. A 70-degree arthroscope is useful but not essential to examine the craniomedial and caudomedial recesses of the joint. A second skin portal, for fluid egress and later instrument access, is made 4 to 5 cm cranial to the arthroscope portal, using a 15-cm spinal needle or catheter stylette to define the path for instrument entry before skin incision.

Visualization of the articular surface of the cranial, lateral, and caudal regions of the hip joint is accomplished with the limb supported in a horizontal position (Fig. 10-5). Manipulation of the limb into a flexed and extended position allows other regions of the femoral head to be viewed. Given the depth of the joint from the skin surface, manipulation of the limb must be done with care, to avoid damage to the arthroscope. Distraction of the limb by axial tension is vital for a complete examination of the hip. This allows the arthroscope to be inserted between the femoral head and the acetabulum. In immature horses, distraction and arthroscope insertion can be accomplished easily and allow

examination of the deeper regions of the joint (Fig. 10-6). In older horses, distraction and increased intraarticular fluid pressures are more important to allow visualization of the femoral head and round ligament of the head of the femur (Fig. 10-7). Joint distraction can be provided by axial tension on the limb from an assistant or by mechanical devices such as a winch attached to the surgery wall. The torso of the horse must be stabilized on the surgery table when distraction techniques are used. An intraoperative decision can be made as to the necessity and degree of mechanical distraction. The use of surgical assistants is necessary for arthroscopy of the hip joint in adults, primarily to manipulate the limb and to provide axial distraction when required.

Instrument access is generally provided through the cranial instrument portal after developing a path to the hip joint through the tendinous insertion of the middle gluteal muscle using a conical obturator. The arthroscope and instrument portals can be exchanged for better examination of the caudal acetabular rim. Utilization of a switching stick or second arthroscope sleeve is vital to allow positive exchange of the arthroscope and instrument portals. The exchange allows entry for rongeurs and curettes through the original arthroscope portal, which can then be directed into the caudal regions of the joint. A long 6-mm diameter egress cannula (Sontec Instruments, Englewood, CO) or a second arthroscope sleeve is suitable for fluid egress after surgical debridement. The use of motorized instruments is possible in small and moderate-sized horses, but use of motorized equipment can be limited by the depth of the joint from the skin surface in adults. Most hand instruments and motorized equipment need to be inserted to the limits of their length. Pressing in on the skin and gluteal musculature occasionally allows an extra 1 to 2 cm of effective length to be garnered from routine surgical instruments. Long rongeurs and long egress cannulae are useful (Sontec Instruments; see Chapter 2). Most surgical triangulation techniques in the hip are difficult. Debridement of cartilage lesions of the femoral head and removal of free bodies and debris within the cranial and caudal recesses of the joint can be achieved with persistence. Lesions in the acetabulum can be more difficult to debride. In smaller horses, examination and debridement of torn portions of the round ligament of the head of the femur can be achieved. Osteochondrosis cysts of the head of the femur and fractures of the caudal acetabular rim are particularly difficult to adequately debride. Instrument entry

caudal to the standard arthroscope entry carries significant risk of damage to the sciatic nerve and should be reserved for cases with caudal acetabular fracture, and only then under previous needle verification of the path, followed by the insertion of a blunt obturator to develop an atraumatic entry.

ARTHROSCOPIC SURGERY OF THE HIP

Femoral Head Cartilage Lesions

Horses with normal radiographs but lameness associated with the hip, as confirmed by intraarticular anesthesia, generally have either focal or more widespread cartilage lesions associated with the femoral head or tearing of the ligament of the head of the femur, or both, when examined arthroscopically. Focal articular cartilage lesions are usually confined to the cranial aspect of the femoral head. Intraarticular debris is occasionally present, most likely originating from the cartilage lesion (Fig. 10-8). Removal of the debris with or without further debridement of the femoral head has improved lameness in three racehorses. More widespread cartilage lesions usually indicate osteoarthritis, and secondary osteophyte formation is often evident over the cranial and caudal perimeter of the acetabulum (Fig. 10-9). In mild and moderate osteoarthritis,

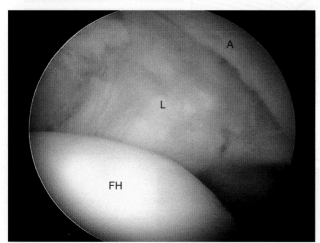

Figure 10-6 Hip distraction in small breed horse. After distraction in a 100-kg miniature horse, additional portions of the femoral head *(FH)* and acetabulum *(A)*, including the ligament *(L)* of the head of the femur (round ligament), become visible and accessible for debridement.

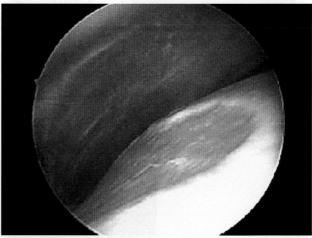

Figure 10-8 A 2-year-old Standardbred racehorse with a cartilage erosion over the cranial portion of the femoral head. The horse returned to successful racing.

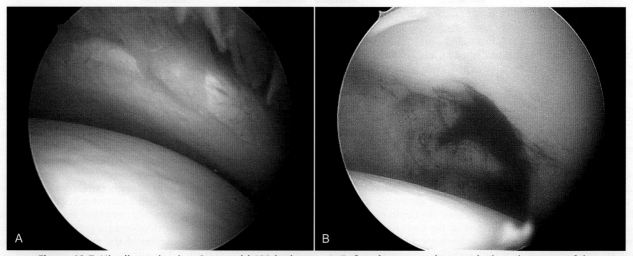

Figure 10-7 Hip distraction in a 2-year-old 480-kg horse. **A,** Before distraction, showing the lateral portions of the femoral head and acetabulum. **B,** With maximal distraction on the limb, revealing the center of the femoral head and the acetabular fossa.

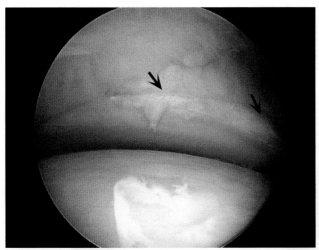

Figure 10-9 Early osteoarthritis in a 1-year-old horse. Cartilage irregularity of the femoral head and osteophytes have developed *(arrows)* along the acetabular perimeter.

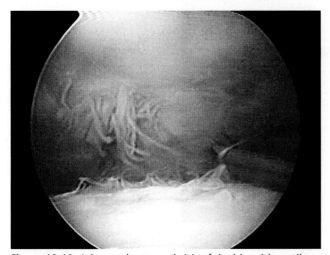

Figure 10-10 Advanced osteoarthritis of the hip with cartilage fibrillation of the acetabular and femoral surfaces. A needle has been inserted caudal to the arthroscope for egress flushing.

most of these osteophytes are not visible on preoperative radiographs. Debridement of cartilage lesions of the femoral head can be accomplished with appropriate manipulation of curettes and rongeurs in combination with axial distraction. A moderate amount of iatrogenic damage to surrounding cartilage is always a possibility during debridement of these lesions. More advanced cases of hip joint osteoarthritis can be assessed by arthroscopy (Fig. 10-10); however, lasting improvement following debridement of fibrillated regions is rare. In humans diagnostic arthroscopy of the hip frequently results in the diagnosis of cartilage injury, including cartilage damage resulting from traumatic subluxation (Yen and Kocher, 2010). In humans the outcome after debridement of cartilage lesions is considerably better when arthritis is minimal compared with more advanced disease. The use of microfracture and chondroplasty both play a role in improving the outcome in more acute cartilage damage in the human hip (Yen and Kocher, 2010). A limited number of cases in the horse have been treated by motorized chondroplasty with return to function. The authors have not utilized microfracture in the hip, but it may have a place for management of focal cartilage lesions after debridement.

Tearing of the Ligament of the Head of the Femur

Fraying and tearing of the ligament of the head of the femur is a relatively common finding during diagnostic arthroscopy of hip joints from small-breed horses but can also be encountered in mature larger-breed animals. Complete rupture of this ligament can occur, and the outlook even with debridement is guarded (Fig. 10-11). Tearing in smaller breeds, particularly miniature horses, can be adequately debrided (Fig. 10-12), and a return of soundness is possible in those cases with incomplete rupture of the ligament (Nixon, 1994). Manipulation of biopsy punch rongeurs and motorized equipment is necessary for complete debridement of the visible portions of the ligament. The accessory ligament of the head of the femur is particularly difficult to visualize, and lesions in this ligament are rarely recognized.

Osteochondrosis and Osteochondritis Dissecans

Debridement of OCD flaps of the femoral head and acetabulum can be accomplished in immature animals. Mature horses can be debrided with more difficulty, particularly lesions involving the lateral half of the femoral head. Lesions in the lateral portion of the acetabulum are also accessible,

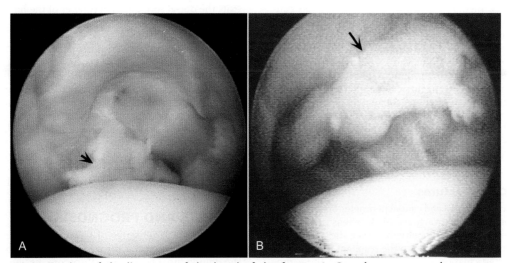

Figure 10-11 Tearing of the ligament of the head of the femur. A, Complete rupture and contraction of the proper ligament of the head of the femur *(arrowhead)*. **B,** Probing of the ligament reveals the free end *(arrow)*. The horse remained lame after surgery.

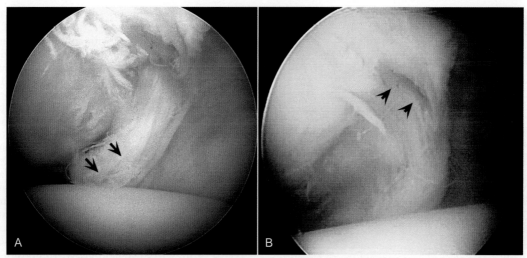

Figure 10-12 Partial tearing of the ligament of the head of the femur. **A,** Partial rupture *(arrows)* of the ligament of the head of the femur in a 4-year-old miniature horse. **B,** Flexion of the hip reveals an additional split in the proximal portion of the ligament of the head of the femur *(arrowheads)*. After debridement the horse was sound for at least 7 years.

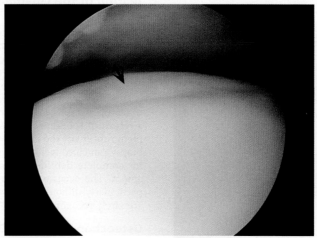

Figure 10-13 Opening of a subchondral cystic lesion of the femoral head *(arrow)*. Adequate debridement of deep cysts is difficult due to limited access of curved instruments.

including most areas up to and including the area of the synovial fossa for insertion of the ligament of the head of the femur. The deeper, more medial, aspects of the femoral head cannot be adequately visualized. In small-breed horses and horses with extensive effusion, the hip joint is easily distracted, allowing better debridement of OCD lesions. Subchondral cystic lesions of the head of the femur can be particularly difficult to debride to the depths of the lesion (Fig. 10-13). Angled curettes and small-angled rongeurs can be effective; however, the depths of the cyst can rarely be adequately debrided. Secondary packing of the debrided cysts with cancellous bone or other graft materials has not been possible. Cartilage lesions associated with the caudal perimeter of the acetabulum may not necessarily represent OCD but can be debrided with long rongeurs.

Acetabular Chip Fractures

Small fractures of the cranial and caudal perimeter of the acetabulum can be removed with rongeurs. More extensive fractures can be removed with some difficulty; however, the outcome is rarely satisfactory, presumably due to the resultant instability of the coxofemoral articulation (Fig. 10-14). Most of these procedures are tedious and time consuming due to the increased depths of the joint from the skin surface. Insertion of instruments

targeting the acetabular rim also places the sciatic nerve at risk, particularly if the instrument rides over the acetabular rim and exits the dorsal (proximal) perimeter of the hip joint.

Infectious Arthritis

Arthroscopy provides an effective means for lavage and debridement of debris from septic hip joints. The voluminous cranial and caudal recesses of the hip joint frequently contain fibrinous and purulent debris, which can be removed by large-bore egress cannulae or retrieved using rongeurs or motorized resectors. Lavage can also be facilitated by a second instrument entry portal for an egress cannula in the caudal recess of the hip joint. Careful insertion of all instruments into the caudal region of the hip is necessary to avoid trauma to the sciatic nerve. Arthroscopic lavage and debridement are considered the standards of care for serious infectious arthritis of the hip joint in man (Lee et al, 2012).

RESULTS AND PROGNOSIS

There are no large series of cases to describe the results of diagnostic or surgical arthroscopy for any of the conditions in the equine hip. Diagnostic arthroscopy has been useful in the treatment of septic hip joints in foals; however, a delay in diagnosis and involvement of other joints is common in foals and

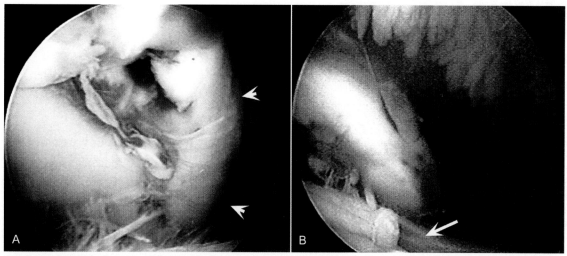

Figure 10-14 Chip fracture of the acetabulum. A, Fractured caudal acetabular rim, showing fracture fragment *(arrowheads)*, the fracture line, and cartilage degeneration in surrounding regions. **B,** An osteotome *(arrow)* is being used to separate the loose fragment for removal.

reduces the likelihood of a sound horse. Diagnostic arthroscopy is also useful to establish the severity of cartilage injury in mild and moderate degenerative OA. Several cases have had focal cartilage injuries that responded particularly well to local debridement. The establishment of a more accurate prognosis is also a useful benefit of hip arthroscopy.

Surgical debridement can be expected to improve the outcome with osteochondrosis and OCD conditions of the hip. Improvement in lameness after debridement of OCD flap lesions on the acetabular perimeter and after debridement of subchondral cysts of the femoral head has been seen. Access for debridement of femoral head lesions depends on the lateromedial location of the cysts within the femoral head. Debridement of relatively shallow cysts can be accomplished, and deeper cysts can be opened to some extent, although debridement is incomplete. In foals and miniature horses, debridement of frayed and torn regions of the ligament of the head of the femur can be easily performed, and at least with incomplete rupture, the results are quite satisfactory. Removal of frayed ligament fibers and lavage of debris from the joint improve the degree of lameness and minimize the likelihood of secondary osteoarthritis. Synovectomy of portions of the accessible synovial membrane also appears to improve the postoperative response in these cases. Complete disruption of the ligament of the head of the femur results in permanent lameness, and long-term improvement after arthroscopy has not been seen. These lesions need further stabilization, and techniques for hip stabilization have not been successful in adult horses.

The prognosis for a horse with hip disease depends on the type of lesion, extent of degenerative OA, and the completeness of lesion debridement. In some circumstances hip arthroscopy has improved the prognosis, whereas in other cases the extent of OA and cartilage damage has prevented a satisfactory outcome. On the basis of limited case experience, arthroscopic debridement of OCD lesions in the hip appears to improve the prognosis, whereas a diagnosis of complete rupture of the head of the ligament of the femur is a predictor of continued lameness. Synovectomy and debridement of portions of incomplete rupture of the ligament of the head of the femur have been useful in providing lasting improvement

in the level of lameness. Removal of chip fractures associated with the acetabular rim is possible; however, significant improvement in outcome is evident only with small fragments. Larger lesions result in destabilization of the articulation and little long-term benefit.

REFERENCES

Baber YF, Robinson AH, Villar RN: Is diagnostic arthroscopy of the hip worthwhile? A prospective review of 328 adults investigated for hip pain, *J Bone Joint Surg (Br)* 81:600–603, 1999.

Barrett EL, Talbot AM, Driver AJ, Barr FJ, Barr AR: A technique for pelvic radiography in the standing horse, *Equine Vet J* 38:266–270, 2006.

Brenner S, Whitcomb MB: Ultrasonographic diagnosis of coxofemoral luxation in horses, *Vet Radiol Ultrasound* 50:423–428, 2009.

Gebruek F, Rotting AK, Stadler PM: Comparison of the diagnostic value of ultrasonography and standing radiography for pelvic-femoral disorders in horses, *Vet Surg* 38:310–317, 2009.

Honnas CM, Zamos DT, Ford TS: Arthroscopy of the coxofemoral joint of foals, *Vet Surg* 22:115–121, 1993.

Lee YK, Park KS, Ha YC, Koo KH: Arthroscopic treatment for acute septic arthritis of the hip joint in adults, *Knee Surg Sports Traumatol Arthros,* Nov 1, 2012 [epub ahead of print].

Miller CL, Todhunter R: Acetabular osteochondrosis dissecans in a foal, *Cornell Vet* 77:75–83, 1987.

Nixon AJ: Diagnostic and operative arthroscopy of the coxofemoral joint in horses, *Vet Surg* 23:377–385, 1994.

Nixon AJ, Adams RM, Teigland MB: Subchondral cystic lesions (osteochondrosis) of the femoral heads in a horse, *J Am Vet Med Assoc* 192:360–362, 1988.

Rose JA, Rose EM, Smylie DR: Case history: acetabular osteochondrosis in a yearling Thoroughbred, *J Equine Vet Sci* 1:173–175, 1981.

Rutkowski JA, Richardson DW: A retrospective study of 100 pelvic fractures in horses, *Equine Vet J* 21:256–259, 1989.

Stashak TS: Diagnosis of lameness. In Stashak TS, editor: *Adams' lameness in horses,* Philadelphia, 1987, Lea and Febiger, pp 150–153.

Trump M, Kircher PR, Furst A: The use of computed tomography in the diagnosis of pelvic fractures involving the acetabulum in two fillies, *Vet Comp Orthop Traumatol* 24:68–71, 2011.

Yen YM, Kocher MS: Chondral lesions of the hip: microfracture and chondroplasty, *Sports Med Arthroscopy* 18:83–89, 2010.

CHAPTER 11

Arthroscopic Surgery of the Distal and Proximal Interphalangeal Joints

Diagnostic and surgical arthroscopy of the distal and proximal interphalangeal joints has developed in parallel with improvements in diagnostic imaging in these areas. The dorsal and palmar/plantar compartments of both joints are amenable to arthroscopic evaluation and treatment. However, the spaces are small and the fields of view are less panoramic than in larger joints. As a result, arthroscopic evaluation is largely uniplanar and is done mainly by lateral movement and rotation of the arthroscope using the lens angle. Additionally, joint distension is limited by adjacent tendon or ligamentous structures that restrict access and maneuverability of both the arthroscope and instruments. These are also invariably in close apposition, which increases the risk of damage to the arthroscopic lens.

ARTHROSCOPY OF THE DISTAL INTERPHALANGEAL JOINT

A technique for diagnostic and surgical arthroscopy of the dorsal compartment of the distal interphalangeal joint (DIP) was described by Boening et al (1990). An approach to and the anatomy of the palmaroproximal and plantaroproximal compartments of the distal interphalangeal joints were reported by Vacek et al (1992) with a modification by Fowlie et al (2011). With the advent of sophisticated imaging modalities, principally magnetic resonance imaging (MRI) and computed tomography (CT), the requirements for diagnostic arthroscopy of the distal interphalangeal joints have declined. However, arthroscopy has an expanded role in treatment. Arthroscopic surgery is indicated in the removal of fragmentation of the extensor process of the distal phalanx and, with some large fragments, arthroscopically guided internal fixation of the process. Fragmentation of the distal (usually abaxial) margins of the middle phalanx can also be removed arthroscopically together with loose bodies from both dorsal and palmar/plantar compartments. Subchondral bone cysts in both distal and middle phalanges and in some cases in the proximal portion of the navicular bone can also be accessed arthroscopically. Parasagittal fractures of both distal and middle phalanges have been reduced and repaired under arthroscopic guidance, and there is a case report of arthroscopically assisted arthrodesis of the distal interphalangeal joint. Avulsions of the joint capsule have been identified and treated, and the suspensory ligaments (collateral sesamoidean ligaments) of the navicular bone can be accessed and divided arthroscopically. Arthroscopy is also the treatment of choice for contaminated and infected distal interphalangeal joints.

Arthroscopic Examination of the Dorsal Pouch of the Distal Interphalangeal Joint

Positioning and Preparation

Arthroscopy can be performed with the horse in dorsal or lateral recumbency, although dorsal is recommended. Arthroscopic examination of the dorsal compartment is facilitated by joint extension, whereas evaluation of the palmar/plantar compartment is optimized by joint flexion. If the dorsal compartment only is to undergo arthroscopy, then the limb may be fixed in an extended position (Fig. 11-1). If both dorsal and palmar/plantar compartments are to be evaluated, the limb can either be flexed by caudal pressure on the carpus

from this position or allowed to hang passively and then extended or flexed as required. The disadvantage of the latter is the need for an assistant.

Because the arthroscopic portals will be close to the hoof, the entire sole and wall surfaces of the foot should be thoroughly cleansed before surgery. Preparation by a thorough hoof trim and scrub, as well as an overnight soak in iodine solution secured with a waterproof barrier, is helpful. During surgery, a further waterproof barrier is created by enclosing the foot in a surgical glove, leaving the coronary band visible as a landmark. The glove can be secured to the hoof with superglue for added watertight seal. Following surgical preparation of the skin, a further sterile barrier can be created by enclosing the gloved hoof in a sterile adhesive bandage. Sterile impervious drapes are then applied (Fig. 11-2). A sterile plastic

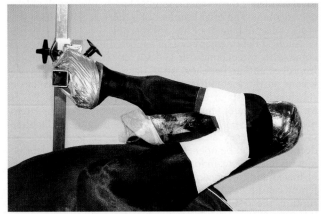

Figure 11-1 Limb positioning. Forelimb positioned with distal joints extended for arthroscopy of the dorsal compartment of the distal interphalangeal joint.

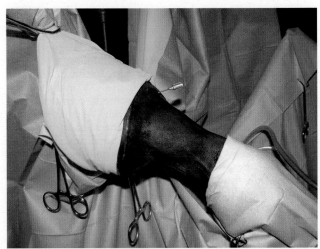

Figure 11-2 Draping for DIP joint arthroscopy. Following application of a sterile adhesive bandage to the foot the surgical field is exposed through a rubberized, fenestrated drape leaving the dorsal coronary band exposed as a landmark.

adhesive antibacterial barrier may be used at the surgeon's discretion. Adhesive plastic drapes can be difficult to develop a good seal against the uneven contours of the palmar/plantar surfaces of the distal limb.

Arthroscopic Technique

The abaxial margins of the common/long digital extensor tendon are key landmarks for arthroscope entry (Fig. 11-3) and are initially palpated (Fig. 11-4A) before distension of the joint using a conventional site of synoviocentesis in either the dorsal or palmar/plantar compartment (Fig. 11-4B). The joint is distended maximally to aid portal location and entry of the arthroscopic cannula. A skin incision is made with a No. 11 or 15 scalpel blade at the previously located abaxial margin of the common/long digital extensor tendon. This should be located proximally in the bulbous outpouching of the dorsal compartment to maximize evaluation and maneuverability within the joint. In adult horses, this is usually between 2 and 3 cm proximal to the coronary band and abaxial to the sagittal midline.

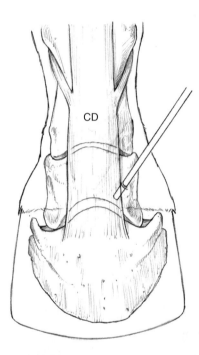

Figure 11-3 Dorsal compartment technique. Diagram of arthroscope position in the dorsal pouch of the distal interphalangeal joint at the commencement of evaluation. CD, Common/long digital extensor tendon.

Once the skin incision has been made, the blade is pushed, in one movement through the joint capsule. The arthroscopic cannula is introduced using a conical obturator. This is passed first perpendicular to the skin using the thumb of the noninserting hand as a friction bridge (Fig. 11-4C), and once the joint has been entered, the inserting hand is lowered to push the sleeve and conical obturator beneath the common/long digital extensor tendon over the condyles of the middle phalanx to the contralateral side of the joint (Fig. 11-4D). The obturator can then be replaced by the arthroscope and the camera with the light cable and fluid ingress line attached (Fig. 11-4E).

For most procedures the most useful instrument portal is made in a similar location to the arthroscopic portal on the contralateral side of the common/long digital extensor tendon (Fig. 11-5). Introduction of an arthroscopic probe to elevate the dorsal joint capsule and its synovium aids arthroscopic evaluation of the joint (Fig. 11-5A). This is then followed by synovial resection or retrieval of fragments with rongeurs (Fig. 11-5B).

Arthroscopic Anatomy

Approximately 30% of the intraarticular anatomy of the distal interphalangeal joint is visible in its dorsal compartment. The principal landmark for orientation is the extensor process of the distal phalanx (Fig. 11-6). Villous synovium overhangs the dorsal rim of the distal phalanx but can readily be elevated with the arthroscopic probe to expose the extensor process and adjacent shallow concavity of the middle phalanx, which is evident between the convex articular surfaces of its condyles. Synovial tissue removal is often performed initially in most DIP joint diagnostic examinations to improve visualization of the articular surfaces. Beneath the villous synovium there is a shallow recess distal to which the joint capsule and common/long digital extensor tendon insert on the dorsal surface of the distal phalanx. By moving the arthroscope medially and laterally while elevating the joint capsule and rotating the lens, the entire dorsal articular rim of the distal phalanx can be visualized. At the medial and lateral margins there are plical folds whose degrees of development vary between individual horses. Slight withdrawal of the arthroscope and palmar/plantar angulation of the lens brings into view the distal dorsal articular surface of the middle phalanx. This has a uniform hyaline cartilage covering. The proximal recess of the joint is filled with thin villous synovium dorsally and palmar/plantarly, where it reflects from the middle phalanx.

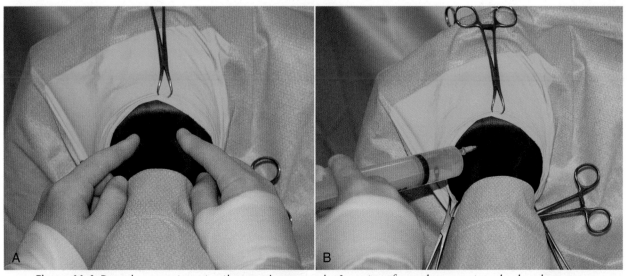

Figure 11-4 Dorsal compartment arthroscopic approach. Insertion of an arthroscope into the dorsal compartment of the distal interphalangeal joint. **A,** Determination of landmarks. **B,** Joint inflation.

Continued

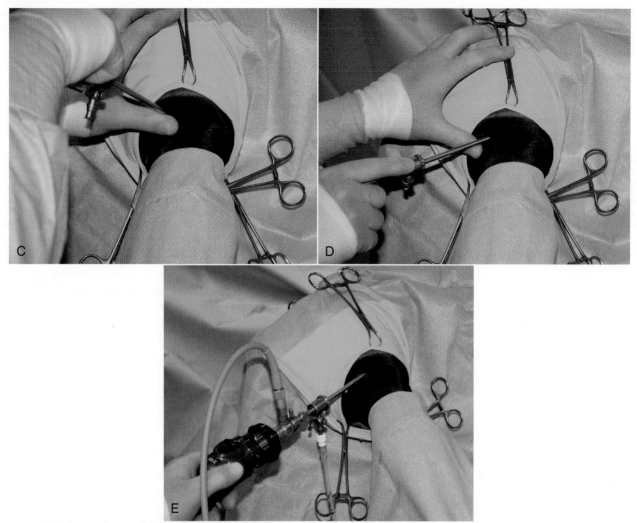

Figure 11-4, cont'd C, Initial entry of the arthroscopic cannula. **D,** Advancement of the arthroscopic cannula to the contralateral side of the joint. **E,** Insertion of the arthroscope and attachment of service lines.

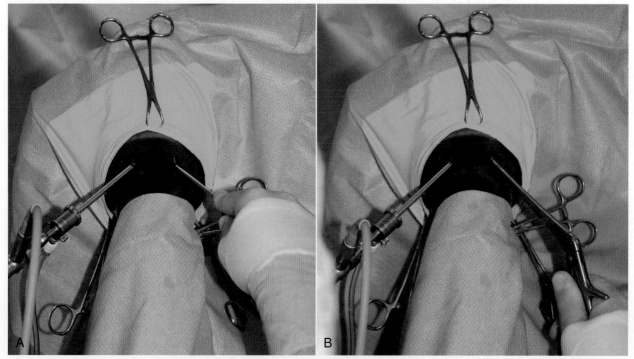

Figure 11-5 Dorsal compartment instrument entry. Arthroscope and instrument portals for the dorsal compartment of the distal interphalangeal joint at similar lateral and medial locations. **A,** An arthroscopic probe used to elevate the joint capsule and synovium. **B,** Introduction of arthroscopic rongeurs.

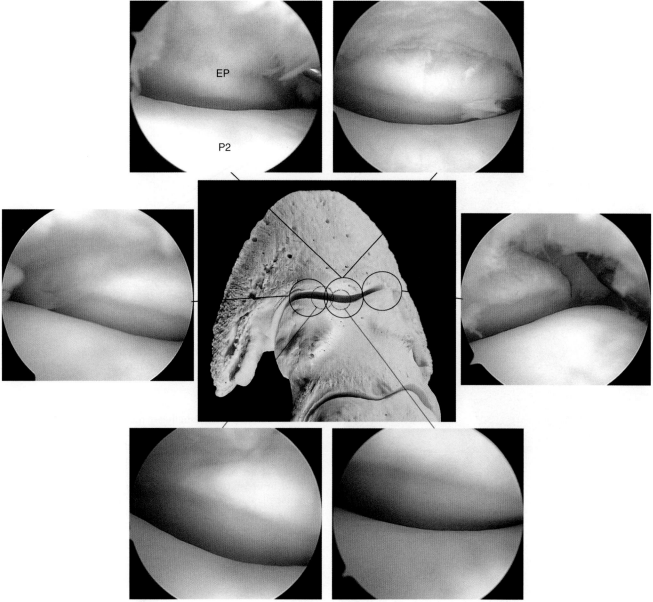

Figure 11-6 Diagnostic arthroscopy of the dorsal compartment of the distal interphalangeal joint. The arthroscope has been inserted in the position shown in Figures 11-3 and 11-4. Lower panels show deeper images of the articular surfaces with the limb extended. *EP,* Extensor process of distal phalanx; *P2,* middle phalanx.

In addition to use of the arthroscopic probe, flexion, extension, and rotation of the hoof will expose additional deeper (palmar/plantar) portions of the articulation.

Arthroscopic Examination of the Palmar/Plantar Pouch of the Distal Interphalangeal Joint

Arthroscopic Technique

Horses may be positioned in either dorsal or lateral recumbency, but dorsal is preferred because this facilitates use of a contralateral instrument portal. The landmarks for location of an arthroscopic portal into the palmar/plantar compartment of the distal interphalangeal joint are the palmar/plantar lateral or medial margins of the middle phalanx, the proximal margin of the collateral cartilage, and the palmar/plantar digital neurovascular bundle. The joint is distended maximally from the dorsal pouch, as described previously (Fig. 11-7). This creates a palpable fluctuant bulge between the palmar landmarks described. A 5-mm vertically orientated skin incision is made in the center

of the outpouching before the joint is penetrated by a stab incision with a No. 11 blade. The arthroscopic cannula is introduced using a conical obturator, first perpendicular to the limb and then directed axially and distally to the contralateral side of the joint (see Figs. 11-7 and 11-8). There is minimal resistance, and the thumb of the noninserting hand should be used as a friction bridge to assist control. The arthroscope can then be inserted (see Fig. 11-7). The original technique (Vacek et al, 1992) involved an arthroscopic portal placed palmar/plantar to the neurovascular bundle (see Fig. 11-8), which carries an increased risk of inadvertent entry to the digital flexor tendon sheath and navicular bursa (Fowlie et al, 2011). An alternative approach in which the incision is placed abaxial (dorsal) to the neurovascular bundle, thereby entering the DIP palmar/plantar pouch between the neurovascular structures and the palmar/plantar surface of the middle phalanx, has been described (Fowlie et al, 2011) and is preferred. The more palmar/plantarly located arthroscopic portal utilizes a skin incision that is similar in location to the

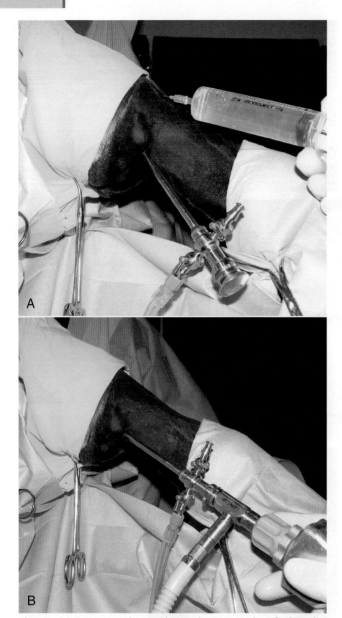

Figure 11-7 Approach to the palmar pouch of the distal interphalangeal joint. A, The joint is distended dorsally and the arthroscope sleeve inserted into the distended palmar pouch located palmar to the digital neurovascular bundle. **B,** The arthroscope is then inserted and examination commenced.

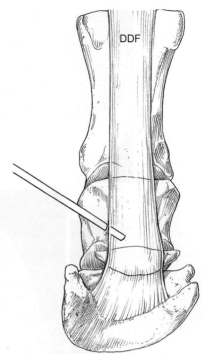

Figure 11-8 Palmar/plantar pouch arthroscopic technique. Diagram of arthroscope position for evaluation of the palmar/plantar distal interphalangeal joint. *DDF,* Deep digital flexor tendon.

Instrument portals usually are made in an identical position on the contralateral side of the limb. Prior insertion of a needle can assist, but it is important that the surgeon also palpates carefully to avoid damage to the neurovascular bundle. Interchange of arthroscope and instrument portals is frequently useful in order to make a comprehensive assessment of the palmar/plantar compartment. Most lesions can be operated in this manner, but occasionally ipsilateral arthroscope and instrument portals are required.

Arthroscopic Anatomy

In most horses, it is not possible to distract the navicular bone from the middle phalanx sufficiently to insert the arthroscope between their articular surfaces. Arthroscopic evaluation is therefore restricted to the proximal rim of the navicular bone, the condyles of the middle phalanx that can be exposed by flexion and extension of the limb, and the adjacent soft tissues (Fig. 11-9). Occasionally, in the authors experience most frequently in hindlimbs, the degree of distraction between the navicular bone and middle phalanx is sufficient to expose a greater portion of their articular surfaces.

The midpoint of the articulation provides the most consistent image and landmark for orientation (see Fig. 11-9) with the arthroscopic lens directed dorsally. The arthroscope can be swept along the entire proximal articular margins in a lateromedial arc. The medial and lateral margins of the navicular bone merge imperceptibly into its suspensory (collateral sesamoidean) ligaments. The differentiation is more readily palpated than visualized. Proximal to the articular cartilage–covered condyles of the middle phalanx is a large area of cortical bone, which is covered by a translucent thin synovium (see Fig. 11-9). Proximal to the navicular bone the voluminous palmar/plantar recess of the joint is filled with villous synovium, which covers the T ligament separating the distal interphalangeal joint from the digital flexor tendon sheath proximally and navicular bursa palmar/plantarly (see Fig. 11-9).

direct approach to the navicular bursa (see Chapter 13) and may be utilized when evaluating and treating horses with concurrent penetration/infection of the navicular bursa and distal interphalangeal joint. The palmar/plantar compartment of the distal interphalangeal joint can also be accessed by a transthecal technique as described for access to the proximal portion of the navicular bursa (Chapter 13), by creating a more dorsally situated window in the T ligament than that described for access to the navicular bursa. If necessary, both structures can be evaluated during the same procedure. This usually necessitates resection of a substantial portion of the T ligament, which does not appear to have any clinically adverse effect.

An Esmarch bandage and tourniquet can be useful in controlling intraoperative bleeding but necessitate careful palpation before portal creation in order to minimize the risk of iatrogenic damage to the adjacent palmar/plantar digital neurovascular bundle.

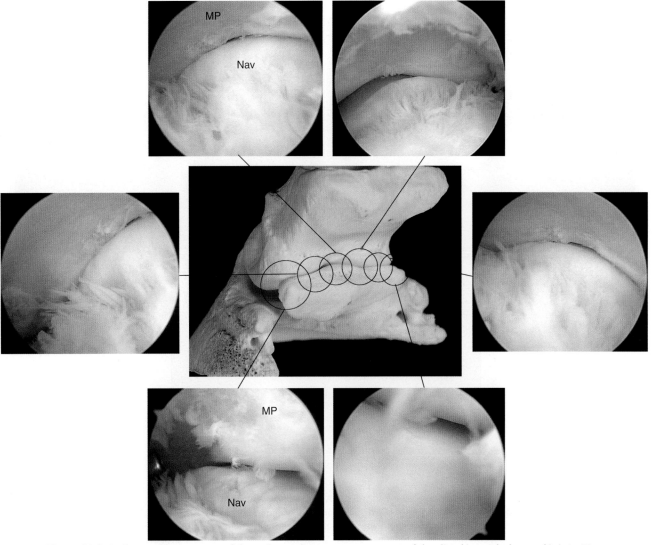

Figure 11-9 Arthroscopic anatomy of the palmar/plantar compartment of the distal interphalangeal joint. *Nav,* Navicular bone; *MP,* middle phalanx.

Postoperative Considerations

The skin portals are closed with simple interrupted sutures. Some surgeons utilize stainless steel skin staples. Postoperative wound hygiene is important. Sterile dressings should incorporate the entire hoof and be maintained until after suture removal. These may be changed at the surgeon's discretion, but it is important that they remain dry. Once wet, from whatever source, the risk of wicking contamination is high. For similar reasons, good postoperative stable hygiene is important both within the hospital and on discharge until wound healing is complete.

Arthroscopic Surgery for Conditions of the Distal Interphalangeal Joint

Osteochondral Fragmentation of the Extensor Process of the Distal Phalanx

Fragmentation of the extensor process of the distal phalanx is common in forelimbs but rare in hindlimbs. The varying presentations and lesion morphology suggest both traumatic and developmental etiologies (Figs. 11-10 and 11-11). Osteochondrosis-related fragments are considered to have more rounded, smoother contours, but differentiation between longstanding traumatic lesions and those with an osteochondrotic etiology is currently impossible. There is a substantial variation in size

and the degree of involvement of the common digital extensor tendon. In some horses the tendon insertion commences close to the proximal articular margin, whereas in others there is a more substantial dorsal recess such that smaller fragments can protrude into the joint with minimal tendon attachment. As a rule of thumb, the larger the fragment in both proximodistal and mediolateral planes, the more substantial the tendon attachment. A complete set of preoperative radiographs provides important information about the size, location, and therefore treatment in individual fractures. Lateromedial and dorsopalmar views are standard; additional projections that are slightly oblique from lateromedial can also be useful. CT may help the decision making with large fractures. The majority of fragmentation of the extensor process of the distal phalanx is amenable to arthroscopic removal as described by Boening (2002). Occasionally, large, nondisplaced or minimally displaced fractures can be repaired by internal fixation.

Arthroscopic Technique. For removal of fragments, a standard dorsal (usually lateral) arthroscopic approach is appropriate and is followed by evaluation of the dorsal compartment. Lesions in the articular cartilage of the middle phalanx are sometimes encountered, apparently as impingement erosions from the fragment. The extensor process of the distal phalanx, particularly if the fragmentation is longstanding, may initially be obscured

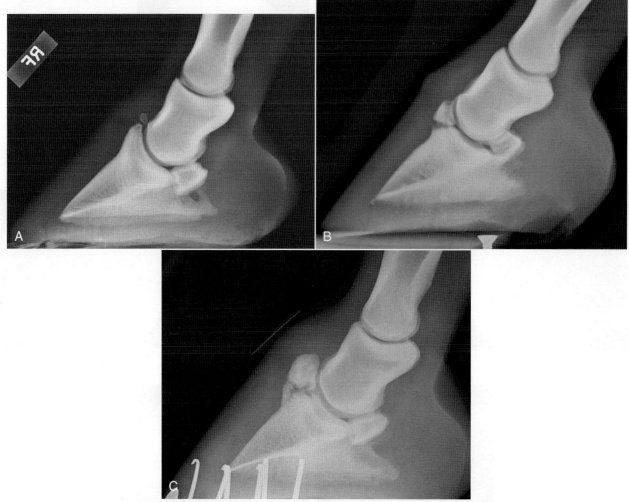

Figure 11-10 Extensor process fragmentation. Lateromedial radiographs of osteochondral fragments from the extensor process of the distal phalanx varying from **A,** a small chronic fragment, possibly a result of osteochondrosis, that have variable impact on the joint, to **B,** large fractures involving most of the extensor process that usually result in symptoms and need fragment removal or internal fixation to recover function, and **C,** massive fractures that are often chronic and may need removal with a bur.

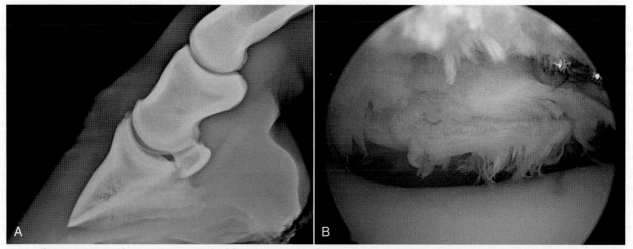

Figure 11-11 Arthroscopic removal of fragmentation of the extensor process of the distal phalanx. A, Latero-medial radiograph demonstrating a smoothly marginated fragment. **B-E,** Arthroscopic images of the fragment identified in **A. B,** Fragment exposed by elevation of the dorsal joint capsule with an arthroscopic probe. There is marked fibril-lation of the overlying cartilage.

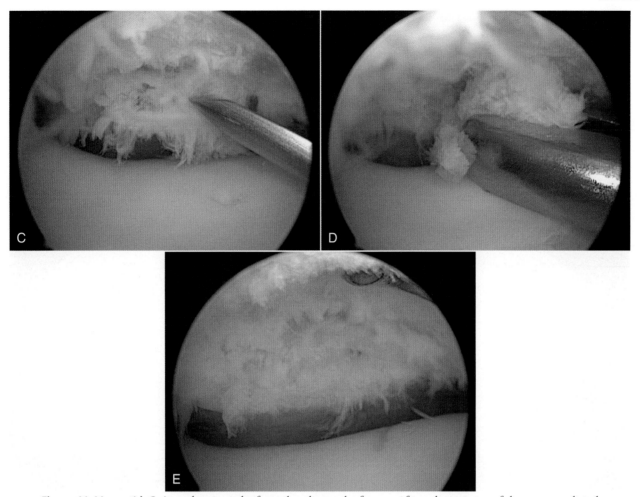

Figure 11-11, cont'd C, An arthroscopic knife used to dissect the fragment from the insertion of the common digital extensor tendon. **D,** Removal of the isolated fragment with arthroscopic rongeurs. **E,** Appearance of the defect following fragment removal and prior to debridement. The dorsal joint capsule and common digital extensor tendon are elevated with an arthroscopic probe.

by overlying proliferative synovium. This is elevated with an arthroscopic probe or resected with a motorized shaver introduced through an instrument portal on the contralateral side of the common digital extensor tendon (Fig. 11-11). A suitable site for the instrument portal is made following insertion of a percutaneous needle. The most frequent error is to place the portal too far proximal, which makes it difficult to establish an instrument trajectory to access the palmar margin of the fracture without impingement on the adjacent middle phalanx. It may be necessary in some cases to perform a localized synovial resection in order to adequately visualize the fracture margins and its attachments prior to dissection and removal. If the tendon attachment is substantial, sharp dissection utilizing a fixed blade knife is the least traumatic means of isolation. If necessary, the fragment can be elevated by insertion of an instrument into the fracture plane (Fig. 11-12). The fragments are removed utilizing arthroscopic rongeurs of a size determined by the individual fracture (see Fig. 11-11). Large fragments may be removed piecemeal. Occasionally, massive, usually longstanding fragments, which are frequently accompanied by distortion of the parent bone, can be debulked using motorized burrs (Fig. 11-13). Although clinical advantages of the latter procedure (Ter Braake, 2005) over arthrotomy (Dechant et al, 2000) have not been demonstrated, the general principles of arthroscopy with, in this instance, preservation of the coronary band suggest that this is likely.

Following fragment removal the fracture bed is debrided. Removal of frayed and extruded common digital extensor

tendon is also appropriate and should be conservative in nature (see Fig. 11-12). It is rarely necessary to address the cartilage lesions on the middle phalanx. During lavage the joint should be reinspected to ensure that all particulate debris is removed before skin portals are closed in a conventional manner.

Occasionally, large or minimally displaced fractures can be repaired by internal fixation under arthroscopic guidance. As in other sites, the fracture margins together with the site and trajectory of the implant are determined radiographically by the insertion of percutaneous needles under arthroscopic guidance (Fig. 11-14).

Postoperative Management. Following fragment removal animals are managed in a manner similar to that recommended for other sites and directions are varied according to individual case characteristics. Horses from which small fragments have been removed and in which minimal debridement has been necessary can return to conditioning exercise between 3 and 6 weeks after surgery. Most surgeons give only perioperative antimicrobial and nonsteroidal antiinflammatory drugs.

Results. Assessment of the results of removal of fragments from the extensor process of the distal phalanx for "preventative" reasons or to enhance sales prospects is impossible to assess. However, there have been several published case series of arthroscopic removal from lame horses. Boening et al (1990) described 14 of 16 lame horses that recovered full athletic function. Lameness due to the fractured extensor process resolved in 9 of 13 horses reported by Crowe et al (2010), although

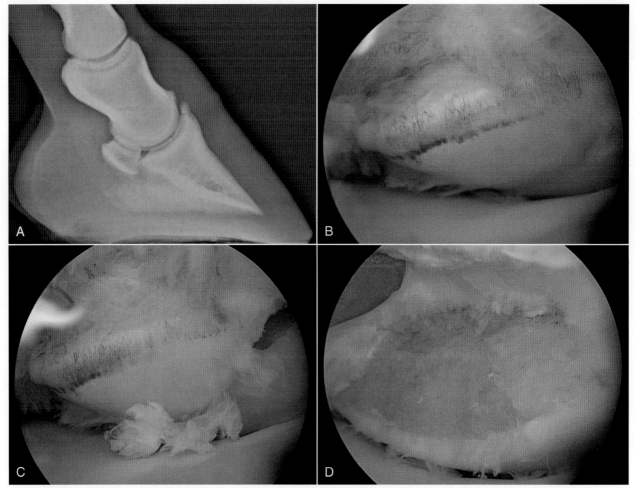

Figure 11-12 Acute chip fracture of the extensor process of the distal phalanx. **A,** Lateromedial radiograph demonstrating a sharp linear fracture line. Note the dorsal soft tissue contours consistent with distension of the distal interphalangeal joint. **B-D,** Arthroscopic images of the fracture depicted in **A. B,** Initial arthroscopic appearance. **C,** Displacement of the fracture with an arthroscopic probe. **D,** The fracture bed following fragment removal and debridement. The common digital extensor tendon is elevated with arthroscopic rongeurs.

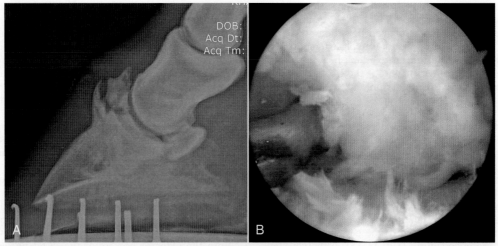

Figure 11-13 Chronic extensor process fracture. A Thoroughbred racehorse with a chronic large extensor process fracture treated by in situ burring before removal. **A,** Lateromedial radiograph showing chronic remodelling of the fracture bed. **B,** Fracture plane is partly identified by probe and periosteal elevator.

3 were unable to compete for unrelated reasons. Ter Braake (2005) reported successful outcomes in 3 of 4 horses with large extensor processes that were removed arthroscopically, which compared favorably with 8 of 14 (57%) of horses with similar fractures removed by arthrotomy (Dechant et al, 2000).

Abaxial Articular Fragments

Abaxial fragments from the middle phalanx commonly are intraarticular with respect to the dorsal or palmar/plantar compartments of the joint, or both (Fig. 11-15), and can be removed arthroscopically (McIlwraith & Goodman, 1989; Vail & McIlwraith, 1992). Such fractures are commonly comminuted. At arthroscopy the fragments are usually hinged onto joint capsule and may also involve the collateral ligaments. A standard, contralateral arthroscopic approach is employed for assessment. Instrument portals are generally more abaxially eccentric and are developed after needle verification of the appropriate location. In some circumstances ipsilateral arthroscope and instrument portals are necessary. Visibility, access, and maneuverability are all limited. The degree of dissection necessary for fragment removal varies but is necessary in almost all cases. If the fractures involves substantial portions of the collateral ligament, then a cast should be considered for anesthetic recovery and support in the immediate postoperative period.

Fragments in the Palmar/Plantaroproximal Pouch of the Distal Interphalangeal Joint

Osteochondral fragments may be identified in the proximal palmar/plantar outpouching of the distal interphalangeal joint, but these are rare (Brommer et al, 2001; Wagner et al, 1982). Etiology is unknown, but fracture from the middle phalanx, detachment of articular cartilage and subsequent endochondral ossification, and osteochondrosis all are possible. Removal utilizing the arthroscopic and instrument portals described earlier is appropriate.

Distal Phalangeal Cysts

Cysts involving the subchondral bone of the distal phalanx are most common in its middle one third (Fig. 11-16 and Fig 11-17). Reported treatments include intraarticular medication, extraarticular evacuation, and arthroscopic debridement and forage. Extraarticular approaches have been complicated by recurrent abscessation and lameness. Story & Bramlage (2004)

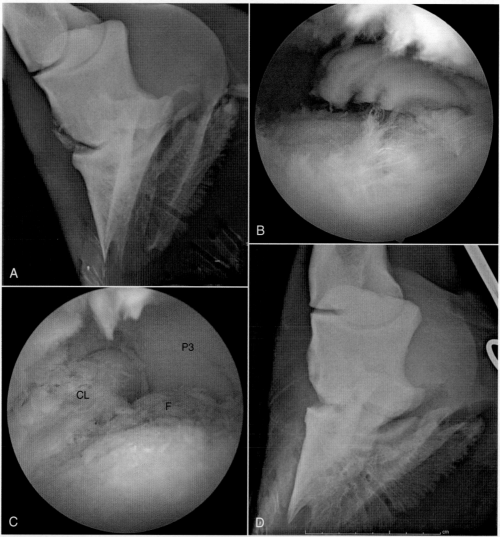

Figure 11-15 Comminuted intraarticular fracture of the distal dorsal surface of the medial condyle of the middle phalanx. **A,** Dorsolateral-palmaromedial oblique radiograph. **B,** Arthroscopic image from a dorsolateral arthroscopic portal demonstrating displaced fragments distomedially. **C,** Arthroscopic image of the fracture bed following fragment removal. Note exposure of an extensive portion of the medial articular surface of the distal phalanx *(P3)* and medial collateral ligament *(CL)*. *F,* Fracture bed in the middle phalanx. **D,** Intraoperative radiograph confirming fragment removal.

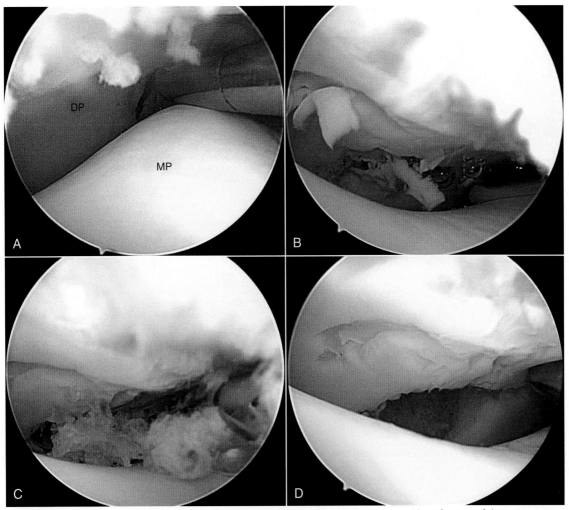

Figure 11-16 Debridement of a subchondral bone cyst of the distal phalanx. **A,** Identification of the cyst opening with a probe. **B,** Cartilage fragmentation of the surface of the cyst during debridement. **C,** Fibromyxoid cyst lining being removed. **D,** Appearance at the completion of evacuation and debridement. *DP,* Distal phalanx; *MP,* middle phalanx.

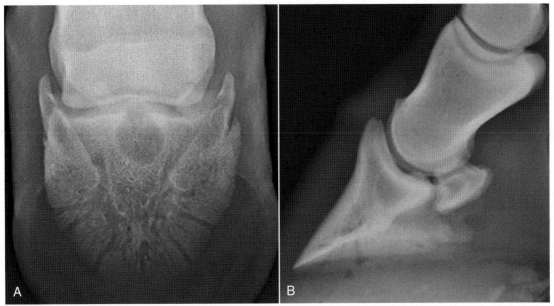

Figure 11-17 Arthroscopic debridement of distal phalanx cysts using second instrument portal for distraction. Dual instrument portals are used in mature horses to allow distal interphalangeal joint distraction and cyst debridement. **A** and **B,** Dorsoproximal–palmarodistal oblique and lateromedial radiographs reveal a large cyst in the more palmar region of the distal phalanx.

Continued

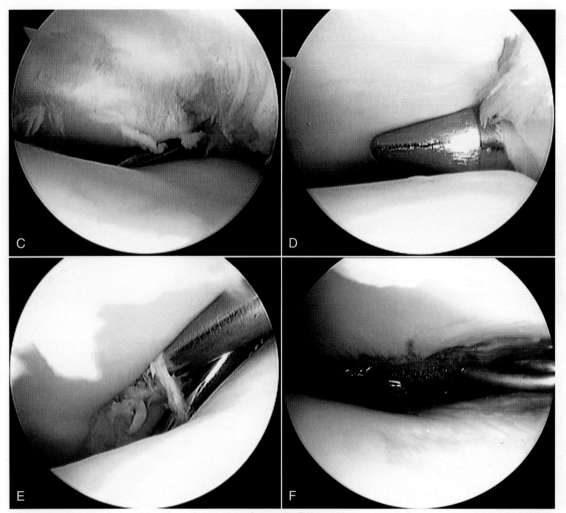

Figure 11-17, cont'd C and **D,** Abaxial insertion of a needle followed by a conical obturator. **E,** A large curved hemostat is used to maintain articular separation while a curved curette is inserted through the standard dorsal instrument portal to debride the cyst. **F,** Injection of cultured mesenchymal stem cell graft after cyst evacuation.

described a dorsal arthroscopic approach for cyst debridement and evacuation.

Surgery is performed in dorsal recumbency using a standard dorsal (in most cases a lateral) approach to the joint. Two instrument portals are necessary, one for joint distraction and the second for treatment. Joint distraction is usually more limited in adults compared with immature animals, and the more palmar/plantar the cyst opening the more difficult this becomes (see Fig. 11-17). A smooth curved hemostat or elevator or blunt obturator is inserted between middle and distal phalanges and rotated or levered to open the joint space. A second instrument portal is used for cyst evacuation and debridement and should be positioned after needle placement to provide the optimum position to allow access. The instrument portal for joint distraction can be made at a more remote location in order to avoid interference while producing the maximum distraction possible; this is generally more abaxial (medial) (Fig. 11-17). Evacuation of the cyst generally requires small curettes. Angled blades on motorized apparatus can also be helpful. If required, the debrided cyst can be filled with cultured mesenchymal stem cells (MSCs) and occasionally with tricalcium phosphate (TCP) in the depths of large cysts (see Fig. 11-17).

Story & Bramlage (2004) reported a successful return to work in 10 of 11 young horses treated by arthroscopic debridement alone. This is considered a considerable improvement compared with results of other treatments.

Middle Phalangeal Cysts

Subchondral bone cysts in the distal extremity of the middle phalanx can open into the distal interphalangeal joint anywhere from the dorsal to the palmar one third of its weight-bearing surface (Fig. 11-18). The communicating canal to cysts dorsal to the center of the convexity of the middle phalanx can be exposed by joint flexion but, unlike the metacarpophalangeal joint, flexion of the distal interphalangeal joint is restricted and more exposure to the central weight-bearing region is not usually possible (see Fig. 11-18). Preoperative application of a toe lever arm to increase the torque on the hoof in order to produce maximum flexion of the distal interphalangeal joint improves access to the communicating canal. Additionally, insertion of a curved hemostat or elevator can distract the distal phalanx enough to view the cyst opening (see Fig. 11-18). Curved curettes are used to debride the cyst contents. Grafts of bone marrow aspirate concentrate or TCP with cultured MSC overlay have been used (see Fig. 11-18). Although case numbers are limited, return to athletic capability is possible.

Cysts of the Proximal Region of the Navicular Bone

Arthroscopic treatment of osseous cyst-like lesions in the proximal region of the navicular bone was reported by Zierz et al (2000). The proximal margin of the navicular bone is visualized utilizing a standard approach to the palmar/plantar compartment of the distal interphalangeal joint. Following cyst identification, a contralateral instrument portal was

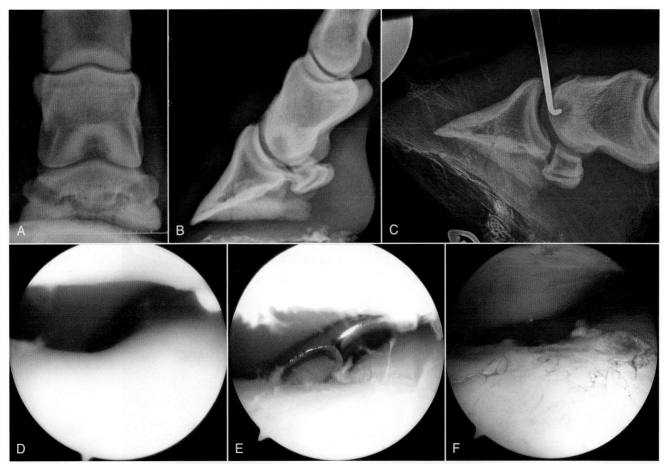

Figure 11-18 Middle phalanx subchondral cyst debridement. **A** and **B,** Dorsopalmar and lateromedial radiographs show a wide communication to the distal interphalangeal joint. **C,** Intraoperative radiograph used to verify cyst entry. **D,** Curved hemostat used for joint distraction and flexion. **E,** Cyst debridement with a curved curette. **F,** Cultured mesenchymal stem cell graft secured in place with platelet-rich plasma.

created and a 4.5-mm drill and sleeve were introduced. A drill tract was created diagonally through the cyst, and the authors reported a loss in drill resistance as the cyst cavity was encountered. Limited follow-up was reported, but two horses were reported to have returned to soundness and work.

Repair of Sagittal Fractures of the Distal Phalanx

Arthroscopic visualization of parasagittal fractures of the distal phalanx has revealed significant fracture disparity and mobility of fragments that disproves the traditional concept of the hoof capsule acting as a stabilizing shell. Arthroscopy allows removal of small comminuted fragments and more importantly guides reduction to ensure articular congruency and anatomic alignment before lag screw fixation.

The surgery is done with the horse in lateral recumbency with the affected limp uppermost. This permits arthroscopic and radiographic guidance. Arthroscope and instrument portals are made in the standard dorsolateral and dorsomedial aspects of the distal interphalangeal joint, although the instrument portal is usually close to the midline to allow direct access to the fracture plane. Any small fragments are removed from the visible portion of the fracture before reduction. Rotating the hoof usually aligns the fracture, which is then repaired using standard lag screw technique. Conventional postoperative management follows.

Repair of Fractures of the Middle Phalanx

Fractures involving the distal articular surface of the middle phalanx can be assessed and managed arthroscopically. As experienced at other sites, this permits detailed evaluation of the articular surface, recognition and removal of radiographically

silent comminution, and assessment and reduction of fracture displacement (Fig. 11-19).

Avulsions of the Joint Capsule

The authors have arthroscopically identified avulsions of the dorsal joint capsule from the middle phalanx. Affected horses have usually exhibited moderate to severe lameness with marked palpable (and sometimes visible) distension of the distal interphalangeal joint. In acute cases there can also be adjacent soft tissue swelling and other acute inflammatory signs. At this time ultrasonography may identify tearing, and MRI is also helpful in identifying the type and extent of injury. Later, irregular new bone may develop on the dorsal diaphysis of the middle phalanx (Fig. 11-20). The arthroscopic appearance of the joint depends on the time post injury, but characteristically the joint cavity extends proximal to its usual confines, exposing a greater portion of the middle phalanx. Treatment includes removal of torn capsular tissue and bone proliferation. Symptomatic benefits have been observed, but long-term follow-up information is not yet available.

Arthroscopically Assisted Arthrodesis

In a case report, accessible articular cartilage was removed arthroscopically from both dorsal and palmar compartments of the joint, followed by lag screw fixation for arthrodesis (Busschers & Richardson, 2006). Surgery was performed in lateral recumbency with a tourniquet. Articular cartilage was removed with curettes and a motorized burr and synovium with a full radius resector. Three 5.5-mm cortical screws were then placed in lag technique with

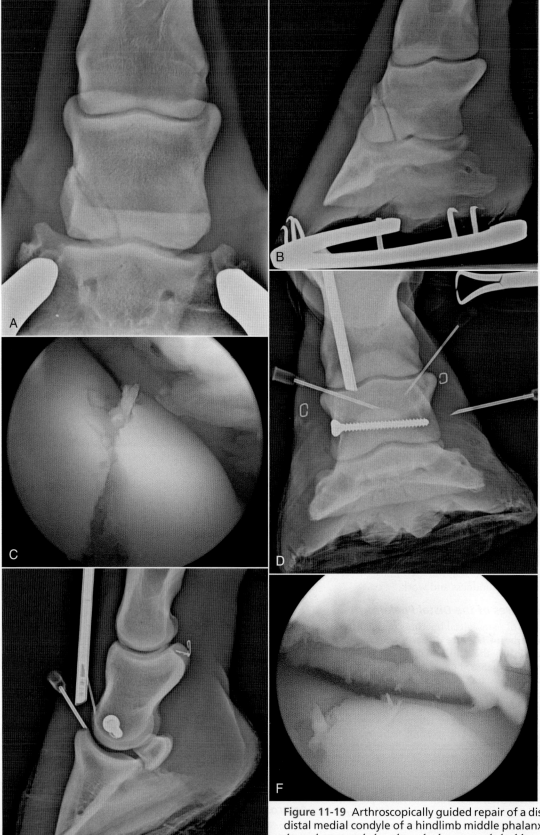

Figure 11-19 Arthroscopically guided repair of a displaced fracture of the distal medial condyle of a hindlimb middle phalanx. **A** and **B,** Preoperative dorsoplantar and dorsolateral–plantaromedial oblique radiographs. **C,** Fracture viewed from a dorsomedial arthroscopic portal. **D** and **E,** Intraoperative dorsoplantar and lateromedial radiographs following reduction and insertion of a 4.5-mm AO/ASIF cortical screw. Note use of percutaneous needles for arthroscopic guidance and stainless steel staples for radiographic alignment. **F,** Arthroscopic appearance of the fracture following reduction and repair.

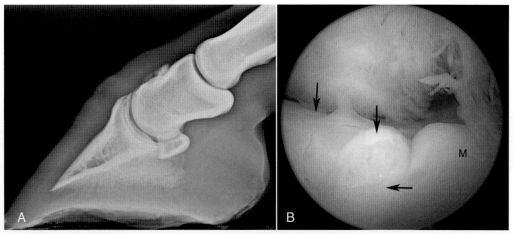

Figure 11-20 Avulsion of the joint capsule. **A,** Lateromedial radiograph demonstrating irregular new bone on the dorsal surface of the middle phalanx. **B,** Arthroscopic appearance. The joint capsule extends proximally along the dorsal surface of the middle phalanx exposing the new bone *(arrows)* proximal to the articular cartilage of the middle phalanx *(M)*. Distal = right; proximal = left.

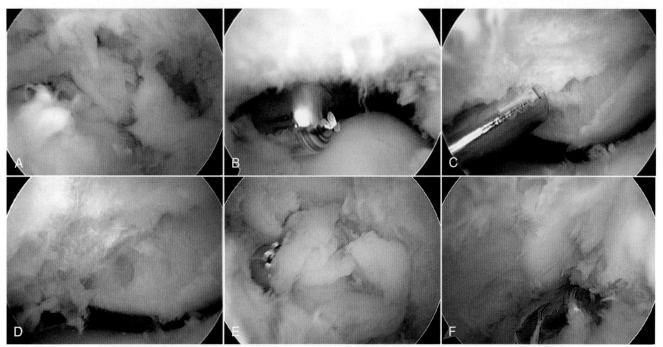

Figure 11-21 Arthroscopic treatment of distal interphalangeal septic arthritis following joint injection in an 8-year-old warmblood. **A,** Initial entry to the dorsal pouch shows considerable purulent debris. **B-D,** Motorized removal of debris reveals an extensor process with bony cavities exposed where infection has entered the bone. **E-G,** Removal of purulent debris from the palmar pouch reveals similar involvement of the palmar surface of the middle phalanx and navicular bone.

Continued

dorsodistal to palmaroproximal orientations through the dorsal hoof wall under fluoroscopic guidance. Arthrodesis was completed by placement of a cancellous bone graft into the dorsal and palmar compartments of the joint. A cast was applied and successful ankylosis and pasture soundness followed.

Transection of the Collateral Sesamoidean (Navicular Suspensory) Ligaments

Sampson et al (2010) described a technique for division of the navicular suspensory ligaments using a hook knife via the palmar pouch of the distal interphalangeal joint. Contralateral arthroscope and instrument portals were employed, and these were interchanged for medial and lateral ligaments. Laceration of a palmar digital vein occurred in 50% of cases. Evaluation of clinical application is pending.

Contamination and Infection

This subject is discussed in detail in Chapter 14. Infection of the distal interphalangeal joint is often a sequel to joint injection or penetrating injuries of the coronary band, heel bulbs, or from solar (street nail) penetrations through the impar ligament. The latter always penetrate through the navicular bursa. Rarely, hematogenous infection can result from bacteremia in foals or even adults when osteomyelitis has not yet developed. Intense therapy including arthroscopy of dorsal and palmar/plantar compartments of the joint is indicated.

Dorsal and palmar/plantar approaches are necessary for assessment, removal of foreign material, devitalized tissue, and purulent material (Fig. 11-21). Extensive lavage is accompanied by fibrinectomy/synovectomy as needed. Continued flushing of both pouches is utilized. The authors vary in their use of antimicrobial delivery by ingress systems and/or

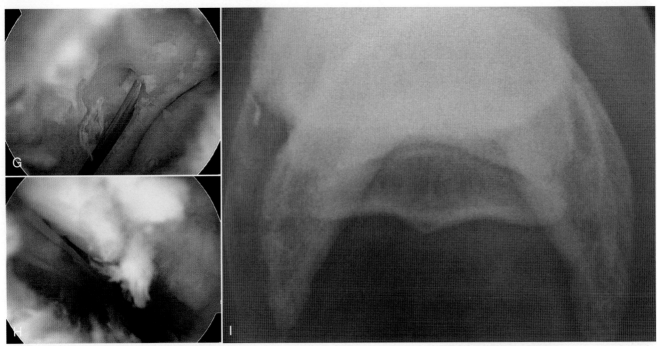

Figure 11-21, cont'd H, Ingress drain in palmar pouch for antimicrobial delivery. **I,** Navicular cystic change evident 6 weeks postoperatively.

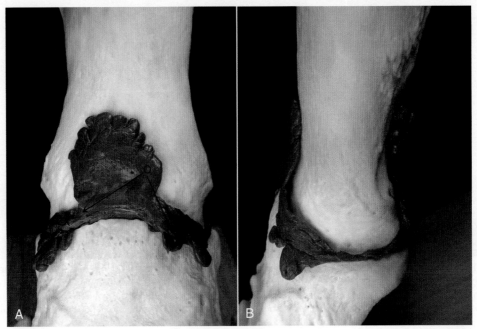

Figure 11-22 Latex injection model showing the proximal interphalangeal (PIP) joint from **(A)** dorsal and **(B)** lateral perspectives. The dorsal PIP joint pouch is small and abaxially constrained by the joint capsule and collateral ligaments. The optimum arthroscopic entry *(O)* allows visualization distally into the contralateral and less optimally the ipsilateral regions *(arrows)* of the dorsal pouch. An instrument portal *(X)* is shown in close proximity to the narrower abaxial portion of the joint. The central arthroscope entry may penetrate the extensor tendon, but this has few consequences and allows improved visualization of both dorsolateral and dorsomedial portions of the joint. *(Latex model images courtesy Dr. R. Radcliffe.)*

regional intravenous perfusion. Systemic antimicrobial drugs are administered in all cases and, when possible, chosen from the results of culture and sensitivity. Absorbable bone cement beads laden with antimicrobial drugs or other sustained release techniques, or both, may also be beneficial. Outcome is often determined by chronicity and the degree of osseous involvement. A complication of chronic distal interphalangeal septic arthritis in adults is navicular cystic degeneration after resolution of the septic process (see Fig. 11-21), which is often accompanied by osteoarthritis. The reason for this is not clear, but continued lameness is often a consequence.

ARTHROSCOPY OF THE PROXIMAL INTERPHALANGEAL JOINT

There are few reports of arthroscopy of the equine proximal interphalangeal (PIP) joint (McIlwraith, 1990; Nixon, 2012; Radcliffe et al, 2008; Schneider et al, 1994), and in all cases

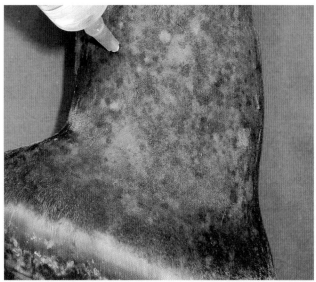

Figure 11-23 Visible distension of the dorsal compartment of the proximal interphalangeal joint after inflation through the palmar pouch.

the numbers are small. One report describes a single case, another group of three Standardbred racehorses in which osteochondral fragments were removed from the dorsal aspect of the joint, and the other group of four horses in which fragments were removed from the palmar/plantar pouch. A recent cadaver study has correlated MRI, contrast arthrography, and arthroscopy of the proximal interphalangeal joint (Kamm et al, 2012). These authors established that 62% of the articular surface can be evaluated arthroscopically; only that area beneath the collateral ligaments is not visible. Methylmethacrylate and latex injection techniques have demonstrated restricted abaxial joint space in both dorsal and palmar/plantar compartments, but a large proximal axial cavity dorsally and voluminous palmar/plantar outpouchings (Fig. 11-22).

Arthroscopy of the Dorsal Pouch of the Proximal Interphalangeal Joint

Technique

The limited space in the dorsal pouch is such that arthroscopic evaluation is uniplanar and accurate location of arthroscopic portals is critical. The range of motion is small and the limb should be fixed in maximal extension. Arthroscopy may be performed in dorsal or lateral recumbency but dorsal is preferred, and use of an Esmarch bandage and tourniquet can be useful but are at the surgeon's discretion. Following application of circumferential impervious drapes, insertion of the arthroscopic cannula is facilitated by maximal distension of the joint (Figs. 11-23 and 11-24). This may be achieved from the dorsal or palmar/plantar aspect but in most cases it is most readily performed through the palmar/plantar pouch using the technique reported by Miller et al (1996), entering 2 to 3 mm proximal to the distal condyle(s) of the proximal phalanx. The dorsal outpouching of the distended joint is palpated on the abaxial margins of the common/long digital extensor tendon (see Fig. 11-24). A 5 mm skin incision is made with a number 11 or 15 blade at the junction of the middle and proximal one thirds of the outpouching at the lateral or medial margin of the tendon (see Fig. 11-24). Portals that are eccentric to this in any direction will limit movement, access, and visibility. Following a stab incision through the thin joint capsule, the arthroscopic sleeve and conical obturator are inserted, at first perpendicular to the limb before the inserting hand is moved in an abaxial and distal arch to push the arthroscopic cannula between the common/long digital

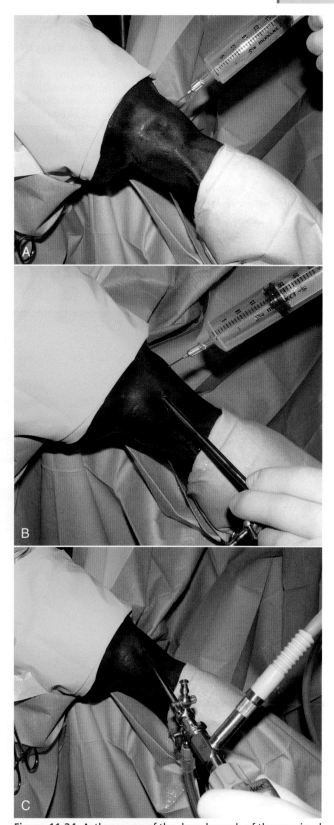

Figure 11-24 Arthroscopy of the dorsal pouch of the proximal interphalangeal joint. **A,** Needle insertion for distension can be done dorsally or in the palmar/plantar pouch. **B,** The skin incision is made abaxial to the extensor tendon, and the arthroscope sleeve inserted obliquely distally and axially. **C,** Insertion of the arthroscope and attachment of the service lines.

extensor tendon and condyles of the proximal phalanx and over to the contralateral side of the joint. Throughout, the thumb of the noninserting hand is used as a friction bridge to control the insertion procedure. The arthroscope and service lines can then be attached (see Fig. 11-24). In most circumstances a contralateral instrument portal is employed. The ideal position is determined by percutaneous needle placement, which again is on the abaxial margin of the extensor tendon, although the proximodistal location may vary. A more distal arthroscopic portal has previously been recommended (Schneider et al, 1994). In the authors' hands this is more restrictive and offers no advantage with respect to visualization (Kamm et al, 2012).

Arthroscopic Anatomy of the Dorsal Pouch of the Proximal Interphalangeal Joint

The easiest location for orientation is the center of the dorsal compartment with the lens angled palmar/plantar, which visualizes the shallow central concavity between the distal condyles of the proximal phalanx and the relatively sharp proximal articular margin of the middle phalanx (Fig. 11-25). Keeping the camera in the same orientation but with left and right angulation of

the arthroscopic lens together with minimal medial and lateral movement visualizes the respective convex condyles of the proximal phalanx and adjacent articular rim of the middle phalanx (see Fig. 11-25). Along the dorsal articular margin of the middle phalanx the synovium is villous, whereas abaxially and beneath the common/long digital extensor tendon it is smooth and avillous. With distal movement of the arthroscopic camera and corresponding angulation of the lens, the proximal dorsal recess is rotated into view. In normal joints this is covered by fine villous synovium, although proliferation in clinical cases is common. The entire proximal margin of the articular cartilage on the distal condyles of the proximal phalanx is visualized (see Fig. 11-25).

Arthroscopy of the Palmar/Plantar Pouch of the Proximal Interphalangeal Joint
Anatomic Considerations

The palmar/plantar pouch of the proximal interphalangeal joint is more spacious axially than abaxially, where it is limited by the palmar/plantar (middle) scutum, palmar/plantar ligaments, and the tendon of insertion of the superficial digital flexor (SDF) (Fig. 11-26). The point of arthroscopic entry

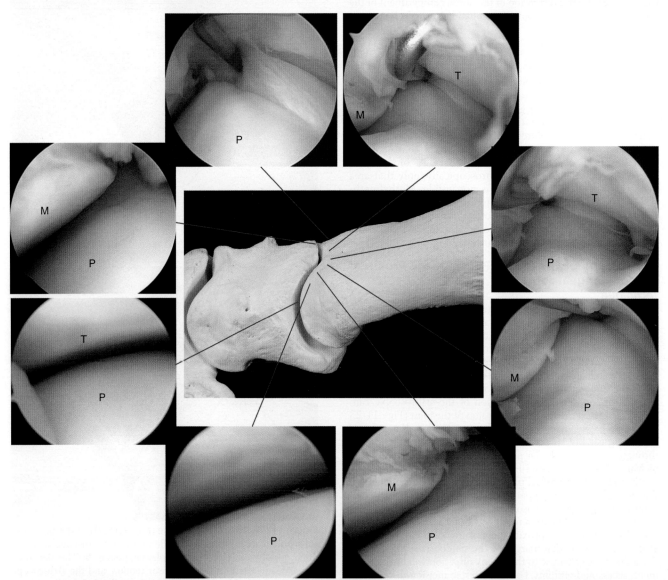

Figure 11-25 Diagnostic arthroscopy of the dorsal compartment of the proximal interphalangeal joint. The arthroscope has been inserted in the position shown in Figure 11-22. Panels on the right were obtained with the proximal interphalangeal joint partially flexed to expose more of the condylar surface of the proximal phalanx. *M,* Middle phalanx; *P,* proximal phalanx; *T,* common/long digital extensor tendon.

must be sufficiently proximal to avoid the SDF insertion. The palmar/plantar scutum is a complete, thick, and rather immovable fibrocartilagenous plate formed by the insertions of the straight distal sesamoidean ligament and the SDF tendon (see Fig. 11-26). The bulk of the palmar/plantar scutum encloses the proximal perimeter of the middle phalanx forming a tight and robust barrier to arthroscope or instrument entry at this level. Shaving of portions of the palmar/plantar scutum to gain access to abaxial fragments has been utilized (Radcliffe et al, 2008), but the extent to which this can be done is not known. Axial fragments can be assessed and dissected free in the void between the two condyles of the proximal phalanx, which maintains a working space.

Arthroscopic Technique

Arthroscopy of the palmar/plantar compartment can be performed in dorsal or lateral recumbency, but dorsal is generally preferred. The forelimbs are positioned with a rolled towel, drape, or similar bulk taped behind the carpus to selectively allow passive and active flexion of the distal limb with support

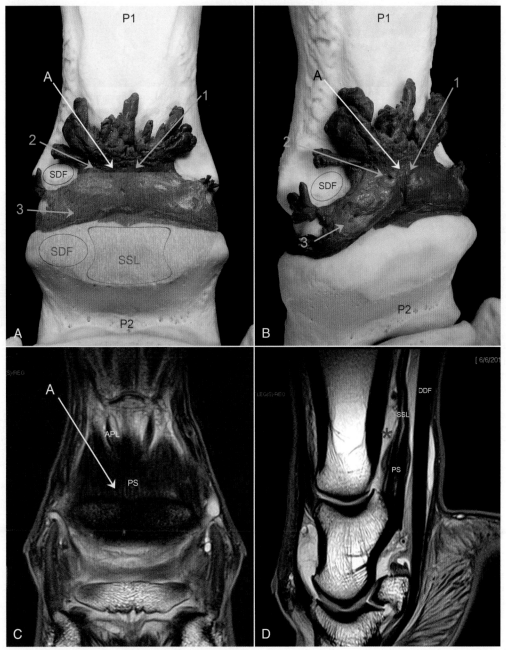

Figure 11-26 Arthroscopic anatomy relevant to the palmar/plantar pouch of the proximal interphalangeal (PIP) joint. **A** and **B,** Latex models show the more spacious axial region and the limited joint space created by the palmar scutum (shaded area) formed by the confluence of the straight sesamoidean ligament *(SSL)* and superficial digital flexor *(SDF)* insertions. Arthroscope entry *(A)* must be proximal to the SDF branch inserting in the palmar epicondyle of the proximal phalanx. Instrument entry is contralateral *(1)*, ipsilateral *(2)*, and rarely distal adjacent to the middle phalanx *(3)*. **C,** Frontal plane magnetic resonance image (MRI) showing the arthroscope entry path *(A arrow)* and broad palmar scutum *(PS)* forming the complete palmar limits to the palmar/plantar pouch of the PIP. The proximal portion of the palmar pouch is also limited by the axial palmar ligament *(APL)*, which arises from the SSL and inserts on the proximal phalanx. **D,** Sagittal MRI showing the confluence of *SSL* with *PS*. The arthroscope entry is marked *(*)*.

Continued

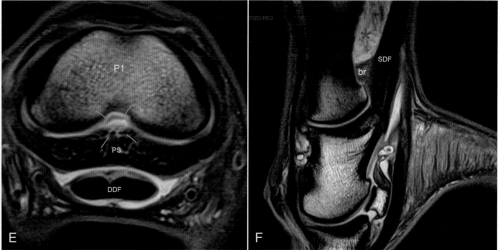

Figure 11-26, cont'd E, Transverse MRI at the level of the middle phalanx palmar/plantar eminence intrusion (blue reference markers) to the PIP joint. Abaxial to this level the dense palmar scutum *(PS)* abuts the articular condyles of the proximal phalanx. **F,** Abaxial sagittal MRI image shows the SDF branch *(br)* inserting on the proximal phalanx. Arthroscope entry *(*)* is always proximal to this insertion. *(Latex model images courtesy Dr. R. Radcliffe.)*

of the foot optional (Fig. 11-27). Hindlimbs passively flex the distal joints because of the reciprocal apparatus, and the foot is supported to prevent excessive flexion. The ease of hindlimb flexion compared with forelimbs may provide improved access to the hindlimb plantar pouch (Radcliffe et al, 2008). The joint is predistended as described earlier (Fig. 11-28). The distended palmar/plantar pouch may be palpated medially and laterally adjacent to the palmar/plantar abaxial margins of the proximal phalanx dorsal to the palmar/plantar digital neurovascular bundles. A 5-mm skin incision is made proximally in the outpouching followed by a stab incision into the joint close to the palmar/plantar margin of the proximal phalanx (see Fig. 11-28). The conical obturator and arthroscopic cannula are then inserted into the palmar/plantar pouch aiming axially and distally (see Fig. 11-28). The arthroscope service lines can then be connected. The most versatile instrument portal is made at a similar location in the contralateral side (Fig. 11-29) and can be varied according to need by prior percutaneous needle insertion. When soft tissue dissection is necessary or anticipated, application of an Esmarch bandage and tourniquet can expedite surgery. However, this requires an increased level of vigilance with respect to location of the adjacent neurovascular bundle.

Arthroscopic Anatomy of the Palmar/Plantar Pouch of the Proximal Interphalangeal Joint

Evaluation of the palmar/plantar compartment commences axially, which provides a consistently recognizable image for orientation (Fig. 11-30). Centrally, there is a marked concavity in the distal palmar/plantar articular surface of the proximal phalanx between its medial and lateral condyles. The articular cartilage of the condyles generally extends farther proximal than this central site, creating the appearance of a notch. Proximal to the hyaline cartilage on the palmar/plantar aspect of the proximal phalanx there is a broad zone of bone covered by a thin translucent and, in the normal joint, avillous layer of synovium. The shallow central eminence of the proximal palmar/plantar margin of the middle phalanx covered by hyaline cartilage is visible at this point. The proximal margin of this blends with the central (axial) portion of the palmar/plantar fibrocartilagenous scutum. Rotation of the arthroscope lens combined with a small amount of advancement/retraction of the arthroscope brings into view the abaxial (medial and

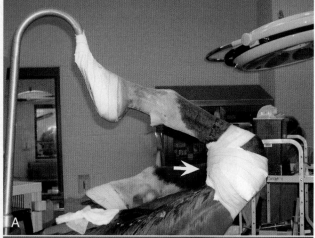
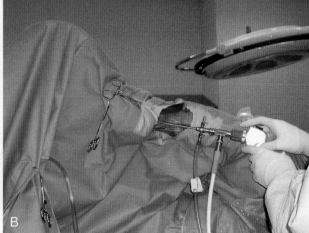

Figure 11-27 Limb positioned for arthroscopy of the palmar proximal interphalangeal joint. **A,** Carpal flexion is limited by a role of firm bandage or towel behind the knee *(arrow).* In this instance the foot is supported. **B,** After application of impervious drapes, windows are created medially and laterally for arthroscope and instrument access.

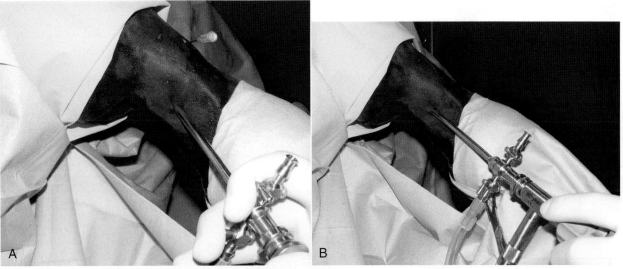

Figure 11-28 Arthroscopic approach to the palmar/plantar compartment of the proximal interphalangeal joint. **A,** With the joint distended the skin incision is made in the proximal portion of the palmar pouch, and the arthroscope cannula inserted obliquely distally and axially. **B,** The arthroscope is inserted to position the tip over the palmar/plantar midline.

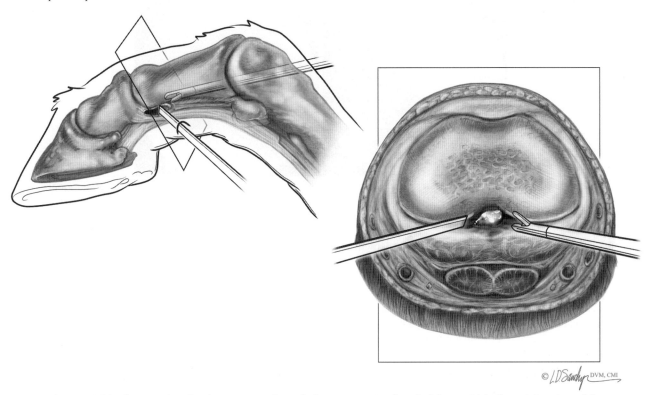

Figure 11-29 Diagram showing instrument triangulation to an osteochondral fragment in the axial region of the palmar/plantar pouch of the proximal interphalangeal joint. The arthroscope and instruments should penetrate the palmar/plantar pouch as far palmar/plantar as possible to allow access to the dorsal surfaces of the fragment and optimize penetration between the cartilage surfaces and the palmar scutum. *(Printed with permission from © Lauren D. Sawchyn, DVM, CMI.)*

lateral) margins of the joint (see Fig. 11-30). The medial and lateral condyles of the proximal phalanx are readily inspected together with the adjacent exposed metaphyseal bone. The medial and lateral palmar/plantar articular margins of the middle phalanx merge imperceptibly into the fibrocartilage of the palmar/plantar scutum (see Fig. 11-30). Slight withdrawal of the arthroscope with proximal angulation of the lens visualizes the spacious proximal outpouching dorsally and proximally, which is lined by fine villous synovium.

Arthroscopic Surgery for Conditions of the Proximal Interphalangeal Joint
Removal of Osteochondral Fragments from the Dorsal Compartment of the Proximal Interphalangeal Joint
Fragmentation of the dorsoproximal articular margin of the middle phalanx is uncommon. Arthroscopic evaluation and treatment of three horses with fragments at this site in hindlimbs were reported by Schneider et al (1994). The authors have seen similar cases, predominantly in hindlimbs, but

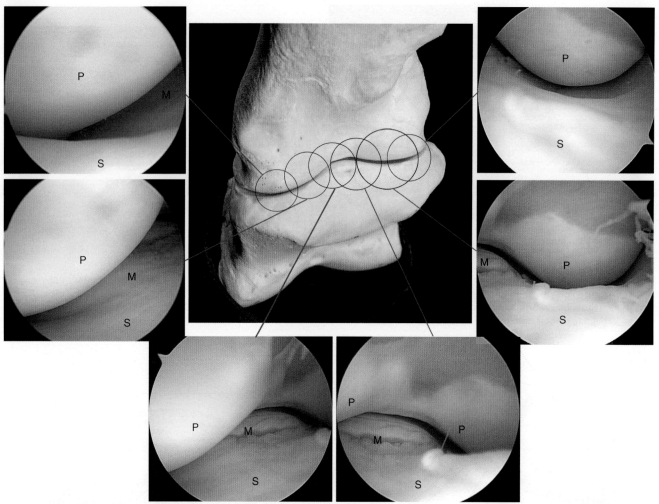

Figure 11-30 Diagnostic arthroscopy images of the palmar compartment of the proximal interphalangeal joint. The arthroscope has been inserted in the position shown in Figures 11-28 and 11-29. *M*, Middle phalanx; *P*, proximal phalanx; *S*, scutum.

several involving the forelimbs. Horses present with lameness and distension of the proximal interphalangeal joint. Fragments can develop at any point on the dorsal articular rim and are identified on lateromedial and/or dorsolateral-plantaromedial oblique or dorsomedial-plantarolateral oblique radiographs. Schneider et al (1994) considered osteochondrosis the most likely etiology in light of the horses' ages (two yearlings and one 2-year-old), but the authors have seen traumatic fragmentation at this site in mature working horses (Fig. 11-31). Central (axial) fragments usually have minimal capsular attachment, whereas abaxial fragments have more substantial capsule adherence, making sharp dissection necessary. Removal utilizes appropriately sized arthroscopic rongeurs and the underlying defect is debrided. In the absence of preexisting degenerative joint disease, the prognosis should be favorable. The three cases reported by Schneider et al (1994) were able to work postoperatively, and this included two Standardbreds that raced 18 and 26 times and a Thoroughbred yearling that entered training as a 2-year-old.

Fragmentation of the dorsodistal articular surface of the proximal phalanx has a similar clinical presentation. Lesions have been reported to be most common medially (Fjordbakk et al, 2007). These authors reported six cases, four involving forelimbs and two hindlimbs, but the authors' cases have all involved hindlimbs. Lesions have only been identified in young animals, but the radiologic and arthroscopic appearance has been more consistent with trauma than an osteochondrosis

(Fig. 11-32), although Fjordbakk et al (2007) considered a developmental etiology most likely. The arthroscopic approach and management is as described for fragmentation of the middle phalanx.

Fragmentation of the Palmar/Plantar Margin of the Middle Phalanx

Fragmentation at this site can have varying amounts of articular involvement. Some fragments are embedded within the palmar/plantar scutum and associated insertions of the superficial digital flexor and straight distal sesamoidean ligament and are entirely extraarticular. Preoperative assessment of the articular proportions and therefore arthroscopic accessibility is usually made on the basis of radiographic location and appearance, distension of the proximal interphalangeal joint, and an ultrasonographic assessment. When available, MRI and CT can also be helpful in determining site of origin.

Asymptomatic axially located fragments are occasionally encountered in prepurchase examination radiographs. Others can be associated with mild lameness, joint distension, and a positive flexion test. Some, frequently larger fragments can occupy a substantial portion of the axial joint space and cause consistent lameness (Fig. 11-33). These and others that are slightly abaxial to this site can be removed arthroscopically using a contralateral portal (see Fig. 11-29). Fragments that are abaxially located are less readily accessed arthroscopically because they are embedded within the palmar/plantar scutum.

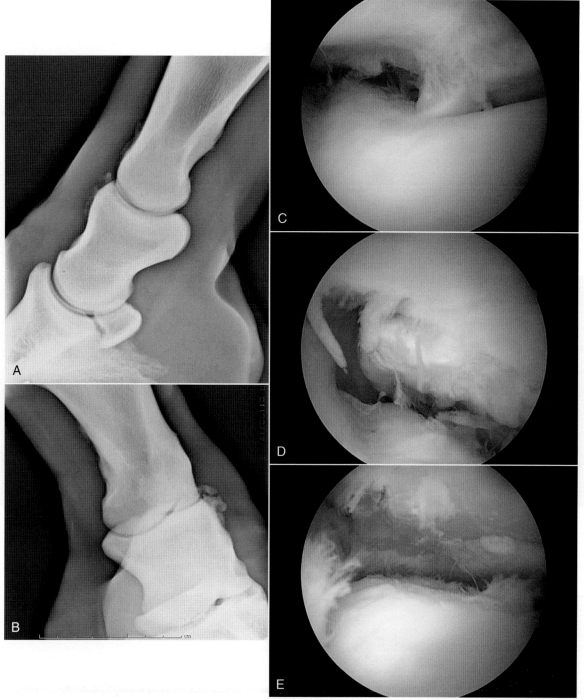

Figure 11-31 Fragmentation of the dorsoproximal articular margin of the middle phalanx in the hindlimb of a show jumper. **A,** Lateromedial and **B,** dorsolateral-plantaromedial oblique radiographs demonstrating dorsal and dorsomedial fragments. **C-E,** Arthroscopic images of the joint imaged in (A) and (B) from a dorsolateral portal. **C,** A small displaced fragment on the sagittal midline. **D,** Large abaxial (medial) fragments. **E,** Arthroscopic appearance following fragment removal and debridement of the middle phalanx.

These appear to be avulsion injuries and in the acute phase can cause marked lameness. The potential benefits of surgery and approach made are determined on an individual case basis but in horses in which the scutum is disrupted, the fragments, which normally would be extraarticular, can become arthroscopically accessible through the fibrocartilage defect (Fig. 11-34).

The palmar/plantar compartment is assessed using the arthroscopic approach and instrument portal described earlier (see Fig. 11-29). In some cases, interchange of arthroscope and instrument portals or use of ipsilateral portals, or both, can be of benefit (Radcliffe et al, 2008). Some large, axial fragments may need to be split with an osteotome or reduced in size by burring (see Fig. 11-33). More abaxial fragments inevitably will require dissection from the palmar/plantar scutum. This is tough, inflexible fibrocartilage and usually requires the use of fixed-blade knives, scissors, and a motorized resector. Intraoperative radiographs or fluoroscopy can be useful aids. In many cases involving abaxial fractures,

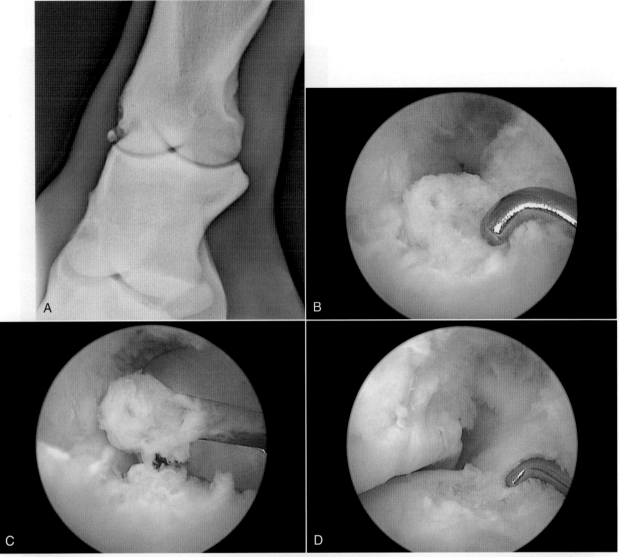

Figure 11-32 Fragmentation of the dorsodistal margin of the proximal phalanx in the proximal interphalangeal joint. **A,** Dorsolateral-plantaromedial oblique radiograph demonstrating fragmentation on the dorsomedial articular margin. **B-D,** Arthroscopic images from a dorsolateral portal. **B,** Fragment identified and manipulated with an arthroscopic probe. **C,** Removal with arthroscopic rongeurs. **D,** Fibrous tissue beneath the fragment covering the defect in the proximal phalanx at completion of debridement.

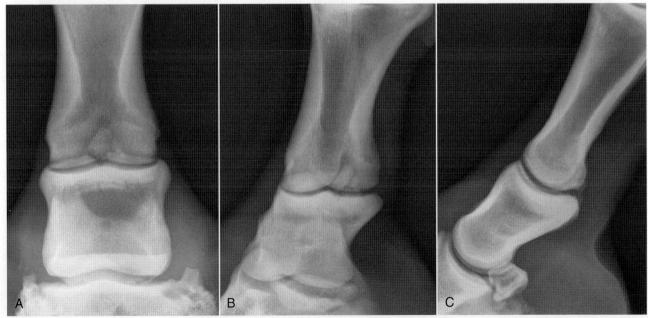

Figure 11-33 Multiple axial palmar fractures originating from the middle phalanx in a 6-year-old Thoroughbred. **A-C,** Radiographs show the site of origin from the palmar perimeter of the middle phalanx and the enlargement to occupy the palmar axial pouch of the proximal interphalangeal joint.

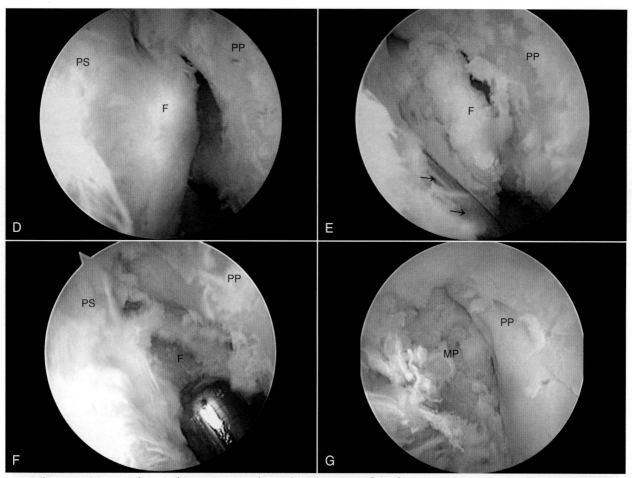

Figure 11-33, cont'd D, Arthroscopic view shows the continuum of the fracture *(F)* and the palmar scutum *(PS),* occupying the axial mid portion of the palmar pouch adjacent to the proximal phalanx *(PP).* **E,** Ipsilateral instrument portal allows a curved, hard-backed blade *(arrows)* to be used to free the fragment from the scutum. **F,** A motorized shaver is used to trim the soft tissues before splitting the fragment with an osteotome using a contralateral portal. **G,** After fragment removal, the bed on the middle phalanx *(MP)* is debrided.

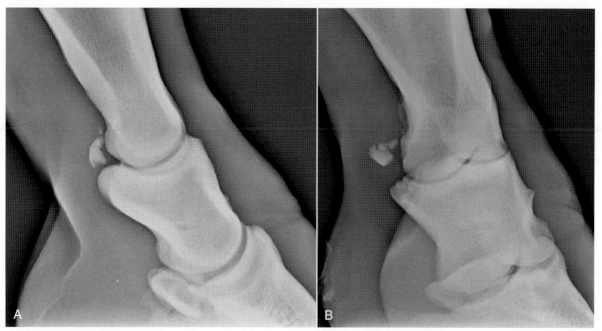

Figure 11-34 Acute, comminuted fracture of the lateral plantar process of the middle phalanx in a 3-day eventer. **A** and **B,** Lateromedial and dorsolateral-plantaromedial oblique radiographs at presentation.

Continued

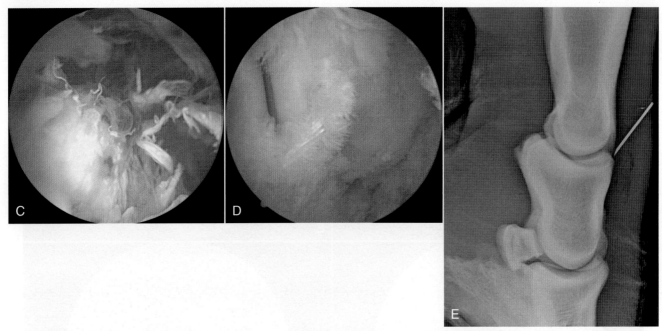

Figure 11-34, cont'd C, Arthroscopic appearance of the fracture site using an ipsilateral portal demonstrating marked disruption of the fibrocartilagenous scutum permitting access to the fracture site. **D,** Arthroscopic appearance following fragment removal and debridement of the fracture bed and disrupted scutum. **E,** Intraoperative radiograph confirming fragment removal. Note the dorsal needle egress.

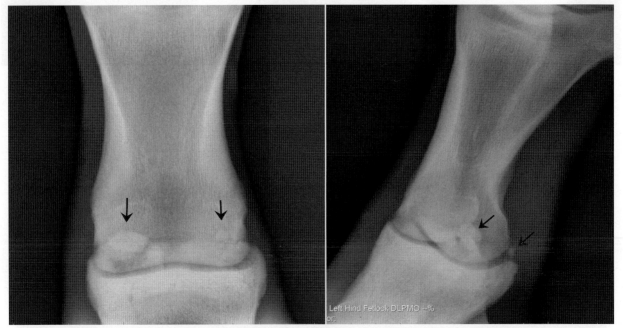

Figure 11-35 Radiographs showing avulsion fractures of the superficial digital flexor tendon and plantar scutum from the abaxial plantar perimeter of a hindlimb middle phalanx *(arrows)*. The fragments are arthroscopically not accessible unless extensive dissection of the plantar scutum, which may have negative consequences, is performed.

a choice has to be made to avoid resecting excessive soft tissue in order to access and remove fragments (Fig. 11-35). There are too few published cases to provide firm guidelines, but common sense suggests that surgeons should avoid disruption of intact palmar/plantar scutum in the pursuit of embedded fragments. Once isolated, fragments are removed with appropriately sized arthroscopic rongeurs before the fracture bed and disrupted soft tissues are debrided in conventional manners. Following joint lavage, skin portals are closed with

simple interrupted sutures and the limb is bandaged in accord with the extent of the injury.

The previous edition of this text described axial fragmentation in the palmar/plantar compartment in five horses affecting four hindlimbs and one forelimb (McIlwraith et al, 2005). The latter and one other were asymptomatic. The remaining horses had lameness referable to this site. Four out of five horses in which fragments were removed arthroscopically were sound post surgery. In one pony, the fragment could not be accessed and this animal remained lame. Radcliffe et al (2008) reported two horses with abaxial hindlimb fragments and two with axial forelimb fragments. All horses were lame before arthroscopic fragment removal, and all four recovered function postoperatively. The abaxial fragments were reported to require considerable soft tissue dissection to permit removal.

REFERENCES

Boening KJ, v. Saldern FC, Leendertse I, Rahlenbeck F: Diagnostic and surgical arthroscoppy of the equine coffin joint, *Proc Am Assoc Equine Pract* 311–317, 1990.

Boening KJ: Arthroscopic surgery of the distal and proximal interphalangeal joints, *Clin Tech Equine Pract* 1:218–225, 2002.

Brommer H, Rijkenhuizen ABM, van den Belt AJM, Keg PR: Arthroscopic removal of an osteochondral fragment at the palmaroproximal aspect of the distal interphalangeal joint, *Equine Vet Educ* 13:294–297, 2001.

Busschers E, Richardson D: Arthroscopically assisted arthrodesis of the distal interphalangeal joint with transarticular screws inserted through a dorsal hoof wall approach in a horse, *J Am Vet Med Assoc* 228:909–913, 2006.

Crowe OM, Hepburn RJ, Kold SE, Smith RK: Long-term outcome after arthroscopic debridement of distal phalanx extensor process fragmentation in 13 horses, *Vet Surg* 39:107–114, 2010.

Dechant JE, Trotter GW, Stashak TS, Hendrickson DA: Removal of large fragments of the extensor process of the distal phalanx via arthrotomy in horses: 14 cases (1992-1998), *J Am Vet Med Assoc* 217:1351–1355, 2000.

Fjordbakk CT, Strand E, Milde AK, Ihler CE and Rorvik AM: Osteochondral fragments involving the dorsomedial aspect of the proximal interphalangeal joint in young horses: 6 cases (1997-2006).

Fowlie JG, O'Neill HD, Bladon BM, O'Meara BO, Prange T, Caron JP: Comparison of conventional and alternative arthroscopic approaches to the palmar/plantar pouch of the equine distal interphalangeal joint, *Equine Vet J* 43:265–269, 2011.

Kamm JL, Goodrich LR, Werpy NM, McIlwraith CW: A descriptive study of the equine proximal interphalangeal joint using magnetic resonance imaging, contrast arthrography and arthroscopy, *Vet Surg* 41:677–684, 2012.

McIlwraith CW, Goodman NL: Conditions of the interphalangeal joints, *Vet Clin North Am Large Anim Pract* 5:161–178, 1989.

McIlwraith CW: Other uses for arthroscopy in the horse. In McIlwraith CW, editor: *Diagnostic and surgical arthroscopy in the horse*, Philadelphia, 1990, Lea & Febiger, p 220.

McIlwraith CW, Nixon AJ, Wright IM, Boening J: Arthroscopic surgery of the distal and proximal interphalangeal joints. *Diagnostic and Surgical Arthroscopy in the Horse*, ed 3, Philadelphia, PA, 2005, Mosby-Elsevier, pp 347–364.

Miller SM, Stover SM, Taylor KT, et al.: Palmaroproximal approach for arthrocentesis of the proximal interphalangeal joint in horses, *Equine Vet J* 28:376–380, 1996.

Nixon AJ: Phalanges and the metacarpophalangeal and metatarsophalangeal joints. In Auer JA, Stick JA, editors: *Equine Surgery*, ed 4, St Louis, 2012, Mosby-Elsevier, pp 1300–1325.

Radcliffe RM, Cheetham J, Bezuidenhout AJ, Ducharme NG, Nixon AJ: Arthroscopic removal of palmar/plantar osteochondral fragments from the proximal interphalangeal joint in four horses, *Vet Surg* 37:733–740, 2008.

Sampson SN, Scheider RK, Gavin PR, Baszler TV, Mealey RH, Zubrod CJ, Marsh CA: Evaluation of an arthroscopic approach for transection of the equine collateral sesamoidean ligament, *Vet Surg* 39:1011–1020, 2010.

Schneider RK, Ragle CA, Carter BG, Davis WE: Arthroscopic removal of osteochondral fragments from the proximal interphalangeal joint of the pelvic limbs in three horses, *JAVMA* 205:79–82, 1994.

Story MR, Bramlage LR: Arthroscopic debridement of subchondral bone cysts in the distal phalanx of 11 horses (1994–2000), *Equine Vet J* 36:356–360, 2004.

Ter Braake F: Arthroscopic removal of large fragments of the extensor process of the distal phalanx in 4 horses, *Equine Vet Educ* 17: 101–105, 2005.

Vacek JR, Welch RD, Honnas CM: Arthroscopic approach and intraarticular anatomy of the palmaroproximal or plantaroproximal aspects of distal interphalangeal joints, *Vet Surg* 4:257–260, 1992.

Vail TB, McIlwraith CW: Arthroscopic removal of an osteochondral fragment from the middle phalanx of a horse, *Vet Surg* 4:269–272, 1992.

Wagner PC, Modransky PD, Gavin PR, Grant BD: Surgical management of subchondral bone cysts of the third phalanx in the horse, *Equine Pract* 4:9–15, 1982.

Zierz J, Schad D, Giersemehl K: Chirurgische Möglichkeiten zur Versorgung von Strahlbeinzysten sowie Strukturdefekten im Strahlbein, *Pferdeheilkunde* 16:171–176, 2000.

CHAPTER 12

Tenoscopy

In recent years tenoscopy has made a major contribution to understanding the pathogenesis of tenosynovitis. This has included identification of previously unreported lesions in all locations. Some have subsequently been identified by other diagnostic techniques, but tenoscopy remains the modality of choice for determination of lesion morphology and it is now a routine part of equine surgical practice. Lesions identified have included intrathecal tearing of tendons and their attachments, which appear to differ in etiology and development from extrathecal flexor tendon tears. In addition, tenoscopy has revealed intrathecal disruption of tendons and ligaments that are normally subsynovial, permitting surgical access to these otherwise obscured tendon surfaces. As a result, rational surgical intervention has replaced symptomatic treatment of tenosynovitis. Finally, tenoscopy has permitted minimally invasive surgical approaches to peritheal structures with the consequential benefits of decreased morbidity, simplified aftercare, and reduced convalescence enjoyed by other endoscopic procedures.

▶ DIGITAL FLEXOR TENDON SHEATH

The digital flexor tendon sheath (DFTS) is a complex synovial cavity housing the superficial digital flexor tendon (SDFT), deep digital flexor tendon (DDFT) and their associated plicae, mesotenons, manicae, and vinculae. It is similar in forelimbs and hindlimbs and extends from the junction of the middle and distal one thirds of the metacarpus/metatarsus to the level of the middle phalanx. Its distal termination is asymmetric, extending dorsally to the level of the T ligament, which separates the DFTS from the navicular bursa and distal interphalangeal joint, while on the palmar/plantar aspect it terminates further proximally as the sheath wall reflects onto the palmar/plantar surface of the DDFT. Palmar/plantar to the metacarpophalangeal/metatarsophalangeal joint, the DFTS passes through an inelastic fetlock or sesamoidean canal created by the palmar/plantar annular ligament (PAL) (Fig. 12-1), the palmar/plantar surface of the proximal sesamoid bones (PSB), and the intervening intersesamoidean ligament (Redding, 1991; Sisson, 1975).

The PAL has consistent transverse (horizontal) fiber orientation and runs between the abaxial margins of the PSB, at which point it blends with the collateral sesamoidean ligaments. The dorsal surface of the PAL is covered by a thin layer of avillous synovium and its smooth surface blends with the fibrocartilage-covered PSB and intervening intersesamoidean ligament (scutum). Over the palmar/plantar aspect of the pastern the DFTS is reinforced by the proximal and distal digital annular ligaments. These are less discrete structures than the PAL. The proximal digital annular ligament is a thin quadrilateral (i.e., X-shaped) sheet located over the palmar/plantar aspect of the proximal phalanx. The corners have fascial attachments to the proximal and distal abaxial eminences of the proximal phalanx. The body and distal margin blend with the DFTS wall where it reflects and cannot be separated from the palmar/plantar surface of the SDFT. The distal digital annular ligament is curved from the level of the distal epiphysis of the proximal phalanx to the distal palmar/plantar boundary of the DFTS where it reflects and is inseparable from the DDFT. When distended, the DFTS protrudes in the areas unenclosed by annular ligaments and these areas in turn provide suitable access portals for insertion of an arthroscope and instruments.

Proximally, the fibrous sheath wall reflects from the metacarpal fascia surrounding the digital flexor tendons. This continues proximodorsally between branches of insertion of the suspensory ligament. From proximal to distal, the dorsal borders of the DFTS are the branches of insertion of the suspensory ligament, proximal scutum (containing the proximal sesamoid bones and intersesamoidean ligament), straight distal sesamoidean ligaments, palmar/plantar fibrocartilaginous scutum of the proximal interphalangeal joint, and the palmar/plantar recess of the distal interphalangeal joint. Except distally, where the DFTS is associated with the distal interphalangeal joint, there is little recognizable fibrous sheath wall and these structures are all subsynovial.

In the proximal recess of the DFTS the SDFT forms a thin smooth ring, the manica flexoria (MF), around the DDFT (Fig. 12-2). The MF has a free distal margin, abaxially blends smoothly with the SDFT, and its proximal margin is continuous with the DFTS wall (Fig. 12-3). A second, less substantial ring (the digital manica) is found at the level of the proximal phalanx (see Fig. 12-8).

The DFTS wall reflects off the palmar/plantar axial surface of the SDFT throughout its length, including the fetlock (sesamoidean) canal, creating a short, robust mesotenon. Distal to the fetlock canal this mesotenon widens such that the sheath wall reflects from the entire palmar/plantar surface of the SDFT (i.e., this surface is outside the synovial cavity). Bifurcation of the SDFT commences at the proximal one third of the proximal phalanx and is complete by mid-diaphyseal level. In the intervening region the central portion of the SDFT thins progressively to produce a distal arch or isthmus between the two branches of insertion (see Fig. 12-3). The latter form the palmar/plantar abaxial margins of the DFTS before inserting via the palmar/plantar scutum of the proximal interphalangeal joint. The straight distal sesamoidean ligament inserts similarly between these branches. Disal to the SDFT bifurcation is a spacious palmar/plantar outpouching of the digital sheath (Fig. 12-4).

In the proximal sheath reflection (just proximal to the MF) the DDFT is attached to the sheath wall medially and laterally by short, thick mesotenons or synovial plicae (Redding, 1993). These have consistent locations but variable morphology, although the lateral plica is generally more substantial and extends farther distally (Fig. 12-5). Distal to the digital manica, further mesotenons (vinculae) attach the DDFT to the dorsal sheath wall over the straight distal sesamoidean ligament (see Figs. 12-3B and 12-8). These are variable in size and number.

Technique

The approach described by Nixon (1990c) offers comprehensive evaluation of the DFTS from a single portal and has become adopted as the standard. Horses may be operated in dorsal or lateral recumbency, but the authors prefer lateral for most procedures. Safe entry into the sheath is facilitated by moderate flexion of the distal joints, whereas neutral fetlock and interphalangeal joint angles are optimal for comprehensive evaluation. Most procedures are facilitated by use of an Esmarch bandage and tourniquet applied to a proximal metacarpal/metatarsal level; placement at distal antebrachial or crural levels usually produces distal joint flexion, which can be counterproductive. All portals are made 3 to 6 mm palmar/plantar to the palmar/plantar digital neurovascular bundles,

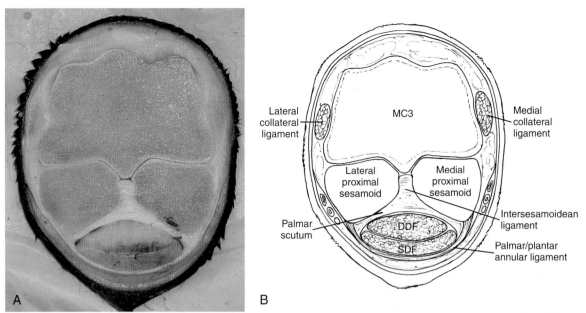

Figure 12-1 A and **B,** Cross section of a forelimb at the level of the fetlock, showing the digital flexor tendon sheath and related structures. *DDF,* Deep digital flexor tendon; *MC3,* third metacarpal bone; *SDF,* superficial digital flexor tendon.

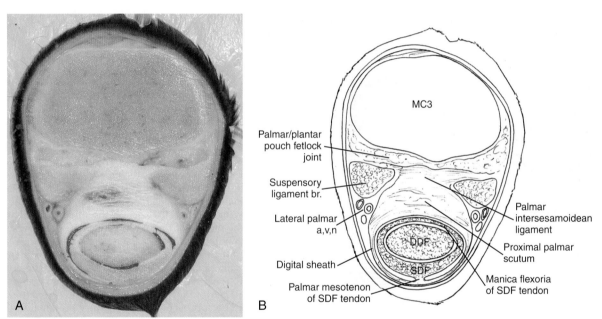

Figure 12-2 A and **B,** Cross section of a forelimb 4 cm proximal to the apices of the proximal sesamoid bones, showing the digital flexor tendon sheath and related structures. *DDF,* Deep digital flexor tendon; *MC3,* third metacarpal bone; *SDF,* superficial digital flexor tendon.

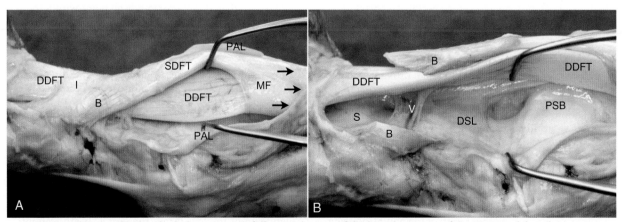

Figure 12-3 A and **B,** Forelimb dissections. **B,** following division of the lateral insertion of the SDFT and digital manica; *DDFT,* deep digital flexor tendon; *MF,* manica flexoria; *PAL,* divided palmar annular ligament; *SDFT,* superficial digital flexor tendon. *B,* Branch of insertion of SDFT; *DSL,* straight distal sesamoidean ligament; *I,* isthmus of SDFT; *arrows,* reflection of MF from digital flexor tendon sheath wall; *PSB,* medial proximal sesamoid bone; *S,* fibrocartilaginous scutum of proximal interphalangeal joint; *V,* vinculae.

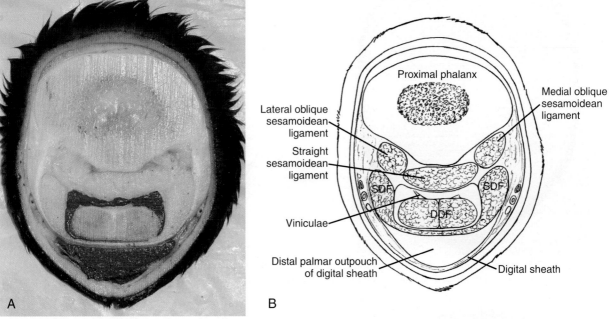

Figure 12-4 A and **B,** Cross section of a forelimb through the distal diaphysis of the proximal phalanx, showing the digital flexor tendon sheath and related structures.

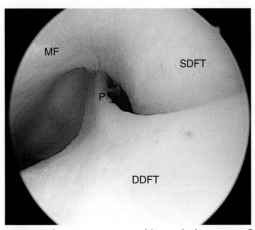

Figure 12-5 Arthroscope positioned beneath the manica flexoria *(MF)* exposing the lateral plica *(P)* of the deep digital flexor tendon *(DDFT)*. *SDFT,* Superficial digital flexor tendon.

the location of which should be ascertained and checked repeatedly when determining the entry portal. All portal locations are symmetric medially and laterally. For ease, the initial arthroscopic portal is made laterally unless preoperative diagnostic information suggests advantages to a medial approach.

The standard initial tensoscopic portal is made into the DFTS outpouching between the PAL and proximal digital annular ligament (Fig. 12-6A). If the sheath is not markedly distended, then identification and entry can be facilitated by further inflation. If possible this should be done at a remote site in order to avoid the potential for local fluid extravasation, which can obscure landmarks. The skin incision is made slightly palmar/plantar to the center of the outpouching and palmar/plantar to the neurovascular bundle. It is continued with a stab incision using a No. 11 or 15 blade sufficient to penetrate only the thin sheath wall. The arthroscopic cannula is then introduced using a conical obturator. This will be met with minimal resistance, and the thumb of the nonintroducing hand should be used as a friction bridge in order to avoid damage to the epitenon of the underlying digital flexor tendons. If

the entry angle is perpendicular to the skin, then this usually places the arthroscopic sleeve dorsal to the DDFT. The sleeve is then directed proximally through the fetlock canal into the proximal dorsal recess of the DFTS (B and C). There should be minimal or no resistance to this maneuver. At this point the conical obturator is replaced by the arthroscope, and light and fluid lines are connected (see Fig. 12-6D).

In chronically thickened digital sheaths, especially where the SDFT has adhered to the sheath, there is real danger of penetrating the lateral edge of the tendon during arthroscope entry. Placing the portal closer to the middle or slightly forward of the middle of the outpouching lessens this risk, while still maintaining a safe distance palmar to the neurovascular structures. If the perimeter of the outpouching is poorly distensible, adhesions should be suspected and a hemostat to allow additional separation of the portal into the sheath may help avoid perforating the adhered SDFT. Alternatively, the sheath can be approached using an entry proximal to the fetlock canal, but this is rarely necessary.

Points of egress for lavage and subsequent instrument portals can be made at ipsilateral or contralateral points avoiding the PAL and digital annular ligaments. It is important to understand that at any proximodistal point within the sheath, the arthroscope can be located at a number of dorsopalmar/plantar positions, each of which will visualize different anatomic structures. A systematic approach is therefore critical to complete evaluation of the sheath and must be prioritized before intervention is undertaken. The authors employ and recommend a "layer-by-layer" approach as described later with the endoscopic anatomy. This necessitates use of the full range of arthroscopic lens angulation, although it is critical that the camera head is maintained in the plane of the limb throughout in order for the surgeon to retain orientation.

Endoscopic Anatomy

Initially the arthroscope should be positioned in the proximal dorsal recess of the sheath (Fig. 12-6C), which is voluminous and lined by villous synovium. Slight withdrawal and dorsal angulation of the lens brings the dorsal sheath wall into view while palmar/plantar angulation images the dorsal surface of the MF. On gradual withdrawal, the distal free margin of the MF

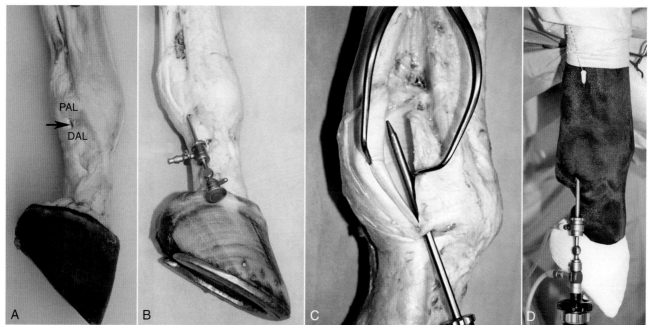

Figure 12-6 Standard tenoscopic approach to the digital flexor tendon sheath. **A,** Dissection specimen with neurovascular bundle removed. The arthroscopic portal *(arrow)* is made between the palmar/plantar annular ligament *(PAL)* and proximal digital annular ligament *(DAL)*. **B,** Dissection specimen with arthroscopic cannula inserted through the standard portal and directed proximally in the digital flexor tendon sheath (DFTS). **C,** Dissection specimen following transaction of the PAL and distraction of the proximal compartment of the DFTS with a Gelpi retractor illustrating initial location of the arthroscopic cannula and conical obturator dorsal to the manica flexoria. **D,** A clinical case in which the arthroscope has been inserted through the standard portal and directed proximally through the fetlock canal. Translumination shows its position in the proximal recess of the DFTS, and a needle has been inserted close to the proximal sheath reflection.

comes into view, which is a key landmark in orientation (Fig. 12-7). This normally is a thin, tapered structure fully enclosing and following the contour of the dorsal surface of the DDFT. Further withdrawal while maintaining the arthroscope in the dorsal regions of the digital sheath images the dorsal surface of the DDFT when viewing palmar/plantarly and the fibrocartilage of the proximal scutum containing the proximal sesamoid bones and intersesamoidean ligament when the arthroscope is rotated to view dorsally (see Fig. 12-7). The intersesamoidean ligament is relatively smooth, but sometimes fine transverse lines are visible. These become most obvious at the distal extent of the fetlock/sesamoidean canal, which is close to the arthroscopic portal. The arthroscope is then inclined to angle the tip distally by raising the camera holding hand in a distal to proximal arc. Immediately distal to the sesamoidean canal the dorsal sheath wall is lined by villous synovium.

As the arthroscope is repositioned to place the tip distal to the entry portal, the digital manica comes into view (Fig. 12-8). Unlike the MF, this is covered by villous synovium. The arthroscope can be manipulated between the digital manica and DDFT and advanced a short distance to image the paired vinculae, which extend between the dorsal surface of the DDFT and sheath wall (see Fig. 12-8). This is generally double but may be asymmetric. In some individuals, the arthroscope can be manipulated past the vinculae, but in others the lack of mobility created by the digital manica precludes this. This is not an issue because the distal dorsal region of the sheath can be evaluated more satisfactorily in the second "sweep" of the sheath.

The arthroscope can now be withdrawn and reoriented proximally in a reverse of the previously described maneuver. When the free margin of the MF is visualized, the tip of the arthroscope should be passed between this and the DDFT. Sometimes this is most readily achieved closer to the

abaxial margin (i.e., reflection of the MF from the SDFT). In the proximal regions of this recess, the medial and lateral plicae (mesotenon) of the DDFT are visualised as thick synovial folds extending between the sheath wall and abaxial margins of the DDFT (see Fig. 12-5). The arthroscope now either can be withdrawn distal to the MF or rotated over the abaxial (usually lateral) margin of the DDFT so that its tip lies between the DDFT and SDFT. With slight distal movement and lens rotation it is possible to visualize both medial and lateral reflections of the MF from the SDFT. While the tip of the arthroscope is maintained between the DDFT and SDFT, it is withdrawn slowly, inspecting the surfaces of both tendons to the level of the base of the fetlock/sesamoidean canal. At this point, the hand holding the arthroscope and the camera moves in a distal to proximal arc so that the tip of the arthroscope is oriented distally. It is then slowly advanced, again rotating the lens en route, to inspect the dorsal surface of the SDFT and palmar/plantar surface of the DDFT (see Fig. 12-8). This is the least encumbered pathway during examination of the distal regions of the digital sheath, without mesotenons or vinculae. Close to the midpoint of the proximal phalanx, the free margin of the SDFT isthmus is visualized (Fig. 12-9A) and, abaxial to this, the dorsal and axial surfaces of the branches of insertion of the SDFT. With further distal advancement of the arthroscope, the palmar/plantar surface of the DDFT is inspected as far as the reflection of the sheath wall onto the DDFT surface (Fig. 12-9B), which also marks the proximal margin of the distal digital annular ligament. With slight withdrawal of the arthroscope, it can then be rotated over the abaxial (lateral) margin of the DDFT so that its tip lies dorsal to the tendon. The arthroscope then can be advanced farther distally beyond the level of the palmar/plantar sheath reflection. This distal dorsal cul-de-sac of the DFTS is usually lined by avillous synovium overlying the so-called

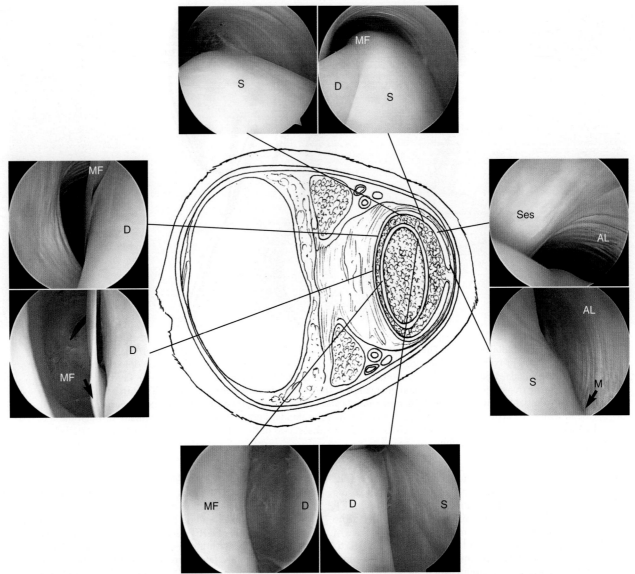

Figure 12-7 Composite tenoscopic view looking proximally, showing multiple regions from dorsal to the flexor tendons to the palmar surface of the sheath. The superficial digital flexor tendon *(S)*, deep digital flexor tendon *(D)*, manica flexoria *(MF)*, palmar/plantar annular ligament *(AL)*, and the lateral proximal sesamoid *(Ses)* are labeled. The sheath cavity on the palmar side of the SDFT *(S)* is divided by the midline attachment of the mesotenon *(M)*, preventing evaluation of the palmaromedial side of the sheath.

T ligament, which consists centrally of the reflections of the fibrous walls of the DFTS, navicular bursa, and distal interphalangeal joint and abaxially of the suspensory ligaments of the navicular bone (Fig. 12-10). While the arthroscope remains dorsal to the DDFT, withdrawal and angulation of the lens dorsally visualizes the synovium overlying the proximal interphalangeal scutum and proximal to this centrally the straight distal sesamoidean ligament and abaxially the surface of the branches of insertion of the SDFT (see Fig. 12-8). If the arthroscope is withdrawn to the level of the entry portal, positioned dorsal to the DDFT and directed distally, this brings into view again the digital manica and vinculae (see Fig. 12-8).

The arthroscope now should be relocated again proximal to the fetlock/sesamoidean canal to lie outside of the MF on the abaxial (usually lateral) surface of the SDFT (see Fig. 12-7). The lens should be angled palmar/plantar to visualize the SDFT as far as the axial reflection of the mesotenon, which extends from the palmar/plantar sheath wall and PAL. In this

location it is not possible to advance the arthroscope farther contralaterally (generally medial) because the sheath wall now reflects from the whole of the palmar/plantar surface of the SDFT (see Fig. 12-7).

For visualization of lesions immediately distal to the arthroscope entry at the base of the sesamoid, the arthroscope may need to be exchanged into a proximal instrument portal, leaving the arthroscopic portal available for instrument entry. In this circumstance it can be an advantage to move the arthroscopic tower so that appropriate line of sight can be maintained to provide coordinated hand movements. It is quite difficult to work effectively if the surgeon is not viewing down the long axis of the arthroscope and onto the video monitor. For digital sheath tenoscopy, an alternative is to have the arthroscopic tower positioned midway between the two positions, therefore midway between the tower near the withers and tower distal to the foot, which for forelimbs would be directly forward of the carpi.

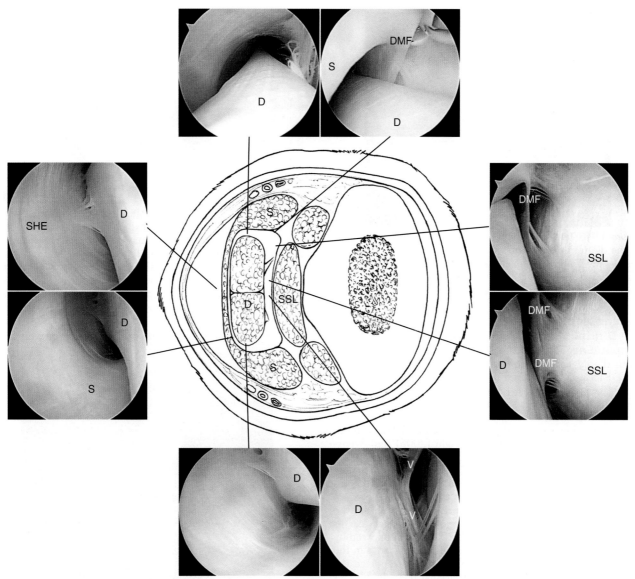

Figure 12-8 Composite tenoscopic view with the arthroscope reversed to view distal regions of the digital flexor tendon sheath. Evaluation between the deep digital flexor tendon *(DDFT)* and superficial digital flexor tendon *(SDFT)* shows the DDFT *(D)* and the terminal portion of the SDFT *(S)* dividing for insertion. Distal to this bifurcation the sheath *(SHE)* is attached to the DDFT in the voluminous palmar/plantar pouch by a small palmar mesotenon. At the proximal phalanx level, a small distal encircling manica called the digital manica flexoria *(DMF)* surrounds the DDFT. Dorsal to the DDFT the vinculae *(V)* attach the DDFT to the sheath.

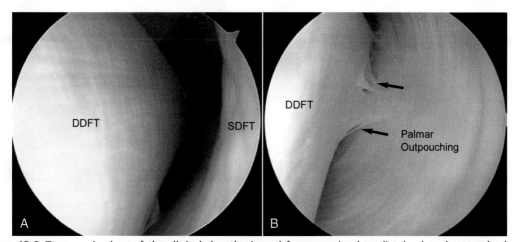

Figure 12-9 Tenoscopic view of the digital sheath viewed from proximal to distal using the standard entry portal. **A,** The bifurcation and isthmus of the superficial digital flexor tendon *(SDFT)* are evident with the deep digital flexor tendon *(DDFT)* continuing distally. **B,** The palmar outpouching of the digital sheath and reflection of the sheath wall onto the DDFT *(arrows)* are evident distal to the SDFT bifurcation.

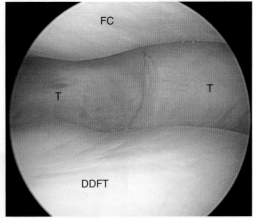

Figure 12-10 Tenoscopic view of the distal dorsal cul-de-sac of the digital flexor tendon sheath *(DFTS)*. Avillous synovium overlies the T ligament *(T)* at the dorsodistal margin of the deep digital flexor tendon (DDFT). *FC,* Fibrocartilage on the palmar/plantar surface of the middle phalanx.

▶ Tenoscopic Treatment of Clinical Conditions in the Digital Sheath
Longitudinal Tears of the Digital Flexor Tendons
Until the advent of tenoscopy, lesions of the DDFT within the DFTS were considered to carry a guarded to poor prognosis (Barr et al, 1995). Lesion morphology was unknown and thus treatment was symptomatic. Tenoscopic identification and treatment of longitudinal tears of the digital flexor tendons has been reported by Wright & McMahon (1999), Wilderjans et al (2003), Smith & Wright (2006), and Arensberg et al (2011). All agree that the most common lesion is a longitudinal tear of the DDFT. Pooled data for these studies provides a reference group of 171 cases with longitudinal tears of the DDFT within the DFTS. Lesions are most common in the forelimbs comprising 135 (79%) of the pooled horses. The most common site of longitudinal tears is on the lateral margin of the DDFT (129, 75%), followed by the medial margin (20, 12%), with a minority of cases in the dorsal and palmar/plantar margins. Two papers reported the ultrasonographic predictability of marginal tears. In a series of 45 cases, Smith & Wright (2006) found a sensitivity, specificity, and positive predictive value (PPV) of 71% and a negative predictive value (NPV) of 55%. In 91 cases reported by Arensberg et al (2011) longitudinal tears of the DDFT were predicted by ultrasound with a sensitivity of 63%, specificity of 75%, PPV of 90%, and NPV of 37%. These contrast with the findings of Edinger et al (2005), who found ultrasound to have poor sensitivity (36.4%) but good specificity and PPV (100%) for lesions of the DDFT within the DFTS. All authors report other nonspecific ultrasonographic changes in affected sheaths, including fluid distension, sheath wall thickening, and thickening of mesotenons and plicae. Both transverse and oblique ultrasonographic examinations are recommended in order to avoid edge-shadowing artifacts produced during transverse acquisition (Edinger et al, 2005; Reef, 1998). Marginal tears of the DDFT occur in all types and uses of horses, although in the Arensberg et al (2011) series, horses that were show jumpers were commonly affected and in another series published by Smith & Wright (2006), racing Thoroughbreds were underrepresented.

Most surgeons (authors included) prefer to perform tenoscopic surgery of the digital sheath with the horse in lateral recumbency with the distal limb free to permit circumferential access and variation of joint angle (Fig. 12-11). In almost all cases, torn tendon fibrils are extruded into the synovial cavity and are identified suspended in the irrigating fluid (Fig. 12-12). In the absence of effective intrinsic mechanisms for

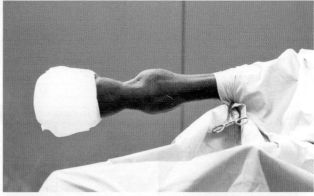

Figure 12-11 Right hindlimb positioned, prepared and draped for tenoscopy of the digital flexor tendon sheath. The limb is supported in the proximal metatarsus. Following thorough hoof cleansing, this is enclosed in a sterile glove to the level of the coronary band. The gloved foot is then further sealed by application of a sterile Vetrap™. The whole distal limb can then be passed through a fenestrated drape to permit circumferential access and to allow limb manipulation during surgery.

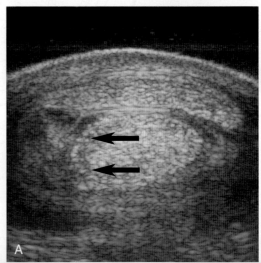

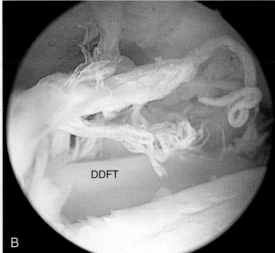

Figure 12-12 Tearing of the lateral margin of the deep digital flexor tendon *(DDFT)*. **A,** Transverse ultrasonograph demonstrating an irregularly truncated lateral margin to the DDFT *(arrows)* with adjacent irregular echoic material. **B,** Tenoscopic image of the area between the manica flexoria and fetlock canal; torn fibers from the lateral margin of the DDFT are extruded and suspended in the irrigating fluid.

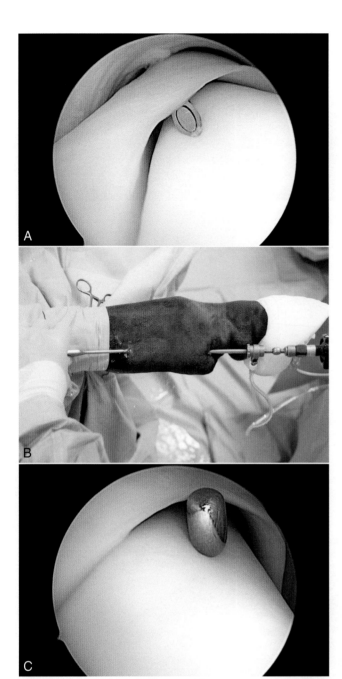

Figure 12-13 Illustration of a proximal instrument portal for longitudinal tears of the deep digital flexor tendon, which requires instruments to pass beneath the manica flexoria and parallel with the tendon **(A).** A suitable location is determined by prior passage of a spinal needle **(B, C).** Instruments can then be passed in this line (i.e., parallel to the long axis of the tendon in order to evaluate and treat lesions).

repair or removal, the principal goal of tenoscopic treatment is removal of torn, extruded tendon tissue to reduce the surface area of exposed disrupted collagenous tissue to the synovial environment. This, it is theorized, should reduce the inflammatory drive and promote development of a viable scar in or over the defect.

Instrument portals are placed according to lesion location. Tears that commence proximally (beneath the MF) require an instrument portal that is made through the most proximal aspect of the sheath to allow passage of instruments beneath the MF parallel with the DDFT (Fig. 12-13). When necessary, the arthroscope and instrument portals are interchanged to optimize accessibility of lesions. Large masses of

torn tendon tissue and granulomata are dissected free with arthroscopic scissors or meniscectomy knives before removal with Ferris-Smith arthroscopic rongeurs. Other extruded material and tendon defects are debrided with suction punch biopsy rongeurs or a motorized synovial sector in oscillating mode with suction applied (Fig. 12-14), or both. This is used to pull the disrupted fibers into the blades, thus avoiding damage to intact tissue. Coblation has been reported as a technique for debridement and smoothing of the fibrillated edges of defects but appears to have a negative impact on outcome (Arensberg et al, 2011). It is therefore not recommended.

When describing marginal tears of the DDFT, the DFTS is considered in three parts: the fetlock canal and those regions proximal and distal to this, accepting that such lesion locations are applicable only to the position and location during surgery. In the series reported by Smith & Wright (2006) approximately 50% of tears were long (i.e., involved two regions, principally the proximal and fetlock canal) and were most common laterally. Short tears were most frequent distal to the fetlock canal and did not exhibit lateral dominance. Clumps of torn tendon fibers at the proximal or distal margins of tears, or both, were commonly capped by granulation tissue with varying degrees of organization (granulomata) (Fig. 12-15). These were reported by Smith & Wright (2006) in 12 of 45 (27%) and by Arensberg et al (2011) in 16 of 78 (20%) of cases. The latter authors recognized synoviosynovial adhesions in 29 of 104 DFTS with longitudinal tears of the digital flexor tendons or MF, or both.

Fourteen of 33 (42%) horses with marginal tears of the DDFT reported by Smith & Wright (2006) returned to previous levels of performance. The negative prognostic features included marked preoperative distension and clinical signs of 15 weeks or longer before surgery. Arensberg et al (2011) combined the results of torn DDFT, SDFT, and MF (although the former dominated) and reported that 37 of 98 (38%) horses returned to preoperative levels of performance. In this series, 71 (72%) had a concurrent palmar annular ligament (PAL) desmotomy. Wright and McMahon (1999) repaired marginal tears of the DDFT by an open approach in 11 horses, 5 of which (45%) returned to working soundness, and it is possible that as minimally invasive techniques for repair evolve that repair may merit reconsideration.

Desmotomy of the PAL, in order to relieve intrathecal restriction, has been advocated in the treatment of complex tenosynovitis of the DFTS (Nixon, 2003). In addition, Wilderjans (2003) reported that transaction of the PAL also improved tenoscopic visualization of the DFTS and mobility within the fetlock/sesamoidean canal when treating horses with tears of the digital flexor tendons. However, this group later amended this recommendation and now performs PAL desmotomy only when this is considered thickened (Arensberg et al, 2011). In comparing the pooled data from Wright & McMahon (1999) and Smith & Wright (2006) with Wilderjans et al (2003) and Arensberg et al (2011), there appears to be no identifiable difference in outcome in cases that do and do not have PAL desmotomy.

Longitudinal tears of the SDFT appear much less common than their DDFT counterparts, comprising 11 of 76 (14%) cases reported by Smith & Wright (2006) and 20 of 135 (15%) cases reported by Arensberg et al (2011). The most common site is distal to the reflection of the MF (Fig. 12-16), although lesions can also occur distally involving the intrathecal portion of the branches of insertion. Proximally, lesions appear to be most common laterally (Arensberg et al, 2011), while distally the medial branch of insertion appears most frequently affected (Smith & Wright, 2006). Instrument access for proximal lesions requires a portal that is abaxial (i.e., outside) the MF. There are inadequate numbers in the literature to assess confidently the current status of ultrasonographic

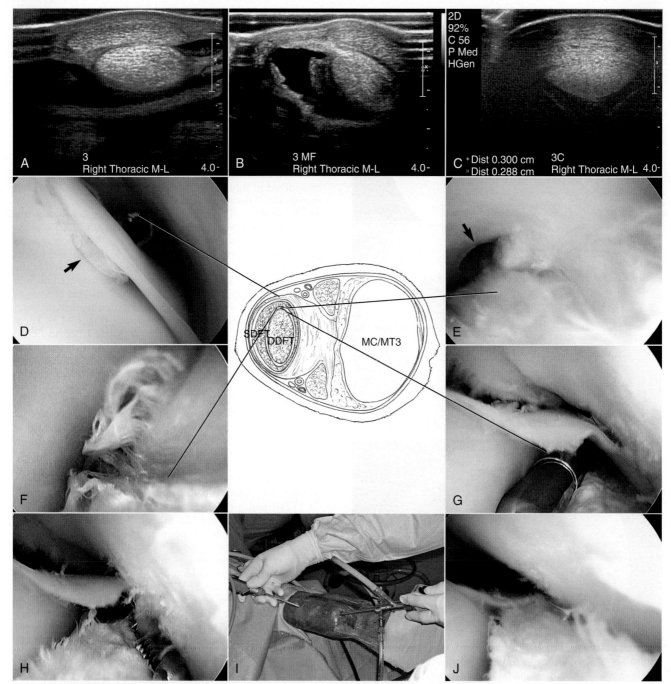

Figure 12-14 Deep digital flexor tendon (DDFT) tear within the confines of the manica flexoria (MF). **A** and **B,** Ultrasonographic images show soft tissue densities originating from the lateral edge of the DDFT. **C,** Concurrent annular ligament thickening. **D,** Arthroscopic view showing torn fibers from the DDFT emerging from beneath the MF *(arrow).* **E-G,** Redirecting the arthroscope back beneath the MF and superficial digital flexor tendon shows the full extent of the deep digital flexor tendon tear, which is debrided with a motorized resector. **H-J,** The motorized resector is positioned beneath the manica to emerge and debride the tear by sweeping across the torn fibers.

identification and prediction of marginal tears of the SDFT, but Edinger et al (2005) found poor correlation between ultrasonographic and tenoscopic examinations of the SDFT within the DFTS.

Tears of the Manica Flexoria

Tears of the MF may be found as solitary lesions or in DFTS with concurrent marginal tears of the DDFT or SDFT (Smith & Wright, 2006). Of 23 cases reported by Smith & Wright

(2006), 17 (74%) occurred in the hindlimbs. Eighteen were complete and 5 were partial; 12 occurred medially, 6 laterally, and the side was not recorded in 5 cases. Most tears occur at or adjacent to the attachment of the manica to the SDFT body, and they may be complete or partial. When complete the MF frequently recoils, hinged on the intact contralateral attachment to the SDFT and proximal sheath wall reflection (Fig. 12-17). The torn margin may then become adherent to the sheath wall. The affected MF commonly is thickened in

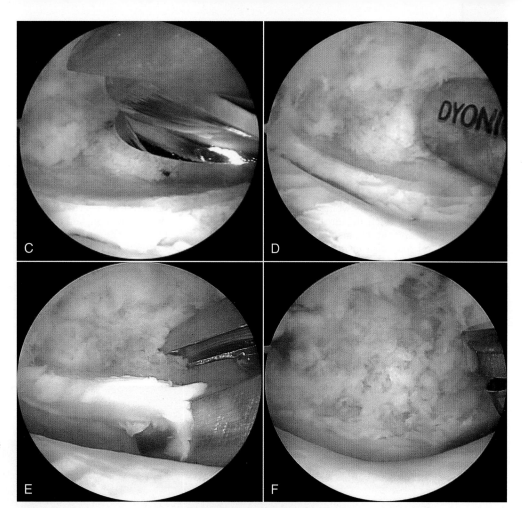

Figure 11-13, cont'd **C** and **D,** Large oval burr (Acromionizer, Smith & Nephew Dyonics, Rapid City, SD) being used to remove the fragment. **E,** Residual cartilage and attached bone removed with rongeurs. **F,** Final appearance of debrided distal phalanx.

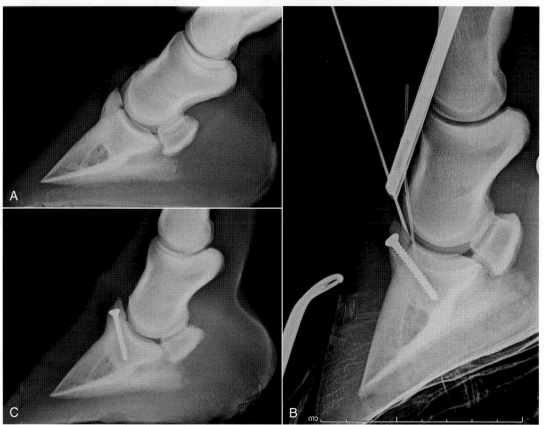

Figure 11-14 Extensor process lag screw fixation. A large acute minimally displaced fracture of the extensor process of the distal phalanx suitable for internal fixation. **A,** Preoperative lateromedial radiograph. **B,** Intraoperative lateromedial radiograph following insertion of a 3.5-mm AO/ASIF cortical screw. **C,** Follow-up radiographs 4 months post surgery before return to training.

chronic cases (Fig. 12-18A). When tears are partial, the congruency between the MF and DDFT may be disturbed, resulting in a space between the two structures (Fig. 12-18B) and sometimes "wrinkling" of the free distal margin of the MF. Transverse

tears are also encountered. These may occur through the MF or as avulsions from the proximal sheath wall.

Partial tears are managed using the same principles and techniques as described for tears of the DDFT. When one margin of the MF is disrupted completely, then total resection is advocated (Smith & Wright, 2006). The opposite, intact margin is divided from the SDFT using arthroscopic scissors or meniscectomy knives (Fig. 12-19A), or both, before the proximal sheath reflection from the MF is similarly sectioned (Fig. 12-19B). This is sometimes aided by creation of a second further distal portal through which the MF can be grasped and stabilized. The free MF can then be grasped with Ferris-Smith arthroscopic rongeurs and removed. In most cases, the MF is sufficiently pliable to be pulled through a standard arthroscopic portal but occasionally enlargement is necessary. Any remaining frayed tissue can be removed using a motorized resector (Fig. 12-19C). In the series reported by Smith & Wright (2006) tears of the MF were predicted ultrasonographically with a sensitivity of 38%, specificity 92%, PPV of 67%, and NPV of 78%. However, the authors now consider that this is likely to underrepresent the current ability of ultrasonography accurately to identify lesions of the MF.

Tears of the MF are considered to have a better prognosis following tenoscopic surgery than marginal tears of the flexor tendons with 10 of 15 (67%) horses returning to preinjury levels of performance in the series reported by Smith & Wright (2006).

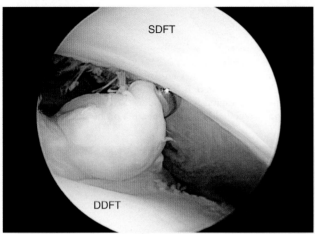

Figure 12-15 A mass of torn tendon fibers at the level of the proximal phalanx bordering the distal margin of a longitudinal tear in the lateral margin of the deep digital flexor tendon *(DDFT)* that commenced beneath the manica flexoria MF (lesion imaged in Fig. 12-12). *SDFT,* Lateral branch of superficial digital flexor tendon and adjacent isthmus.

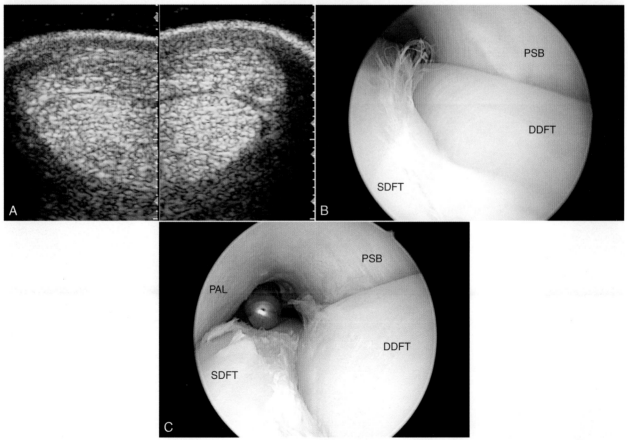

Figure 12-16 A longitudinal tear of the medial margin of the superficial digital flexor tendon *(SDFT)*. **A,** Transverse ultrasonographs imaging the lateral *(left)* and medial margins of the SDFT demonstrating a bulbous medial margin and poorly marginated anechoic to hypoechoic defect dorsomedially. **B** and **C,** Tenoscopic views of the lesion identified in **(A)** using a medial approach through the standard arthroscopic portal with the arthroscope located within the sesamoidean canal. **B,** before and **C,** following debridement with a motorized resector. *PAL,* Palmar annular ligament; *PSB,* medial proximal sesamoid bone. Note that for such lesions the resector is introduced abaxial to the manica flexoria.

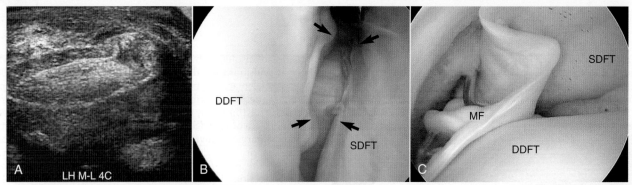

Figure 12-17 Torn manica flexoria *(MF)*. A, Transverse ultrasonographic image shows an irregular mass adjacent to the lateral border of deep digital flexor tendon *(DDFT)* where the MF has recoiled. **B,** Tenoscopic image with the arthroscope passed from lateral to medial between the DDFT and superficial digital flexor tendon *(SDFT)* shows an MF tear along its medial attachment to SDFT body *(arrows)*. **C,** Laterally recoiled free MF beneath a probe showing slack tissue before resection.

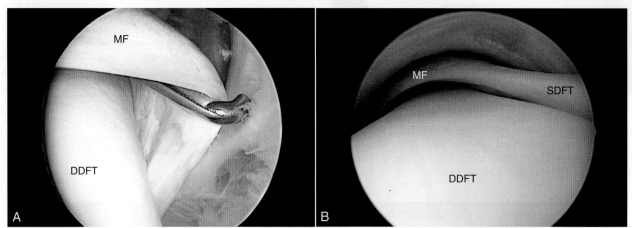

Figure 12-18 A, Thickened manica flexoria *(MF)* associated with chronic tearing. Tenoscopic image with a probe elevating the thickened MF. **B,** Tenoscopic image from a lateral arthroscopic portal demonstrating increased space between the MF and deep digital flexor tendon *(DDFT)* produced by a medial tear/avulsion of the MF from the superficial digital flexor tendon *(SDFT)*.

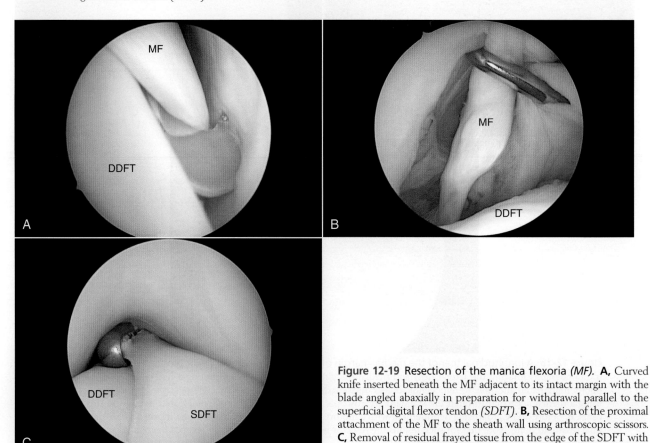

Figure 12-19 Resection of the manica flexoria *(MF)*. A, Curved knife inserted beneath the MF adjacent to its intact margin with the blade angled abaxially in preparation for withdrawal parallel to the superficial digital flexor tendon *(SDFT)*. **B,** Resection of the proximal attachment of the MF to the sheath wall using arthroscopic scissors. **C,** Removal of residual frayed tissue from the edge of the SDFT with a motorized resector. *DDFT,* Deep digital flexor tendon.

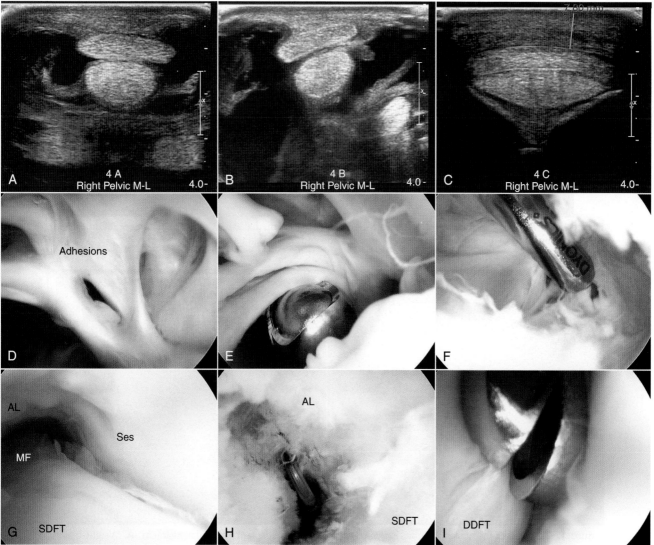

Figure 12-20 Deep digital flexor tendon *(DDFT)* linear tear with secondary adhesions and palmar/plantar annular ligament (PAL) constriction. **A** and **B,** Transverse ultrasonographic images show marked fluid distension, tenosynovial masses, and poorly defined manica. **C,** Thickened PAL and digital sheath fibrous layers (7.8 mm) add to constriction. **D-F,** Adhesions between flexor tendons and dorsolateral sheath wall and removal with a synovial resector. **G** and **H,** Freehand division of PAL *(AL)* with a radiofrequency probe; landmarks include the proximal lateral sesamoid bone *(Ses)* and manica flexoria *(MF)*. **I,** A shallow tear in the lateral edge of the DDFT is then debrided.

Complex Tenosynovitis

The term *complex tenosynovitis* is used to describe lesions involving two or more structures in and/or adjacent, to the DFTS; usually the PAL and at least one other (Fortier et al, 1999; Edinger et al, 2005; Fortier, 2005; Owen et al, 2008). The etiology (ies) is (are) obscure but it may result from chronic, self perpetuating simple tenosynovitis. Chronic low grade inflammation with accompanying tendon sheath fluid accumulation, sheath fibrosis, secondary PAL constriction and deformation of the DDFT and to a lesser extent the SDFT, are all common features (Fig. 12-20). Tenosynovial mass and adhesions from the sheath to the SDFT and MF are a later feature. Adhesions and synovial proliferative masses are typically located in the dorsal recesses of the proximal sheath (see Fig. 12-20) (Fortier et al, 1999; Fortier, 2005). Synovial proliferative masses can be secondary to sheath wall or tendon disruption but with chronicity determination of the primary lesion can be difficult. Adhesions are usually synoviosynovial but some can involve the digital flexor tendons. Synovial proliferative masses have a fibrovascular stroma commonly containing haemosiderophages with a similar appearance to chronic proliferative

(villonodular) synovitis and to granulomas described at the end of tendon tears. Most originate from the sheath wall but some may eminate also from the digital flexor tendons. Straight and curved motorized synovial resectors, with relatively wide cutting apertures and active suction, facilitate entry of tissue to the cutting blade (see Fig. 12-20). Biopsy punch rongeurs, biopsy cutting forceps, retractable blades, and arthroscopic scissors can also be useful for removal of masses. The biopsy punch rongeur is useful for removal of adhesions (Fig. 12-21); however, motorized resectors provide more efficient soft tissue mass removal. A large-bore biopsy punch rongeur (6 mm; Sontec Instruments, Englewood, CO) may improve mass removal where the synovial resector aperture is too small to accommodate large, dense, fibrous masses. Additionally, with large masses, a second instrument portal may be required to provide tension on the mass while it is severed at its base and removed using hand instruments. To access lesions beneath the MF, the instrument portal can be continued through the manica directly over the lesion, but the preferred technique is creation of a proximal instrument portal where the manica blends with the sheath wall reflection

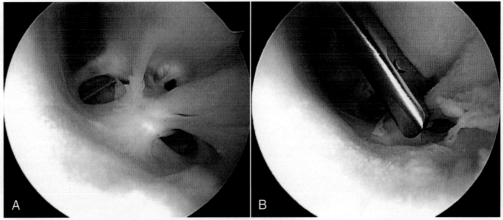

Figure 12-21 A, Adhesions between the flexor tendons and the dorsomedial aspect of the digital flexor tendon sheath. **B,** Arthroscopic biopsy punch rongeurs being used to divide and remove adhesions.

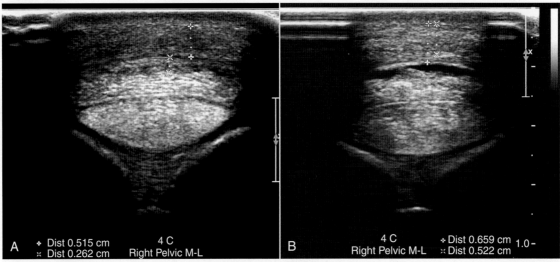

Figure 12-22 Transverse ultrasonographic examination of a thickened plantar annular ligament. **A,** Weight-bearing examination shows enlarged palmar/plantar annular ligament (PAL) with indistinct border to the junction with the superficial digital flexor tendon *(SDFT)*. **B,** Limb flexion allows separation of the SDFT from the digital flexor tendon sheath and PAL.

as described earlier. Bleeding from the sheath and surface of the tendons after mass resection can be profuse, and a tourniquet becomes more important as disease chronicity increases. Adding epinephrine (1000 units per liter) to the lavage fluid often provides further hemostasis. In most circumstances, the PAL is transected after removal of tendon sheath masses. However, if movement through the fetlock canal is restricted, the PAL should be divided early. This also expedites a thorough examination of the tendon sheath contents, including tendons and attachments. Fortier et al (1999) reported observations on 25 cases. Treatment in all cases was by tenoscopic removal of synovial masses, adhesiolysis, and PAL desmotomy, which is generally advocated in such cases (Nixon, 2002a). Ten cases involved forelimbs and 16 hindlimbs. Cosmesis was improved in 22 of 25 horses. Eighteen of 25 (72%) were sound when working between 1.5 and 7 years (mean 3.4 years) postoperatively. There were negative relationships between duration of clinical signs, presence of synovial masses, and functional outcome.

Palmar/Plantar Annular Ligament Desmitis and Desmotomy

The palmar/plantar annular ligament (PAL) has long been implicated in the pathogenesis of DFTS tenosynovitis, and has been considered by some to be largely responsible for the self-perpetuating nature of the condition (Adams, 1974; Gerring & Webbon, 1984). In some cases there is a primary desmitis (McGhee et al, 2005; Verschooten & Picavet, 1986) or desmopathy (Owen et al, 2008) of the PAL, whereas in others its involvement is secondary to tenosynovitis of the DFTS (Fortier et al, 1999). Differentiation is sometimes not clear and hence the term PAL syndrome (Gerring & Webbon, 1984) may be applicable. McGhee et al (2005) and Owen et al (2008) highlighted the differentiation between primary lesions and injuries of the PAL and thickening of the area that may result from clinical tenosynovitis of the DFTS. Whether a pathogenetic contribution of the latter leads to changes in the PAL is debatable. Desmotomy in such cases may be performed in the belief that removal of constriction contributes to sheath homeostasis or to improve tenoscopic access and visibility in the sesamoidean canal (Fortier, 2005; Fortier et al, 1999). Ultrasonographic differentiation between the PAL and thickening of the DFTS wall, adjacent subcutis, and perithecal connective tissue (Fig. 12-22) is often imprecise (Arensberg et al, 2011; Edinger et al, 2005; Fortier et al, 1999; Owen et al, 2008). Flexing the limb and squeezing fluid from the distal regions of the digital sheath are both effective at separating the SDFT from the annular ligament and sheath covering and can allow a more accurate measure of the contribution of this structure to fetlock canal

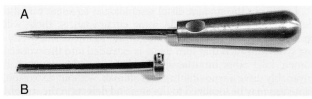

Figure 12-23 Obturator **(A)** and slotted cannula **(B)** for palmar/plantar annular ligament transection. A 90-degree blade works well to sever the ligament, pulling it across the fibers.

constriction (see Fig. 12-22). Thickness beyond 4 mm is considered to indicate potential PAL constriction.

Desmotomy of the PAL may be performed tenoscopically or by extrathecal techniques. Endoscopic PAL desmotomy is performed abaxially between the proximal sesamoid bone and palmar/plantar reflection of the sheath wall from the PAL to the SDFT. There are two basic techniques; the first involves use of a slotted cannula (Hawkins & Moulton, 2002; Nixon et al, 1993), and the second "free-hand" division. Both have protagonists. The former is based on and uses instruments designed for treatment of carpal tunnel syndrome in man (Fig. 12-23) (Chow, 1989 & 1990; Hawkins & Moulton, 2002). Use of the slotted cannula provides advantages in the most chronic and overtly constricted fetlock canal cases. Once appropriately positioned, accurate and complete division of the PAL is assured, compared with free-hand division in these cases, where consistent visual guidance of the desmotomy may be limited. The decision on free-hand or slotted cannula techniques can be made during the initial examination of the sheath.

Placement of the slotted cannula is critical to facilitate insertion of the arthroscope and angle blade. The proximal entry portal should be dorsal in the DFTS and the distal exit portal palmar/plantar (Fig. 12-24), to allow the arthroscope and blade to clear the heel bulbs (this can be particularly difficult in breeds with short pasterns and large feet such as cobs). The cannula is inserted from proximal to distal under arthroscopic visualization (see Fig. 12-24A). The insertion path must be external to the MF to avoid iatrogenic severance. As the slotted cannula and its ribbed obturator near the distal portal, the tip of the arthroscope is retracted 5 mm into its sleeve, to create a docking portal for the obturator of the slotted cannula (Fig. 12-25). This is then advanced, pushing the arthroscope and sleeve out of the tendon sheath and allowing the slotted cannula to exit the arthroscopic skin portal (see Fig. 12-24B). The ribbed obturator is then removed from the slotted cannula, and the unsheathed arthroscope inserted to view and confirm positioning with respect to the flexor tendons, sesamoid surface, and PAL. The slot in the cannula is then oriented to open directly toward the PAL before the 90-degree angle blade is inserted and drawn across the fibers of the PAL to sever the full thickness of the ligament (see Fig. 12-24C & D). Complete division is verified by external palpation of the blade tip beneath the skin, transillumination of light from the arthroscope through the skin, and direct visual evidence of a lack of remaining ligament fibers along the path of the transection. Hemorrhage is flushed from the cannula and tendon sheath, and in most cases the arthroscope is reinserted to inspect the desmotomy for further exploration or surgical procedures, within the DFTS. Reinsertion of the arthroscope sheath with obturator can be expedited by using the slotted cannula as a guide, docking into the exposed slotted cannula, and pushing both units back into the sheath. Once further exploration and masses, adhesions, or tears in the flexor tendons are treated, the instruments are removed and skin portals are closed in a routine manner.

The "free-hand" technique involves a standard arthroscopic portal and creation of an ipsilateral proximal instrument portal abaxial to the MF. The proximal and distal margins of the PAL are usually tenoscopically discernible, but if there is any

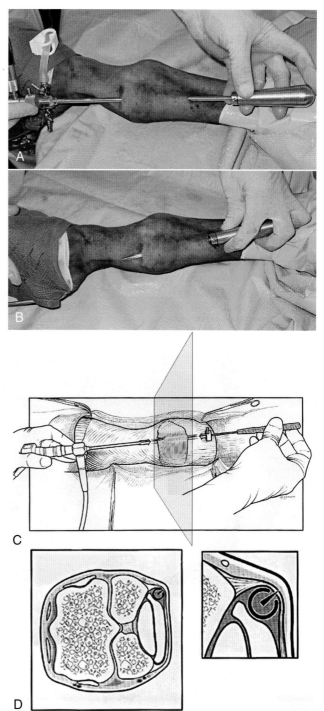

Figure 12-24 Tenoscopically assisted annular ligament division using a slotted cannula. **A,** The instrument portal for placing the cannula is dorsal in the proximal region of the sheath, to allow the cannula to angle through the fetlock canal and avoid the bulbs of the heel. **B,** The obturator and cannula are exteriorized at the arthroscope portal, and the oburator is removed. **C,** With the unsheathed arthroscope viewing the 90-degree blade, the annular ligament fibers are severed by drawing the blade out of the slotted cannula. **D,** Cross-sectional view showing the position and orientation of the blade.

doubt then the margins can be marked by percutaneous needle placement. The optimal axial-abaxial site of transection is midway between the proximal sesamoid bone and sheath wall reflection to the SDFT and again, if required, percutaneous needles can be used as a guide. A curved meniscectomy knife is the instrument of choice (Wilderjans et al, 2003), but a (right-angled) blade can also be used (Fig. 12-26A and B). The cut is made distal to proximal. Division of the mediolaterally oriented fibers of the PAL is readily visualized, and the appearance of loose connective tissue indicates completion. On occasions, it can be advantageous to switch arthroscope and instrument portals in order to confirm complete distal desmotomy because the distal margin of the PAL is close to the standard arthroscopic portal.

McCoy & Goodrich (2012) describe use of a radiofrequency probe for tenoscopically guided PAL desmotomy using the same approach as the free-handed hook knife technique including proximal-distal portal interchange. Radiofrequency probes vary in the consistency of division without char, and the ideal settings seal minor vessels and cut without PAL discoloration (Fig. 12-26C). The principal advantage of radiofrequency probe use is hemostasis in cases in which a tourniquet is not employed. Comparison of clinical outcomes between techniques is pending.

Access to Extrathecal Structures

A transthecal approach to the navicular bursa and palmar/plantar compartment of the distal interphalangeal joint is described in Chapter 13.

Lesions in the straight distal sesamoidean ligament can also be accessed via the DFTS. In some circumstances, these will disrupt the palmar/plantar surface of the ligament and overlying synovium such that torn tissue is extruded into the synovial lumen. Like other intrathecal tears, lesions of this nature will invariably drive a synovitis. In other animals, without distension, lameness may be localized to the area and defects in the straight distal sesamoidean ligament identified ultrasonographically. If required, access for installation of regenerative therapies or debridement, or both, can be achieved tenoscopically.

External Trauma Involving the Digital Flexor Tendon Sheath

The principles of management of penetrating injuries of DFTS are discussed in Chapter 14, but a number of features particular to this site are highlighted here. The complex, layered anatomy of the DFTS (as described earlier) necessitates meticulous tenoscopic evaluation in cases with penetrating wounds because foreign material can migrate and lodge at any site. This may be at multiple foci, and thorough preoperative ultrasonographic examination is critical for identification and surgical planning. This is particularly important with numerous foreign body entries such as porcupine quill penetration (Fig. 12-27). Wounds can be used as sites for instrument entry,

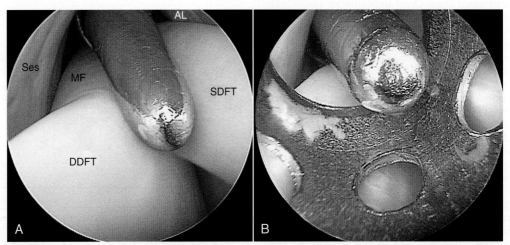

Figure 12-25 A, Tenoscopic view looking proximal, showing the slotted cannula and obturator being inserted superficial to the manica flexoria *(MF)* along the lateral margins of the superficial digital flexor tendon *(SDFT)* and deep digital flexor tendon *(DDFT)*. The flexor surface of the lateral sesamoid *(Ses)* and the palmar/plantar annular ligament *(AL)* provide the other essential landmarks. **B,** After clearing the MF with the slotted cannula, the arthroscope is withdrawn 5 mm into the sleeve, to provide a docking port for the cannula and obturator. The obturator then pushes the arthroscope sleeve from the sheath.

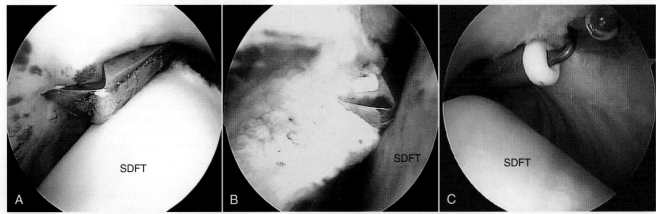

Figure 12-26 Free-hand division of the palmar/plantar annular ligament. **A,** A right-angled blade can be used under direct arthroscopic guidance. **B,** Depth and completeness of division are immediately verified. **C,** Radiofrequency probes also provide a clean and efficient mechanism for free-hand division.

but additional portals commonly are necessary in order to access remote foreign material. When debriding lesions of the digital flexor tendons or fibrocartilage around the proximal sesamoid bones, it is important to recognize that sharp margination between viable and nonviable tissue is rarely obvious and excessive debridement should be avoided.

Fraser & Bladon (2004) reported 39 horses with wounds involving the DFTS, which were all treated by tenoscopy. In follow-up of 7 or more months post surgery, 15 of 16 (94%) that had no concurrent tendon damage returned to their previous or intended use. Twelve of 16 (75%) with lacerations of the SDFT also returned to function, while 5 of 6 horses with lacerations of the SDFT and DDFT were euthanized and the remaining horse was paddock sound only. Four of the 33 (12%) horses that survived the first surgery required a second procedure. Overall, surgery performed within 36 hours of injury carried a better prognosis than that carried out after this time.

Postoperative Care

Skin portals are generally closed with simple interrupted sutures of monofilament nonabsorbable sutures, which are removed between 10 and 14 days postoperatively. Horses usually receive perioperative, antimicrobials and nonsteroidal antiinflammatory drugs at the surgeon's discretion. Counterpressure bandaging is generally recommended for between 2 and 4 weeks after surgery. Some authors advocate intrathecal hyaluronan to aid tendon repair and to prevent adhesion formation (Amiel et al, 1989; Gaughan et al, 1991). Administration

following skin closure and again 10 to 14 days postoperatively has been recommended (Fortier, 2005; Nixon, 2002). In cases where adhesions have been resected or are likely consequences of the primary lesion, direct intrathecal injection of tissue plasminogen activator (tPA) has been recommended. A case report suggests a dose of 500 ug, given every day for 3 injections may diminish adhesions by fibrinolysis (Judy, 2009).

Most horses receive gradually ascending controlled exercise programs, varied empirically by lesion severity and clinical response. Horses with marginal tears of the digital flexor tendons and tears of the MF reported by Smith & Wright (2006) returned to work between 3 and 18 (mean 7.4) months postoperatively. Wilderjans (2003) and Arensburg et al (2012) followed similar gradually ascending postoperative protocols, recommending a return to work not less than 8 months postoperatively.

▶ TENOSCOPY OF THE CARPAL SHEATH

The carpal sheath of the digital flexor tendons is described as beginning 8 to 10 cm proximal to the carpus (Sisson, 1975) or 6 to 8 cm proximal to the antebrachiocarpal joint (Leach et al, 1981). Throughout its course it envelops the SDFT and DDFT including their myotendinous junctions. The SDFT and DDFT are closely related through the carpal sheath and have a common and extensive mesotenon that extends from the caudomedial aspect of the tendons and attaches to the caudal aspect of the carpal sheath (Figs. 12-28, 12-29, and 12-30). This effectively prevents circumferential evaluation of the sheath. The radial head of the DDF originates

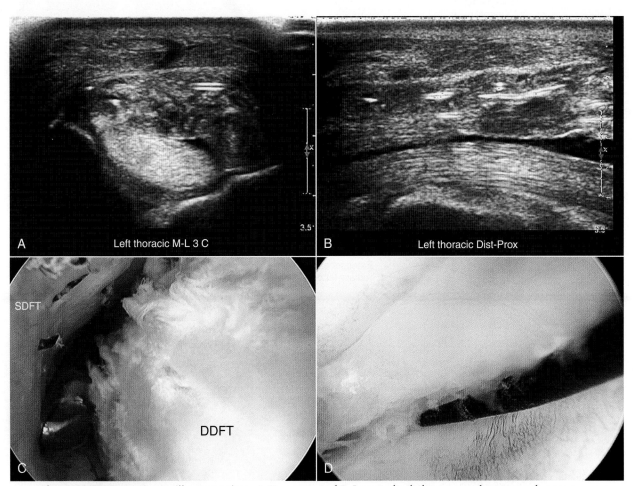

Figure 12-27 Porcupine quill penetration. **A,** Transverse and **B,** Longitudinal ultrasonographic images show numerous quills buried among the deranged superficial digital flexor tendon *(SDFT)*. **C,** Tenoscopic image shows quills perforating completely through the SDFT and subsequent surface damage to the deep digital flexor tendon *(DDFT)*. **D,** The quills are individually drawn from the tendon using Ferris-Smith and punch biopsy rongeurs.

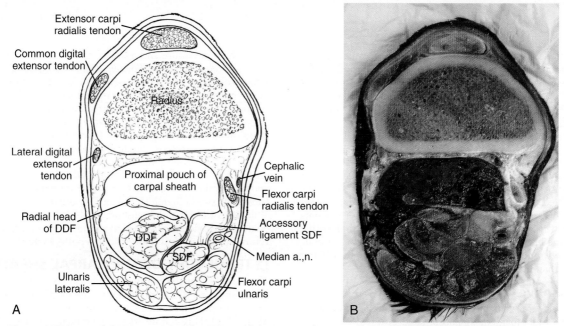

Figure 12-28 A and **B,** Cross-sectional anatomy of the proximal region of the carpal sheath and adjacent structures 8 cm proximal to the accessory carpal bone.

Labels in Figure 12-28 A:
Extensor carpi radialis tendon
Common digital extensor tendon
Radius
Lateral digital extensor tendon
Proximal pouch of carpal sheath
Cephalic vein
Radial head of DDF
Flexor carpi radialis tendon
Accessory ligament SDF
DDF
SDF
Median a.,n.
Ulnaris lateralis
Flexor carpi ulnaris

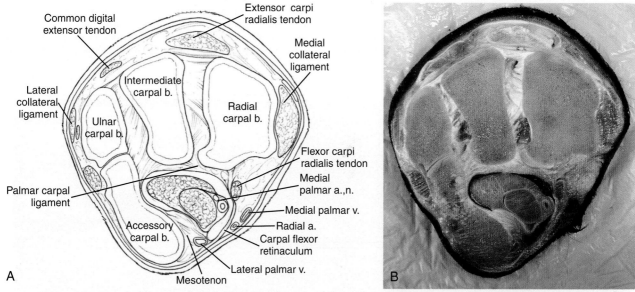

Figure 12-29 A and **B,** Cross-sectional anatomy of the carpal sheath and adjacent structures at the level of the proximal row of carpal bones.

Labels in Figure 12-29 A:
Common digital extensor tendon
Extensor carpi radialis tendon
Medial collateral ligament
Lateral collateral ligament
Intermediate carpal b.
Radial carpal b.
Ulnar carpal b.
Flexor carpi radialis tendon
Medial palmar a.,n.
Palmar carpal ligament
Medial palmar v.
Radial a.
Accessory carpal b.
Carpal flexor retinaculum
Lateral palmar v.
Mesotenon

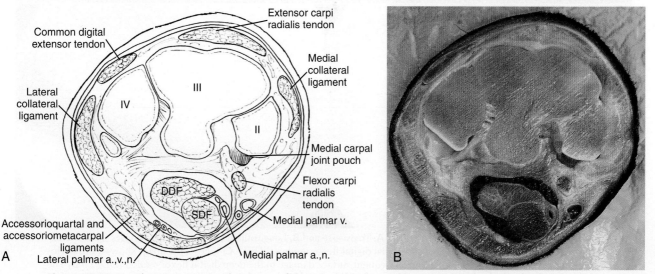

Figure 12-30 A and **B,** Cross-sectional anatomy of the carpal sheath and adjacent structures at the level of the distal row of carpal bones.

Labels in Figure 12-30 A:
Common digital extensor tendon
Extensor carpi radialis tendon
Medial collateral ligament
Lateral collateral ligament
III
IV
II
Medial carpal joint pouch
Flexor carpi radialis tendon
DDF
SDF
Medial palmar v.
Accessorioquartal and accessoriometacarpal ligaments
Lateral palmar a.,v.,n.
Medial palmar a.,n.

principally from the middle of the caudal surface of the radius, and in the carpal sheath a separate mesotenon reflects from the caudal medial sheath wall. The tendon of insertion of the radial head blends with that of the humeral and ulnar heads of the DDF in the proximal compartment of the sheath.

The proximal medial wall of the carpal sheath is covered by avillous synovium and has a barely perceptible indentation formed by the accessory ligament of the SDF (ALSDF) (Fig. 12-31). Cranially (adjacent to the radius) the tendon of insertion of flexor carpi radialis lies medial to this while caudally (beneath the thicker part of the accessory ligament) lie the median artery and nerve (see Fig. 12-28). These adjacent structures are important when considering desmotomy or evaluation of tearing of the ALSDF.

The synovium in the proximal recess of the sheath is villous. This extends over the lateral wall as far as the accessory carpal bone. Fine villi are usually also seen on the synovium covering the thick periosteum of the caudal radius, which forms the cranial margin of the proximal pouch. Within the carpal canal the dorsal boundary of the carpal sheath is the palmar carpal ligament while its lateral and caudolateral margin is the accessory carpal bone. The carpal flexor retinaculum forms the medial boundary (see Fig. 12-29). This is thickest dorsally and thins palmarly. It contains the radial artery and medial palmar vein and tendon of insertion of flexor carpi radialis. At this level the medial palmar artery and nerve are within the common mesotenon of the SDFT and DDFT (see Fig. 12-29). Throughout the region of the carpal canal the synovium is avillous, but distally the sheath wall is lined by

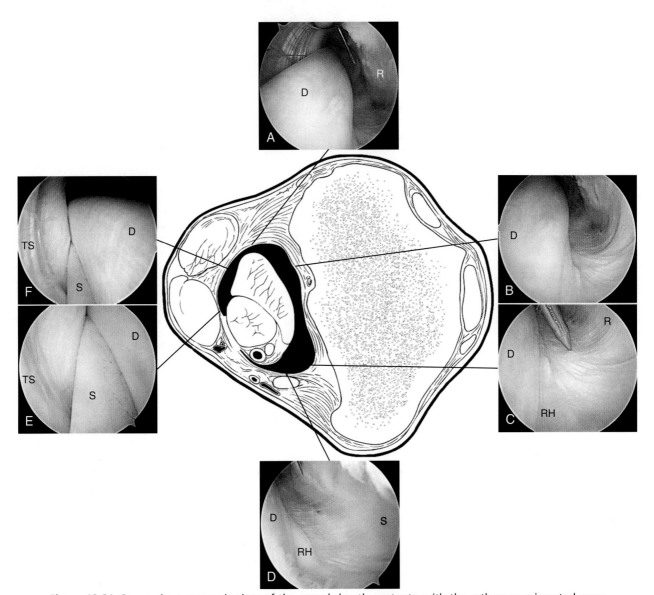

Figure 12-31 Composite tenoscopic view of the carpal sheath contents, with the arthroscope inserted proximolaterally. The deep digital flexor tendon (DDFT) *(D)* is the only visible tendon on the lateral side of the flexor tendon bundle. Repositioning the arthroscope more cranially shows the caudal aspect of the radius *(R)*, including the slight prominence of the closed distal physis, the cranial aspect of the DDFT, and the radial head of the DDF *(RH)*. **C** shows an instrument pressing on the intrusion of the distal limits of the accessory ligament of the superficial digital flexor over the medial wall of the sheath. The DDFT and the caudal aspect of the radius are also visible. The arthroscope can be positioned caudally to reveal the caudal surfaces of the DDFT and SDFT *(S)*, as well as the caudal surface of the tendon sheath *(TS)*.

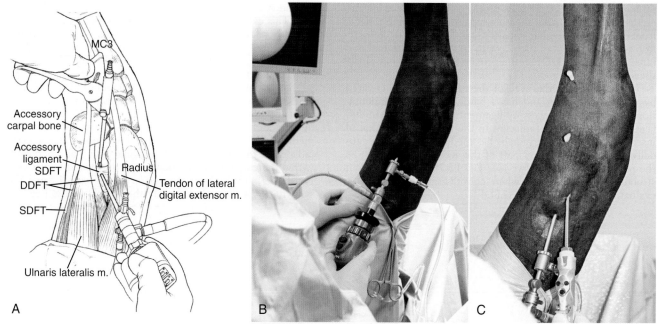

Figure 12-32 A-C, Tenoscopic approach to the carpal sheath. The standard entry point is made proximolaterally, leaving the remaining area free for instrument portals to approach the caudal aspect of radius, carpal canal and contents, or accessory ligament of the superficial digital flexor. *DDFT,* Deep digital flexor tendon; *MC3,* third metacarpal bone; *SDFT,* superficial digital flexor tendon.

villous synovium. Distal to the accessory carpal bone, the carpal sheath becomes slightly more voluminous (see Fig. 12-30), but it remains much narrower than the proximal pouch.

Tenosynovitis of the carpal sheath can result from osteochondroma of the caudal distal radius (Held et al, 1988; Lee et al, 1979; Nixon, 2002a; Southwood et al, 1997; Squire et al, 1992; Stahre & Tufvesson, 1967; Wright & Minshall, 2012); exostosis of the caudal margin of the bony remnant of the distal radial physis (Nixon et al, 2004); tearing of the accessory ligament of the SDF (Nixon et al, 2004); fractures of the accessory carpal bone (Dyson & Dik, 1995; Nixon et al, 2004); superficial digital flexor tendonitis (Dyson & Dik, 1995); incomplete rupture of the DDFT (Dik, 1990); and tearing of the radial head of the DDF (Minshall & Wright, 2012). Tenoscopy also offers a minimally invasive approach to desmotomy of the accessory ligaments of the SDF (Southwood et al, 1999) and DDF (Caldwell et al, 2011) and for treatment of carpal tunnel syndrome (Textor et al, 2003).

The most distensible portion of the carpal sheath is its proximolateral pouch centered over the distolateral antebrachium between the ulnaris lateralis (caudally) and lateral digital extensor (cranially). When intact, the thick carpal retinaculum obscures/restrains medial distension. Distension can also usually be appreciated in the proximal metacarpus but if subtle is obscured by the metacarpal fascia.

Technique

The authors routinely use variations of the standard proximolateral approach to the carpal sheath as described by Southwood et al (1998). This technique allows evaluation of the entire proximal portion of the carpal sheath, including the carpal canal, but provides limited access to the metacarpal region of the sheath. Insertion of the arthroscope into the distal region of the carpal sheath improves examination of this area (Cauvin et al, 1997).

Surgery can be performed with the horse in dorsal recumbency or in lateral recumbency with the affected limb uppermost. Dorsal recumbency is generally preferred by the authors. It has obvious advantages for bilateral evaluation

and significantly reduces intraoperative hemorrhage. Lateral recumbency facilitates tenoscopy through the distolateral (metacarpal) portal. In both situations, the carpus is positioned in slight (≈ 15- to 20-degree) flexion. The carpal sheath is distended with 50 to 60 mL of lactated Ringer solution and the arthroscope entry portal is made laterally, 6 to 8 cm proximal to the remnant of the radial physis. This allows examination of the carpal sheath, while leaving the region between the arthroscope entry and the distal physis of the radius available for instrument entry (Fig. 12-32).

Initial examination from the lateral approach reveals the caudal aspect of the radius and the lateral portion of the DDFT, which at this level obscures most of the SDFT (see Fig. 12-31). The SDFT can be examined later by rolling the DDFT with a probe, but this exposes only small portions of the tendon; complete examination of the SDFT is difficult using the lateral approach. The common mesotenon for the SDFT and DDFT attaches to the caudomedial aspect of the carpal sheath and effectively prevents examination of the SDFT over its caudal and medial surfaces. In the more distal regions of the carpal sheath, the SDFT emerges, although better examination of this tendon is provided through a palmarolateral portal 4 to 6 cm distal to the accessory carpal bone (Cauvin et al, 1997).

Maneuvering the arthroscope to examine the more proximal regions of the carpal sheath reveals the radial head of the DDF coursing from its aponeurosis on the DDFT cranially to curve and expand into its origin on the caudal aspect of the radius (see Fig. 12-31). The ALSDF (proximal check ligament) can also be identified within the medial wall of the carpal sheath immediately cranial to the radial head of the DDF but can be more clearly defined by using an instrument to probe for the intrusion of the ligament into the sheath (see Fig. 12-31). The arthroscope can then be redirected to more caudal regions of the carpal sheath, examining the caudal surface of the DDFT and a small portion of the SDFT (see Fig. 12-31). It can also be inserted a small distance between the SDFT and DDFT before encountering the common mesotenon joining the tendons.

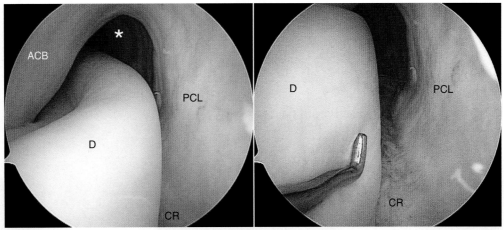

Figure 12-33 Tenoscopic views of the carpal canal from a proximolateral arthroscope portal with the arthroscope pointed distally. The lateral and dorsal surfaces of the deep digital flexor tendon *(D)*, the palmar aspect of the carpal joints overlaid by the palmar carpal ligament *(PCL)*, the accessory carpal bone *(ACB)*, and the narrowing of the sheath at the carpometacarpal joint *(asterisk)* are visible. The fibers of the carpal flexor retinaculum *(CR)* are evident traversing palmarly from the palmar carpal ligament to their insertion on the ACB.

Further distally examination of the craniomedial carpal sheath reveals the transversely oriented fibers of the carpal flexor retinaculum, forming the medial boundary to the carpal canal (Fig. 12-33). The proximal and distal limits of the retinaculum are not as distinct as the intrusion formed by the proximal check ligament. The proximal border of the retinaculum can be recognized only by the adjacent caudal protuberance of the physeal scar of the radius. The distal border of the retinaculum can be determined by digital pressure over the palmaromedial portion of the carpal sheath, which can easily be indented only beyond this distal margin. The distal regions of the carpal sheath can be examined beyond the level of the carpometacarpal joint, but mobility distal to this level is restricted. Examination of the most distal regions of the carpal sheath can be performed by inserting the arthroscope palmarolaterally in the proximal metacarpus (Cauvin et al, 1997). This can be difficult with the horse in dorsal recumbency, but the limb should be prepared and draped to enable use of this portal if needed. The portal is made palmar to the lateral palmar vein and extends through the metacarpal fascia and sheath wall. The arthroscopic cannula and conical obturator are inserted dorsal to the DDFT and directed proximally. The arthroscope portal can also be made in the palmaromedial surface of the sheath at this level, but with the horse in dorsal recumbency, manipulating the arthroscope becomes even more difficult.

▶ Tenoscopic Treatment of Conditions in the Carpal Sheath

Radial Osteochondroma

Solitary (monostotic) osteochondroma in the horse are most common on the caudal aspect of the distal metaphysis of the radius (Held et al, 1988; Lee et al, 1979; Lundvall & Jackson, 1976; Southwood et al, 1997; Squire et al, 1992; Stashak, 2002). They are thought to result from separation of a portion of the metaphyseal growth plate margin creating an island of chondrogenic tissue, capable of endochondral ossification, that is carried into the metaphysis with growth of the bone (Thompson, 2007; Thompson & Pool, 2002). In mature osteochondroma, endochondral ossification may be complete such that little or no cartilage remains.

Most present in young adult horses; in a series of 22 horses with caudal distal radial osteochondroma reported by Wright & Minshall (2012), there was an age range of 2 to 6 (mean 2.8) years. When clinically significant, osteochondroma present, or

have a history of distension of the carpal sheath. Lameness is frequently variable, often recurrent, and accompanied by distension of the carpal sheath. Of the 25 osteochondroma cases reported by Wright & Minshall (2012), 22 occurred in the central and 2 in the lateral one third of the radius; one was at the junction of the central and medial one thirds. The distance between the distal metaphyseal growth plate and the center of the osteochondroma varied between 7 and 33 (mean 19) mm and appeared unrelated to the animal's age. Most are single, sharply pointed protuberances and may be proximally inclined or perpendicular to the radial diaphysis (see Fig. 12-34A). They are of variable size, and clinical signs appear to result from impingement on the overlying DDFT and subsequent tenosynovitis. Impingement on the DDFT can usually be identified ultrasonographically using a curved array probe with the limb in a semiflexed position (Wright & Minshall, 2012).

Surgery is performed in dorsal recumbency using the standard proximolateral arthroscopic portal described earlier. The sheath usually contains sanguineous or xanthochromic fluid with proliferative synovium, which frequently contains hemosiderin deposits. The osteochondroma protrude through the synovium of the carpal sheath, with their sloping margins covered to varying degrees by synovium and the underlying periosteum of the caudal radius (Fig. 12-34). Impingement lesions on the overlying DDFT usually take the form of longitudinal tears of varying length and depth aligned with the osteochondroma (see Fig. 12-34). A site for a suitable lateral instrument portal in the proximal pouch of the carpal sheath is ascertained by using a percutaneous 18-gauge spinal needle to target the osteochondroma and adjacent DDFT lesion. The authors' preference is to remove extruded torn tendon tissue first before dealing with the osteochondroma. This is most efficiently undertaken using a synovial resector in oscillating mode with suction applied. Small osteochondromas can be removed by gripping in arthroscopic rongeurs and fracturing from the caudal radius, while larger masses should first be cleaved with an osteotome (see Fig. 12-34). When cleaved from the caudal radius the osteochondroma frequently remains hinged on adjacent synovium and periosteum from which it can be torn or cut before it is retrieved with appropriately sized arthroscopic rongeurs. Any remaining irregular bone is then debrided with a closed-cup curette or bone rasp until uniform cortical bone is seen (see Fig. 12-34). Adjacent tags of periosteum and synovium are removed with the motorized

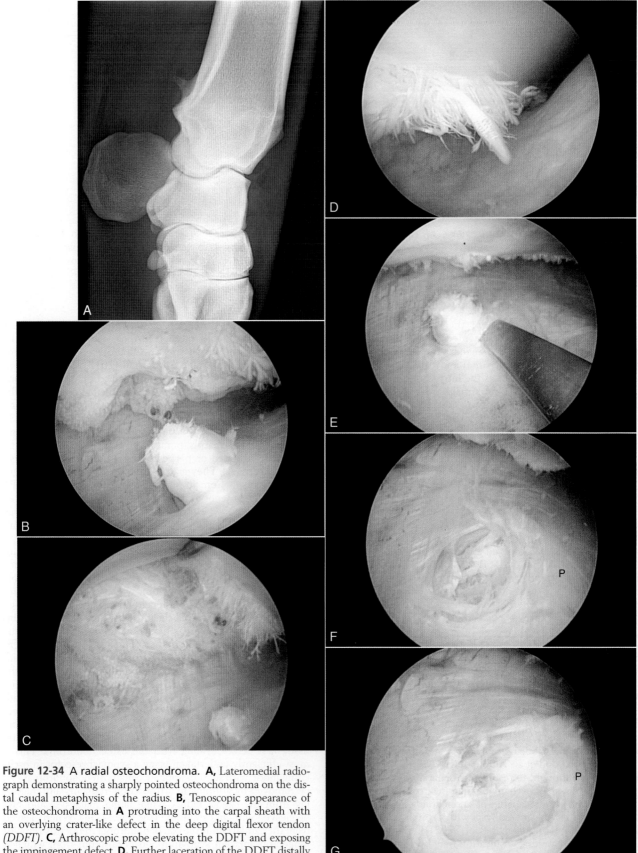

Figure 12-34 A radial osteochondroma. **A,** Lateromedial radiograph demonstrating a sharply pointed osteochondroma on the distal caudal metaphysis of the radius. **B,** Tenoscopic appearance of the osteochondroma in **A** protruding into the carpal sheath with an overlying crater-like defect in the deep digital flexor tendon *(DDFT)*. **C,** Arthroscopic probe elevating the DDFT and exposing the impingement defect. **D,** Further laceration of the DDFT distally within the carpal canal. **E,** Osteotome used to cleave the osteochondroma from the caudal radius. **F,** Caudal radius immediately following removal of the osteochondroma. Note the thick periosteal surface *(P)*, which is highly vascular. **G,** Appearance following debridement of the osteochondroma base to well organized cortical bone and removal of adjacent, frayed periosteum.

synovial resector. The sheath is then lavaged, paying particular attention to the proximal recess, which in dorsal recumbency becomes the dependent point in which debris generally accumulates. Skin portals are closed routinely.

The prognosis for return to function after osteochondroma removal is excellent. All horses reported by Wright & Minshall (2012) returned to work. Thirteen of 19 racing Thoroughbreds raced postoperatively. The time from surgery to the first race varied between 4 and 18 (mean 7) months, and those that had raced preoperatively performed at similar or improved postoperative levels. No evidence of recurrence was reported in any of the cases.

Radial Physeal Exostoses

Radial physeal exostoses are removed using a similar technique to that for radial osteochondroma (Nixon, 2002; Nixon et al, 2004). Most clinically relevant radial physeal exostoses involve protrusion of one or two caudally directed physeal remnants (Fig. 12-35). The shape varies from sharp to irregular and blunted. Damage to the cranial surface of the DDFT appears as linear fraying, similar to that developing with sharp osteochondromas, and penetrates a variable depth into the tendon depending on the height of the exostosis. Damage to the DDFT can be extensive, including excoriation of the epitenon, linear fiber laceration, and surface proliferation (see Fig. 12-35). Removal of the physeal exostoses can be accomplished using an osteotome, or small spikes can be removed using a motorized burr. The bony bed is generally smoothed using a burr, curette, or rasp. Damage to the DDFT is debrided to healthy tendon using motorized synovectomy equipment or biopsy punch rongeurs, or both. An assessment of the degree of fibrosis and potential constriction of the carpal canal is warranted after removal of radial physeal exostoses. Additionally, any deeper tendonitis lesions may cause expanded flexor tendon volume within the carpal canal, complicating the syndrome and making the need for carpal retinaculum release more likely (Nixon et al, 2004; Textor et al,

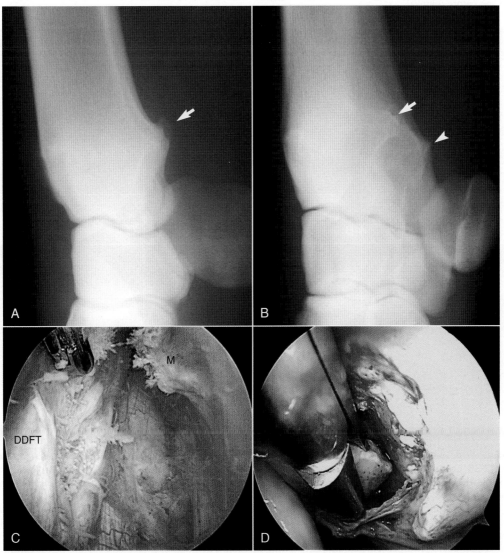

Figure 12-35 Caudal radial physeal exostoses. **A,** A lateromedial radiograph of the distal radius of a horse with persistent carpal sheath effusion and lameness. The exostoses appear as sharp bony *(arrow)* spikes that protrude a variable distance toward the carpal sheath. **B,** A dorsolateral-palmaromedial oblique radiograph is used to separate the axial, potentially harmful, exostoses *(arrow)*, from the abaxial (palmarolateral) exostosis *(arrowhead)* that is beyond the limits of the carpal sheath and its contents and thus unlikely to cause lameness. **C,** A medially positioned caudal exostosis *(M)* arising from the physeal remnant causing focal damage to the deep digital flexor tendon *(DDFT)*. A biopsy rongeur is being used to debride the tendon. **D,** An osteotome has been used to separate the spike, which is being removed in rongeurs. Hemorrhage was profuse and gas distension is being used to allow better visualization.

Continued

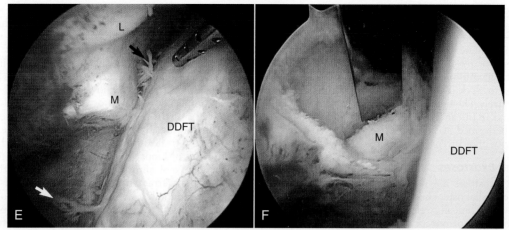

Figure 12-35, cont'd E, A different case showing a pair of intruding exostoses, one lateral *(L)* and one medial *(M)*. The DDFT has erosions and epitenal proliferation *(arrow)*. **F,** The medial spike has been separated from the radius with an osteotome before removal.

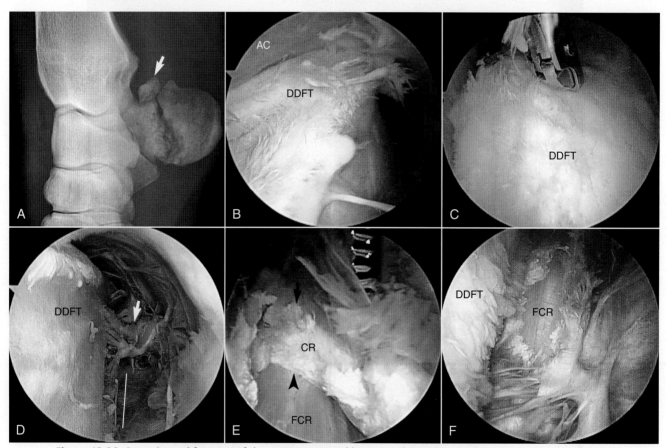

Figure 12-36 Comminuted fracture of the accessory carpal bone involving the antebrachiocarpal joint and the carpal sheath. A, Radiograph shows a chronic vertical fracture of the accessory carpal bone, with a discrete articular fragment *(arrow)*. **B,** Tenoscopic view of deep digital flexor tendon *(DDFT)* damage associated with irregular bony edges and callus from the displaced vertical fracture. **C,** Debridement of the DDFT damage. **D,** Other consequences of the tenosynovitis include adhesions *(arrow)* between DDFT and carpal retinaculum and carpal tunnel constriction. *Line* indicates location of retinaculum release to relieve constriction. **E,** Carpal tunnel release showing extremely thickened (between *arrows*) carpal retinaculum *(CR)* during division. The incision is located over the flexor carpi radialis *(FCR)* tendon. **F,** Completed carpal tunnel release and adhesiolysis.

2003). Postoperative radiographs need to be carefully scrutinized to differentiate the removed exostoses from those more abaxially located, the latter of which do not enter the carpal sheath or cause lameness (see Fig. 12-35). The prognosis is generally excellent, with all 10 horses returning to work in one report (Nixon et al, 2004).

Fractures of the Accessory Carpal Bone

Frontal plane or comminuted fractures of the accessory carpal bone disrupt the carpal canal and frequently create open communication with the carpal sheath. The two principal consequences of the latter are the impingement of fracture fragments and edges on the adjacent DDFT (Fig. 12-36), and

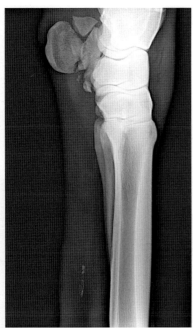

Figure 12-37 Lateromedial radiograph of a comminuted frontal plane fracture of the accessory carpal bone. Comminuted fragments are evident as far distally as the mid metacarpus in the most distal cul-de-sac of the carpal sheath.

release of comminuted fragments into the sheath lumen. The latter can gravitate to the most dependent (distal) cul-de-sac, and a lateromedial radiograph imaging the middle one third of the metacarpus is necessary in order to determine their presence (Fig. 12-37). Laceration of the DDFT by displaced fracture fragments is common and of varying degrees of severity. Removal of the offending bone and torn tendon tissue is believed to contribute to case outcome, but the optimum time for interference is yet to be determined. Comminuted accessory carpal bone fragments can also involve the proximodorsal articular surface and complicate the lameness by antebrachiocarpal joint disease (see Fig. 12-36). Approaches to remove articular fragments through palamarolateral arthroscopy portals can then be followed by carpal sheath tenoscopy. Subcutaneous fluid leakage complicates this approach; however, expression of free fluid from the fascial planes between approaches often defines landmarks to continue the surgery on the carpal sheath.

Horses are operated on in dorsal recumbency with a standard proximolateral tenoscopic approach. The surgeon should be cognizant that fracture fragments which preoperatively have been identified in the distal cul-de-sac of the sheath may now, under the influence of gravity, migrate proximally. Removal of loose fragments should be performed first while visibility is optimal. Torn and extruded tendon fibers can then be removed using standard techniques (see Fig. 12-36). In acute fractures, protruding fragments can also be removed using lateral instrument portals distal or proximal to the accessory carpal bone, or in some circumstances provided by percutaneous needle placement through the fracture plane. In longstanding cases protuberant "spiked" margins of the fracture may protrude into the sheath lumen causing trauma to the DDFT. The spikes should be removed using a motorized burr to prevent ongoing trauma.

Tears of the Radial Head of the Deep Digital Flexor

Tears of the radial head of the DDF have been reported as a specific cause of tenosynovitis of the carpal sheath (Minshall & Wright, 2012). The degree of lameness and distension of the carpal sheath appear variable. Ultrasonography demonstrated

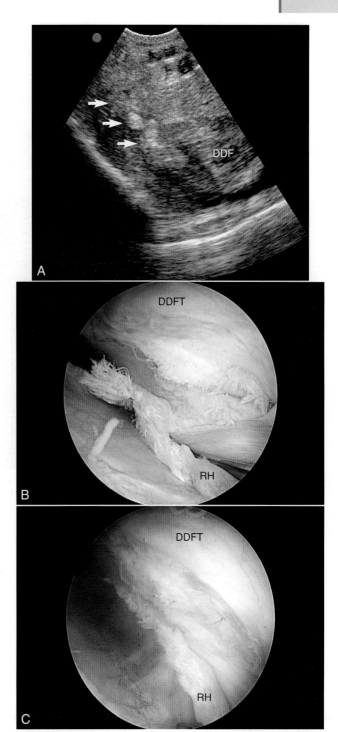

Figure 12-38 Torn radial head of the deep digital flexor. **A,** Ultrasonograph demonstrating irregular echogenic material *(arrows)* suspended in a distended carpal sheath adjacent to the deep digital flexor *(DDF)* adjacent to its musculotendinous junction. **B,** Tenoscopic image of the area imaged in **A** demonstrating tearing/avulsion of the radial head of the DDF *(RH)* from the principal tendon. **C,** Tenoscopic appearance following removal of the torn tissue.

intrathecal disorganized echogenic material adjacent to the DDF, close to the proximal sheath reflection, and in the region of the radial head of the DDF in 9 of 11 cases (Fig. 12-38). Using standard tenoscopic technique, the lesion is invariably located at the junction of the radial head with the DDF. In some cases torn tendon fibrils are extruded into the sheath lumen and readily visible at initial inspection (see Fig. 12-38). In other horses, the lateral surfaces of the mesotenon and

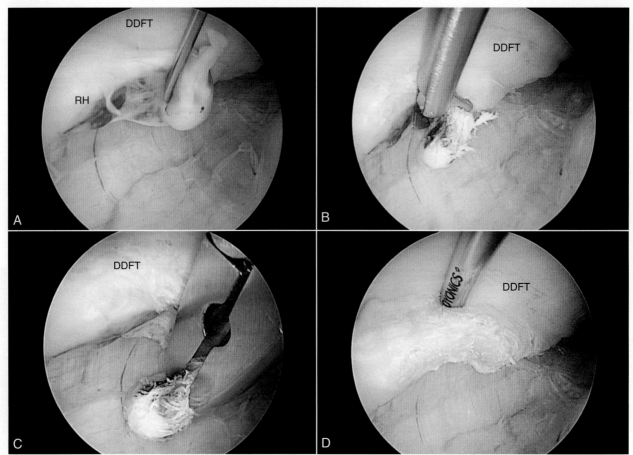

Figure 12-39 A, Granulomatous mass associated with the distal margin of a tear/avulsion of the radial head of the deep digital flexor tendon *(DDF) (RH)*. **B,** Division with arthroscopic scissors. **C,** Removal with arthroscopic rongeurs. **D,** Appearance of the lesion following debridement. *DDFT,* Deep digital flexor tendon.

epitenon of the radial head of the DDF are intact, but when these are elevated with an arthroscopic probe in order to assess its cranial surface, a breach in the radial head surface layers is evident and through this torn fibrils can be seen. Frequently in such cases, fibrils that have avulsed from their insertion recoil proximally within the epitenon and perimysium. Occasionally, bundles of torn tendon tissue may be covered by granulation tissue with varying degrees of organization. These granulomatous masses can be sectioned with arthroscopic scissors and removed with arthroscopic rongeurs (Fig. 12-39). In most cases, disrupted tendon tissue is readily removed using a 4-mm synovial resector in oscillating mode and suction applied. Occasionally, when debriding recoiled musculotendinous tissue, vessels of sufficient size to produce intrathecal hemorrhage, and thus to obscure visibility, can be encountered. Recently one of the authors (IMW) has used an esmarch bandage and tourniquet when operating on carpal sheaths in which intrathecal hemorrhage might be anticipated. Use of epinephrine in the distending fluid has been helpful to avoid tourniquet use for most small vessel hemorrhage.

Following routine postoperative care, horses receive graduated ascending controlled exercise programs. In the series reported by Minshall & Wright (2012) all horses returned to work. The time between surgery and the first race for 8 of 10 racing Thoroughbreds varied between 6 and 17 (mean 8.8) months, and postoperative performances were equal to preinjury levels.

Tearing of the Deep and Superficial Digital Flexors

Although not yet documented in the literature, the authors have recognized intrathecal tears of the DDFT, SDFT, and also disruption of the ALSDF within the carpal sheath. All present with similar clinical features, including lameness, sheath distension, and ultrasonographic evidence of intrathecal adventitious echogenic material. Commonly, there is evidence of hemorrhage within the carpal sheath. Tenoscopic appearance is highly variable, and in some cases multiple structures may be involved. Most tears are situated in the proximal recess of the carpal sheath, at or close to the musculotendinous junctions of DDF and SDF. Some may culminate in carpal canal syndrome due to volume expansion, as described later. Treatment of the visible tear by debridement, injection of ultrasonographically deeper tendonitis with biologics such as PRP or cultured stem cells, and carpal canal release by division of the carpal retinaculum are all logical, but none are supported by published literature.

Tearing of the ALSDF can usually be predicted ultrasonographically. From a tenoscopic perspective, the most common site of tearing is caudally through the thickest portion of the ligament (Fig. 12-40). Treatment has followed the basic principles of removal of extruded material with the goal of creating a smooth surface over the disrupted tendon fibers. Caution is necessary when dealing with the ALSDF to avoid trauma to the underlying median artery and nerve, which can be exposed (see Fig. 12-40). Additional injections of PRP or cultured stem cells, or both, to the residual deeper disrupted regions of the ALSDF have been used.

▶ Desmotomy of the Accessory Ligament of the Superficial Digital Flexor (Proximal Check Ligament)

The accessory ligament of the SDF (ALSDF) is slightly wedge shaped in cross section; thinner distally and thicker

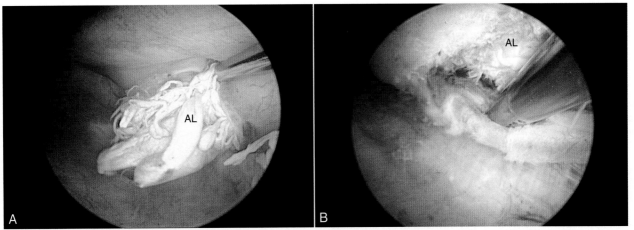

Figure 12-40 A, Tenoscopic appearance of an intrathecal tear of the accessory ligament of the superficial digital flexor *(AL)* with torn fibers protruding laterally into the sheath lumen. **B,** Exposure of the median artery, elevated with an arthroscopic probe, at the distal margin of the debrided tear.

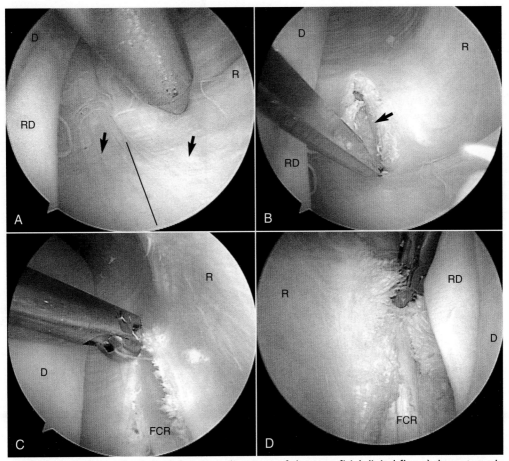

Figure 12-41 Tenoscopic proximal check (accessory ligament of the superficial digital flexor) desmotomy in a left leg. **A,** Landmarks for identification of the distal limit of the ligament *(arrows)* include the radial head of the deep digital flexor *(RD)*, the caudal aspect of the radius *(R)*, the cranial aspect of the deep digital flexor tendon DDFT *(D)*, and the intrusion of the check ligament body *(arrows)*. The line indicates the transection pathway. **B,** Commencement of transection with a curved serrated blade exposes the underlying tendon of flexor carpi radialis *(FCR) (arrow)*. **C,** Biopsy punch rongeurs (Dyovac 5.2) provide an effective cutting instrument, exposing more of the FCR. **D,** With arthroscope and instrument portals reversed, the view from distal to proximal shows the more robust proximal ligament being cut with biopsy rongeurs.

proximally where it sometimes contains a large nutrient artery that arises as a direct caudal branch of the underlying median artery. From a tenoscopic perspective, the ALSDF extends proximally from the level of the distal radial physeal remnant and the aponeurosis/junction of the radial head with the body of the DDF (Fig. 12-41). The ALSDF is entirely extrasynovial and forms a slight intrusion to the medial sheath wall, which extends from the landmarks described earlier to beyond the normal proximomedial reflection of the carpal sheath wall.

The two principal indications for desmotomy are superficial digital flexor tendonitis and metacarpophalangeal flexural deformity. The goal in both is the elongation of the bone-to-bone (origin to insertion) unit of the SDF (Hogan & Bramlage, 1995). Varying degrees of success have been reported in the former (Bramlage & Hogan, 1996; Fulton et al, 1994; Hawkins & Ross, 1995; Hogan & Bramlage, 1995). Its use in Thoroughbreds has declined in recent years, although it remains more commonly employed in Standardbreds. The authors also consider tearing of the ALSDF as an indication for desmotomy when the degree of disruption is marked.

The technique is a variation of one originally described by Southwood et al (1999), and although it can be accomplished using lateral recumbency, it is now increasingly done bilaterally, necessitating dorsal recumbency. The arthroscope is placed proximolaterally in the sheath, as described earlier. This allows identification of important landmarks including the radial head of the DDF (see Fig. 12-41), the cranial edge of the DDFT, the caudal aspect of the radius, and the proximal reflection of the carpal sheath. The distal border of the ALSDF is usually level with the junction of the radial head of the DDF with the main body of the DDFT. Instrument entry is made 4 to 6 cm distal to the arthroscope, through the lateral portion of the carpal sheath. The ALSDF is subsynovial and is probed with a blunt instrument to verify its distal limit. The ligament can then be severed using a curved serrated blade (Sontec Instruments, Centennial, CO); straight serrated blade (3 mm, Acufex–Smith & Nephew, Mansfield, MA); or a 90-degree angled radiofrequency probe (Arthrex, Naples, FL; Stryker Endoscopy, San Jose, CA), commencing at its distal border and severing across the fibers in a distal to proximal direction (see Fig. 12-41). As the ALSDF is severed proximally, it becomes thicker. The body of the structure is located beyond the proximal reflection of the carpal sheath, and this portion is more cleanly and quickly severed using a biopsy punch rongeur or radiofrequency probe. These instruments provide better visualization of the proximal extent of the ligament, as well as any contained vasculature (evident in ≈25% of horses). Bleeding from the artery contained within the ALSDF is reduced with horses in dorsal recumbency and usually can be controlled using fluid pressure to allow completion of the surgery. Alternatively, it can be stopped using bipolar laparoscopic cautery forceps (Linvatec, Largo, FL) or application of a hemostatic clip (Ligaclip, US Surgical, Norwalk, CT). Penetration of the thin sheath surrounding the flexor carpi radialis tendon is routine during division of the ALSDF (see Fig. 12-41), and the tendon is an important landmark because it defines the medial end point for the dissection (Nixon, 1990a). Exchange of arthroscope and instrument portals is often useful to improve visualization during division of the more proximal regions of the ligament. With experience, it is generally easier to perform the entire surgery with the arthroscope placed in the more distal instrument portal. The instrument and arthroscope tend to follow a similar plane, making triangulation more difficult during the latter portion of the surgery. The proximal fibers of the ALSDF can be identified and divided using biopsy rongeurs. Use of a radiofrequency probe (Stryker Endoscopy, San Jose, CA, or Arthrex, Naples, FL) has been helpful to divide the ALSDF more cleanly (Fig. 12-42), although for this reason, it can be difficult to see the depths of the division between the closely apposed divided edges, particularly in the proximal region of the check ligament.

David et al (2011) reported monopolar electrosurgical tenoscopic desmotomy in 33 horses. Nonetheless, severe intrathecal hemorrhage occurred in 6 and mild intrathecal hemorrhage in another 6 horses. All severe hemorrhage came from the nutrient artery and was subsequently controlled by the use of the electrosurgical probe in coagulation mode. Drainage of clear fluid from skin portals was reported in 22 of 33 (67%)

horses. In the authors' experience this is unusual and may be associated with the use of 1.5% glycine as the irrigating fluid.

Desmotomy of the Accessory Ligament of the Deep Digital Flexor

Caldwell et al (2011) described a tenoscopic approach for desmotomy of the accessory ligament of the DDF (ALDDF). This utilized a distomedial arthroscopic portal into the carpal

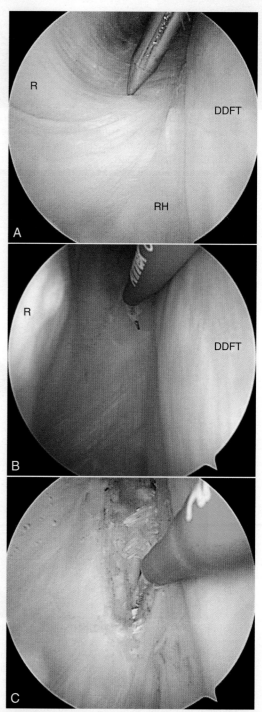

Figure 12-42 Radiofrequency probe being used to sever the accessory ligament of the superficial digital flexor (proximal check ligament) in a right leg. **A,** Defining the distal edge of the ligament. **B,** 90-degree radiofrequency probe. **C,** Drawing the probe from distal to proximal cuts through the ligament and exposes the tendon of the flexor carpi radialis. *DDFT,* Deep digital flexor tendon; *R,* radius; *RH,* radial head of deep digital flexor.

sheath modified from that described by Cauvin et al (1997), at the level of the junction of the middle and proximal thirds of the metacarpus. A contralateral instrument portal is created at the same level in the sheath. The authors used a 6400 Beaver blade (Becton-Dickinson, Franklin Lakes, NJ) for desmotomy in cadaveric limbs and experimental horses. Dorsal recumbency was recommended. The limb was positioned in approximately 20 degrees of carpal flexion for arthroscope entry to the sheath, followed by distal limb extension to place the ALDDF under tension and facilitate transection. The lateral side of the ALDDF was sectioned in this manner before arthroscope, and instruments were interchanged for division

of the medial side of the ligament. Complete division could be confirmed by identification of loose areolar tissue overlying the suspensory ligament and by separation of the cut ends of the accessory ligament on manual extension of the distal interphalangeal joint (Fig. 12-43). Tenoscopic division of the ALDDF requires practice because the entry is to a much less distensible portion of the carpal sheath, and the arthroscope tip and cutting blades are always in close proximity. One of the authors (AJN) favors placing the arthroscope in a portal proximal to the accessory carpal bone to view distally while inserting a needle to verify an appropriate distal medial arthroscopic portal (see Fig. 12-43). Transillumination also

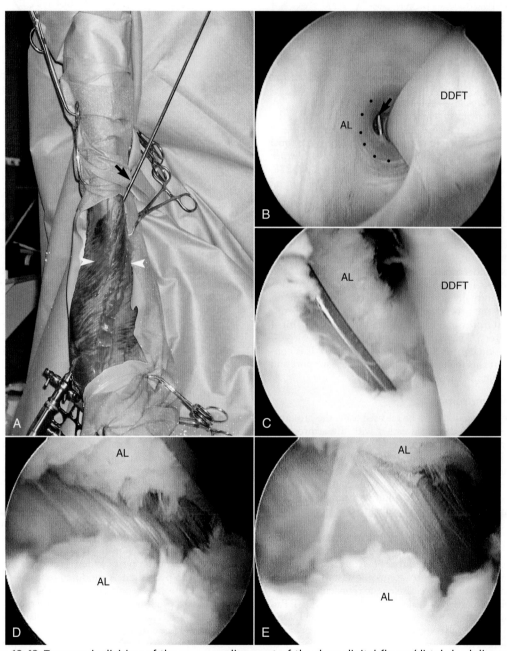

Figure 12-43 Tenoscopic division of the accessory ligament of the deep digital flexor (distal check ligament). **A,** A proximal arthroscopic portal provides transillumination to identify distal medial and lateral entry sites *(white arrows)*. **B,** Viewing distally from the proximal entry, the termination of the carpal sheath can be seen, including the deep digital flexor tendon *(DDFT)* and intrusion of its accessory (check) ligament *(dotted line)*; a preplaced needle *(arrow)* guides instrument entry and dissection. **C,** Beginning of desmotomy, viewed from a proximal arthroscopic portal showing accessory ligament fibers *(AL)* beginning to spread. **D** and **E,** Visually complete desmotomy is confirmed by flexion **(D)** and extension **(E)** of the foot to tense the DDFT and separate the divided check ligament fibers.

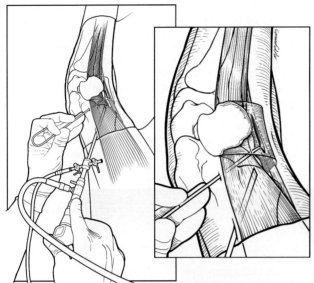

▶ **Figure 12-44** Drawing of tenoscopic carpal canal release in the right limb, with the arthroscope inserted in the proximolateral aspect of the carpal sheath and instrument portal 1 cm proximal to the accessory carpal bone. *(From Textor, JA, Nixon, AJ, Fortier, LA. Tenoscopic release of the equine carpal canal, Vet Surg. 32, 278-284, 2003, with permission of publisher.)*

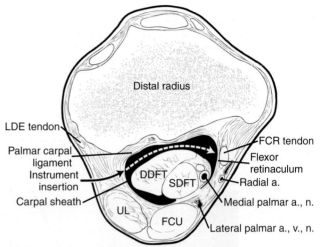

Figure 12-45 Cross-sectional drawing of the carpal canal at the level of instrument insertion. A serrated blade is inserted along the path as shown and drawn across the fibers of the carpal retinaculum. *(Textor, JA, Nixon, AJ, Fortier, LA. Tenoscopic release of the equine carpal canal, Vet Surg. 32, 278-284, 2003, with permission of publisher.)*

helps define medial and lateral regions of the carpal sheath at the site of ALDDF division. A second arthroscopic cannula or a switching stick can then be inserted under arthroscopic control and the lateral portal made after needle verification. This approach to assisted entry is particularly useful when both accessory ligaments (ALSDF and ALDDF) are being divided and provides a minimally invasive approach to both ligaments.

At the end of the procedure, skin portals were closed routinely and counterpressure bandages were maintained for 4 weeks post surgery. The authors reported minimal surgical morbidity and good cosmesis (Caldwell et al, 2010). It is considered likely that this technique will gain clinical support and adaptation into equine surgical practice.

Carpal Tunnel Syndrome

The carpal flexor retinaculum can be released using the proximal tenoscopic access portal described earlier with the arthroscope directed distally (Fig. 12-44) (Textor et al, 2003). Identification of the fibers of the carpal flexor retinaculum that form the medial aspect of the carpal tunnel is accomplished using digital pressure followed by insertion of a percutaneous needle to define the distal and proximal extent of the retinaculum. A lateral instrument portal is then made 10 to 15 mm proximal to the accessory carpal bone. This should be defined by prior insertion of a spinal needle to verify sufficient angulation for instrument access to the distal aspect of the retinaculum. If the incision is made immediately adjacent to the accessory carpal bone, it can be difficult to insert instruments obliquely to access the distal portion of the retinaculum. Arthroscopic release of the retinaculum is performed in the visible portion cranial to the SDFT and DDFT. Partial flexion of the carpus is used to allow retraction of the DDFT within the carpal canal and exposure of the visible fibers of the carpal retinaculum. The incision in the retinaculum is made 5 to 10 mm caudal to its confluence with the palmar carpal ligament, which forms the palmar surface of the carpal joints (Fig. 12-45). Transection is confirmed by entry into the tendon sheath of the flexor carpi radialis. This is a major landmark in safely performing carpal retinaculum release. Severing the surpal retinaculum more caudally risks perforation of the radial artery or medial palmar vein. The palmar retinaculum predominantly runs on the deep

surface of the flexor carpi radialis tendon, although there are some portions that are superficial (medial) to this tendon (Textor et al, 2003). The retinaculum is divided with a curved serrated blade or radiofrequency probe, cutting from the distal edge proximally until 1 cm beyond the proximal border of the accessory carpal bone. The carpal sheath is then probed to ensure there are no thickened areas containing residual fibers of the carpal retinaculum, either proximally or distally. The flexor carpi radialis tendon should be visible throughout the entire transected area (Fig. 12-46).

If necessary, the dissection can be continued superficial (medial) to the flexor carpi radialis tendon, by retraction of this tendon cranially and division of the superficial lamina of the flexor retinaculum (see Fig. 12-46). The decision whether to continue the dissection through this thin medial portion of the carpal retinaculum is based on the degree of relief of the carpal canal, which can be assessed by increases in the ease of movement of the arthroscope and in viewable structures within the carpal canal. Severing the medial portion of the retinaculum can be done safely because the radial artery is approximately 7 mm caudal to the flexor carpi radialis tendon. However, the medial palmar vein is only 2 to 4 mm caudal to this site, and careful dissection is necessary to avoid perforating this vessel.

In clinical cases, the carpal sheath and flexor retinaculum have been thickened predominantly on the deep (inner) portion, forming the visible interior layer of the retinaculum overlying the flexor carpi radialis tendon. Division of only this portion of the retinaculum has been adequate to resolve carpal canal symptoms in 2 horses (Textor et al, 2003) and a further 11 horses operated on since then. However, a larger case series has not been published. A modified tenoscopic technique was described in a case report by Byron et al (2010). This utilized the standard proximolateral arthroscope portal (described earlier) with a lateral instrument portal distal to the accessory carpal bone (Cauvin et al, 1997).

Secondary carpal canal syndrome, developing as a result of radial physeal exostoses, myotendinosis or tendonitis of the contained flexor tendons, may also benefit from division of the carpal retinaculum, using the same rationale as described for treating flexor tendonitis within the confines of the palmar annular ligament at the fetlock (Nixon, 1990b). The procedure is simple, has few risks of wound-healing complications, and if necessary can be added to other procedures during the

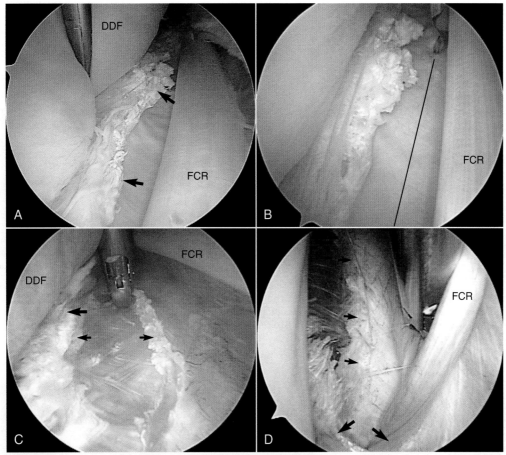

Figure 12-46 Tenoscopic view (proximal to distal, left limb) of division of both the inner and outer layers of the flexor retinaculum. **A,** Division of the heavier inner layer of the retinaculum *(arrowheads)* has exposed the flexor carpi radialis tendon (FCR). **B,** The FCR tendon is retracted cranially, exposing the outer layer of the retinaculum (line indicates division site). **C,** Division of the thin outer layer with biopsy rongeurs, showing retraction of the outer layer edges *(thin arrows)* and the thicker inner layer edge *(arrowhead)*. **D,** Retraction of the FCR tendon and divided inner layer *(arrowheads)* reveals the cut edge of the outer layer *(small arrows)* and the underlying dark dermal tissues. In clinical cases, division of the thin outer layer appears unnecessary.

tenoscopic examination and treatment of disorders of the carpal sheath contents.

Postoperative Care

The use of tenoscopic techniques to evaluate the carpal sheath and address specific pathology has minimized wound healing complications and the need for extended wound support by bandaging. Return to an active walking program is therefore rapid, and the extent of layoff from work is then dictated only by the pathology of the tendons themselves rather than the surgical procedure. Animals are usually given perioperative antimicrobial drugs. Intrathecal NaHA (20 to 40 mg) is commonly used, both at surgery and 2 to 3 weeks later. Follow-up intravenous NaHA may also be useful, commencing 4 to 6 weeks after suture removal. Bandages are used to keep the arthroscope and instrument portals covered for the first 5 to 10 days after surgery. This usually consists of light bandages and adhesive elastic bandage. Additional surgical sponges in the bandage directly over the portals help control leakage. Most horses undergoing tenoscopic procedures of the carpal sheath show little lameness beyond the initial day of surgery. Intrathecal analgesics such as bupivacaine can be used during surgery but generally are unnecessary in the control of postoperative pain. Nonsteroidal antiinflammatory agents are usually given for 2 to 3 days after surgery.

Horses are confined to the stall for the initial 1 to 2 days after surgery, and small periods of hand walking are then instituted. A balance is necessary between an early return to walking exercise and healing of carpal sheath structures. Adhesions associated with surgery in the carpal sheath appear to be rare.

▶ TENOSCOPY OF THE TARSAL SHEATH

The tendon of insertion of the lateral digital flexor (LDFT), which comprises the combined deep and superficial heads of the deep digital flexor, is invested by a synovial sheath as it traverses the tarsus. Although there are other tendon sheaths associated with the tarsus, this is usually referred to as the tarsal sheath. It has been variously described in mature horses as ranging from 16 to 20 cm (Cauvin, 2003; Cauvin et al, 1999) and 21 to 32 cm (Dik & Merkens, 1987; Hago & Vaughan, 1986) long. It commences near the musculotendinous junction of the lateral digital flexor in the distal caudal aspect of the crus. At this level the tarsal sheath forms a large pouch surrounding the LDFT and interposed between this and the common calcaneal tendon. When distended this pouch is largest laterally. At the level of the tarsocrural joint, the two synovial structures are separated only by their synovial and thin fibrous walls (Fig. 12-47). Further distally, the tarsal sheath is separated from the remaining tarsal joints by thick fibrocartilaginous tissue. At the level of the sustentaculum tali, the tarsal sheath is enclosed by a thick transversely orientated ligament, the tarsal flexor retinaculum,

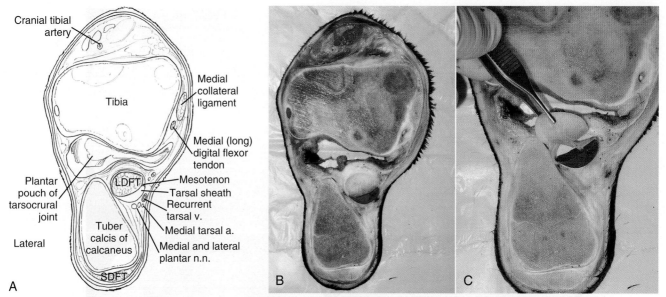

Figure 12-47 Cross-sectional study at the level of the proximal region of the tarsal sheath. **A,** Labeled diagram of **B.** The sheath cavity contains red latex. **C,** Same cross section with lateral digital flexor tendon *(LDFT)* retracted to show medial mesotenon attachment from the LDFT to the tarsal sheath wall.

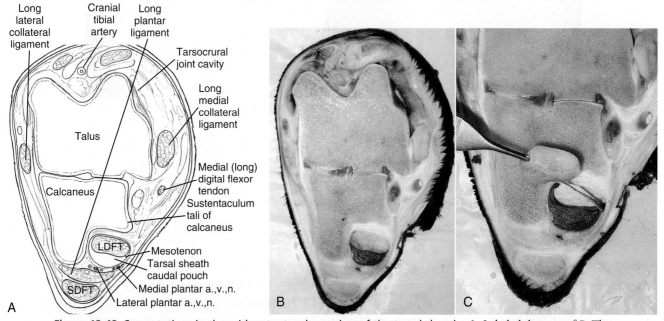

Figure 12-48 Cross sections in the mid sustentacular region of the tarsal sheath. **A,** Labeled diagram of **B.** The sheath cavity contains red latex. **C,** Same cross section with lateral digital flexor tendon *(LDFT)* retracted to show medial mesotenon attachment from the LDFT to the tarsal sheath wall.

in addition to both superficial and deep tarsal fascia (Fig. 12-48). The flexor retinaculum does not enclose the proximal and distal recesses of the sheath, which, therefore, are more voluminous (Cauvin, 2003; Cauvin et al, 1999; Dik & Merkens, 1987). The tarsal sheath terminates distally as a recess dorsomedial to the deep digital flexor tendon in the proximal third of the metatarsus (Fig. 12-49).

There are no major neurovascular structures within the tarsal sheath but several associated with its outer, fibrous layers (see Figs. 12-47 and 12-48). Proximally the medial and lateral plantar nerves, medial tarsal artery, and recurrent tarsal vein are located in the caudomedial fibrous layers (see Fig. 12-47). Further distally, the plantar nerves and vessels run within the tarsal flexor retinaculum in the plantar two thirds of its width.

The sheath is lined by parietal synovial membrane, which is villous in the proximal and distal outpouchings. The membrane reflects caudally/plantarly to wrap around the tendons, leaving a thin but continuous mesotenon along the caudo/plantaromedial aspect of the tendon (Fig. 12-50). There are several small vinculae in the proximal recesses of the sheath. As the LDFT approaches the sustentaculum tali, the tarsal sheath becomes visibly narrowed by the flexor retinaculum forming the tarsal tunnel. The recurrent tarsal vein is in a more medial location (see Fig. 12-47) and is susceptible to injury when making instrument portals into the proximal pouch. More distally, at the level of the sustentaculum tali, the medial and lateral plantar nerves, arteries, and veins are located plantarly, deep in the fibrous layers of the tarsal sheath, but also within the confines of the

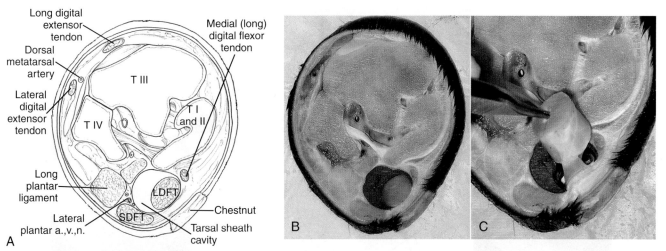

Figure 12-49 Cross sections at the level of the distal row of tarsal bones. **A,** Labeled diagram of **B.** The sheath cavity contains red latex. **C,** Same cross section with lateral digital flexor tendon *(LDFT)* retracted to show the plantaromedial mesotenon attachment from the LDFT to the tarsal sheath wall. *SDFT,* Superficial digital flexor tendon.

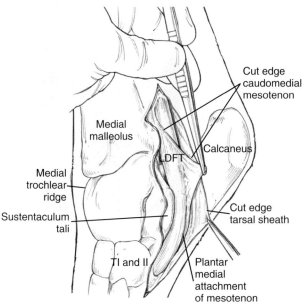

Figure 12-50 Drawing of the medial aspect of the tarsal sheath, showing arthroscopically relevant anatomic structures. The caudomedial mesotenon separates the entire medial approach to the tarsal sheath to cranial/dorsal and caudal/plantar approaches.

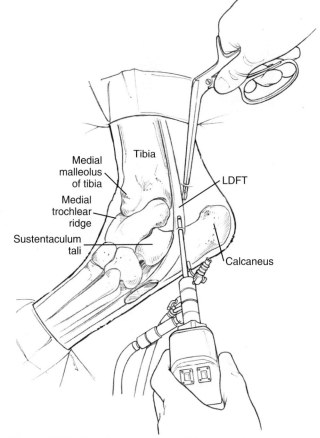

Figure 12-51 Standard centromedial approach to the tarsal sheath, with the arthroscope directed proximally. The entry portal is located 2 cm proximal to the proximal palpable edge of the sustentaculum tali, approximately level with the medial malleolus. *LDFT,* Lateral digital flexor tendon.

tarsal flexor retinaculum (see Fig. 12-48). Distally, the chestnut overlies the tarsal sheath medially and has to be avoided. The lateral plantar neurovascular structures are positioned along the plantarolateral perimeter of the termination of the sheath and are relatively protected (see Fig. 12-49).

The principal indication for tenoscopy of the tarsal sheath is tenosynovitis. This may be associated with tearing of the enclosed LDFT, mesotenon, tenosynovial masses, intrathecal fragmentation of the sustentaculum tali, and contamination or infection. It is also involved in endoscopic evaluation and treatment of proximally located synoviocoeles (Minshall & Wright, 2012).

Technique

Several approaches to the tarsal sheath have been described, but the preferred arthroscopic entry is a central medial portal made 1 to 2 cm proximal to the sustentaculum tali (Fig. 12-51). This permits visualization of both proximal and distal regions of the sheath (Cauvin et al, 1999). A choice of entry either cranial or caudal to the mesotenon of the LDFT is required to gain arthroscope entry to the proximal outpouching. The selection depends on preoperative ultrasound assessment of the primary lesions. Similarly, instrument portals can be made in the proximal outpouching either caudal or cranial to the mesotenon, although cranial is often preferred due to the predominance of masses and adhesions in the cranial region of the proximal

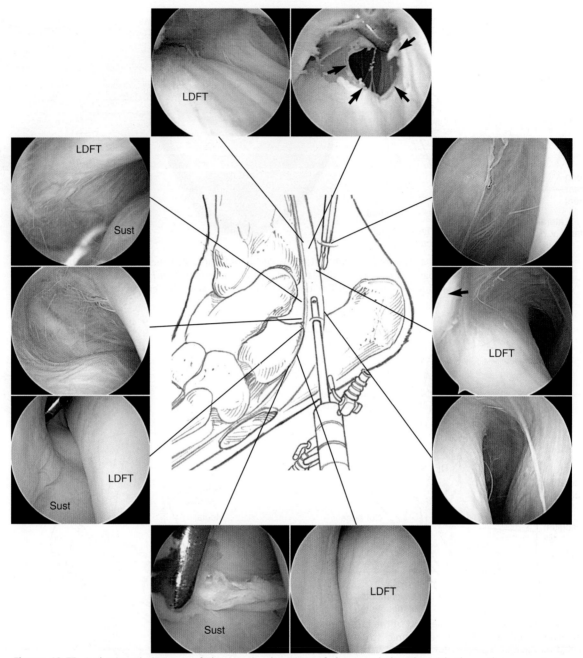

Figure 12-52 Arthroscopic images of the proximal region of the tarsal sheath, with the arthroscope entry cranial/dorsal to the mesotenon. The lateral digital flexor tendon *(LDFT)* is readily visible, with the caudal and caudomedial aspect of the sheath and its contents obstructed by a mesotenon, which can be perforated with an instrument *(arrows)* to allow examination of the caudomedial regions. The alignment of the LDFT over the sustentaculum tali *(Sust)* can be readily seen.

pouch. Examination and debridement of the visible portions of the LDFT and many areas of the sustentaculum tali can be performed using instrument portals directly over or immediately distal to the sustentaculum tali.

The central medial approach can be performed with the horse in dorsal or lateral recumbency with the limb extended. Hemorrhage is reduced by using dorsal recumbency, and a tourniquet is useful when using lateral recumbency because the affected limb is down. The tarsal sheath is distended with saline if it is not already markedly distended. The voluminous outpouching of the proximomedial aspect of the tarsal sheath is readily palpated. A skin incision is made in the distal region of this proximal outpouching, approximately level with the medial malleolus of the tibia. The arthroscope sleeve is inserted in a proximal direction to

commence the examination in the cranial cul-de-sac of the proximal region of the tarsal sheath (see Fig. 12-51). The mesotenon of the LDFT originates from the caudo/plantaromedial border of the tendon and provides a barrier to complete examination of the caudal and medial portions of the tarsal sheath (see Fig. 12-50). However, this layer is relatively thin and can be perforated, in several areas if necessary, allowing the arthroscope to view the caudal portions of the proximal pouch of the tarsal sheath. Instrument portals can be made cranial or caudal to the mesotenon as determined by lesion location.

With the arthroscope directed proximally, the LDFT and proximal reflection of the tarsal sheath are evident (Fig. 12-52). The mesotenon and medial and cranial/dorsal surfaces of the LDFT are readily examined. Redirection of the

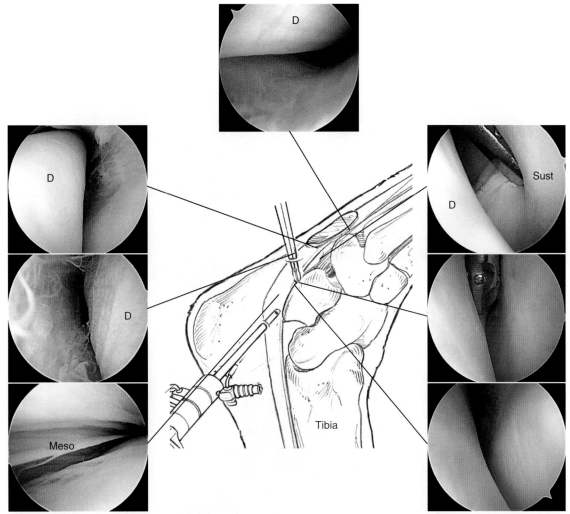

Figure 12-53 Redirection of the arthroscope inserted in the centromedial portal to view the distal region of the tarsal sheath. Composite shows the lateral digital flexor tendon *(LDFT) (D)* coursing over the sustentaculum *(Sust)* and the LDFT in the plantar regions *(left panels).* The mesotenon *(Meso)* is evident, attaching to the medial side of the LDFT. Regions of the dorsal surface of the LDFT and the weight-bearing region of the sustentaculum are evident in the right panels.

arthroscope more distally reveals the LDFT as it curves over the sustentaculum tali (see Fig. 12-52). Limited portions of the fibrocartilage surface of the sustentaculum can also be examined. The LDFT can be retracted after an instrument portal is made, which improves access to the caudolateral surface of the sustentaculum (see Fig. 12-52). The medial extremity of the sustentaculum is extrasynovial and cannot be viewed tenoscopically. This area is also the most frequent site for bony exostosis and fragmentation, which may then have to be removed using an open approach. Preoperative planning using ultrasound or computed tomography may assist in making the determination for tenoscopic or open approaches. Over the sustentaculum the tarsal sheath is confined by the tarsal flexor retinaculum, which stabilizes the LDFT (see Fig. 12-52). Redirection of the arthroscope allows the LDFT to be viewed as it curves distally (Fig. 12-53). When the arthroscope entry has been made cranial to the mesotenon, the sustentaculum and dorsal surface of the LDFT are readily examined. Advancing the arthroscope farther distally allows examination of the remainder of the sustentaculum and the LDFT as it courses toward the distal termination of the sheath. The medial mesotenon is thicker and somewhat compressed within the tarsal canal (see Fig. 12-53), and to facilitate examination of the distal regions of the LDFT and sustentaculum, sequential entry both dorsal and plantar to the mesotenon allows complete assessment of the LDFT surfaces and the weight-bearing surfaces of the sustentaculum.

A distomedial approach to the tarsal sheath is less frequently necessary (Fig. 12-54). The retinaculum of the tarsal sheath is more dense distally, and the chestnut provides a problem for sterile skin preparation. However, examination of this area is occasionally necessary, and a skin incision can be made 1 to 2 cm proximal to the level of the chestnut over the medial aspect of the distended tarsal sheath (see Fig. 12-54). The LDFT can then be seen as it courses over the distal portions of the sustentaculum tali. Surgical procedures in the distal limits of the tarsal sheath are more difficult, due to the small volume of the tarsal sheath at this level and the overlying retinaculum. Additionally, the converging medial digital flexor tendon and check (accessory) ligament immediately distal to the tarsal sheath narrow the sheath as the distal limits are approached.

▶ Tenoscopic Treatment of Conditions in the Tarsal Sheath
Tearing of the Lateral Digital Flexor Tendon
Intrathecal tearing of the LDFT can occur at any level within the tarsal sheath but appears to be most common just proximal and at the level of the sustentaculum tali. In contrast to

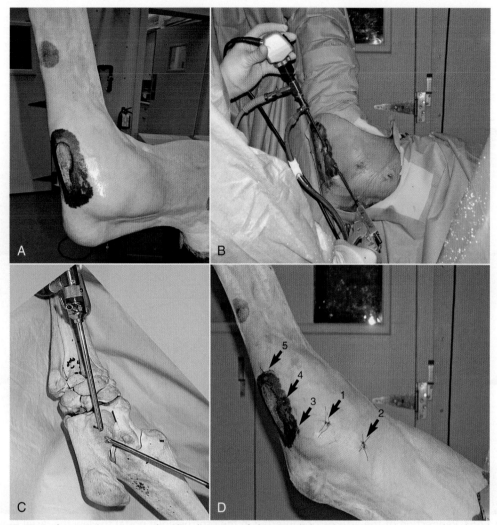

Figure 12-54 Arthroscopic entry to the distal aspect of the tarsal sheath. **A,** Horse positioned in dorsal recumbency for tenoscopy, showing marked effusion, which outlines the extent of the tarsal sheath proximally and distally. **B,** Arthroscope inserted immediately proximal to the chestnut with an instrument portal over the proximal aspect of the sustentaculum tali. Notice the examination using the centromedial arthroscopic portal and proximal instrument portal have been completed (skin incisions remain). **C,** Reference points illustrated on a skeleton. **D,** Sutured portals showing the five portals required for complete assessment and debridement of the lesions in this severe case. The portals are numbered according to sequence utilized, starting proximally and working distally.

tears of the flexor tendons within the digital flexor and carpal sheaths, tears of the LDFT are often long and relatively deep and do not necessarily follow a strict linear alignment (Fig. 12-55). Disruption of the epitenon occasionally spirals along the length of the tear. The appearance of torn and extruded tissue is similar to that seen elsewhere and is managed with the same principles and techniques (see Fig. 12-55). To date, no series have been published to document in detail the findings and results.

Tenosynovial Masses and Adhesion Resection

Ultrasonographic evaluation of cases with chronic tarsal sheath distension frequently reveals tenosynovial masses within the sheath (Fig. 12-56). Further inflammation and advancing fibrosis of the tarsal sheath are believed to restrict the free range of motion of the LDFT within the tarsal sheath. Mineralization is a late complication of chronic disease and can involve portions of the mesotenon, as well as the surface layers of the LDFT. Removal of most tenosynovial masses can be accomplished using the central medial approach to the tarsal sheath (see Fig. 12-56). After a thorough examination, an 18-gauge

7.5-cm spinal needle is used to define the most appropriate portal for mass removal. The neurovascular structures caudal/plantar to the tarsal sheath can be avoided by penetration with arthroscope and instruments immediately adjacent to the cranial-caudal midline, allowing entry either side of the mesotenon. This provides access for mass removal and debridement of the medial surfaces of the LDFT (see Fig. 12-56). Masses can involve the inner layers of the tarsal sheath (see Fig. 12-56B) or become more pendulous and float between the LDFT and the tarsal sheath lining (Fig. 12-56E). With chronic disease, the tarsal sheath can become quite thick, and examination of the sheath contents can be slow and tedious. High ingress fluid pressure frequently results in subcutaneous fluid accumulation, making the surgical exploration more difficult. A gradual increase in the areas available for examination can be accomplished using motorized resection of proliferative synovium. Masses can be removed with scissors and rongeurs, biopsy punch rongeurs, motorized resection (Fig. 12-56), or radiofrequency probes, depending on the density of the masses. Large masses and mineralized areas may need a second instrument portal to allow the mass to be stabilized before transection at

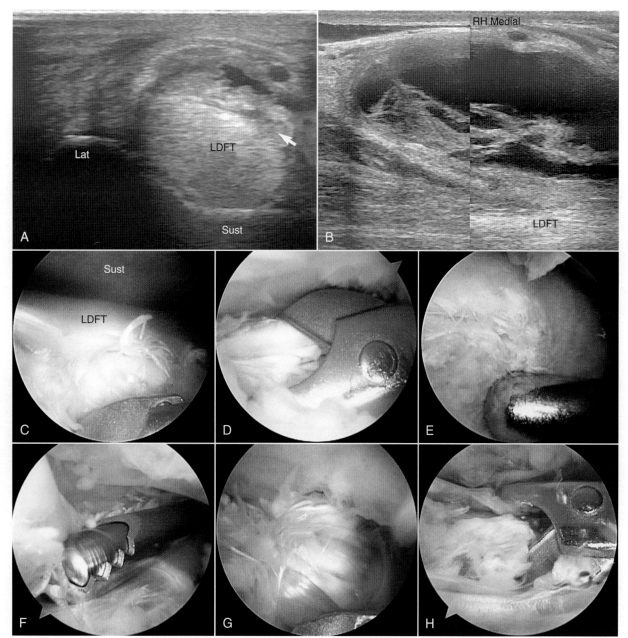

Figure 12-55 Lateral digital flexor tendon *(LDFT)* tear with chronic tarsal sheath tenosynovitis. **A,** Transverse ultrasonographic image at the level of the sustentaculum tali *(Sust)* and shows a surface tear *(arrow)* with chronic granuloma formation on medial aspect of LDFT, and tenosynovial proliferation. **B,** Longitudinal ultrasonographic view shows marked tenosynovial mass formation and fluid distension. **C,** Assessment of LDFT split. **D,** Trimming edge of LDFT split with biopsy rongeurs. **E,** Final debridement with synovial resector. **F,** Continuing tear distal to the sustentaculum. **G** and **H,** Trimming the tear and granuloma on LDFT distal to sustentaculum tali.

its base. Mineralized masses generally result from dystrophic mineralization of chronic lesions and are more common in the tarsal sheath than the equivalent syndromes in the carpal sheath. Their location can be determined by presurgical ultrasonographic examination. Motorized resection of masses and surface proliferation of the LDFT can be associated with hemorrhage. Tourniquet application proximal to the tarsal sheath may be helpful, but most hemorrhage is controlled by the pressure of the ingress fluid and addition of epinephrine. Distension with gas is an alternative if bleeding continues to hamper the diagnostic examination and further mass removal.

Masses and mineralization can extend down to the terminal portions of the tarsal sheath, and a second arthroscope and/or instrument entry in the distal medial recess of the

sheath may be required. After removal of masses, the sheath is flushed before routine skin closure. Intrathecal administration of NaHA and tPA may be helpful in reducing reformation of tendon sheath adhesions.

Debridement of the Sustentaculum Tali

The sustentaculum tali is prone to trauma over its plantaromedial aspect, resulting in bone proliferation within or adjacent to the insertion of the retinaculum on the calcaneus. Some wounds also cause contamination or infection of the tarsal sheath. The most medial areas of bone proliferation are beyond the medial extremity of the tarsal sheath. Resection of accessible proliferative bone and debridement of the LDFT-bearing surfaces of the sustentaculum can be accomplished using the central medial arthroscope

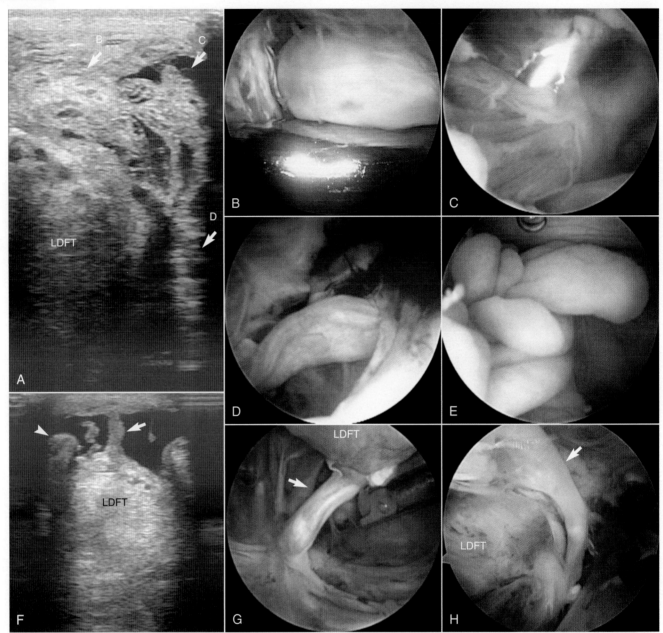

Figure 12-56 Tenosynovial masses and adhesions in tarsal sheath. **A,** Ultrasonographic transverse image showing lateral digital flexor tendon *(LDFT)* covered in soft tissue proliferation. The mesotenon is contained within the proliferation. *Arrows* with letters *B, C,* and *D* correspond to subsequent tenoscopic images of various masses and adhesion shown in panels (**B** to **E**). **F,** Ultrasound image obtained distal to chestnut showing intact LDFT and more filamentous adhesions *(arrows)* seen in tenoscopic panels **G** and **H**.

entry, with instrument portals made directly over the sustentaculum. Alternatively, and sometimes additionally, the distomedial portal (see Fig. 12-54), is required for arthroscope entry, to allow complete examination of the medial edges of the sustentaculum and the lateral perimeter of the tarsal tunnel as it curves proximally. Fragmented or infected foci in the sustentaculum can be removed or debrided, using hand instruments. Further details concerning the principles of treating contaminated or infected lesions are provided in Chapter 14.

Synoviocoeles Associated with the Tarsal Sheath

Tearing of the tarsal sheath wall can result in the formation of synoviocoeles (Minshall & Wright, 2012). These occur on the caudodistal crus between the tibia and tendons of insertion of gastrocnemius and SDFT proximally and the calcaneus distally, and they may be asymmetric (Fig. 12-57). The swellings contain fluid with varying quantities of irregular echogenic material, and communication with the tarsal sheath may be recognized ultrasonographically (Fig. 12-58). Synoviocentesis usually reveals viscid xanthochromic synovial fluid.

Endoscopy has revealed a smooth avillous synovial lining and communication between the cavity and the cranially situated tarsal sheath. The defects in the tarsal sheath wall have been consistently located caudally, close to the proximal reflection of the tarsal sheath onto the LDFT (Minshall & Wright, 2012). The defects were transverse (mediolateral) or "D" shaped usually revealing the enclosed LDFT (Fig. 12-59). The arthroscope can be passed through the defect and into the tarsal sheath and advanced as far distally as the sustentaculum tali. No other defects have been identified

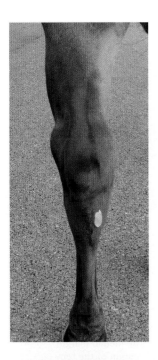

Figure 12-57 Clinical appearance of a synoviocoele associated with the proximal tarsal sheath.

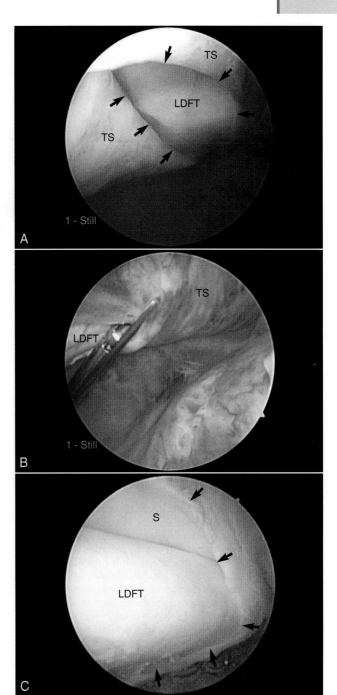

Figure 12-59 Endoscopic images of a synoviocoele (proximal to left). **A,** D-shaped defect in the tarsal sheath wall (→). **B,** Distal elongation of the defect by division of the sheath wall with arthroscopic scissors introduced through a contralateral portal. *LDFT*, Lateral digital flexor tendon; *TS*, tarsal sheath wall. **C,** Endoscopic appearance at completion of surgery. The lateral digital flexor tendon sheath wall has been divided to the distal margin of the synoviocoele (→) exposing a length of tendon (LDFT) and tarsal sheath synovium *(S)*. *(From Minshall, GJ., Wright IM. Synoviocoeles associated with the tarsal sheath: Description of the lesion and treatment in 15 horses Equine Vet J. 44:71-75, 2012, with permission.)*

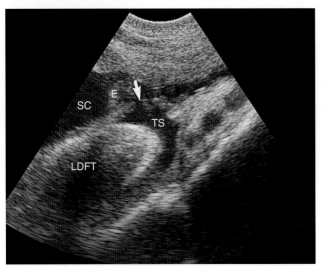

Figure 12-58 Transverse ultrasonographic image obtained using a curved array probe and medial approach with the limb semiflexed, caudal to the left. *E*, Echogenic material; *LDFT*, lateral digital flexor tendon; *SC*, synoviocoele; *TS*, tarsal sheath; →, defect in sheath wall. *(From Minshall, GJ., Wright IM. Synoviocoeles associated with the tarsal sheath: Description of the lesion and treatment in 15 horses Equine Vet J. 44, 71-75, 2012, with permission.)*

within affected tarsal sheaths. Treatment consists of removal of fibrinoid deposits within the synoviocoele, using ipsilateral and/or contralateral instrument portals, for arthroscopic rongeurs. Minshall & Wright (2012) reasoned that the defect in the sheath wall may create a valve effect. To prevent this, the communication between the cavity and the sheath wall is enlarged by distal division using arthroscopic scissors to the level of the proximal margin of the sustentaculum tali (see Fig. 12-59). The free edges produced are then resected further with a motorized synovial resector in an oscillating mode with suction applied to draw tissue into the blade. At the end of the procedure the whole caudal/plantar margin of the LDFT is visible from the level of the sustentaculum tali to the proximal limit of the original defect (see Fig. 12-59). After lavage

and evacuation of the cavity, skin portals are closed routinely and a counterpressure bandage is applied. Varying periods of box rest are followed by an ascending exercise program. Of 15 horses reported, 10 returned to work with little or no visible swelling, 1 was able to work at a lower level, and 2 had recurrence of swelling on return to work. In one animal, swelling

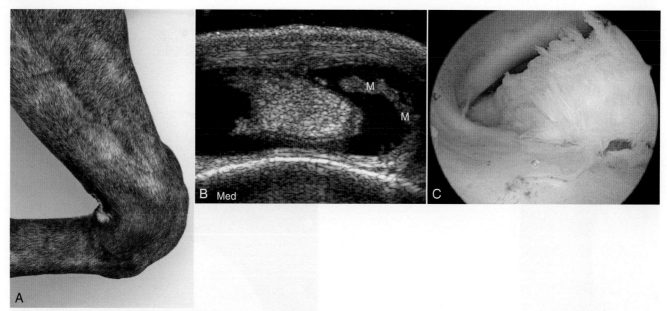

Figure 12-60 Tenosynovitis of the carpal sheath of extensor carpi radialis. **A,** Clinical appearance. **B,** Transverse ultrasonograph demonstrating distension, suspended irregular echogenic material and disruption of the medial margin of the tendon. The mesotenon *(M)* is markedly thickened. **C,** Tenoscopic appearance of the medial margin of the tendon demonstrating an irregular longitudinal tear with extrusion of torn fibers.

returned within 1 week of surgery and then increased in size; this horse later underwent an open ablation procedure.

Postoperative Care

Wound healing complications associated with tenoscopic evaluation of the tarsal sheath are generally minimal, and exercise can usually be initiated once skin sutures are removed. Horses respond to tenoscopic surgery of the tarsal sheath differently, and some can be quite lame postoperatively. This can be controlled at the time of surgery by intrathecal deposition of bupivacaine at the time of closure, while postoperative pain relief is provided with nonsteroidal antiinflammatory agents. Horses with disease processes involving the sustentaculum tali frequently also have damage to the dorsal surface of the LDFT and are more lame than horses with primary tenosynovitis. In such cases, follow-up medication to the tarsal sheath is more likely to be necessary and includes intrathecal NaHA and follow-up intravenous NaHA. Postoperative intrathecal tPA (500 µg) has been used routinely on days 2, 3, and 4 by one of the authors (A.J.N.). Adhesion formation or reformation is frequent in the tarsal sheath, and aggressive medication, bandaging, and early exercise are vital. Repeat ultrasonographic examination is also useful in these cases to assess return of tenosynovial masses and to evaluate tendon healing.

TENOSCOPY OF THE CARPAL EXTENSOR TENDON SHEATHS

The extensor tendon sheaths are prone to injury due to their location on the dorsal aspect of the limb (Mason, 1977; Platt & Wright, 1997). Blunt trauma can result in variable degrees of tendonitis and chronic effusion of the sheath (Fig. 12-60A). A small number of these cases do not spontaneously resolve but progress to develop intrathecal adhesions and soft tissue masses. This can involve the sheath of the extensor carpi radialis, the common digital extensor (CDE), or rarely the lateral digital extensor or extensor carpi obliquus. Lameness is variable, but restricted carpal flexion is common. Ultrasonographic evaluation commonly reveals areas of fibrinous and fibrous tissue deposition, considerable amounts of free fluid, and quite often relatively normal tendon fiber architecture. In some cases tenoscopy is undertaken to improve the cosmetic appearance of the limb. The presence of infection usually results in more severe lameness. Hunters are predisposed to thorn penetration of the forelimb extensor sheaths, which can lead to obvious lameness and the need for more aggressive surgical and medical therapy (Platt & Wright, 1997). The carpal sheaths of extensor carpi radialis (ECR) and CDE are both amenable to tenoscopic evaluation and treatment. The most frequent indications are persisting tenosynovitis after trauma to the sheath, tearing of the associated contained tendon, and tendon sheath infection.

Horses are operated in dorsal recumbency with the limb(s) extended (Fig. 12-61). The arthroscope portal to the affected extensor sheath is generally made toward the proximal or distal extremity of the sheath, depending on ultrasonographic evidence of the more severely affected region, which is reserved for the instrument portal. This provides good evaluation of the length of each sheath, although circumferential passage of the arthroscope is limited by substantial mesotenons in both. The mesotenon of the ECR is situated on the dorsolateral surface. Commonly, there are two separate tendons within the carpal sheath of CDE representing the insertions of the large humeral and smaller radial heads. Each has a mesotenon attached to its dorsomedial surface. Instrument portals are made as needed to allow rongeur and motorized resector access for soft tissue debridement. The aims of debridement include removal of proliferative masses and reestablishment of free motion of the affected tendon. Synovectomy should be used judiciously in an attempt to reduce fluid accumulation in the sheath.

Marginal tears and partial ruptures, including granuloma formation, have been identified and treated in a similar manner to those affecting the flexor tendons in the carpal and digital flexor tendon sheaths (see Fig. 12-60). These cases have presented with lameness, distended sheaths, reduced flexion, and ultrasonographic evidence of tendon disruption. Infected

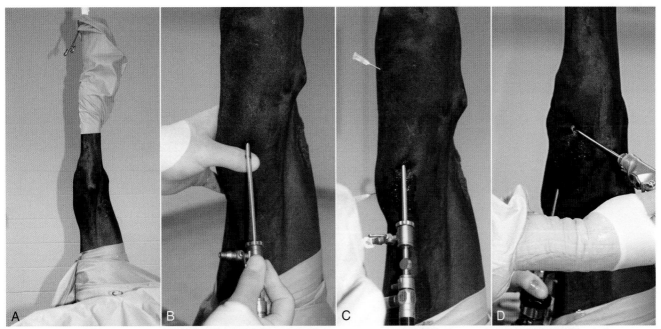

Figure 12-61 Tenoscopy of the extensor carpi radialis sheath. A, Horse in dorsal recumbency with limb extended. **B,** Insertion of the arthroscopic cannula proximomedially. **C,** Evaluation of the sheath with needles placed at potential instrument portal sites. **D,** Insertion of a motorized synovial resector into a distal medial portal.

extensor sheaths are treated by debridement, lavage and instillation of antibiotic delivery drains, or depot forms of antibiotic-laden cements. The dorsal mesotenon generally dictates the need for instrument entry on both lateral and medial sides of the ECR tendon to allow complete debridement and flushing of the sheath. Up to four entry points can be required to allow lateral and medial arthroscope and instrument access for complete evaluation and debridement.

Results of open treatment of chronic extensor sheath tenosynovitis are fair to good in the limited series of cases in the literature (Mason, 1977; Platt & Wright, 1997). In the authors' experience, tenoscopic treatment of the sheaths of the ECR and CDE, has allowed more focused debridement with good resolution of lameness. Cosmetic appearance after debridement of most distended extensor sheaths can be substantially improved, although some residual fibrosis can persist.

TENOSCOPY OF THE TARSAL EXTENSOR SHEATHS

The tarsal sheaths of the long digital extensor (LDE) and tibialis cranialis (TC) are both amenable to tenoscopic evaluation. Dorsal recumbency is recommended with the limb positioned in extension. Unless distended (Fig. 12-62), the sheaths are ill defined. The LDE sheath is most superficial, although it is covered by thick dorsal tarsal fascia and three dorsal annular ligaments. Unless markedly distended, entry is facilitated by further distension, which generally is most readily achieved between the middle and distal annular ligaments. Arthroscopic portals may be made medially and/or laterally, avoiding the annular ligaments. Complete evaluation requires both approaches because circumferential evaluation is prohibited by a plantar mesotenon. Cases of traumatic tenosynovitis of the LDE sheath have been treated by debridement (Fig. 12-63). Longitudinal tears of the LDE and tears of the tendon sheath

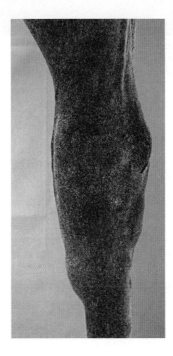

Figure 12-62 Distension of the tarsal sheaths of the long and lateral digital extensor tendons.

wall, including traumatic confluence with the lateral digital extensor tendon sheath, have also been identified and treated tenoscopically.

The tendon of insertion of tibialis cranialis lies plantar to the LDE and peroneus tertius within the extensor bundle. It has a short tendon sheath that extends from the musculotendinous junction. There is a plantar mesotenon and, in some animals, confluence with the cunean bursa has been identified.

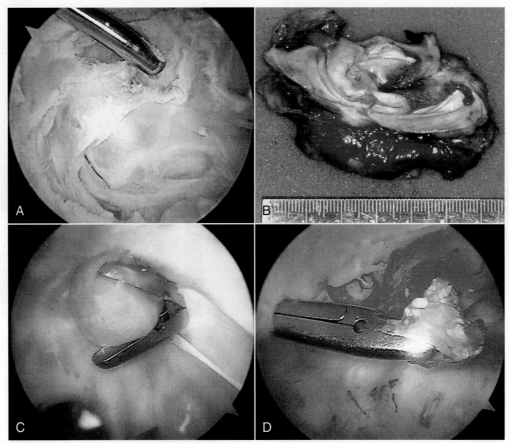

Figure 12-63 Tenoscopic removal of tenosynovial masses within the long digital extensor sheath. **A,** Removal of a mass from the long digital extensor sheath. **B,** The large mass after removal. **C,** Removal of a smaller mass. **D,** Free fragments of fibrin and tenosynovial mass being removed.

REFERENCES

Adams OR: Constriction of the palmar (volar) or plantar annular ligament of the fetlock in the horse, *Vet Med/Small An Clin* 69: 327–329, 1974.

Amiel D, Ishizue K, Billings E, et al.: Hyaluronan in flexor tendon repair, *J Hand Surg* 14A:837–843, 1989.

Arensberg L, Wilderjans H, Simon O, Dewulf J, Boussauw B: Nonseptic tenosynovitis of the digital flexor tendon sheath caused by longitudinal tears in the digital flexor tendons: A retrospective study of 135 tenoscopic procedures, *Equine Vet J* 43:660–668, 2011.

Barr ARS, Dyson SJ, Barr FJ, O'Brien JK: Tendonitis of the deep digital flexor tendon in the distal metacarpal/metatarsal region associated with tenosynovitis of the digital sheath in the horse, *Equine Vet J* 27:348–355, 1995.

Bramlage LR, Hogan PM: Career results of 137 Thoroughbred racehorses that have undergone superior check ligament desmotomy for treatment of tendinitis, *Proc Am Assoc Equine Pract* 42:162–163, 1996.

Byron CR, Benson BM, Karlin WM, Stewart AA: Modified tenoscopic method for carpal flexor retinaculum release in a horse, *Vet Surg* 39:239–243, 2010.

Caldwell FJ, Waguespack RW: Evaluation of a tenoscopic approach for desmotomy of the accessory ligament of the deep digital flexor tendon in horses, *Vet Surg* 40:266–271, 2011.

Cauvin ER: Tarsal sheath. In Ross MW, Dyson SJ, editors: *Diagnosis and Management of Lameness in the Horse*, Philadelphia, 2003, WB Saunders, pp 687–692.

Cauvin ER, Tapprest J, Munroe GA, May SA, Schramme MC: Endoscopic examination of the tarsal sheath of the lateral digital flexor tendon in horses, *Equine Vet J* 31:219–227, 1999.

Cauvin ERJ, Munroe GA, Boyd JS: Endoscopic examination of the carpal flexor tendon sheath in horses, *Equine Vet J* 29:459–466, 1997.

Chow JC: Endoscopic release of the carpal ligament for carpal tunnel syndrome: Long-term results using the Chow technique, *Arthroscopy* 15:417–421, 1999.

Chow JCY: Endoscopic release of the carpal ligament: A new technique for carpal tunnel syndrome, *Arthroscopy* 5:19–24, 1989.

David F, Laverty S, Marcoux M, Szoke M, Celeste C: Electrosurgical tenoscopic desmotomy of the accessory ligament of the superficial digital flexor muscle (proximal check ligament) in horses, *Vet Surg* 40:46–53, 2011.

Dik KJ: Radiographic and ultrasonographic imaging of soft tissue disorders of the equine carpus, *Tijdschr Diergeneeskd* 115:1168–1174, 1990.

Dik KJ, Dyson SJ, Vail TB: Aseptic tenosynovitis of the digital flexor tendon sheath, fetlock and pastern annular ligament constriction, *Vet Clin North Am Equine Pract* 11:151–162, 1995.

Dik KJ, Merkens HW: Unilateral distension of the tarsal sheath in the horse: A report of 11 cases, *Equine Vet J* 19:307–313, 1987.

Dik KJ, Van Den Belt AJM, Keg PR: Ultrasonographic evaluation of fetlock annular ligament constriction in the horse, *Equine Vet J* 23:285–288, 1991.

Dyson SJ, Dik KJ: Miscellaneous conditions of tendons, tendon sheaths and ligaments, *Vet Clin N Am: Equine Pract* 11:315–337, 1995.

Edinger J, Möbius G, Ferguson J: Comparison of tensoscopic and ultrasonographic methods of examination of the digital flexor tendon sheath in horses, *Vet Comp Orthop Traumatol* 4:209–214, 2005.

Edwards GB: Changes in the sustentaculum tali associated with distension of the tarsal sheath (thoroughpin), *Equine Vet J* 10:97–102, 1978.

Fortier LA: Indications and techniques for tenoscopic surgery of the digital flexor tendon sheath, *Equine Vet Educ* 17:218–224, 2005.

Fortier LA, Nixon AJ, Ducharme NG, Mohammed HO, Yeager A: Tenoscopic examination and proximal annular ligament desmotomy for treatment of equine "complex" digital sheath tenosynovitis, *Vet Surg* 28:429–435, 1999.

Fraser BSL, Bladon BM: Tenoscopic surgery for treatment of lacerations of the digital flexor tendon sheath, *Equine Vet J* 36:528–531, 2004.

Frees KE, Lillich JD, Gaughan EM, DeBowes RM: Tenoscopic-assisted treatment of open digital flexor tendon sheath injuries in horses: 20 cases (1992–2001), *J Am Vet Med Assoc* 220:1823–1827, 2002.

Fulton IIC, MacLean AAA, O'Reilly JJL, et al.: Superior check ligament desmotomy for treatment of superficial digital flexor tendonitis in Thoroughbred and Standardbred horses, *Aust Vet J* 71:233–235, 1994.

Gaughan EM, Nixon AJ, Krook LP, et al.: Effects of sodium hyaluronate on tendon healing and adhesion formation in horses, *Am J Vet Res* 52:764–773, 1991.

Gerring EL, Webbon PM: Fetlock annular ligament desmotomy: A report of 24 cases, *Equine Vet J* 16:113–116, 1984.

Hago BED, Vaughan LC: Radiographic anatomy of tendon sheaths and bursae in the horse, *Equine Vet J* 18:102–106, 1986.

Hago BED, Plummer JM, Vaughan LC: Equine synovial tendon sheaths and bursae: An histological and scanning electron microscopical study, *Equine Vet J* 22:264–272, 1999.

Hawkins JF, Moulton JS: Arthroscope-assisted annular desmotomy in horses, *Equine Vet Educ* 14:252–255, 2002.

Hawkins JF, Ross MW: Transection of the accessory ligament of the superficial digital flexor muscle for the treatment of superficial digital flexor tendinitis in Standardbreds: 40 cases (1988–1992), *J Am Vet Med Assoc* 206:674–678, 1995.

Held JP, Patton CS, Shires M: Solitary osteochondroma of the radius in three horses, *J Am Vet Med Assoc* 193:563–564, 1988.

Hogan PPM, Bramlage LLR: Transection of the accessory ligament of the superficial digital flexor tendon for treatment of tendinitis: Long term results in 61 Standardbred racehorses (1985–1992), *Equine Vet J* 27:221–226, 1995.

Judy CE: *Personal communication.*

Kretzschmar BH, Desjardins MR: Clinical evaluation of 49 tenoscopically assisted superior check ligament desmotomies in 27 horses, *Proc 47th Ann Conv Am Assoc Equine Pract* 47:484–487, 2001.

Leach D, Harland R, Burko B: The anatomy of the carpal sheath of the horse, *J Anat* 133:301–307, 1981.

Lee HA, Garnt BD, Gallina AM: Solitary osteochondroma in a horse: A case report, *J Equine Med Surg* 3:113–115, 1979.

Lundvall RL, Jackson LL: Periosteal new bone formation of the radius as a cause of lameness in two horses, *J Am Vet Med Assoc* 168:612–613, 1976.

MacDonald MH, Honnas CM, Meagher DM: Osteomyelitis of the calcaneus in horses: 28 cases, *J Am Vet Med Assoc* 194:1317–1323, 1989.

McCoy AM, Goodrich LR: Use of a radiofrequency probe for tenoscopic-guided annular ligament desmotomy, *Equine Vet J* 44:412–415, 2012.

McGhee JD, White NA, Goodrich LR: Primary desmitis of the palmar and plantar annular ligaments in horses: 25 cases (1990–2003), *J Am Vet Med Assoc* 226:83–86, 2005.

McIlwraith CW: Osteochondromas and physeal remnant spikes in the carpal canal, *Proc 12th Ann ACVS Symposium* 12:168–169, 2002a.

McIlwraith CW: Tenosynovitis; diseases of joints, tendons, ligaments and related structures. In Stashak TS, editor: *Adams' lameness in horses*, Philadelphia, 2002b, Lippincott, Williams & Wilkins, pp 630–633.

Malark JA, Nixon AJ, Skinner KL, Mohammed H: Characteristics of digital flexor tendon sheath fluid from clinically normal horses, *Am J Vet Res* 53:1292–1294, 1991.

Mason TA: Chronic tenosynovitis of the extensor tendons and tendon sheaths of the carpal region in the horse, *Equine Vet J* 9:186–188, 1977.

Minshall GJ, Wright IM: Synoviocoeles associated with the tarsal sheath: Description of the lesion and treatment in 15 horses, *Equine Vet J* 44:71–75, 2012.

Minshall GJ, Wright IM: Tenosynovitis of the carpal sheath of the digital flexor tendons associated with tears of the radial head of the deep digital flexor: Observations in 11 horses, *Equine Vet J* 44:76–80, 2012.

Moro-oka T, Miura H, Mawatari T, et al.: Mixture of hyaluronic acid and phospholipid prevents adhesion formation on the injured flexor tendon in rabbits, *J Orthop Res* 18:835–840, 2000.

Nixon AJ: Superficial flexor tendinitis. In White NA, Moore JN, editors: *Current practice of equine surgery*, Philadelphia, 1990a, JB Lippincott, pp 441–448.

Nixon AJ: Annular ligament constriction. In White NA, Moore JN, editors: *Current practice of equine surgery*, Philadelphia, 1990b, JB Lippincott, pp 435–440.

Nixon AJ: Endoscopy of the digital flexor tendon sheath in horses, *Vet Surg* 19:266–271, 1990c.

Nixon AJ: Arthroscopic surgery of the carpal and digital tendon sheaths, *Clin Techn Equine Pract* 1:245–256, 2002a.

Nixon AJ: Medical and surgical therapy for tendinitis, *Proc ACVS Symposium* 12:161–164, 2002b.

Nixon AJ, Sams AE, Ducharme NG: Endoscopically assisted annular ligament release in horses, *Vet Surg* 22:501–507, 1993.

Nixon AJ, Schachter BL, Pool RR: Exostoses of the caudal perimeter of the radial physis as a cause of carpal synovial sheath tenosynovitis and lameness in horses: 10 cases (1999–2003), *J Am Vet Med Assoc* 224:264–270, 2004.

Owen KR, Dyson SJ, Parkin TDH, Singer ER, Krisoffersen M, Mair TS: Retrospective study of palmar/plantar annular ligament injury in 71 horses: 2001-2006, *Equine Vet J* 40:237–244, 2008.

Platt D, Wright IM: Chronic tenosynovitis of the carpal extensor tendon sheaths in 15 horses, *Equine Vet J* 29:11–16, 1997.

Ragland III WL: Localized nodular tenosynovitis in the horse, *Pathol Vet* 5:436–441, 1968.

Redding WR: Ultrasonographic imaging of the structures of the digital flexor tendon sheath, *Comp Cont Educ* 13:1824–1832, 1991.

Redding WR: Evaluation of the equine digital flexor tendon sheath using diagnostic ultrasound and contrast radiography, *Vet Radiol Ultrasound* 34:42–48, 1993.

Reef VB: Artifacts. In Reef VB, editor: *Equine diagnostic ultrasound*, Philadelphia, 1998, WB Saunders, pp 24–38.

Santschi EM, Adams SB, Fessler JF, Widmer WR: Treatment of bacterial tarsal tenosynovitis and osteitis of the sustentaculum tali of the calcaneous in five horses, *Equine Vet J* 29:244–247, 1997.

Sisson S: Equine mycology. In Getty RG, editor: *The Anatomy of the Domestic Animals* 5th edn, Philadelphia, 1975, WB Saunders, pp 376–453.

Smith MRW, Wright IM, Minshall GJ, Dudhia J, Verheyen K, Heinegard D, Smith RKW: Increased cartilage oligomeric matrix protein concentrations in equine digital flexor tendon sheath synovial fluid predicts intrathecal tendon damage, *Vet Surg* 40:54–58, 2011.

Smith MRW, Wright IM: Non-infected tenosynovitis of the digital flexor tendon sheath: A retrospective analysis of 76 cases, *Equine Vet J* 38:134–141, 2006.

Southwood LL, Stashak TS, Fehn JE, Ray C: Lateral approach for endoscopic removal of solitary osteochondromas from the distal radial metaphysis in three horses, *J Am Vet Med Assoc* 210:1166–1168, 1997.

Southwood LL, Stashak TS, Kainer RA: Tenoscopic anatomy of the equine carpal flexor synovial sheath, *Vet Surg* 27:150–157, 1998.

Southwood LL, Stashak TS, Kainer RA, Wrigley RH: Desmotomy of the accessory ligament of the superficial digital flexor tendon in the horse with use of a tenoscopic approach to the carpal sheath, *Vet Surg* 28:99–105, 1999.

Squire KRE, Adams SB, Widmer WR, Coatney RW, Habig C: Arthroscopic removal of a palmar radial osteochondroma causing carpal canal syndrome in a horse, *J Am Vet Med Assoc* 201:1216–1218, 1992.

Stahre KRE, Tufvesson G: Volar, supracarpal exostoses as causes of lameness in the horse, *Nord Vet Med* 19:356–361, 1967.

Stanek C, Edinger H: Rontgendiagnostick bei der striktur des fesselringbandes bzw. durch das fesselringband beim pferd, *Pferdeheilkunde* 6:125–128, 1990.

Stashak TS: The forearm (antebrachium). In Stashak TS, editor: *Adams' lameness in horses* 5th edn, Philadelphia, 2002, Lippincott, Williams & Wilkins, pp 864–879.

ter Braake F, Rijkenhuizen ABM: Endoscopic removal of osteochondroma at the caudodistal aspect of the radius: An evaluation in 4 cases, *Equine Vet Educ* 13:90–93, 2001.

Textor JA, Nixon AJ, Fortier LA: Tenoscopic release of the equine carpal canal, *Vet Surg* 32:278–284, 2003.

Thompson K: Tumors and tumor-like lesions of bones. In Maxie MG, editor: *Jubb, Kennedy and Palmer's pathology of domestic animals*, 5th edn, Edinburgh, 2007, Elsevier, pp 110–130.

Thompson KG, Pool RR: Tumors of bones. In Meuten DJ, editor: *Tumors in domestic animals*, 4th edn, Ames, 2002, Iowa State Press, pp 245–317.

Van Pelt RW: Inflammation of the tarsal synovial sheath (Thoroughpin) in horses, *J Am Vet Med Assoc* 155:1481–1488, 1969.

Van Pelt RW, Riley Jr WF, Tillotson PJ: Tenosynovitis of the deep digital flexor tendon in horses, *Can Vet J* 10:235–243, 1969.

Verschooten F, Picavet TM: Desmitis of the fetlock annular ligament in the horse, *Equine Vet J* 18:138–142, 1986.

Verschooten F, Picavet TM: Desmitis of the fetlock annular ligament in the horse, *Vet Ann* 28:98–101, 1988.

Watrous BJ, Dutra FR, Wagner PC, Schmotzer WB: Villonodular synovitis of the palmar and plantar digital flexor tendon sheaths and the calcaneal bursa of the gastrocnemius tendon in the horse, *Proc AAEP* 33:413–428, 1987.

Weiss C, Levy HJ, Denlinger J, Suros JM, Weiss HE: The role of Nahylan in reducing postsurgical tendon adhesions, *Bull Hosp Joint Dis Orthop Instit* 46:9–15, 1986.

Welch RD, Auer JA, Watkins JP, Baird AN: Surgical treatment of tarsal sheath effusion associated with an exostosis on the calcaneus of a horse, *J Am Vet Med Assoc* 196:1992–1994, 1990.

Wereszka MM, White II NA, Furr MO: Factors associated with outcome following treatment of horses with septic tenosynovitis: 51 cases (1986-2003), *J Am Vet Med Assoc* 230:1195–1200, 2007.

Wilderjans H, Boussauw B, Madder K, Simon O: Tenosynovitis of the digital flexor tendon sheath and annular ligament constriction syndrome caused by longitudinal tears in the deep digital flexor tendon: A clinical and surgical report of 17 cases in Warmblood horses, *Equine Vet J* 35:270–275, 2003.

Wright IM, McMahon PJ: Tenosynovitis associated with longitudinal tears of the digital flexor tendons in horses: A report of 20 cases, *Equine Vet J* 31:12–18, 1999.

Wright IM, Minshall GJ: Clinical, radiological and ultrasonographic features, treatment and outcome in 22 horses with caudal digital radial osteochondromata, *Equine Vet J* 44:319–324, 2012.

CHAPTER 13

Bursoscopy

Synovial bursae are closed sacs, found interposed between moving parts or at points of unusual pressure. They may be congenital or acquired. Congenital bursae are located in constant positions. They may be subfascial, subligamentous, submuscular, or subtendinous. The latter are most common and are found between tendons and bones at points where the tendon direction changes. The bursal side of the tendon and bone are fibrocartilaginous, and in most circumstances the bursal margins are lined with villous synovium. In a classical work, translated by Ottaway & Worden (1940), Müller (1936) described 22 congenital subtendinous bursae in the horse. The principal congenital bursae of clinical importance (from an endoscopic perspective) are the calcaneal bursa, the intertubercular (bicipital) bursa, and the podotrochlear (navicular) bursa.

Acquired, also called reactive, functional, or pathologic bursae, are formed after birth. They are most common over osseous prominences and may be subcutaneous. They are considered to have a traumatic etiology and to follow synovial metaplasia within encapsulated seromas or hematomas. The most frequent sites of acquired bursae are subcutaneous or subfascial over the calcaneus and olecranon and either subcutaneously or between the extensor tendons and fibrous joint capsule of the metacarpophalangeal and metatarsophalangeal joints.

All bursae are amenable to evaluation with standard arthroscopic equipment and the usual principles of fluid distension with triangulation of arthroscope and instruments apply. In congenital bursae, portals are made abaxial to associated tendons. Endoscopy has resulted in identification of previously unreported lesions. It appears that bursae respond to aseptic insult in a manner similar to tendon sheaths but, as yet, little is known about healing of the fibrocartilaginous surfaces. Response to open wounds or other introduction of contaminants is common to all synovial cavities. However, as might be expected with their constituent tissues, with establishment of infection, the response of congenital bursae has some features in common with tendon sheaths and some, with diarthrodial joints.

Indications for endoscopy of congenital bursae include lameness referable to the bursa, investigation of bursal distension, contamination, and infection. Some lesions will have radiologic or ultrasonographic changes, or both, but there is invariably bursal distension. Since the last edition of this book further publications have highlighted the contribution of endoscopy to the understanding and management of lesions. The principle indications for endoscopy of acquired bursae are still contamination and infection, but evacuation and resection of both developing and established synovial linings can, in some circumstances, result in resolution.

CALCANEAL BURSA

There are two congenital calcaneal bursae (Fig. 13-1). The principal, intertendinous bursa (B. calcanea subtendinea m. flexoris digit superficialis) lies beneath the superficial digital flexor (SDF) tendon which, together with its fibrocartilagenous cap, forms the plantar margin of the bursa. Cranially/dorsally it is bordered by the tendon of insertion of gastrocnemius, the fibrocartilage covered proximal plantar calcaneus, and the long plantar ligament. In its middle one third,

the abaxial margins are formed by the medial and lateral extensions of the fibrocartilaginous cap of the SDF and its conjoined tendinous calcaneal insertions (Fig. 13-2). In the proximal and distal one thirds, medial and lateral margins of the bursa are lined by villous synovium. A smaller congenital bursa, the gastrocnemius or deep calcaneal bursa is found proximally, cranial to the tendon of insertion of gastrocnemius (bursa tendinis m. gastrocnemii). The two bursae consistently communicate. Latex injection studies have suggested that this always occurs medially and in 50% of cases laterally (Post et al, 2007); the authors' endoscopic experience suggests consistent lateral and inconsistent medial communication.

Technique

Endoscopy of the calcaneal bursae may be performed with the horse in lateral or dorsal recumbency, with the limb in an extended position. Application of an Esmarch bandage and tourniquet at proximal crural level can be of assistance. The most comprehensive evaluation of the principal bursa is obtained from a distal arthroscopic portal using a modification of the technique described by Ingle-Fehr & Baxter (1998). Safe insertion of the arthroscopic cannula with a conical obturator in situ is optimized by maximal distension of the bursa. This can be achieved at any point, but when the bursa is minimally distended, separation of the SDF tendon and long plantar ligament, with firm finger and thumb pressure, creates a safe and confident point of entry (Fig. 13-3).

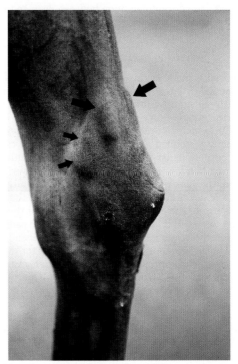

Figure 13-1 Distention of the calcaneal bursae; the principal or intertendinous bursa dorsal to the superficial digital flexor tendon *(large arrows)* and deep bursa dorsal to the gastrocnemius tendon *(small arrows).*

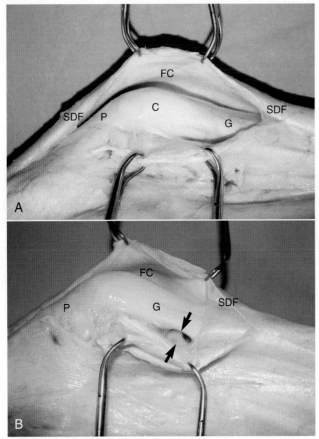

Figure 13-2 Dissection of the (intertendinous) bursa. **A,** Medially and **B,** laterally following division of the calcaneal insertions of the superficial digital flexor *(SDF)* tendon, which are secured in towel clamps. *C,* Calcaneus; *FC,* fibrocartilaginous cap of SDF; *G,* tendon of insertion of gastrocnemius; *P,* long plantar ligament; ➜, lateral communication between deep and principal (intertendinous) calcaneal bursae.

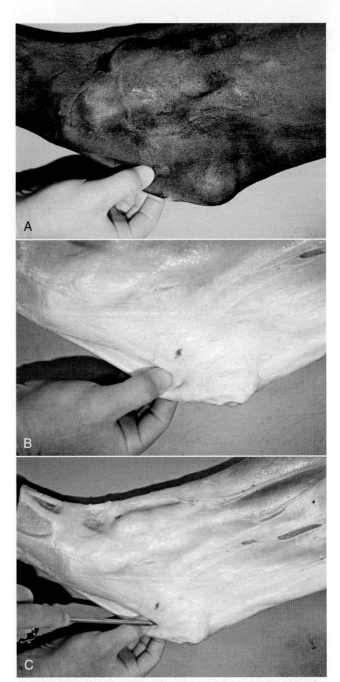

Figure 13-3 Introduction of arthroscopic cannula into the calcaneal bursa via a distolateral portal demonstrated on a cadaver limb. **A** and **B,** Separation of superficial digital flexor *(SDF)* of the long plantar ligament. **C,** Introduction of the cannula and conical obturator dorsal to the SDF directed proximally and axially beneath SDF fibrocartilage.

A skin portal is made at this level with a No. 11 blade. Entry can be medial or lateral, and this can be varied according to preoperative diagnostic information. It is important that the site of arthroscopic entry is distal to the calcaneal insertion of the SDF, which can readily be delineated when the bursa is maximally distended. As in other locations, the cannula is inserted perpendicular to the skin using the thumb on the noninserting hand as a friction bridge. As the synovial cavity is entered, the inserting hand can be moved distally and the arthroscopic sleeve advanced proximally beneath the fibrocartilaginous cap of the SDF until the full length of the cannula has been inserted (Fig. 13-4A). At this point the cannula will lie between the tendons of insertion of the SDF and gastrocnemius. The arthroscope can then be inserted for evaluation of the bursa. This approach provides thorough examination of the principal bursa from a single portal. It permits complete endoscopic evaluation of the subsynovial portion of the ipsilateral calcaneal insertion of the SDF but does not allow complete evaluation of the contralateral insertion. This necessitates creation of a similar portal on the opposite side of the limb. Communication between principal bursa and that cranial to the tendon of insertion of gastrocnemius can be identified (laterally) from this location, but entry of the arthroscope into this bursa requires a surtal proximal to the calcaneus (Fig. 13-4B). This is made proximal to the lateral margin of the fibrocartilaginous cap of the SDF and permits

evaluation of the deep calcaneal bursa and also passage of the arthroscope to and from this into the principal calcaneal bursa (Fig. 13-5). As a result of the communication, evaluation and treatment (evacuation) of the deep (gastrocnemius bursa) is considered particularly important in the management of contaminated and infected bursae. Instrument portals may be created at appropriate locations as determined by lesions identified within the bursa. These may be proximal (see Fig. 13-4C) or distal to the fibrocartilaginous cap and calcaneal insertions of the SDF and may be ipsilateral or contralateral to the arthroscope.

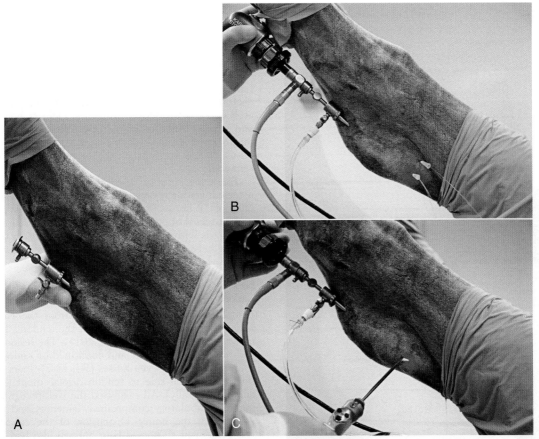

Figure 13-4 Arthroscopy of calcaneal bursa using a distolateral arthroscopic portal. **A,** Arthroscopic cannula inserted between the fibrocartilage of the SDF and calcaneus into the proximal recess. **B,** Transillumination of the proximal cul-de-sac of the calcaneal bursa. Caudal egress needle placed into the principal (intertendinous) bursa and cranial needle into the lateral communication between this and the deep calcaneal bursa illustrating the site of entry for arthroscopic evaluation of the same. **C,** Instrument portal into the proximal cul-de-sac of the calcaneal bursa.

Endoscopic Anatomy

Most arthroscopic movement within the bursa is two dimensional, and systematic evaluation requires rotation of the arthroscope in order to utilize its lens angle effectively. The proximal recess of the principal calcaneal bursa contains villous synovium, and at this level evaluation of the medial, caudal, and lateral surfaces of the tendon of insertion of gastrocnemius is possible. Laterally, communication with the deep calcaneal bursa is invariably recognized; this is bordered by villous synovium. Longitudinal fiber orientation is identifiable in the proximal portion of the SDF tendon. Distal to this the SDF tendon widens markedly to form the fibrocartilaginous cap over the apex of the calcaneus. This occupies the middle one third of the bursa. The fibrocartilaginous surface is relatively amorphous, although a few transverse lines sometimes are visible. At the medial and lateral margins of the calcaneus the fibrocartilaginous cap of the SDF can have slight proximodistally oriented indentations. Abaxially from these points, if the arthroscope is passed to the side of the calcaneus, the subsynovial portion of the calcaneal insertions of the SDF is tendinous. The fiber orientation visible at the abaxial margins of the bursa appears to reflect from the calcaneus and mark the plantar margins of the insertion. Returning to the midline and rotating the arthroscope lens dorsally images the caudal/plantar insertion of the gastrocnemius, which blends imperceptibly into the fibrocartilage at the apex of the calcaneus. The arthroscope is withdrawn farther, and while the lens

remains in this orientation, the junction between the fibrocartilage of the calcaneus and smooth origin of the long plantar ligament is discernible. In order to visualize the distal portion of the bursa, it is now necessary for the hand holding the arthroscope to be raised and rotated proximad such that the tip of the arthroscope is directed distally. The plantar surface of the long plantar ligament can then be followed into the distal recess. Synovium becomes increasingly villous as the arthroscope is moved distally. By rotating the lens to a plantar orientation, subsynovial alignment can once again be identified in the SDF tendon.

Evaluation of the deep calcaneal bursa from a proximolateral portal permits examination of the cranial/dorsal surface of the tendon of insertion of the gastrocnemius. This has ill-defined longitudinal fiber organization with a smooth reflection of the bursal surface at its calcaneal insertion. A small amount of villous synovium is evident abaxially.

Clinical Application

Tearing of the Calcaneal Insertions of the Superficial Digital Flexor

The calcaneal insertions of the superficial digital flexor are substantial structures whose dorsal margins are subsynovial with respect to the principal calcaneal bursa. Their calcaneal insertions provide the caudal arm to the reciprocal apparatus (Dyce et al, 1996; Sisson, 1975). Wright & Minshall (2011) described intrathecal tearing of the tendinous portions of the calcaneal insertions of the SDF as the sole identifiable lesion

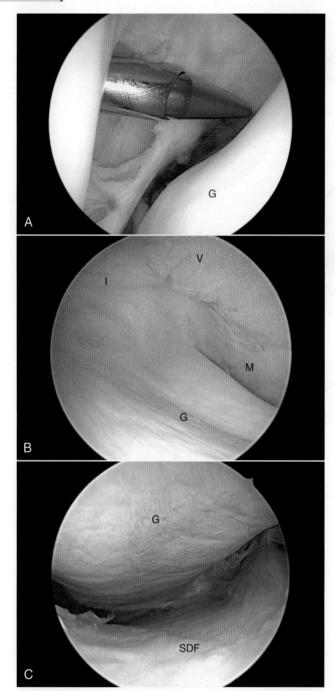

Figure 13-5 Arthroscopic evaluation of the deep calcaneal bursa. **A,** Arthroscopic cannula and conical obturator introduced at the site of needle placement shown in Figure 13-4B passing cranial to the tendon of insertion of gastrocnemius. **B,** Arthroscopic view in the deep calcaneal bursa. **C,** Withdrawal of the arthroscope to relocate to the intertendinous bursa. *G,* Tendon insertion of gastrocnemius; *I,* insertion of gastrocnemius; *M,* medial wall of deep calcaneal bursa; *SDF,* tendon of insertion of superficial digital flexor; *V,* villous synovium cranially in deep calcaneal bursa.

in 12 lame horses with distended calcaneal bursae. Medial and lateral insertions were equally affected; 9 of 12 lesions were predicted by ultrasonography. In all cases, torn fibrils were extruded into the bursa. Granulomatous tissue covered torn stumps in 5 horses (Fig. 13-6). Tears varied in proximodistal

length and axial/abaxial thickness, but all were partial. In some cases the tears revealed a bilayered structure to the tendinous insertion. In 2 horses tears were full thickness resulting in loss of bursal integrity and visible communication with an adjacent (subcutaneous) bursa.

Treatment in all cases involved removal of disrupted tendinous tissue. Large masses were resected using meniscectomy knives or scissors and removed with appropriately sized arthroscopic rongeurs. Defects were debrided, and smaller bundles of disrupted fibers removed using a motorized synovial resector with suction applied (see Fig. 13-6). When appropriate, other fibrinoid debris was also removed.

Following routine perioperative management, horses received gradually ascending controlled exercise programs. Nine of 12 horses returned to work at or greater than their previous level of performance. This included four racing Thoroughbreds with time intervals from surgery to the first race varying between 7 and 10 months. No postoperative complications were reported.

▶ Unstable Subluxation of the Superficial Digital Flexor Tendon

Unstable subluxation of the SDF from the calcaneus has been associated with disruption of the tendon's fibrocartilaginous cap (Wright & Minshall, 2011). The lesion was identified ultrasonographically and confirmed by endoscopy of the principal bursa in seven horses (Fig. 13-7). Tears occurred on the contralateral side to tendon displacement (six medially and one laterally). All exhibited the well-recognized signs of marked ambulatory compromise, lameness, and anxiety that accompany the injury. Distension of the calcaneal bursae was evident in all horses. Four animals also had an adjacent, acquired (subcutaneous) bursa that communicated with the congenital bursae.

Surgery can be performed in dorsal or lateral recumbency, using arthroscopic portals that are either contralateral or ipsilateral to the torn tissue, but the latter is technically easier. Use of an Esmarch bandage and tourniquet to a proximal crural level is recommended. In the reported series, all horses with unstable subluxation of the SDF tendon had extensive proximodistally oriented defects in the fibrocartilage cap. The defects involved almost the entire proximodistal length of the fibrocartilage, and in each case there was proximally and distally a bridge of intact tissue. When the tendon was manually repositioned onto the calcaneus, defects in the fibrocartilage cap were reduced, and when the tendon subluxated, the defects opened. Bridges of tissue proximally and distally restricted further abaxial displacement of the tendon, and thus it was reasoned they prevented progression to stable subluxation. The fibrocartilage defect was full (dorsoplantar) thickness in all cases creating a breach in the bursal wall and communication with an acquired (subcutaneous) fluid-filled space. In acute cases the fibrocartilage defect was irregular (see Fig. 13-7), whereas in longstanding cases the margins were rounded and covered partially by fibrous tissue or were margined by clumps of fibrillated fibrocartilage (Fig. 13-8).

Treatment is aimed at creation of a stable subluxation by resection of the proximal and distal attachments to the torn abaxial portion of the fibrocartilage cap. This is performed with meniscectomy knives and scissors. The detached portion of fibrocartilage then remains anchored by the tendinous portion of the calcaneal insertion of the SDF to the calcaneus. This may also be partially torn but requires sharp dissection with similar instruments. The resultant mass can then be removed. The bulk of tissue is invariably substantial and may require further division. However, if the fibrocartilaginous tissue is grasped firmly with large rongeurs or similar grasping equipment, it frequently will compress

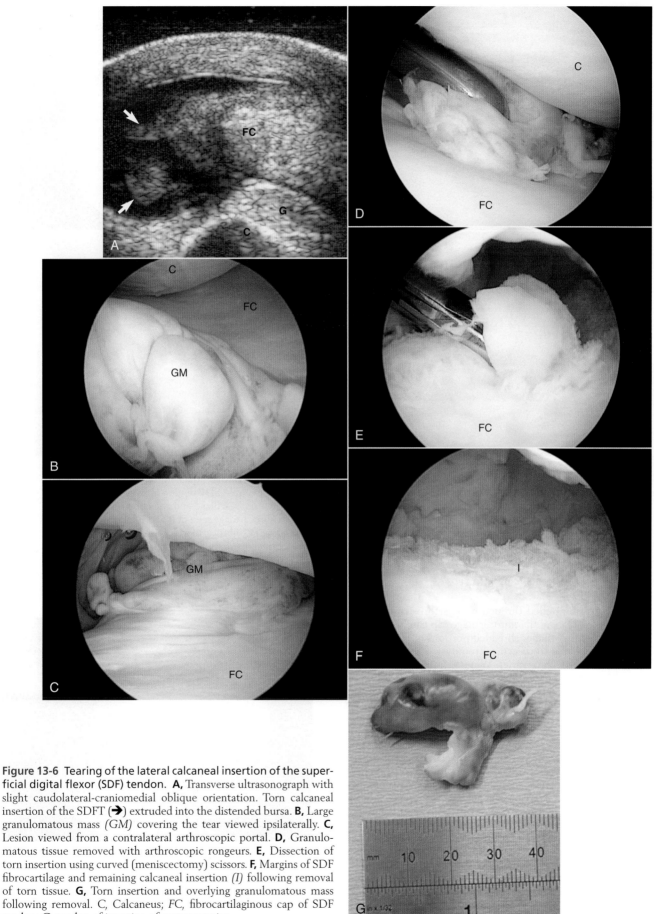

Figure 13-6 Tearing of the lateral calcaneal insertion of the superficial digital flexor (SDF) tendon. **A,** Transverse ultrasonograph with slight caudolateral-craniomedial oblique orientation. Torn calcaneal insertion of the SDFT (➜) extruded into the distended bursa. **B,** Large granulomatous mass *(GM)* covering the tear viewed ipsilaterally. **C,** Lesion viewed from a contralateral arthroscopic portal. **D,** Granulomatous tissue removed with arthroscopic rongeurs. **E,** Dissection of torn insertion using curved (meniscectomy) scissors. **F,** Margins of SDF fibrocartilage and remaining calcaneal insertion *(I)* following removal of torn tissue. **G,** Torn insertion and overlying granulomatous mass following removal. C, Calcaneus; *FC*, fibrocartilaginous cap of SDF tendon; *G*, tendon of insertion of gastrocnemius.

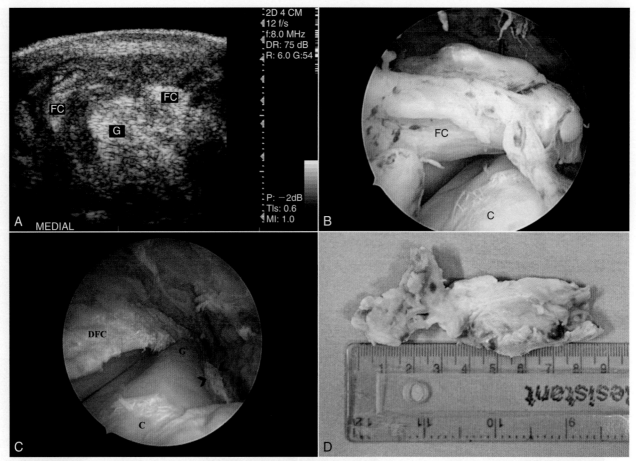

Figure 13-7 A, Transverse ultrasonographic image obtained using a linear probe proximal to the *calcaneus* demonstrating a full-thickness defect in the fibrocartilage with lateral displacement of that attached to the superficial digital flexor *(SDF)* tendon. **B,** Ipsilateral (medial) endoscopic view of acutely disrupted SDF tendon fibrocartilage imaged in **A. C,** Similar endoscopic image to **B** following removal of the disrupted fibrocartilage and resection of the calcaneal insertion of the SDF tendon and debridement of both. **D,** Mass of torn fibrocartilage seen in **A** and **B** following removal. C, Calcaneus; *DFC,* resected and debrided fibrocartilage of SDF tendon; *FC,* fibrocartilage of SDF tendon; G, tendon of insertion of gastrocnemius; >, proximal margin of resected and debrided medial calcaneal insertion of SDF tendon. *(Reproduced from Equine Veterinary Journal with permission.)*

sufficiently to be pulled through most arthroscopic portals. In some cases, tears in the fibrocartilage cap can be markedly irregular, creating smaller shredded portions of fibrocartilage that are amendable to piecemeal removal. The mediolateral location of the defects varies. When relatively abaxial, the natural curvature of the fibrocartilage cap may still restrict free contralateral displacement of the tendon. When this occurs, further axial resection of the fibrocartilage cap is indicated until the tendon and remaining fibrocartilage cap can readily be displaced and remain in this (usually lateral) location. Such dissection can be undertaken using sharp cutting equipment or alternatively with a large (5.5-mm) full radius synovial resector. Once stable subluxation has been achieved, tissue margins are debrided to reduce exposure of disrupted collagenous tissue (see Fig. 13-7). Organized blood clots and fibrinoid debris are removed from both congenital and acquired bursae.

The authors reported relief and creation of stable subluxation in all horses. Six of seven horses returned to work, of which four were considered to have returned to their previous level of performance. Two horses subsequently sustained similar injuries to their contralateral limbs 23 and 30 months post surgery. Both were managed in a similar manner and again returned to athletic function.

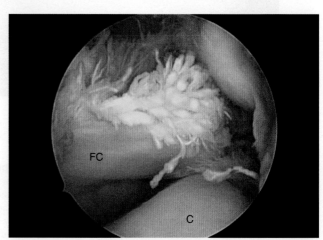

Figure 13-8 Medial endoscopic image of the calcaneal bursa in a horse with unstable (lateral) subluxation of the superficial digital flexor (SDF) tendon for 13 weeks. The axial margin of the fibrocartilage defect is covered with clumps of fibrillated tissue. C, Calcaneus; *FC,* SDF tendon fibrocartilage. *(Reproduced from Equine Veterinary Journal with permission.)*

Osteolytic Lesions of the Calcaneus

Regions of osteolysis in the calcaneal tuber have been reported by Ingle-Fehr & Baxter (1998) and Bassage et al (2000). Affected animals present with distension of the calcaneal bursa and lameness that is responsive to intrathecal local analgesia. Radiographs, principally flexed plantaroproximal-plantarodistal oblique projections, demonstrate radiolucencies in the proximal plantar margin or apex of the calcaneal tuber, or both. Ultrasonography confirms distension of the calcaneal bursa and may also reveal disruption of the proximal plantar margin of the calcaneus. At endoscopy, there may be discoloration of the calcaneal fibrocartilage with soft, crumbling, and apparently degenerate bone exposed by use of a blunt probe. Removal of the degenerate bone and debridement has resulted in return to soundness, but the number of cases is small and thus confident prognostication is difficult. The etiology of such lesions is unknown. Previous authors have tentatively suggested that these may be avulsion injuries of the plantar ligament (Ingle-Fehr & Baxter, 1998) or gastrocnemius (Bassage et al, 2000). However, in the authors' experience, defects have occurred between these two structures beneath the fibrocartilage on the plantar surface of the apex of the calcaneus.

Traumatic Fragmentation of the Calcaneus

External trauma, usually as a result of falls or kicks from other horses, may result in intrathecal fragmentation of the calcaneal tuber. These may be open or closed. Most fractures are identified radiographically and, when the apex of the calcaneus is involved, flexed plantaroproximal-plantarodistal oblique (skyline) projections are most useful.

Endoscopy is most readily performed with ipsilateral arthroscope and instrument portals. When accompanied by wounds, the surgeon should look diligently for the presence of hair and foreign material. Fragments are removed with appropriately sized arthroscopic rongeurs, and the fracture bed is debrided with curettes. In some instances foreign material may be embedded in bone. Lesions should be debrided using the same principles as applied with osteochondral fragmentation in diarthrodial joints, but fibrocartilaginous margins always appear less sharply demarcated than their hyaline counterparts.

INTERTUBERCULAR (BICIPITAL) BURSA

The intertubercular bursa is found between the tendon of origin of biceps brachii and the cranial margin of the humerus (Fig. 13-9). The bursa envelops the medial and lateral margins of the tendon in the manner of a tendon sheath and in foals appears to extend farther cranially than in adults. Proximal to the humerus it is separated from the scapulohumeral joint by their fibrous capsules and an intervening fat pad. Unlike dogs, the bicipital bursa rarely communicates directly with the scapulohumeral joint. The cranial margin of the humerus bears three tubercles: lateral (greater), medial (lesser), and an intermediate tubercle. The overlying tendon is bilobed and indented markedly by the intermediate tuberosity. The medial lobe is slightly larger than its lateral counterpart. A tendinous band from pectoralis ascendens envelops the tendon and bursa in the region of the humeral tuberosities. Over the humeral tuberosities the biceps tendon is partly cartilaginous and presents a smooth fibrocartilaginous bursal surface. The musculotendinous junction of the biceps brachii lies in the distal portion of the bursa, which terminates just proximal to the deltoid tuberosity of the humerus.

Lameness localized to the bicipital bursa is uncommon, and therefore indications for endoscopy are correspondingly few.

Technique

Endoscopy is performed with the horse in lateral recumbency, with the affected limb uppermost and positioned parallel to the ground (Fig. 13-10). Surgeons should stand in front of the

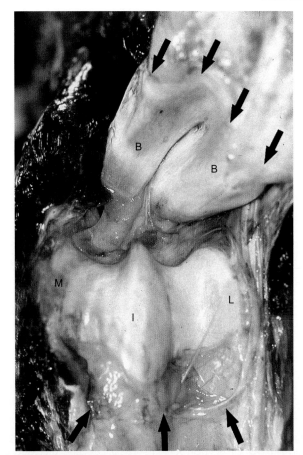

Figure 13-9 Left bicipital bursa open by distal division and reflection of biceps brachii. The distal margins of the bursa are marked by *arrows*. Fibrocartilage covers the lateral *(L)* intermediate *(I)*, and medial *(M)* tuberosities of the humerus and the lobes of the adjacent bicipital tendon *(B)*.

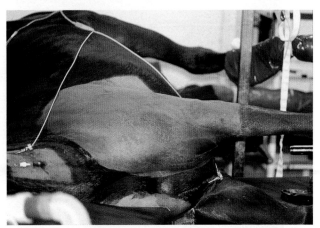

Figure 13-10 Horse positioned for endoscopy of the left bicipital bursa.

limb with the arthroscope tower on the opposite side of the horse. In the majority of circumstances a distal arthroscopic portal, as described by Adams & Turner (1999) (Fig. 13-11), is most suitable but evaluation of the proximal recess requires an additional lateral arthroscopic portal. Generally, pathologic bursae are distended and there is no advantage to further distension. A skin portal is made using a No. 11 or 15 blade over the craniolateral margin of the humerus 2 to 3 cm proximal to the deltoid tuberosity. Using a conical obturator, the arthroscopic

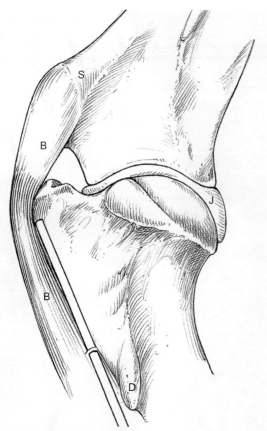

Figure 13-11 Distal endoscopic approach to the bicipital bursa. *B*, Tendon of origin of biceps brachii; *D*, deltoid tuberosity of humerus; *J*, scapulohumeral joint; *S*, supraglenoid tubercle of scapula.

cannula is directed axially and proximally through the brachiocephalicus muscle and between the cranial margin of the humerus and tendon of origin of biceps brachii (Fig. 13-12). Entry to the bursa is usually accompanied by flow of synovial fluid from the cannula, and this is advanced proximally before the arthroscope is inserted. Instrument portals can be made laterally at any point along the bursal length. An additional arthroscopic portal may be made proximal to the lateral tuberosity of the humerus using a percutaneous 1.2 × 90 mm (18-ga × 3.5-inch) needle as a guide. If necessary, arthroscopy and instrument portals can be interchanged (Fig. 13-12). The bicipital bursa permits only a small amount of craniocaudal movement; evaluation therefore requires rotation of the arthroscopic lens throughout the examination in order to visualize all possible surfaces. At the end of the diagnostic and surgical procedures, skin portals are closed in a routine manner and the wounds protected by oversewing swabs or gauze pads as stent bandages.

Endoscopic Anatomy

Proximal to the humeral tuberosities the bursal synovium is villous and covers the supraglenoid tubercle of the scapula, the origin of biceps brachii, and the voluminous bursal recess cranial to the scapulohumeral joint. At this level, the proximal portion of the biceps brachii tendon has visible fiber orientation (Fig. 13-13). Withdrawing the arthroscope provides visualization of the lateral tuberosity and later (abaxial) side of the intermediate tuberosity of the humerus. These and the overlying biceps brachii tendon are covered with smooth fibrocartilage (Fig. 13-14). The tight interdigitation of the tendon and the cranial surface of the humerus precludes evaluation of the medial tubercle and axial side of the intermediate tubercle of the humerus from this position. Abaxial to the lateral margin of the lateral tubercle of the humerus there is a cover of fine synovial villi through which tendinous bands from pectoralis

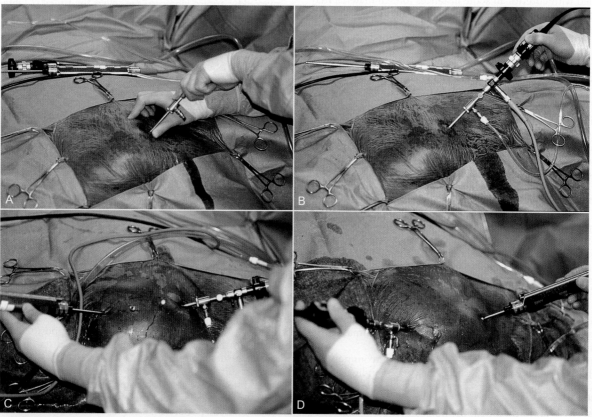

Figure 13-12 Endoscopy of the bicipital bursa **(A)** use of a conical obturator to enter the bursa distally. **B,** Commencing evaluation of the bursa. **C,** Use of a proximal instrument portal; percutaneous needles mark other potential sites for instrument portals. **D,** Reversal of arthroscope and instrument portals.

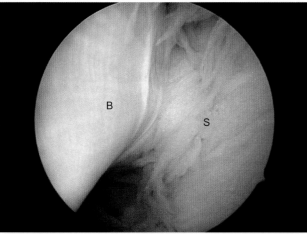

Figure 13-13 Endoscopic view of the proximal recess of the bicipital bursa. The synovium *(S)* is villous and the tendon of biceps brachii *(B)* has visible fiber orientation.

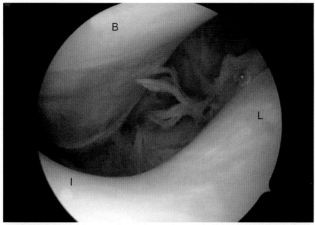

Figure 13-14 Endoscopic view of the proximal margins of the fibrocartilage covered surfaces of the lateral *(L)* and intermediate *(I)* tubercles of the humerus and overlying biceps brachii tendon *(B)*.

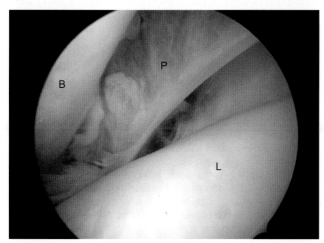

Figure 13-15 Synovial plica *(P)* is visible adjacent to the abaxial margin of the lateral tuberosity of the humerus *(L)*; *B*, Bicipital tendon.

ascendens are seen perpendicular and attaching to the lateral tuberosity. With further withdrawal of the arthroscope, a synovial plica is visible at the lateral margin of the intertubercular groove (Fig. 13-15). At this level the arthroscope can be inserted between the biceps brachii tendon and fibrocartilagenous surface of the humerus as far axial only as the intermediate tubercle

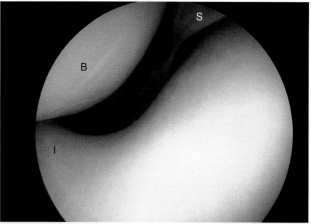

Figure 13-16 Arthroscope position between the bicipital tendon *(B)* and cranial surface of the humerus illustrating the axial limit of visibility. *I*, Intermediate tubercle of humerus; *S*, lateral synovial plica.

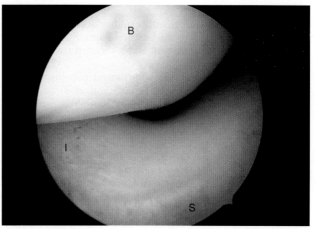

Figure 13-17 Endoscopic view of the distal margin of the humeral fibrocartilage. *B*, Lateral lobe of the bicipital tendon; *I*, intermediate tubercle of the humerus; *S*, synovium on the cranial surface of the humerus.

(Fig. 13-16). Approaching its distal margin the fibrocartilage is slightly irregular (Fig. 13-17). Beyond this point the cranial surface of the humerus and biceps brachii tendon and musculotendinous junction are covered by villous synovium (Fig. 13-18). In the distal recess it is possible to visualize also a small area of the fibrocartilage medial to the intermediate tubercle (see Fig. 13-18) and to push the arthroscope axially to obtain limited visualization of the distal medial lobe of the tendon. Utilizing a proximolateral arthroscopic portal, the most proximal margin of the intermediate tubercle and a small portion of the medial lobe of the tendon can be visualized (Fig. 13-19).

Clinical Application

Endoscopy of the bicipital bursa has been used in the investigation of lameness referable to this site and to treat intrathecal fragmentation of the supraglenoid tubercle of the scapula and lateral tubercle of the humerus, injuries of the bicipital tendon, and management of contaminated and infected bursae.

Fragmentation of the Supraglenoid Tubercle and Lateral Tuberosity of the Humerus

Most fractures of the supraglenoid tubercle of the scapula produce large fragments that involve the articular surface of the shoulder, approximate to the physeal line, and compromise a substantial portion of the origin of biceps brachii. Occasionally,

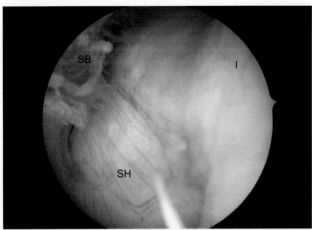

Figure 13-18 Endoscopic view of the distal recess. *I*, Distal margin of the intermediate tubercle of the humerus; *SB*, synovium covering the musculotendinous junction of biceps brachii; *SH*, synovium covering the cranial surface of the humerus.

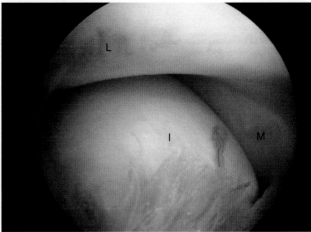

Figure 13-19 Endoscopic view from a proximolateral arthroscope portal. *I*, Proximal margin of the intermediate tubercle of the humerus; *L*, lateral; *M*, medial lobes of the bicipital tendon.

smaller more proximal fragments can displace distally and are intrathecal with respect to the bicipital bursa. Such fragments can be visualized and removed, and associated tissues can be debrided endoscopically.

Intrathecal fragmentation of the lateral tuberosity of the humerus results from external trauma and in some cases is associated with penetrating wounds. Radiologic signs can be subtle but are frequently highlighted by craniomedial-caudolateral oblique projections. Ultrasonography may also image fragmentation at this site and confirm bursal distension (Fig. 13-20). Fractures can be assessed, fragments removed, and fracture beds debrided from the arthroscopic position described earlier. In the presence of a penetrating wound, this may be used as an instrument portal or the portal can be created using percutaneous needles as positional guides. Fractures can have limited bursal communication and be more extensive extrathecally. This does not preclude endoscopic removal and debridement but requires careful control of fluid flow in order to limit extravasation in and adjacent to the fracture site, which will compromise visualization. Fragments may be removed, and fracture beds may be debrided using appropriately sized arthroscopic instruments, but access to motorized equipment is essential.

Lesions of the Bicipital Tendon

Ultrasonographic examination of the tendon of origin of biceps brachii and its associated bursa has been described by Crabill et al (1995), Tnibar et al (1999), and Pasquet et al (2008). Traumatic injuries of the tendon are most common laterally (Pasquet et al, 2008). Partial rupture of the tendon involving the lateral lobe can follow blunt trauma or falls, or both. These may be identified ultrasonographically and are accompanied by marked bursal distension (see Fig. 13-20). Disruption of the lateral lobe can be identified at endoscopy and detached tissue removed using a combination of hand and motorized equipment, in line with general surgical principles. Spadari et al (2009) reported complete rupture of the lateral lobe of the biceps brachii tendon in one horse, which was diagnosed ultrasonographically. This was confirmed by endoscopy and the bursa was debrided; little clinical improvement was reported. In this case, the extensive nature of the lesions precluded treatment, but endoscopy was considered diagnostically useful.

The authors have seen lame horses with loss of humeral fibrocartilage and fibrillation of the adjacent bicipital tendon. Other identified lesions have included rupture of the lateral

wall of the bursa and intrathecal tearing of the bicipital tendon. These cases have been treated endoscopically by debridement of torn or detached tissues, or both.

Osseous Cystlike Lesions

Osseous cystlike lesions involving the bursal margins of the humerus have been reported by Ramzan (2004), Arnold et al (2008), and Little et al (2009). The case reported by Arnold et al (2008) involved the lateral margin of the intermediate tubercle of the humerus. Bursal communication was identified endoscopically in an area of infolded fibrocartilage, and there was marked fibrillation of the adjacent bicipital tendon. The cyst was debrided under endoscopic guidance, and the horse returned to working soundness 8 months postoperatively. Little et al (2009) reported osseous cystlike lesions on the intermediate tubercle in four and lateral tubercle in one horse. All were managed by intrathecal medication with corticosteroids resulting in a return to soundness in work. Cases reported by Ramzan (2004) were not treated. Endoscopic treatment is clearly feasible and, on current evidence, is indicated in cases that are refractory to medical management.

Contamination and Infection

Ultrasonography is a sensitive indicator of an infected bicipital bursa. The echogenicity of the bursal contents depends on the cellular and proteinaceous nature of the fluid. Osteolysis may also be identified in some cases (Pasquet et al, 2008). Endoscopic evaluation and treatment of an infected bursa has been described by Tudor et al (1998). The authors have endoscopically managed contaminated and infected bicipital bursae, including cases with infected osteitis/osteomyelitis of the humeral tuberosities. The use of proximal and distal arthroscope and instrument portals is necessary to evaluate and evacuate infected tissues. Treatment follows the principles detailed in Chapter 14.

PODOTROCHLEAR (NAVICULAR) BURSA

The dorsal margins of the navicular bursa are, from distal to proximal, the distal sesamoidean impar ligament, the palmar/plantar fibrocartilage of the navicular bone, the navicular suspensory ligaments, and the intervening "T" ligament. The latter lacks directional fiber organization and consists of little more than the fibrous capsules of the distal interphalangeal joint, digital flexor tendon sheath, and navicular bursa. The

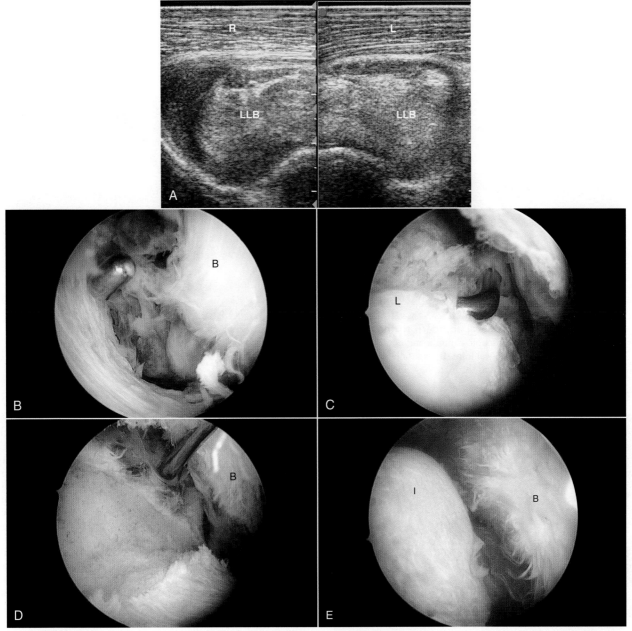

Figure 13-20 Fragmentation of the lateral tuberosity of the humerus with partial rupture of the adjacent lateral lobe of the bicipital tendon. **A,** Transverse ultrasonographs imaging right *(R)* and left *(L)* bicipital bursae. On the right there is loss of mass and infrastructure with irregular margination of the lateral lobe of the bicipital tendon *(LLB)*, a distended bursa, and irregular osseous reflection to the lateral tuberosity and groove of the humerus. **B,** Hemorrhage in the proximal lateral cul-de-sac adjacent to the irregularity of the origin of the bicipital tendon *(B)*. A synovial resector introduced at the beginning of debridement. **C,** Probing fragmentation of the lateral tuberosity *(L)* and groove of the humerus. **D,** Lateral tuberosity and groove of the humerus following removal of fragmentation and debridement of the defect. **E,** Fibrillation of the distal medial lobe of the bicipital tendon and adjacent intermediate tubercle of the humerus in the distal bursa.

dorsal surface of the deep digital flexor (DDF) tendon forms the palmar/plantar margin of the bursa.

Techniques

There are two separate techniques, each with distinct indications, for endoscopic evaluation of the navicular bursa: (1) transthecal technique and (2) a direct approach.

Transthecal Technique

A transthecal approach to the navicular bursa was reported briefly in the third edition of this book (Fig. 13-21). It is the most useful approach for evaluation and treatment of aseptic bursae, particularly when tearing of the dorsal surface of the DDF tendon has been identified by magnetic resonance imaging (MRI) or is a clinical differential. This use has been reported by Smith et al (2007) and by Smith and Wright (2012).

The horse is positioned in dorsal recumbency with passive flexion of the distal joints. This is readily achieved by placing a conforming pad (such as a roll of cotton wool cut or broken in half) between the distal antebrachium and proximal metacarpus (Fig. 13-22). An Esmarch bandage and tourniquet are

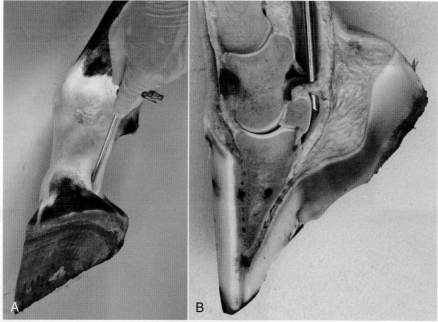

Figure 13-21 Transthecal approach to the navicular bursa illustrated in cadaver limbs. **A,** Location and trajectory of the arthroscopic cannula and conical obturator dorsal to the deep digital flexor tendon at the level of the proximal interphalangeal joint. **B,** Sagittally sectioned limb demonstrating passage of an arthroscope dorsal to the deep digital flexor tendon and through the T ligament into the proximal bursal recess.

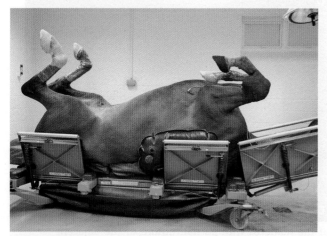

Figure 13-22 Horse positioned for a transthecal endoscopy of the left fore navicular bursa.

applied. Following surgical preparation of the pastern, a sterile foot wrap is applied to the level of the coronary band. The foot is passed through a fenestrated drape, and the latter is secured at the level of the fetlock, leaving the distal limb free and suspended (see Fig. 13-23A). Lateral and medial approaches are similar, and for ease of description a lateral approach is described.

The digital flexor tendon sheath is distended sufficiently to delineate the outpouching between the digital annular ligaments. The lateral palmar digital neurovascular bundle is palpated and its palmar margin ascertained. A skin incision suitable for an arthroscopic portal is made over the distended digital flexor tendon sheath at the level of the proximal interphalangeal joint, just palmar to the neurovascular bundle. This places the arthroscopic portal distal to the vinculae, which extend between the dorsal surface of the DDF tendon and the sheath wall at the level of the insertion of superficial digital

flexor tendon and straight distal sesamoidean ligament (Fig. 13-23). A stab incision with a No. 11 blade is made into the digital flexor tendon sheath at the dorsal margin of the DDF tendon. An arthroscopic cannula and obturator are passed dorsal to the DDF tendon, first perpendicular to the limb and then directed distally and medially to lie adjacent to the T ligament (see Fig. 13-23). The obturator is then withdrawn and the arthroscope inserted into the sleeve. When correct location is confirmed and, following palpation of the medial neurovascular bundle, a percutaneous needle is placed medially in a similar location to the lateral arthroscopic portal. An instrument portal is created, taking care not to traumatize the neurovascular bundle, and an arthroscopic probe is inserted (see Fig. 13-23F and G; Fig. 13-24B and C). One of the authors (A.J.N.) prefers to make the instrument portal dorsal to the neurovascular bundle to reduce the possibility of trauma to the medial palmar digital nerve during repeated instrument insertion. The probe then follows a similar trajectory to the proximal margin of the T ligament, which is palpated on the dorsal margin of the DDF tendon (see Fig. 13-24D).

A portal into the navicular bursa is created by division of the T ligament along the dorsal margin of the DDF tendon. This is most readily achieved with sharp fixed-blade meniscectomy knives, banana knives, or curved beaver blade and completed by arthroscopic scissors (see Chapter 2). The incision in the T ligament is started near the midline of the DDF tendon, using the subtle crease between the lateral and medial lobes of the DDF tendon to define the entry. It is important that the incision is made as close to the dorsal margin of the DDF tendon as possible; a slightly dorsal incision will extend into the body of the T ligament, while farther dorsally this will extend into the palmar compartment of the distal interphalangeal joint (see Fig. 13-24E). In order to evaluate fully the navicular bursa, the portal should be made as wide as possible (Fig. 13-24F). It therefore should extend medially and laterally to the insertions of the navicular suspensory ligaments, which creates a portal that is approximately 40 mm wide (see Fig. 13-28C). Frayed tissue created by the incision in the

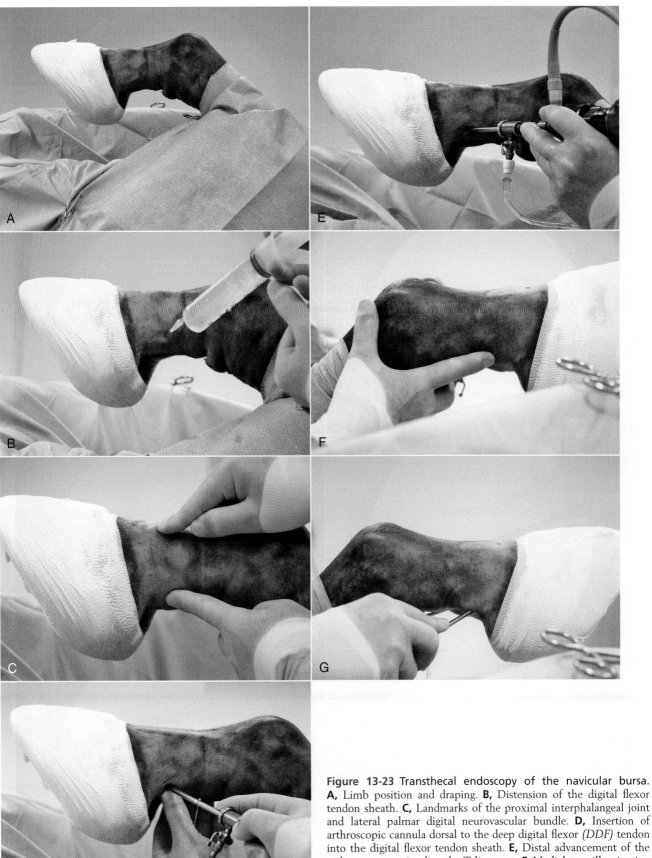

Figure 13-23 Transthecal endoscopy of the navicular bursa. A, Limb position and draping. **B,** Distension of the digital flexor tendon sheath. **C,** Landmarks of the proximal interphalangeal joint and lateral palmar digital neurovascular bundle. **D,** Insertion of arthroscopic cannula dorsal to the deep digital flexor *(DDF)* tendon into the digital flexor tendon sheath. **E,** Distal advancement of the arthroscope to visualize the T ligament. **F,** Medial transillumination and determination of the instrument portal site. **G,** Introduction of a probe medially in preparation for creating a portal into the navicular bursa.

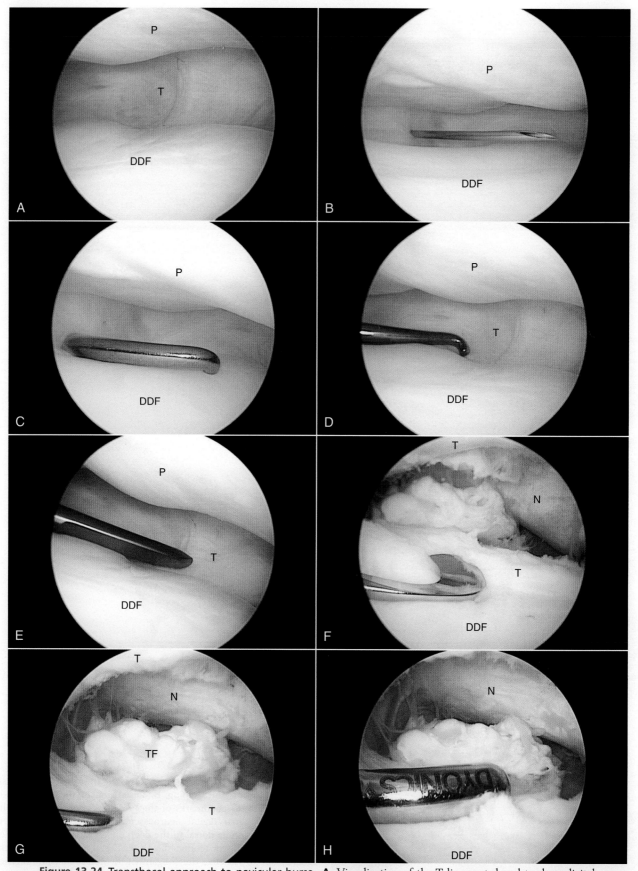

Figure 13-24 Transthecal approach to navicular bursa. **A,** Visualization of the T ligament dorsal to deep digital flexor *(DDF)* tendon. **B,** Introduction of a percutaneous needle to determine a suitable contralateral instrument portal. **C,** Introduction of an arthroscopic probe. **D,** Palpation of the T ligament with the arthroscopic probe. **E,** Commencement of division of the T ligament adjacent to the dorsal surface of the DDF tendon using a straight meniscectomy knife. **F,** Enlargement of the portal into the navicular bursa using a curved meniscectomy knife. Abnormal tissue is seen in the proximal (medial) bursa. **G,** Torn fibers from the medial lobe of the DDF tendon recoiled into the proximal medial cul-de-sac of the bursa. **H,** Removal of the torn fibers with a motorized synovial resector.

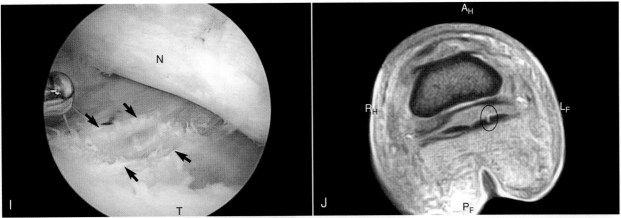

Figure 13-24, cont'd I, Inspection of the site following removal of the torn fibers. **J,** A transversely orientated magnetic resonance image of this case before surgery at a level just distal to the T ligament and within the proximal recess of the navicular bursa. This image is from a T2*-weighted gradient echo pulse sequence. Lateral is to the left. There is fluid distension of the navicular bursa and linear high signal demarcating a parasagittal split within the dorsal margin and body of the medial lobe of the DDF tendon (circled). *N,* Navicular bone, *arrows* demarcate the tear in the medial lobe of the DDFT; *P,* palmar surface of the middle phalanx; *T,* T ligament; *TF,* torn tendon fibers.

T ligament can be removed using a motorized synovial resector with suction applied.

Once a clear communication between the navicular bursa and digital flexor tendon sheath has been produced, a probe can be introduced through the portal created and evaluation of the bursa commenced. This approach optimizes evaluation of the proximal two thirds of the bursa, including the entirety of the proximal bursal recess. This site is important because it represents the most common location for intrabursal tears of the DDF tendon and extrusion of torn fibers, which usually recoil to this location (Smith et al, 2007; Smith & Wright, 2012). The arthroscopic trajectory produced by the transthecal approach (see Fig. 13-21B) compromises free passage of the arthroscope and instruments into the distal one third of the bursa. This can be improved by careful flexion of the distal limb with the arthroscope in situ and using an arthroscopic probe to place palmar pressure onto the dorsal surface of the DDF tendon. Adding a second instrument portal more distal to the arthroscope entry allows a probe to be inserted to retract the DDF tendon palmarly and improve access to the distal region of the navicular bone and adjacent DDF tendon. However, because of the convex palmar/plantar contour to the navicular bone, evaluation of the distal portion of the bursa, including the impar ligament, is still inferior to that achieved with the direct approach (described next). The authors recommend use of the transthecal approach for evaluation and treatment of aseptic navicular bursae, but if access to the most distal regions of the bursa is required, then this can be supplemented by subsequent direct approach.

In the transthecal technique both medial and lateral approaches are equally possible, and arthroscope and instrument portal interchange is recommended when biaxial lesions are present within the bursa. In cases in which a medial or lateral lesion is identified before surgery (usually by MRI), then contralateral arthroscope and ipsilateral instrument portals are appropriate. If, following lesion identification interchange is desirable, then this can be achieved without difficulty. For this reason, the authors recommend inclusion of a second arthroscopic cannula within a standard instrument set.

No untoward sequelae of the transthecal technique have been identified or reported (Smith & Wright, 2012). Perhaps surprisingly, postoperative distension of the digital flexor tendon sheath has not been identified. In a small number of cases in which a revisionary transthecal approach has been

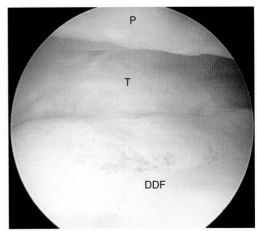

Figure 13-25 Healed T ligament 13 months post transthecal desmotomy. *DDF,* Deep digital flexor tendon; *P,* palmar middle phalanx; *T,* T ligament. *(Courtesy of M.R.W. Smith.)*

undertaken, there has been healing of the portal created in the T ligament with smooth, well-organized scar tissue (Fig. 13-25; Smith M.R.W. personal communication, 2012).

Direct Approach

The direct approach was described by Wright et al (1999) and Cruz et al (2001). Subsequently, a modified direct approach through the distal digital flexor tendon sheath was reported by Rossignol & Perrin (2003). The horse may be in either dorsal or lateral recumbency. The former facilitates triangulation and use of medial and lateral arthroscope and instrument portals. Lateral recumbency is favored for investigation and treatment of solar penetrations. Distal limb joints should be positioned in slight flexion. Use of an Esmarch bandage and tourniquet is recommended. The direct approach described by Wright et al (1999) is recommended for evaluation and treatment of penetrating injuries to the navicular bursa or treatment of infected navicular bursae. It avoids (patent) penetration of other synovial cavities and permits advancement of the arthroscope to the most distal portions of the bursa including the impar ligament, where most penetrating injuries occur.

A 5-mm skin incision is made proximal to the collateral cartilage on the abaxial margin of the DDF tendon, palmar/plantar to the digital neurovascular bundle. The arthroscopic cannula with a conical obturator is introduced and advanced distally and axially along the dorsal surface of the DDF tendon to enter the bursa at approximately the midpoint of the middle phalanx. As the bursa is entered, there is usually a loss of resistance to advancement of the cannula. The obturator is then withdrawn and replaced by the arthroscope (Fig. 13-26).

Using this technique, it is important that the surgeon considers the alignment of the DDFT in relation to the position of the limb and adjusts the trajectory of the arthroscopic cannula accordingly. If the trajectory is too dorsal, then it is likely that the arthroscopic sleeve will pass through the T ligament and into the palmar/plantar compartment of the distal interphalangeal joint. In such circumstances, the sleeve should be withdrawn and realigned in a more palmar/plantar direction before it is advanced again distally. Excessive horizontal (axial) orientation of the arthroscopic sleeve can also result in penetration of the digital flexor tendon sheath. In this event the sleeve should be withdrawn and the arthroscope replaced by the conical obturator, before the cannula is advanced again with a more abaxial and distal trajectory.

An instrument portal can be created using a similar technique on the contralateral side of the limb following a trajectory established by prior insertion of a 1.2- × 90-mm (18-gauge × 3.5-inch) stiletted spinal needle. The trajectory of the arthroscope, with the direct approach, offers much improved evaluation of the middle and distal portions of the navicular bursa (see Fig. 13-26B and Fig. 13-27) compared with the transthecal technique. However, it is inferior in examining the proximal bursal cul-de-sac when the T ligament is resected with the transthecal approach (Figs. 13-21B, 13-24I, and Fig. 13-28C and G).

Haupt & Caron (2010) compared direct and transthecal approaches in cadaver forelimbs. Using the direct approach, the navicular bursa was successfully entered at the first attempt in 12 of 16 limbs. These authors determined that an average of

approximately 60% of the medial lateral width of the bursa could be assessed from a single portal. Iatrogenic penetration of the distal interphalangeal joint occurred in five limbs, either during entry or during surgical manipulation. The transthecal approach resulted in the entry of navicular bursa in all 16 limbs, although in 7 there was unintentional penetration of the distal interphalangeal joint during dissection of the T ligament. The authors estimated that 80% of the width of the bursa is visible using this technique. This is not correct. Width assessment is determined by the size of the communication created through the T ligament. If this is extended to the suspensory ligaments of the navicular bone (ligamenta sesamoidea collaterale), then the whole mediolateral width can be accessed from a single arthroscopic portal.

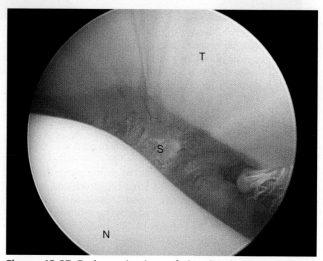

Figure 13-27 Endoscopic view of the distal navicular bursa using the direct approach. *N*, Smooth fibrocartilage covered palmar surface of the navicular bone; *S*, villous synovium between the DDFT and impar ligament; *T*, deep digital flexor tendon.

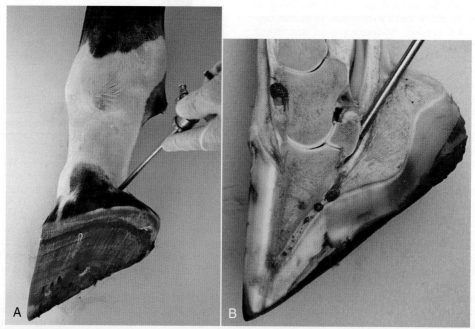

Figure 13-26 The direct approach to the navicular bursa demonstrated on cadaver limbs. **A,** Position of the arthroscopic portal at the proximal margin of the collateral cartilage adjacent to the dorsal surface deep digital flexor tendon. **B,** Arthroscope introduced into the navicular bursa demonstrating direct trajectory and position of the arthroscope permitting evaluation of the distal two thirds of the navicular bursa.

The authors' conclusion that iatrogenic damage to bursal surfaces is reduced by the transthecal approach appears valid.

LESIONS OF THE DEEP DIGITAL FLEXOR TENDON

Smith & Wright (2012) reported transthecal endoscopic evaluation of aseptic navicular bursae in the forelimbs of 114 lame horses. Lesions were identified in 92 horses (105 bursae). These involved a variety of skeletally mature nonracing horses. Seventy nine (86%) were affected unilaterally. In 71 (68%) limbs there were no significant radiologic abnormalities. Ultrasonography demonstrated abnormalities in 13 of 41 (32%) legs. Lesions involving the dorsal surface of the DDF tendon were identified in 48 of 55 (87%) legs that underwent MRI (51 low and 4 high field strength) (Figs. 13-24J and 13-28A). Additionally, CT identified disruption of the dorsal surface of the DDF tendon in 7 of 8 (88%) horses in which this was performed. Lesions of the DDF tendon were identified endoscopically in 103 of 105 (98%) bursae. The most common lesions were sagittal tears, which were seen in 87 (83%) bursae; 24 were classified as small and 63 as extensive. All involved the tendon proximal to the navicular bone (with the limb flexed) and extended variable distances distally. Torn tissue was extruded into the bursae and tended to recoil proximally, frequently presenting as a bundle of torn fibers covered by hemorrhage or granulation tissue adjacent to the T ligament (Fig. 13-24F-H and Fig. 13-28B, D, and E). Tears were usually wider proximally and narrowed as they extended distally. Less commonly, extruded torn tendon fibrils were evident along the margins of the tear. Large strands of torn tendon occasionally were found adherent to the T ligament, collateral sesamoidean ligaments, or contralateral lobe of the DDF tendon. Fibrinous synovio-synovio adhesions were occasionally seen.

In all cases the torn tissue was removed. Large granulomatous masses and bundles of torn tendon were sectioned using meniscectomy scissors before removal with arthroscopic rongeurs. Smaller masses and torn fibers at the lesion margins were removed using a motorized synovial resector with suction applied (Figs. 13-24H and I; 13-28F and G). Tears were medial in 36%, lateral in 32%, and both medial and lateral in 31% of bursae. Thirty-eight of 56 (68%) lesions of the DDFT identified endoscopically were correctly predicted by low-field MRI. A further 10 lesions were predicted by MRI but could not be corroborated endoscopically. Low-field MRI predicted 4 of 16 bursae, which contained endoscopically identifiable adhesions.

Follow-up was available for 84 cases at greater than 6 months and 74 horses at greater than 12 months post surgery. Of these 51 (61%) were sound and working with 35 (42%) performing at a level equal or greater than achieved before surgery. Twelve (14%) were performing at lower levels at the owner's choice, and 13 (15%) had been unable

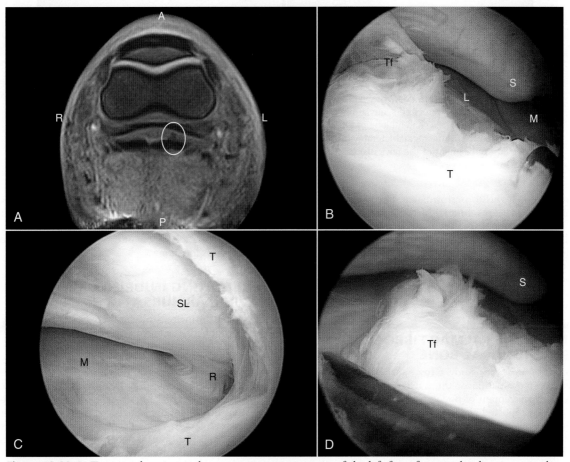

Figure 13-28 A, Transversely orientated magnetic resonance image of the left front foot at a level just proximal to the proximal border of the navicular bone and within the proximal recess of the navicular bursa. This image is from a T2*-weighted gradient echo pulse sequence. Lateral is to the right. There is moderate fluid distension of the navicular bursa and an irregular mass of tissue of intermediate to low signal protruding from the dorsal margin of the lateral lobe of the DDFT (circled). **B,** Tearing of the lateral lobe of the deep digital flexor *(DDF)* tendon visualized from an ipsilateral arthroscopic portal on sectioning the T ligament. **C,** Opening the T ligament medially to the abaxial margin of the navicular bursa. **D,** Organized hemorrhage covering the torn tissue protruding from the lateral lobe of the DDF tendon.

Continued

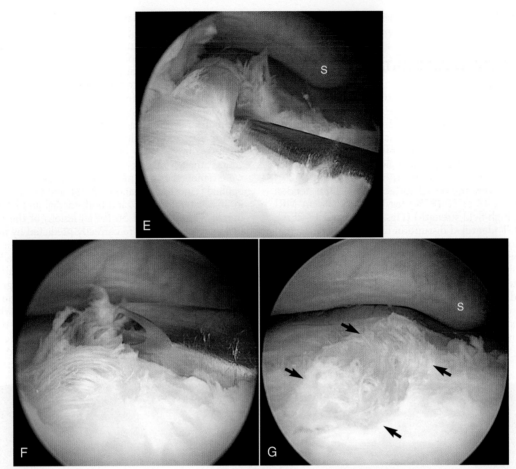

Figure 13-28, cont'd E, Arthroscopic probe penetrating the organized hemorrhage into the DDF tendon tear. **F,** Removal of the torn tissue with a motorized synovial resector. **G,** Appearance of the defect following removal of torn tissue and debridement of the defect. *L*, Lateral lobe of DDFT; *M*, medial lobe of DDFT; *R*, reflection at the bursal margins; exposure indicates that the whole medial-lateral width of the bursa has been evaluated; *S*, sagittal ridge of navicular bone; *SL*, medial suspensory ligament of the navicular bone; *T*, T ligament; *Tf*, torn fibers from DDFT; ➜ = margins of the defect following debridement.

to reach previous levels of performance. Thirty-four horses were classified as failures, but 10 of these were sound and working with additional treatment (8 receiving daily nonsteroidal antiinflammatory drugs and 2 following palmar digital neurectomy). Horses with extensive tears were less likely (56%) to be sound and working compared with those with small tears (82%) and less likely to return to work at their previous levels of performance (34% and 58%, respectively).

LESIONS OF THE PALMAR FIBROCARTILAGE AND SUBCHONDRAL BONE

On the basis of a cadaver study, Cruz et al (2001) suggested that endoscopic evaluation of the navicular bursa might be useful in the management of podotrochlear lesions. Rossignol & Perrin (2003) reported endoscopic evaluation of six horses with lesions involving the palmar fibrocartilage, subchondral bone or both, although no surgical interference was reported. In a further three cases presented later, these authors undertook adhesiolysis and debridement of lesions on the palmar surface of the navicular bone and all three returned to work (Rossignol & Perrin, 2004).

The authors have treated only a few such cases. Access to lesions is feasible with a transthecal approach preferred for lesions in the proximal two thirds of the bursa and a direct approach for lesions in the distal one third. The space for instrument manipulation is limited and demands close control to avoid iatrogenic damage, particularly if curettage is undertaken. There are currently inadequate numbers to provide accurate evaluation of its contribution to the management of lesions in this location.

PENETRATING INJURIES OF THE NAVICULAR BURSA

The general principles of the management of contamination and infection of the navicular bursa are similar to those of other synovial cavities described in Chapter 14. However, at this site there are a number of features that merit particular attention. The most common etiology is a self-sealing solar puncture, which commonly introduces foreign material and causes varying degrees of damage to adjacent structures. The navicular bursa may be punctured by penetrating wounds in the palmar/plantar one half of the solar surface of the foot. The risk and site of bursal penetration are determined by the length of the penetrating object and its trajectory. In order to reach the navicular bursa, there must be a penetrating wound in the DDF tendon and, in some circumstances, perforating objects may continue also proximally through the T ligament and into the digital flexor tendon sheath or, more commonly, distally through the impar ligament and into the distal interphalangeal joint. In a series of 57 horses, 22 had concurrent involvement of the distal interphalangeal joint and 3 had

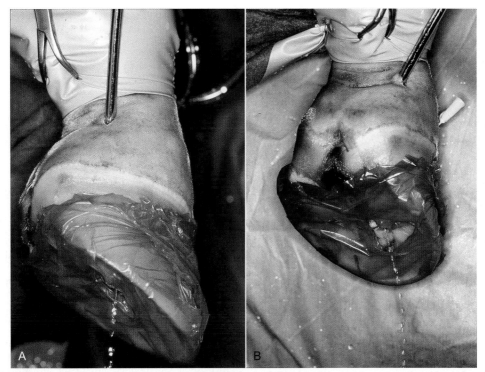

Figure 13-29 A and **B,** Direct approach to the navicular bursa following a penetrating wound just lateral to the apex of the frog.

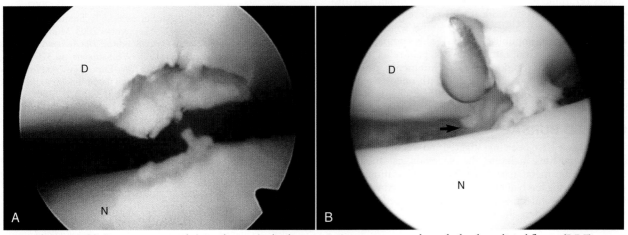

Figure 13-30 Puncture wounds into the navicular bursa. A, Acute puncture through the deep digital flexor *(DDF)* tendon with a full-thickness defect in the adjacent navicular fibrocartilage. **B,** Probe introduced through a penetrating wound in the DDF tendon with adjacent puncture of the impar ligament (➔). *D,* Deep digital flexor tendon, *N,* navicular bone.

penetration of the digital flexor sheath (Wright & Smith, unpublished data).

The bursa is evaluated using the direct approach described earlier. In acute cases, there may be drainage of fluid from the puncture as soon as the bursa is inflated (Fig. 13-29). Thorough evaluation of the bursa should be performed in all cases to include identification of the puncture wound (Fig. 13-30) and detection of foreign material (Fig. 13-31). In 57 cases the puncture wound was identified and accessed in 53 (93%), and there was intrathecal foreign material in 14 (25%) horses. Penetrating objects may produce defects in the navicular fibrocartilage and underlying palmar/plantar subchondral bone. Instruments are generally introduced through the penetrating wound (see Fig. 13-30B). From this site, removal of foreign material and pannus together with debridement of

contaminated and infected tissues may be performed following the principles described in Chapter 14. The DDF tendon is debrided by rotating a motorized synovial resector around its circumference while suction is applied.

If necessary, the palmar/plantar compartment of the distal interphalangeal joint and the digital flexor tendon sheath can be evaluated and treated by redirecting the arthroscopic cannula, with a conical obturator in situ from the same skin portal. The dorsal compartment of the distal interphalangeal joint is approached in a conventional manner. In some cases, it can be useful to introduce the arthroscopic sleeve using a conical obturator into the puncture tract in order that this can be assessed arthroscopically for the presence of foreign material, devitalized tissue, or both, that may not have been recognized from an intrathecal location.

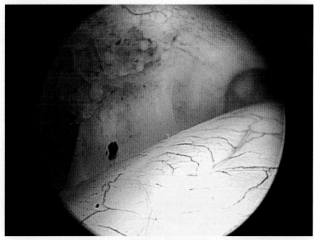

Figure 13-31 Small pieces of wood lodged in the proximal recess of the navicular bursa following a distal penetrating wound.

At the end of the procedure, arthroscopic and/or instrument skin portals are closed routinely. Unless there is undermining of laminar tissues, solar punctures receive minimal debridement before the foot is enclosed in a counterpressure bandage. Of the 16 cases reported originally (Wright et al, 1999) 10 (63%) became sound and returned to a preinjury level of performance. This was later expanded to 15 of 27 (55%) horses (Wright, 2002) and has now been updated to 30 of 56 (54%) of horses returning to preinjury levels of performance. A further 9 horses were able to work at a lower level, 4 were usable following neurectomy, 5 were retired, and 8 were destroyed (Wright and Smith, unpublished data). This compares favorably in terms of survival, return to work, pain relief, reduced postoperative nursing and medical requirements, period of hospitalization, and complication rate with open "streetnail" surgical techniques (Honnas et al, 1995; Richardson et al, 1986; Steckel et al, 1989) and is now the treatment of choice.

ACQUIRED BURSAE

Acquired bursae have been investigated and treated endoscopically at several sites, including the olecranon, calcaneus, and proximal plantar metatarsus. In each of these locations aetiologic tissue tearing has been identified and removed with good clinical responses. Infective processes are managed in accord with the principles described in Chapter 14.

REFERENCES

Adams MN, Turner TA: Endoscopy of the intertubercular bursa in horses, *J Am Vet Med Assoc* 214:221–225, 1999.
Arnold CE, Chaffin MK, Honnas CM, Walker MA, Heite WK: Diagnosis and surgical management of a subchondral bone cyst within the intermediate tubercle of the humerus in a horse, *Equine Vet Educ* 20:310–315, 2008.
Bassage II LH, Garcia-Lopez J, Gurrid EM: Osteolytic lesions of the tuber calcanei in two horses, *J Am Vet Med Assoc* 217:710–716, 2000.
Crabill MR, Chaffin MK, Schmitz DG: Ultrasonographic morphology of the bicipital tendon and bursa in clinically normal Quarter Horses, *Am J Vet Res* 56:5–10, 1995.

Cruz AM, Pharr JW, Bailey JV, Barber SM, Fretz PB: Podotrochlear bursa endoscopy in the horse: A cadaver study, *Vet Surg* 30:539–545, 2001.
Dyce KM, Sack WO, Wensing CJG: The hindlimb of the horse. In *Textbook of Veterinary Anatomy*, ed 2, Philadelphia, 1996, WB Saunders, pp 611–630.
Haupt JL, Caron JP: Navicular bursoscopy in the horse: A comparative study, *Vet Surg* 39:742–747, 2010.
Honnas CM, Crabill MR, Mackie JT, Yarbrough TB, Schumacher J: Use of autogenous cancellous bone grafting in the treatment of septic navicular bursitis and distal sesamoid osteomyelitis in horses, *J Am Vet Med Ass* 206:1191–1194, 1995.
Ingle-Fehr JE, Baxter GM: Endoscopy of the calcaneal bursa in horses, *Vet Surg* 27:561–567, 1998.
Little D, Redding WR, Gerard MP: Osseous cyst-like lesions of the lateral intertubercular groove of the proximal humerus: A report of 5 cases, *Equine Vet Educ* 21:60–66, 2009.
Müller F: Schleimbeutel und Sebnenscheiden des Pferdes, *Arch wiss prackt Tierheilk* 70:351–370, 1936.
Ottaway CW, Worden AN: Bursae and tendon sheaths of the horse, *Vet Rec* 52:477–483, 1940.
Pasquet H, Coudry V, Denoix J- M: Ultrasonographic examination of the proximal tendon of the biceps brachii: Technique and reference images, *Equine Vet Educ* 20:331–336, 2008.
Post EM, Singer ER, Clegg PD: An anatomic study of the calcaneal bursae in the horse, *Vet Surg* 36:3–9, 2007.
Ramzan PHL: Osseous cyst-like lesion of the intermediate humeral tubercle of a horse, *Vet Rec* 154:534–536, 2004.
Richardson GL, O'Brien TR, Pascoe JR, Meagher DM: Puncture wounds of the navicular bursa in 38 horses: A retrospective study, *Vet Surg* 15:156–160, 1986.
Rossignol F, Perrin R: Tenoscopy of the navicular bursa: Endoscopic approach and anatomy, *J Equine Vet Sci* 23:258–265, 2003.
Rossignol F, Perrin R. Navicular bursoscopy: Technique and results. In *12th ESVOT Congress*, 10–12th September 2004, Munich, 180–182.
Sisson S: Equine myology. In Getty R, editor: *The Anatomy of Domestic Animals*, ed 5, Philadelphia, 1975, WB Saunders, pp 376–453.
Smith MRW, Wright IM, Smith RKW: Endoscopic assessment and treatment of lesions of the deep digital flexor tendon in the navicular bursa of 20 lame horses, *Equine Vet J* 39:18–24, 2007.
Smith MRW, Wright IM: Endoscopic evaluation of the navicular bursa; observations, treatment and outcome in 93 cases with identified pathology, *Equine Vet J* 44:339–345, 2012.
Spadari A, Spinella G, Romagnoli N, Valentini S: Rupture of the lateral lobe of the biceps brachii tendon in an Arabian horse, *Vet Comp Orthop Traumatol* 22:253–255, 2009.
Steckel RR, Fessler JF, Huston LC: Deep puncture wounds of the equine hoof: A review of 50 cases, *Proc Am Assoc Equine Pract* 35:167, 1989.
Tnibar MA, Auer JA, Bakkali S: Ultrasonography of the equine shoulder: Technique and normal appearance, *Vet Radiol Ultrasound* 40:44–57, 1999.
Tudor RA, Bowman KF, Redding WR, Tomlinson JC: Endoscopic treatment of suspected infectious intertubercular bursitis in a horse, *J Am Vet Med Assoc* 213:1584–1585, 1998.
Wright IM, Phillips TJ, Walmsley JP: Endoscopy of the navicular bursa: A new technique for the treatment of contaminated and septic bursae, *Equine Vet* 31:5–11, 1999.
Wright IM: Endoscopy in the management of puncture wounds to the foot, *Proc Eur Coll Vet Surg* 11:107–108, 2002.
Wright IM, Minshall GJ: Injuries of the calcaneal insertions of the superficial digital flexor tendon in 19 horses, *Equine Vet J* 44:136–142, 2011.

CHAPTER 14

Endoscopic Surgery in the Management of Contamination and Infection of Joints, Tendon Sheaths, and Bursae

Diarthrodial joints, tendon sheaths, and bursae are closed spaces with a similar mesenchymal synovial lining that produces and maintains a selective physical, cellular, and biochemical environment. The principles of synovial contamination and infection are similar for each of these cavities. Contamination results from the introduction of microorganisms and can occur through open wounds or self-sealing punctures, by hematogenous spread, local extension of a perisynovial infection, or iatrogenically. Open wounds and self-sealing punctures may also introduce foreign material. In humans, bacterial inoculation is more commonly hematogenous than direct (Mathews & Coakley, 2008); although this holds true in equine neonates, the reverse applies in all other horses.

Low fluid shear conditions in synovial cavities and influx of host matrix proteins both promote bacterial adherence (García-Arias et al, 2011; Shirtliff and Mader, 2002). Infection follows when the microorganisms reproduce and colonize the synovial cavity. The principal potentiating factors for establishing infection are considered to be the presence of foreign material or devitalized tissue, or both; the nature and number of contaminating organisms; and immunologic compromise, particularly in young animals. Following colonization of the synovium, a combination of bacterial pathogenicity and host-immune response leads to the release of a variety of enzymes and free radicals, which result in massive inflammation and ultimately destruction of the tissues in the synovial cavity. The acute inflammatory response following inoculation of microorganisms is characterized by a rapid influx of inflammatory cells, predominately neutrophils (Bertone & McIlwraith, 1987). A plethora of destructive enzymes has been detected in synovial fluid from infected joints, including collagenase, caseinase, lysozyme, elastase, cathepsin G, and gelatinase (Palmer & Bertone, 1994; Spiers et al, 1994). These appear to originate both from invading neutrophils and activated synoviocytes. Together with other inflammatory mediators, such as eicosanoids, interleukins, and tumor necrosis factor (Bertone et al, 1993), and the disturbed synovial environment in joints, these trigger production of degradative enzymes by chondrocytes (such as stromelysin, aggrecanase, collagenase, and gelatinase). There is also reduced proteoglycan synthesis (Palmer & Bertone, 1994). The effusion generated by infection increases intraarticular pressure, which in turn reduces tissue perfusion and further compromises synovium and cartilage (García-Aria et al, 2011).

Established infection frequently results in the production of an intrasynovial fibrinocellular conglomerate (pannus). This may cover foreign material and devitalized tissue and act as a nidus for bacterial multiplication; it is rich in inflammatory cells, degradative enzymes, and free radicals. It is also a barrier to synovial membrane diffusion, thus compromising further intrasynovial nutrition and limiting access for circulating antimicrobial drugs. The quantity and nature of pannus appear to be dependent on the type and number of infecting organisms, and its production is also enhanced by the presence of foreign material. Its presence has been associated with increasing duration of clinical signs, presence of osteochondral lesions, and presence of osteomyelitis (Wright et al, 2003).

The objectives in treating contamination and infection are similar for all synovial structures: removal of foreign material, debridement of contaminated/infected and devitalized tissue, elimination of microorganisms, removal of destructive enzymes and free radicals, promotion of tissue healing, and restoration of a normal synovial environment. A number of techniques that include use of drains (Jackman et al, 1989), through-and-through lavage (Koch, 1979; Wereszka et al, 2007), open surgery (Baxter, 1996; Bertone et al, 1992; Chan et al, 2000; Honnas et al, 1991a; Rose & Love, 1979; Schneider et al, 1992a), and endoscopy (Bertone et al, 1992; Carmalt & Wilson, 2005; Fraser & Bladon, 2004; Frees et al, 2002; McIlwraith, 1983; Wright et al, 1999, 2003; Wereszka et al, 2007) have been described. Variations of these techniques have also been described. These include open surgery followed by insertion of closed suction (McIlwraith, 1983) or open passive (Santschi et al, 1997) drains or by open drainage (Bertone et al, 1992; Schneider et al, 1992a) and endoscopy followed by closed suction drainage (LaPointe et al, 1992; Ross et al, 1991), continuous closed irrigation-suction systems (Kuo et al, 2011), fenestrated drains (Honnas et al, 1991b), or creation of an open draining wound (Bertone, 1999).

In all species, delayed or suboptimal management leads to permanent disability and all authors agree that prompt removal of purulent material is important (García-Arias et al, 2011; Mathews & Coakley, 2008; Wright & Scott, 1989). In treating joint infection in humans, arthroscopy is considered to offer several advantages over lavage and arthrotomy, including improved visualization, identification of foreign material and infected or devitalized tissue, and access to a larger area of synovial surfaces (Dory & Wantelet, 1985; Jackson, 1985; Kuo et al, 2011; Parisien & Shaffer, 1990). Arthroscopy is reported to ensure an efficiently evaluated, cleaned, debrided, and decompressed joint with minimal morbidity, reduced period of hospitalization, and maximal functional recovery compared with other treatments (Bussière & Beaufils 1999; Ivey & Clark, 1985; Jarrett et al, 1981; Parisien & Shaffer, 1990; Skyhar & Mubarak, 1987; Smith, 1986; Stutz et al, 2000; Thiery, 1989; Vispo Seara et al, 2002; Wirtz et al, 2001).

Four stages of joint infection have been reported in man (Gächter, 1985, cited by Stutz et al, 2000):
- Stage I: turbid fluid, hyperemic synovium, possible petechial bleeding, no radiologic changes
- Stage II: severe inflammation, fibrinous deposition, purulent fluid, no radiologic changes
- Stage III: thickening of the synovial membrane, villous adhesions and compartment formation, no radiologic changes
- Stage IV: aggressive pannus with infiltration of the cartilage, possibly undermined cartilage, radiologic signs of subchondral osteolysis, possible osseous erosions, and cysts

These stages are related to but do not follow precisely temporal categorization. Vispo Seara et al (2002) adopted this classification and recommended the following arthroscopic treatment protocols for each category:
- Stage I: thorough irrigation of all joint compartments
- Stage II: removal of fibrin and clots, sometimes also with a limited synovectomy followed by I (earlier)

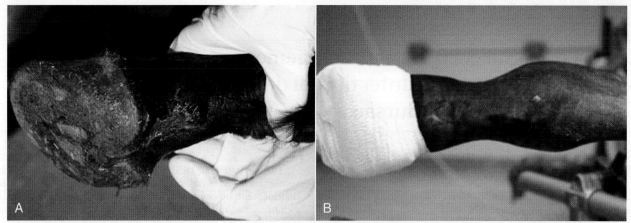

Figure 14-1 Penetrating wound into a hindlimb digital flexor tendon sheath. **A,** At presentation. **B,** Horse positioned in lateral recumbency with the affected limb uppermost and foot enclosed in a sterile wrap in order to permit circumferential access to the sheath.

- Stage III: as II, but with resection of adhesions and subtotal synovectomy
- Stage IV: as earlier but including removal of detached cartilage and debridement of osseous lesions

The Gächter classification has correlated with functional results (Yanmiş et al, 2009). Stutz et al (2000) and Vispo Seara et al (2002) also reported correlation between the stage of the disease process, prognosis, and the number of arthroscopic procedures required. Like all attempts to categorize clinical disease, this classification suffers from oversimplification. Nonetheless, it provides a useful comparative guide.

When an open synovial cavity is encountered or intrasynovial foreign material is detected within, then no other diagnostic tests are necessary to establish the presence of contamination or infection. In the absence of these, a number of features are important but none should be seen as diagnostically exclusive. These include synovial fluid white cell count (WCC) and protein content for which widely varying guidelines have been reported and limitations identified (Dykgraaf et al, 2007; Frees et al, 2002; Madison et al, 1991; Mathews et al, 2007; Trumble, 2005; Wereszka et al, 2007). In addition to radiologic features indicating osseous involvement, radiographic examination can also reveal the presence of gas, soft tissue swelling and elimination of fat pad shadows, presence of radiodense foreign material, and other features consistent with contamination and infection. Ultrasonography can identify distended synovial cavities and provide valuable information regarding the nature of their content. In the acute phase, affected fluid can be anechoic, but as protein and cellular levels increase, it becomes increasingly echoic. Similarly, there will be thickening and proliferation of synovium, frequently with irregular adventitious intrathecal strands. Later, fibrous capsules will also become involved. Ultrasonography is also the most sensitive modality for detection of intrathecal and perithecal foreign material, and careful examination of all synovial cavities that are accompanied by open wounds or punctures is critical. This can, particularly in the acute phase, be confounded by the presence of intrathecal and perithecal air. Ultrasonography will also provide a valuable preoperative guide to the presence of concurrent soft tissue injuries or compromise, or both. When there is extensive perisynovial soft tissue swelling, ultrasonography also can provide a valuable guide for synoviocentesis.

It is salutary that a systematic review of the literature on the management of suspected infected joints in man concluded that the most reliable standard for diagnosis was "the

level of clinical suspicion of a physician experienced in the diagnosis and management of rheumatic disease" (Mathews et al, 2007).

TECHNIQUES

Evaluation

Most contaminated and infected synovial cavities are amenable to endoscopic evaluation and surgery. Occasionally, there will be sufficient capsular disruption to preclude inflation but in some individuals, even if there is marked tissue loss on one aspect of the limb, other synovial compartments may be treated endoscopically. In most cases, even when there are substantial defects, sufficient inflation can usually be achieved with high fluid flow rates to effectively evaluate and treat the cavity. The absence of adequate synovial space precludes the use of endoscopy in few sites, the most frequently affected examples being the centrodistal (distal intertarsal) and tarsometatarsal joints.

Endoscopy is performed under general anesthesia, and the patient should be positioned to permit all-round access to the affected synovial cavity(ies) (Fig. 14-1). Esmarch bandages and tourniquets are recommended for distal limbs. Generally, there is a greater degree of inflammation and soft tissue involvement than in other endoscopic procedures and control of hemorrhage improves the efficiency of the procedures significantly.

In most cases, initial evaluation of the synovial cavity is made utilizing standard endoscopic portals as described in preceding chapters. It is important in all circumstances to evaluate fully each structure and thus to use all available portals, examining dorsal and palmar/plantar or cranial and caudal compartments, and also, whenever appropriate, evaluating each cavity from both medial and lateral sides. If a tourniquet is used, the surgeon should take particular care in the creation of portals (especially into the digital flexor tendon sheath) because neurovascular bundles are less readily appreciated and iatrogenic damage is possible.

An initial lavage of the cavity is usually necessary in order to clear discolored synovial fluid. A thorough systematic evaluation should follow, examining the whole intrasynovial environment and, in turn, all of the contained structures. Particular attention should be paid to the vicinity of wounds (Fig. 14-2).

Acute synovial infection is characterized endoscopically by marked synovial hyperemia (Fig. 14-3). This is followed by villous enlargement and proliferation (Fig. 14-4). In cases with more established infection, villi can appear in areas that are

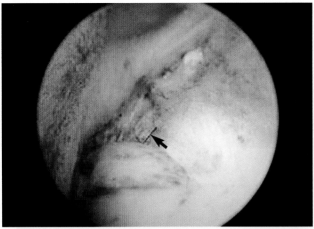

Figure 14-2 Acute penetrating wound into a forelimb digital flexor tendon sheath resulting from an "interference" injury during racing. Hair *(arrow)* is visible protruding through the wound into the sheath lumen.

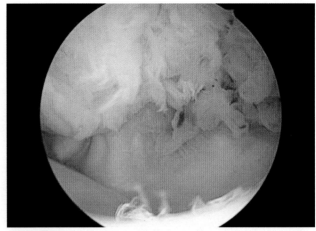

Figure 14-4 Swollen and proliferative villi in the palmar pouch of an infected metacarpophalangeal joint.

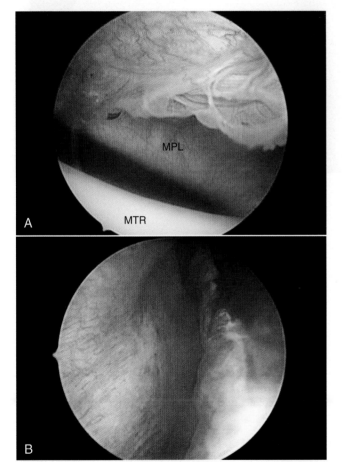

Figure 14-3 Hyperaemia associated with acute synovial infection. **A,** Femoropatellar joint of a foal. *MPL,* Medial patellar ligament; *MTR,* medial trochlear ridge of femur. **B,** Proximal digital flexor tendon sheath following a penetrating wound.

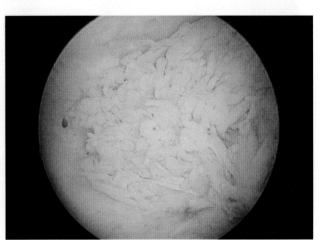

Figure 14-5 Proliferation of short blunt villi distally in the intertrochlear groove of the talus in a tarsocrural joint with longstanding infection.

intact, chronic tenosynovitis is characterized by synovial proliferation and adhesion formation, whereas if it is disrupted there is usually rapid intratendinous collagenolysis (Fig. 14-7). The features of chronic infective bursitis are similar to both infected arthritis and tenosynovitis.

Pannus is usually identified first over areas of villous synovium and, as it increases in mass, villi become obscured (Fig. 14-8A). If the infective process continues, pannus will also cover avillous synovium and in some advanced cases it also covers articular cartilage and tendon surfaces (Fig. 14-8B).

Foreign Material

In the presence of open wounds or self-sealing punctures, the surgeon should be aware of the potential presence of foreign material within the synovial cavity. Frees et al (2002) found intrasynovial foreign material in 4/20 (20%) of tenoscopically investigated wounds involving the digital flexor tendon sheath, whereas Wright et al (2003) documented foreign material in 41 of 95 (43%) horses with wounds or punctures into synovial cavities that were investigated endoscopically. In the latter series, foreign material was predicted preoperatively in only 15% of animals (Fig. 14-9). The majority are free floating, but the foreign material may also be adherent to pannus or synovium, embedded in osteochondral lesions

normally devoid of such (Fig. 14-5). In the absence of osteochondral defects, chronic joint infection is characterized by cartilage degeneration, but if subchondral bone is breached, then infected osteitis/osteomyelitis may result. Subchondral bone can also sequestrate (Fig. 14-6) and can be both the cause of or result from an infected joint. If the epitenon is

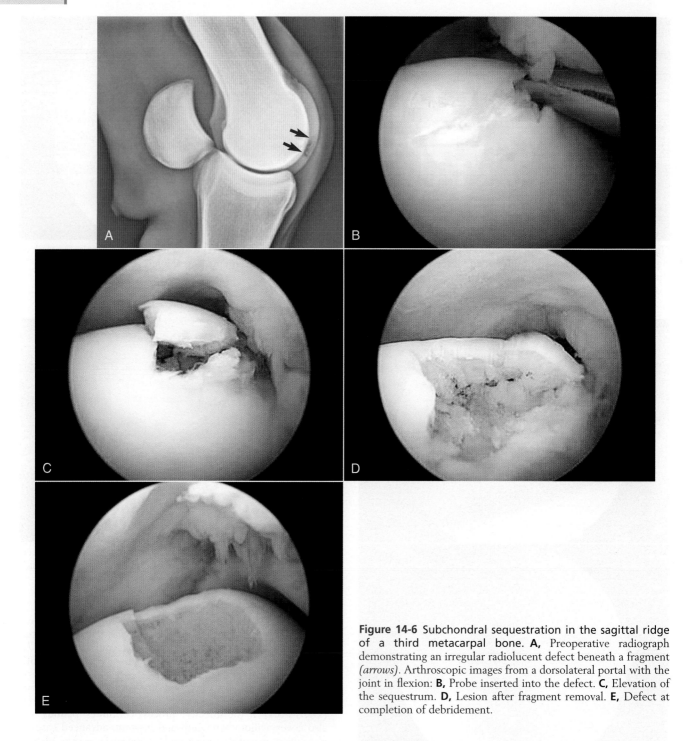

Figure 14-6 Subchondral sequestration in the sagittal ridge of a third metacarpal bone. **A,** Preoperative radiograph demonstrating an irregular radiolucent defect beneath a fragment *(arrows).* Arthroscopic images from a dorsolateral portal with the joint in flexion: **B,** Probe inserted into the defect. **C,** Elevation of the sequestrum. **D,** Lesion after fragment removal. **E,** Defect at completion of debridement.

or found in penetrating wounds. The most common contaminants are hair and wood (Fig. 14-10). An association has been demonstrated in man between the presence of foreign material and the development of infected synovitis following penetrating wounds (Reginato et al, 1990). Foreign material acts as a nidus for and is a potent perpetuator of infection. It also causes physical and biochemical irritation within the synovial environment. Meticulous evaluation of the whole synovial cavity is imperative when there is a wound or puncture because foreign material (including hair), often in small pieces, can migrate anywhere. Large pieces may be removed with Ferris-Smith rongeurs, small pieces by a motorized synovial resector, and if embedded in bone, curettes may be necessary.

Debridement

In the series reported by Wright et al (2003), 51 of 121 (42%) horses had endoscopically identifiable osseous or chondral lesions, of which only 25 (49%) were predicted before endoscopy. Fragmentation may be removed with rongeurs. Foreign material may be embedded in the fracture bed, and debridement of contaminated or infected fracture sites is invariably appropriate. Foci of osteitis/osteomyelitis are generally debulked with rongeurs before debridement with curettes (Fig. 14-11). Motorized burrs are rarely indicated. When debriding chondral or osteochondral defects in bursae, the surgeon should be cognizant that fibrocartilagenous margins will invariably be less well defined than their hyaline counterparts in diarthrodial joints (Fig. 14-12).

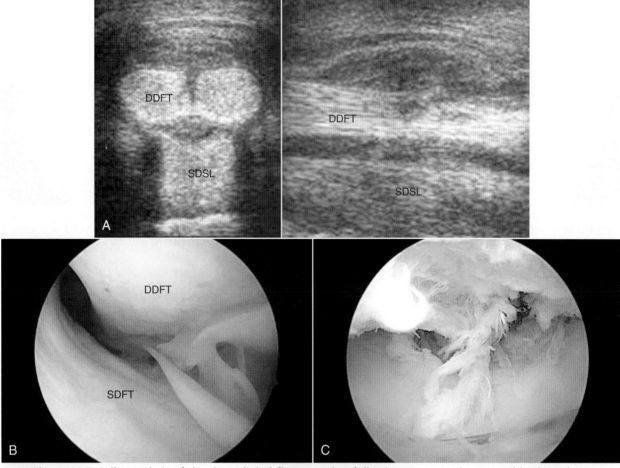

Figure 14-7 Collagenolysis of the deep digital flexor tendon following a penetrating wound in the palmar pastern. **A,** Transverse and longitudinal ultrasonographs. **B,** Strands of purulent material extending from the lesion **C,** Lesion following removal of overlying pannus revealing marked loss of infrastructure with no recognizable organization. *DDFT,* Deep digital flexor tendon; *SDFT,* isthmus of superficial digital flexor tendon; *SDSL,* straight distal sesamoidean ligament.

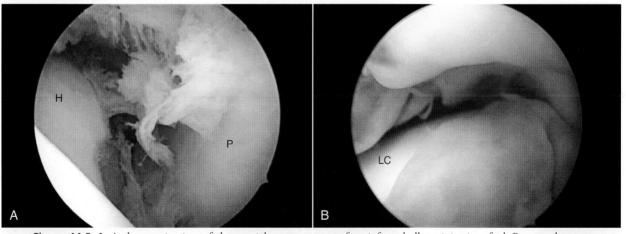

Figure 14-8 A, Arthroscopic view of the cranial compartment of an infected elbow joint in a foal. Pannus obscures entirely the villous synovium of the cranial joint capsule. *H,* Medial condyle of humerus; *P,* pannus. **B,** Dorsal aspect of a chronically infected metacarpophalangeal joint with organized pannus covering the entire dorsal synovium and extending over the lateral condyle *(LC)* of the third metacarpal bone.

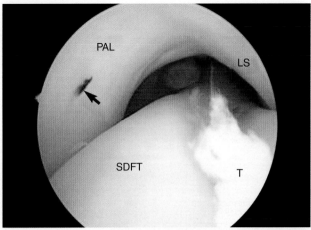

Figure 14-9 Penetration of a forelimb digital flexor tendon sheath by a thorn, which was not identified preoperatively. *Arrow,* thorn; *LS,* lateral proximal sesamoid bone; *PAL,* palmar annular ligament; *SDFT,* superficial digital flexor tendon; *T,* tendon laceration.

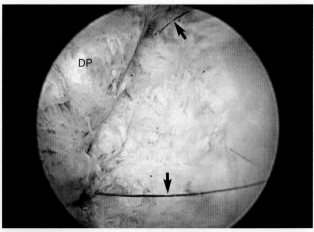

Figure 14-10 Puncture wound into the dorsal metacarpophalangeal joint adjacent to the dorsal plica *(DP)* depositing hair *(arrows)* and particulate debris into the joint.

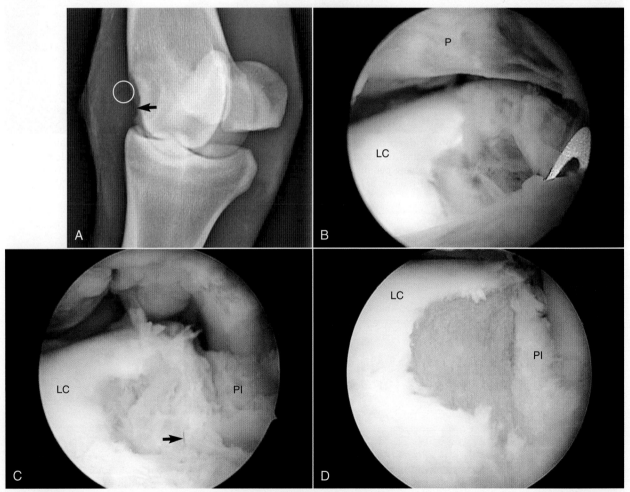

Figure 14-11 Infected osteitis of the lateral condyle of the third metatarsal bone following a penetrating wound into the metatarsophalangeal joint. **A,** Dorsomedial-plantarolateral oblique radiograph demonstrating displaced fragments (circled) proximal to the lesion *(arrow).* **B,** Arthroscopic appearance of the defect in the lateral condyle of the third metatarsal bone before debridement. **C,** Defect in the lateral condyle of the third metatarsal bone after debulking with rongeurs. **D,** Lesion at the end of debridement. *LC,* Lateral condyle of third metatarsal bone; *P,* pannus overlying dorsal synovium; *arrow,* hair embedded in the defect; *Pl,* abaxial plica.

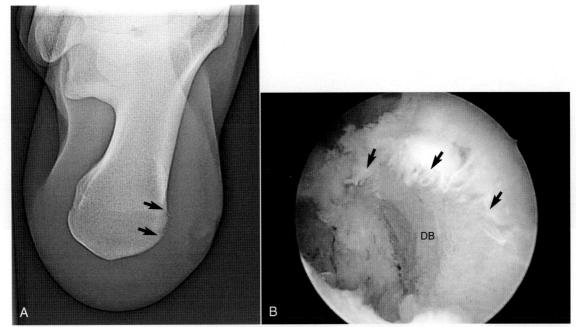

Figure 14-12 Focus of infected osteitis of the calcaneus. **A,** Flexed plantaroproximal-plantarodistal oblique projection demonstrating soft tissue swelling consistent with distension of the calcaneal bursae and irregular osteolysis proximolaterally in the calcaneus *(arrows)*. **B,** Arthroscopic image following lesion debridement. *DB,* Debrided bone; arrows, irregular fibrocartilage margin.

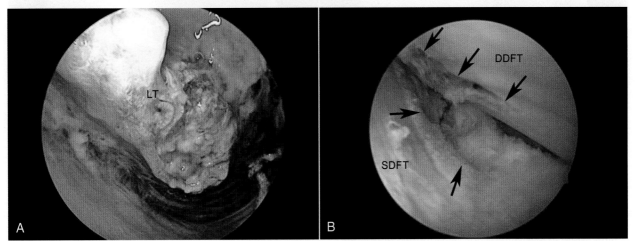

Figure 14-13 Laceration of the superficial digital flexor tendon within the forelimb digital flexor tendon sheath illustrated in Figure 14-2. **A,** Protrusion of lacerated tendon tissue into the sheath lumen *(LT)*. **B,** Lesions in the superficial digital flexor tendon *(SDFT)* and deep digital flexor tendon *(DDFT)* following debridement. Arrows, debrided lesions.

Penetrating wounds and punctures of tendon sheaths and bursae may result in defects in the associated tendons (Fig. 14-13A), and frequently articular wounds will also traumatize periarticular ligaments; an incidence of 34% has been documented (Wright et al, 2003). Removal of detached contaminated and infected tissue is appropriate and may be achieved with a motorized synovial resector (Fig. 14-13B). Occasionally, discrete detached pieces of tendon or ligament are removed more satisfactorily by sharp dissection using arthroscopic scissors or knives.

Piecemeal removal of pannus with rongeurs preserves underlying synovium. This can be time consuming but whenever possible is the technique of choice (Fig. 14-14). When pannus is widespread, use of a motorized synovial resector may be required, although this almost invariably results in at least partial synovial resection. The authors' preference in

motorized resectors, for safety and efficiency, is an enclosed, serrated blade (Fig. 14-15A). This is used in oscillating mode with suction applied to draw material into the blade. Angled blades are also available and can be useful in some areas. Sometimes pannus can be stripped from synovium with suction applied to an open resector sleeve without engaging the blades (Fig. 14-15B). Intermittent blade movement is necessary to clear the apparatus, but this technique can help to preserve synovium.

It is suggested that synovium may harbor bacteria, sequester inflammatory cells, release potent inflammatory mediators, and be a source of immunologic components of inflammation (Riegels-Nielson et al, 1991; Riegels-Nielson & Jensen, 1984). Synovectomy has therefore been proposed to be of benefit in treating infected arthritis (Bertone et al, 1992; Ross et al, 1991), although some surgeons consider its use should be limited

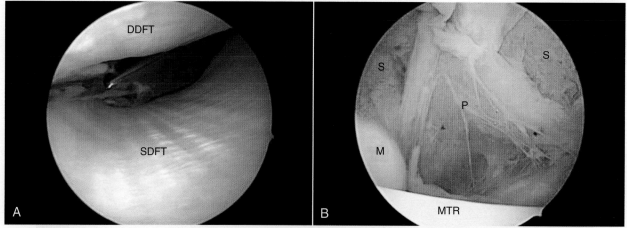

Figure 14-14 Piecemeal removal of pannus with arthroscopic rongeurs. **A,** Retrieval of pannus from between the superficial *(SDFT)* and deep *(DDFT)* digital flexor tendons in the proximal digital flexor tendon sheath. **B,** Dorsal aspect of the tarsocrural joint in a foal in which pannus has been partially removed piecemeal with rongeurs illustrating the synovial-sparing effect. *M,* Medial malleolus of tibia; *MTR,* medial trochlear ridge of talus; *P,* pannus; *S,* villous synovium in the regions from which pannus has been removed.

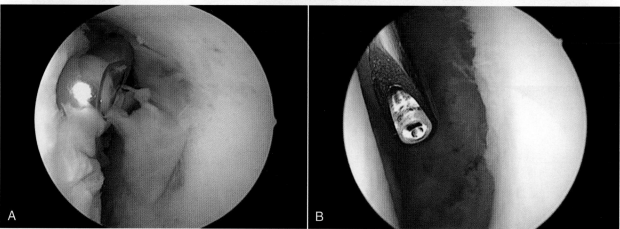

Figure 14-15 Removal of pannus with a motorized synovial resector. **A,** Suction applied to draw pannus into the resector blades. **B,** Open resector sleeve used to remove pannus by suction alone.

(Parisien & Shaffer, 1990). The authors generally remove contaminated/infected synovium that is adjacent to wounds and punctures. More extensive resection is performed in the presence of marked pannus deposits, which are usually associated with long-standing infective processes. Regeneration of normal villous synovium does not occur following synovectomy (Doyle-Jones et al, 2002; Theoret et al, 1996), but the clinical implication of this and potential compromise compared with the benefits of synovectomy have not been determined.

Lavage

Lavage is visually directed, high pressure, and should be performed thoroughly until all areas of the synovial cavity are visibly clean (Gaughan, 1994; Smith, 1986; Thiery, 1989). The fluid of choice is sterile buffered polyionic solution (Baird et al, 1990; Bertone et al, 1987a), and this should be delivered by a pump system capable of rates in excess of 500 mL/min. It is important to move the arthroscope, and thus the fluid ingress, repeatedly to all parts of the cavity in order to produce effective lavage. The surgeon should be aware of all synovial sulci because, without individual attention, fluids will frequently flow over or past pockets of debris in these sites. This is particularly important in tendon sheaths, where, in addition to moving around the tendons, the arthroscope should be insinuated

between these structures. The mechanical action of flushing removes small, free-floating debris; debulks microorganisms; and reduces the load of destructive radicals and enzymes. Lavage is also thought to raise the pH from the acidic environment produced by infective processes. This in turn improves the action of several antimicrobial drugs, including aminoglycosides (McIlwraith, 1983). Effective lavage invariably requires multiple ingress and egress portals. In animals with wounds or punctures, these may also serve as instrument and egress portals.

Potential additives to lavage fluid include antimicrobial drugs, antiseptics, dimethyl sulfoxide, and fibrinolytics. Antimicrobial preparations used by the authors include a combination of sodium benzylpenicillin (2.5×10^6 IU) with gentamicin sulfate (250 mg), or alternatively ceftiofur sodium (500 mg) or amikacin sulfate (500 mg) added to the final liter of lavage fluid. There is no objective evidence to support the use of antimicrobial drugs in this manner, although administration of an aqueous antimicrobial on completion of lavage has been suggested to be of benefit (Nixon, 1990). Antiseptic solutions appear to offer no advantages over buffered polyionic solution (Bertone et al, 1986) and, even in dilute concentrations, may produce synovial irritation (Bertone et al, 1986; Wilson et al, 1994). Dimethyl sulfoxide has been recommended as part of the final lavage (Bertone 1996, 1999; Frees et al, 2002). Its efficacy has not been evaluated experimentally and no demonstrable clinical benefits have been documented, but deleterious effects on equine cartilage matrix metabolism have been reported (Matthews et al, 1998; Smith et al, 2000). Intermittently, the use of fibrinolytics has been mentioned in the human literature (Jackson, 1985), but fibrinolytics are uncommonly employed in veterinary medicine. With the advent of endoscopic removal of fibrinoid deposits, their use largely appears superfluous.

Wound Management

Arthroscope and instrument portals are closed routinely. Traumatic wounds are debrided or (preferably) excised to a clean/contaminated state, and then if possible these are also closed. This is based on the premise that endoscopic surgery can thoroughly cleanse synovial cavities and that a closed wound minimizes the risk of further or secondary contamination or infection, or both. These principles contrast with those of others in the literature (Baxter, 1996; Gibson et al, 1989; Schneider et al, 1992a) who advocate open management of infected synovial cavities in order to maintain decompression. Such alternatives include closed suction drainage (LaPointe et al, 1992; Ross et al, 1991), fenestrated drains (Honnas et al, 1991b), or creation of an open draining wound (Bertone, 1999), techniques that the authors also advocate in cases of chronic recalcitrant infection. Solar punctures are debrided, dressed, and managed as open wounds. Traumatic wounds elsewhere in which soft tissue loss precludes closure should be debrided as rigorously as if closure were to be effected. The wound is then dressed, and the limb immobilized while second intention healing ensues.

When wound healing will be optimized by limb immobilization, casts may be fitted. When possible, counterpressure should be applied to all sites: this limits extravascular exudation of fluid, promotes primary wound healing, and reduces pain (Bertone, 1999; Nixon, 1990). It can be applied effectively to the distal limb with layered compressed cotton wool (as used in constructing a Robert Jones bandage). Commercial, tailored elasticized bandages are effective on the carpus and tarsus, whereas in the proximal limb stent bandages may be oversewn.

Antimicrobial Therapy

Conventional culture and susceptibility testing of synovial fluid can be, and frequently is, unrewarding (Annear et al, 2011; Bertone et al, 1987; Frees et al, 2002; Lescun et al, 2006a; Madison, 1991; Schneider et al, 1992b; Wereszka et al, 2007). Blood culture medium enrichment appears superior to other techniques of bacterial isolation (Dumoulin, 2010). Ideally microbiological samples should be taken before antimicrobial therapy (Bertone et al, 1987; Lescun et al, 2006a), but even in this scenario, empirical treatment is necessary before results are available. There appears to be no difference in culture rates between synovial fluid and membrane (Bertone et al, 1987; Madison et al, 1991), and submission of both together with any recovered pannus is recommended.

Lescun (2011) highlighted the well-recognized clinical dictum that "in vitro bacterial suscepitibility does not equal in vivo antimicrobial efficacy." This is also influenced by bacterial location, tissue perfusion, antimicrobial penetration, presence of foreign material, local environmental conditions, presence of bacterial biofilms, etc. (Clutterbuck et al, 2007; Freeman et al, 2009). Systematic reviews and meta-analysis of antimicrobial use as performed in man (Mathews et al, 2007; Stengel et al, 2001) are not available in the veterinary literature. However, the applicability of such is questionable due to the multiorganism nature of infections that follow traumatic innoculation, which makes monotherapy unlikely to be optimal.

Systemic antimicrobial treatment is necessary in all cases of synovial infection and can be supplemented by local administration techniques. These include direct intrasynovial injection or depots, regional intravenous or intraosseous perfusion, and continuous intrasynovial infusion. All have been shown to achieve local antimicrobial levels in excess of systemic administration (Beccar-Varela et al 2011; Farnsworth et al, 2001; Haerdi-Landerer et al 2010; Lescun et al, 2000; Lescun et al 2006a&b; Meagher et al 2006; Werner et al, 2003; Whitehair et al, 1992b), but their potential contribution has been questioned (Kuo et al, 2011). Meta-analysis in man of antimicrobials used in treating infected joints revealed no clinical or bacteriologic advantage of one therapeutic regimen over another (Stengel et al, 2001). Choices should be made on the basis of the likely etiologic organism(s). This can be modified if clinical response is unsatisfactory, and results of culture and susceptibility suggest viable alternatives.

A contemporary, comprehensive review of antimicrobial alternatives in treating the infected synovial cavity is outwith the scope of this book. When synovial contamination has a hematogenous etiology, single organisms may be responsible for infection. However, horses that develop synovial infection following wounds are likely to have multiple bacterial involvement (Schneider et al, 1992b). Reported bacterial studies and susceptibility patterns suggest that a cephalosporin/aminoglycoside combination is likely to be most efficacious but that most organisms are likely to be susceptible to a synergistic combination of penicillin and an aminoglycoside (Moore et al, 1992; Schneider et al, 1992b; Snyder et al, 1987).

Determination of an appropriate duration of antimicrobial administration is difficult. The authors prioritize clinical signs of response and continue antimicrobial administration until there is a consistent improvement in lameness, together with reduced synovial distension, adjacent soft tissue swelling, surface temperature, and engorgement of visible draining veins and lymphatics. The use of sequential synovial fluid analysis has also been advocated (Bertone, 1999), although in the authors' experiences it has proved inferior to close clinical observation. Largely on the basis of the experiences of experimental joint infection (Bertone et al, 1987b), other authors have employed or recommended protracted administration of antimicrobial drugs (Frees et al 2002; Gaughan, 1994; Gibson et al, 1989; Honnas et al, 1991b). In a review of 121 cases of synovial contamination and infection treated endoscopically, there was a mean period of antimicrobial administration of 13 days (Wright et al, 2003). A shorter period of antimicrobial administration required with arthroscopic treatment of infected joints compared with other techniques has also been reported in man (Smith, 1986).

POSTOPERATIVE CARE

Nonsteroidal antiinflammatory drugs have been advocated in the treatment of synovial infection to provide analgesia and to limit deleterious effects of inflammatory mediators on the synovial environment (Baxter, 1996; Bertone & McIlwraith, 1987; Cook & Bertone, 1998; Gaughan, 1994; Schneider 1999). There is some support for the concept in an experimental rabbit model (Smith et al, 1997). However, in this experiment, the treatment comparisons were only between administration of antimicrobial drugs or administration of antimicrobial and antiinflammatory drugs; there was no surgical decompression or lavage, etc. Evidence that systemically administered therapeutic doses of nonsteroidal antiinflammatory drugs suppress deleterious effects of intrasynovial inflammatory mediators is lacking (May & Lees, 1996). These drugs may partially lessen release of factors involved in joint tissue breakdown (Lee et al, 2003), but administration of nonsteroidal antiinflammatory drugs effectively obviates use of clinical parameters, particularly lameness, in determining response to treatment (Gaughan, 1994; McIlwraith, 1983). Current opinion in assessing potential benefits of postoperative administration of nonsteroidal antiinflammatory drugs is therefore divided. This is reflected in the diversity of clinical use in the authors' practices, although all use nonsteroidal antiinflammatory drugs for provision of perioperative analgesia.

Intermittently, the use of other, adjunctive medicaments have also been recommended, principal of which is postoperative intrasynovial hyaluronan. Benefits have been reported in an experimental model of tarsocrural infection (Brusie et al, 1992), and it has been advocated in clinical cases of infected tenosynovitis (Frees et al, 2002; Gaughan, 1994; Nixon 1990).

Movement is necessary for restoration of a normal synovial environment, and endoscopy permits an early return to exercise (Frees et al, 2002; Nixon, 1990; Vispo Seara, 2002). The association between immobilization and cartilage degeneration has been well documented (Josza et al, 1987; Kallio et al, 1988; Palmoski et al, 1979; Videman, 1981). Benefits from early instigation of exercise, in the form of continuous passive motion, have been demonstrated in experimental models (Salter et al, 1981) and reported in clinical cases in man (Parisien & Shaffer, 1990; Perry et al, 1992). Dynamic loading counteracts effects of inflammatory mediators, such as bacterial lipopolysaccharide, on chondrocyte metabolism, and it is suggested that this may have contributed to successful management of articular infection (Lee et al, 2003). Whenever possible, the authors recommend walking exercise to commence immediately after surgery and a graduated, controlled exercise program follows in line with tissue compromise.

POSTOPERATIVE MONITORING

Close clinical monitoring is critical in the immediate postoperative period. Because most synovial structures will be enclosed in bandages at this time, pain is the most sensitive indicator of response to treatment. In the face of progressive lameness or lack of clinical improvement, complete case reevaluation, including repeated radiographs, ultrasonographs, and synoviocentesis, is always merited. If potential reasons for relapse or lack of response can be identified, then management can be changed in a logical manner. Because endoscopy maximizes intrasynovial evaluation, this is also indicated in recurrent or recalcitrant cases. Repeated endoscopy has proved useful in detecting and removing foreign material, infected bone, and intraarticular sequestra that were not present or identified at the first surgery (Wright et al, 2003). When no satisfactory explanation for a poor response or relapse has been identified, then lack of susceptibility of the causative organisms to the current antimicrobial regimen should be considered and modification is frequently appropriate. It always remains possible that infecting organisms are susceptible but that they have not been exposed to the antimicrobial drugs at an appropriate level; nonetheless, a change in regimen is usually made at this time.

▶ RESULTS AND PROGNOSIS

Results of endoscopic surgery in treating clinical cases of contaminated and infected synovial cavities have been reported by a number of authors (Frees et al, 2002; Fraser & Bladon 2004; Gibson et al, 1989; LaPointe et al, 1992; Ross et al, 1991; Schneider et al, 1992a; Steel et al, 1999; Wereszka et al, 2007; Wright et al, 1999, 2003). Arthroscopy and partial synovial resection were reported to be inferior to arthrotomy and open drainage in the treatment of experimentally induced infection of tarsocrural joints (Bertone et al, 1992). However, this experiment does not reflect many features found in clinical cases of synovial contamination and infection. Arthrotomy was also associated with an increased risk of secondary infection by other organisms and postoperative fibrosis and required a greater degree of postoperative care. The senior

author of this report subsequently recommended endoscopy as a primary line of therapy (Bertone, 1999). Frees et al (2002) reported 18 of 20 (90%) cases surviving and 14 (70%) returning to athletic soundness following tenoscopic treatment of contaminated and infected digital flexor tendon sheaths. A retrospective analysis of 121 cases of contaminated and infected synovial cavities treated endoscopically reported a 90% survival rate, with 81% of animals returning to their preoperative level of performance. Negative prognostic indicators included involvement of the navicular bursa, the presence of marked pannus, and the presence of osteochondral lesions (Wright et al, 2003). Neither of these studies found a correlation between the duration of clinical signs before endoscopy and case outcome. In a comparable series of 192 cases treated by combinations of lavage, open surgery, drainage, intrasynovial antimicrobial drugs, and systemic antimicrobial drugs, 73% of 126 animals older than 6 months of age and 45% of foals younger than 6 months of age survived and 56% of 52 adult horses returned to performance (Schneider et al, 1992b).

Fraser & Bladon (2004) reported tenosocopic treatment of 39 horses with wounds involving a digital flexor tendon sheath. Fifteen of 16 (94%) horses that were devoid of tendon damage returned to their previous use. Twelve of 16 (75%) with concurrent wounds of the superficial digital flexor tendon also returned to preinjury use. In contrast only 1 of 6 animals that lacerated both superficial and deep digital flexor tendons survived. In this study treatment within 36 hours of injury carried a significantly better prognosis for return to work than those that underwent tenoscopy after this time. In a comparative study, Wereszka et al (2007) documented 41 cases of infected digital flexor tendon sheaths in a series of 51 horses with tendon sheath infections. Twenty underwent tenoscopy and 26 received through-and-through needle lavage. Outcome was influenced by the time between injury and treatment with horses treated within 1 day more likely to survive than those that underwent treatment more than 10 days following injury. In this series there was no significant difference in outcome between the two procedures but horses with concurrent tendon damage and/or marked pannus deposits had poorer prognoses. Thirty-seven of 51 (73%) horses survived more than 1 year, and of these 21 (57%) returned to preinjury levels of performance and a further 16 (43%) were able to function at a reduced level.

The authors believe that management of contaminated and infected synovial cavities is optimized by endoscopic treatment. This permits thorough evaluation, with appropriate debridement, effective lavage, and minimal tissue trauma. Multiple synovial cavities may be treated simultaneously, there is early pain relief, few complications, and minimal postoperative care. Animals are able to make an early return to exercise, and the prognosis appears to be better than with other reported regimens.

REFERENCES

Annear MJ, Fuur MO, White NA: Septic arthritis in foals, *Equine Vet Educ* 23:422–431, 2011.

Baird AM, Scruggs DW, Watkins JP, et al.: Effect of antimicrobial solution on the palmar digital tendon sheath in horses, *Am J Vet Res* 51:1488–1494, 1990.

Baxter GM: Instrumentation and techniques for treating orthopaedic infections in horses, *Vet Clin N Am Equine Pract* 12:303–335, 1996.

Beccar-Varela AM, Epstein KL, White CL: Effect of experimentally induced synovitis on amikacin concentrations after intravenous regional limb perfusion, *Vet Surg* 40:891–897, 2011.

Bertone AL: Infectious arthritis. In McIlwraith CW, Trotter GW, editors: *Joint disease in the horse*, Philadelphia, 1996, WB Saunders, pp 397–409.

Bertone AL: Update on infectious arthritis in horses, *Equine Vet Educ* 11:143–152, 1999.

Bertone AL, Davis DM, Cox HU, et al.: Arthrotomy versus arthroscopy and partial synovectomy for treatment of experimentally induced arthritis in horses, *Am J Vet Res* 53:585–591, 1992.

Bertone AL, McIlwraith CW: A review of current concepts in the therapy of infectious arthritis, *Proc Am Asso Equine Pract* 32: 323–339, 1987.

Bertone AL, McIlwraith CW, Jones RL, et al.: Povidone-iodine lavage treatment of experimentally-induced equine infectious arthritis, *Am J Vet Res* 48:712–715, 1987a.

Bertone AL, McIlwraith CW, Jones RL, et al.: Comparison of various treatments for experimentally induced equine infectious arthritis, *Am J Vet Res* 48:519–529, 1987b.

Bertone AL, McIlwraith CW, Powers BE, et al.: Effect of four antimicrobial lavage solutions on the tarsocrural joint in horses, *Vet Surg* 15:305–315, 1986.

Bertone AL, Palmer JL, Jones J: Synovial fluid inflammatory mediators as markers of equine synovitis, *Vet Surg* 22:372–373, 1993.

Brusie RW, Sullins KE, White NA, et al.: Evaluation of sodium hyaluronate therapy in induced septic arthritis in the horse, *Equine Vet J* 11(Suppl):18–23, 1992.

Bussiére F, Beaufils P: Apport de l'arthroscopie au traitement des arthritis septiques à pyogères banals du genom de l'adulte: a propos de 16 cas, *Revue de Chirurgie Orthopédique* 85:803–810, 1999.

Carmalt JL, Wilson DG: Arthroscopic treatment of temporomandibular joint sepsis in a horse, *Vet Surg* 34:55–58, 2005.

Chan CC, Murphy H, Munroe GA: Treatment of chronic digital septic tenosynovitis in 12 horses by modified open annular ligament desmotomy and passive open drainage, *Vet Rec* 147:388–393, 2000.

Clutterbuck AL, Woods EJ, Knottenbelt DC, Clegg PD, Cochrane CA, Percival SL: Biofilms and their relevance to veterinary medicine, *Vet Microbiol* 121:1–17, 2007.

Cook VL, Bertone AL: Infectious arthritis. In White NA, Moore JN, editors: *Current technique in equine surgery and lameness*, ed 2, Philadelphia, 1998, WB Saunders, pp 381–385.

Dory MA, Wantelet MJ: Arthroscopy in septic arthritis, *Arthritis Rheum* 28:198–203, 1985.

Doyle-Jones PS, Sullins KE, Saunders GK: Synovial regeneration in the equine carpus after arthroscopic, mechanical or carbon dioxide laser synovectomy, *Vet Surg* 31:331–343, 2002.

Dumoulin M, Pille F, van den Abeele A-M, Boyen F, Boussauw B, Oosterlinck M, Pasmans F, Gasthuys F, Martens A: Use of blood culture medium enrichment for synovial fluid culture in horses: A comparison of different culture methods, *Equine Vet J* 42:541–546, 2010.

Dykgraaf S, Dechant JE, Johns JL, Christopher MM, Bolt DM, Snyder JR: Effect of intrathecal amikacin administration and repeated centesis on digital flexor tendon sheath synovial fluid in horses, *Vet Surg* 36:57–63, 2007.

Farnsworth KD, White NA, Robertson J: The effect of implanting gentamicin impregnated polymethylmethacrylate beads in the tarsocrural joint of the horse, *Vet Surg* 30:126–131, 2001.

Fraser BSL, Bladon BM: Tenoscopic surgery for treatment of lacerations of the digital flexor tendon sheath, *Equine Vet J* 36:528–531, 2004.

Freeman K, Woods E, Welsby S, Percival SL, Cochrane CA: Biofilm evidence and the microbial diversity of horse wounds, *Can J Microbiol* 55:197–202, 2009.

Frees KE, Lillich JD, Gaughan EM, DeBowes RM: Tenoscopic-assisted treatment of open digital flexor tendon sheath injuries in horses: 20 cases (1992–2001), *J Am Vet Med Assoc* 220:1823–1827, 2002.

Gächter A: *Der Gelenkinfekt Inform Arzt* 6:35–43, 1985.

García-Arias M, Balsa A, Martín Mola E: Septic arthritis, *Best Pract Res Clin Rheumatol* 25:407–421, 2011.

Gaughan EM: Wounds of tendon sheaths and joints in horses, *Comp Cont Educ Prat Vet* 16:517–529, 1994.

Gibson KT, McIlwraith CW, Turner AS, et al.: Open joint injuries in horses: 58 cases (1980-1986), *J Am Vet Med Assoc* 194:398–404, 1989.

Haerdi-Landerer MC, Habermacher J, Wenger B, Suter MM, Steiner A: Slow release antibiotics for treatment of septic arthritis in large animals, *Vet J* 184:14–20, 2010.

Honnas CM, Schumacher J, Cohen ND, et al.: Septic tenosynovitis in horses: 25 cases (1983–1989), *J Am Vet Med Assoc* 199:1616–1622, 1991a.

Honnas CM, Schumacher J, Watkins JP, et al.: Diagnosis and treatment of septic tenosynovitis in horses, *Comp Cont Educ Pract Vet* 13:301–311, 1991b.

Ivey M, Clark R: Arthroscopic debridement of the knee for septic arthritis, *Clin Orthop Rel Res* 199:201–206, 1985.

Jackman BR, Baxter GM, Parks AH, et al.: The use of indwelling drains in the treatment of septic tenosynovitis, *Proc Am Assoc Equine Pract* 35:251–257, 1989.

Jackson RW: The septic knee–arthroscopic treatment, *Arthroscopy* 1:194–197, 1985.

Jarrett MP, Grossman L, Sadler AH, et al.: The role of arthroscopy in the treatment of septic arthritis, *Arthritis Rheum* 24:737–739, 1981.

Josza L, Jarrinen M, Kannus P, et al.: Fine structural changes in the articular cartilage of the rat's knee following short-term immobilisation in various positions: A scanning electron microscopic study, *Int Orthop*(II)129–133, 1987.

Kallio PE, Michelsson JE, Bjorkenheim JM: Immobilisation leads to early changes in hydrostatic pressure of bone and joint. A study on experimental osteoarthritis in rabbits, *Scand J Rheumatol* 17:27–32, 1988.

Koch DB: Management of infectious arthritis in the horse, *Comp Cont Educ Pract Vet* 1:545–550, 1979.

Kuo C-L, Chang J-H, Wu C-C, Shen P-H, Wand C-C, Lin L-C, Shen H-S, Lee C-H: Treatment of septic knee arthritis: Comparison of arthroscopic debridement alone or combined with continuous closed irrigation-suction system, *J Trauma* 71:454–459, 2011.

LaPointe JM, Laverty S, LaVoie JP: Septic arthritis in 15 Standardbred racehorses after intra-articular injection, *Equine Vet J* 24:430–434, 1992.

Lee MS, Ikenove T, Trindale MCD, et al.: Protective effects of intermittent hydrostatic pressure on osteoarthritic chondrocytes activated by bacterial endotoxin in vitro, *J Orthop Rel Res* 21:117–122, 2003.

Lescun TB: Orthopaedic infections; laboratory testing and response to therapy, *Equine Vet Educ* 23:127–129, 2011.

Lescun TB, Adams SB, Wu CC, Bill RP: Continuous infusion of gentamicin into the tarsocrural joint of horses, *Am J Vet Res* 61:407–412, 2000.

Lescun TB, Vasey JR, Ward MP, Adams SB: Treatment with continuous intrasynovial antimicrobial infusion for septic synovitis in horses: 31 cases (2000-2003), *J Am Vet Med Ass* 228:1922–1929, 2006a.

Lescun TB, Ward MP, Adams SB: Gentamicin concentrations in synovial fluid and joint tissues during intravenous administration or continuous intravenous administration or continuous intra-articular infusion of the tarsocrural joint of clinically normal horses, *J Am Vet Med Ass* 67:409–416, 2006b.

McIlwraith CW: Treatment of infectious arthritis, *Vet Clin North Am Large Anim Pract* 5:363–379, 1983.

Madison JB, Sommer M, Spencer PA: Relations among synovial membrane histopathologic findings, synovial fluid cytologic findings, and bacterial culture results in horses with suspected infectious arthritis: 64 cases (1979-1987), *J Am Vet Med Assoc* 198:1655–1661, 1991.

Mathews CJ, Kingsley G, Field M, Jones A, Weston VC, Phillips M, Walker D, Coakley G: Management of septic arthritis: A systematic review, *Ann Rheum Dis* 66:440–445, 2007.

Mathews CJ, Coakley G: Septic arthritis: Current diagnostic and therapeutic algorithm, *Curr Opin Rheumatol* 20:457–462, 2008.

Matthews GL, Engler SJ, Morris EA: Effect of dimethylsulfoxide on articular cartilage proteoglycan synthesis and degradation, chondrocyte viability and matrix water content, *Vet Surg* 27:438–444, 1998.

May SA, Lees P: Nonsteroidal anti-inflammatory drugs. In McIlwraith CW, Totter GW, editors: *Joint disease in the horse Philadelphia*. WB Saunders, 1996, pp 223–237.

Meagher DT, Latimer FG, Sutter WW, Saville WJA: Evaluation of a balloon constant rate infusion system for treatment of septic arthritis, septic tenosynovitis, and contaminated synovial wounds: 23 cases (2002-2005), *J Am Vet Med Assoc* 228:1930–1934, 2006.

Moore RM, Schneider RK, Kowalski J, Bramlage LR, Mecklenburg LM, Kohn CW: Antimicrobial susceptibility of bacterial isolates from 233 horses with musculoskeletal infection during 1979-1989, *Equine Vet. J* 24:450–456, 1992.

Nixon AJ: Septic tenosynovitis. In White NA, Moore JN, editors: *Current practice of equine surgery*, Philadelphia, 1990, JB Lippincott, pp 451–455.

Palmer JL, Bertone AL: Joint structure, biochemistry and biochemical disequilibrium in synovitis and equine joint disease, *Equine Vet J* 26:263–277, 1994.

Palmoski M, Perricore E, Brande KD: Development and reversal of a proteoglycan aggregation defect in normal canine knee cartilage after immobilisation, *Arthritis Rheum* 22:508–517, 1979.

Parisien JS, Shaffer B: Arthroscopic management of pyarthrosis, *Clin Orthop Rel Res* 275:243–246, 1990.

Perry CR, Hulsey RE, Mann FE, et al.: Treatment of acutely infected arthroplasties with incision, drainage and local antibiotics delivered via an implantable pump, *Clin Orthop* 281:216–223, 1992.

Reginato AJ, Ferreiro JL, O'Connor CR, et al.: Clinical and pathologic studies of twenty-six patients with penetrating foreign body injury to the joints, bursae and tendon sheaths, *Arthritis Rheum* 33:1753–1762, 1990.

Riegels-Nielson P, Frinodt-Møller N, Sørensen M, et al.: Synovectomy for septic arthritis. Early versus late synovectomy studied in the rabbit knee, *Acta Orthop Scand* 62:315–318, 1991.

Riegels-Nielson P, Jensen JS: Septic arthritis of the knee. Five cases treated with synovectomy, *Acta Orthop Scand* 55:657–659, 1984.

Rose RJ, Love DN: Staphylococcal septic arthritis in three horses, *Equine Vet J* 2:85–89, 1979.

Ross MW, Orsini JA, Richardson DW, et al.: Closed suction drainage in the treatment of infectious arthritis of the equine tarsocrural joint, *Vet Surg* 20:21–29, 1991.

Salter RB, Bell RS, Keeley FW: The protective effect of continuous passive motion on living articular cartilage in acute septic arthritis: An experimental investigation in the rabbit, *Clin Orthop* 159:223–247, 1981.

Santschi EM, Adams SB, Foster JF, et al.: Treatment of bacterial tarsal tenosynovitis and osteitis of the sustentaculum tali of the calcaneus in five horses, *Equine Vet J* 29(3):244–247, 1997.

Schneider RK, Bramlage LR, Mecklenburg LM, Kohn CW, Gabel AA: Open drainage, intra-articular and systemic antibiotics in the treatment of septic arthritis/tenosynovitis in horses, *Equine Vet J* 24:443–449, 1992a.

Schneider RK, Bramlage LR, Moore RM, Mecklenberg LM, Kohn CW, Gabel AA: A retrospective study of 192 horses affected with septic arthritis/tenosynovitis, *Equine Vet J* 24:436–442, 1992b.

Schneider RK: Orthopaedic infections. In Auer JJ, Stick JA, editors: *Equine surgery*, ed 2, Philadelphia, 1999, WB Saunders, pp 727–735.

Shirtliff ME, Mader JT: Acute septic arthritis, *Clin Microbiol Rev* 15:527–544, 2002.

Skyhar MJ, Mubarak SJ: Arthroscopic treatment of septic knees in children, *J Pediatr Orthop* 7:47–651, 1987.

Smith CL, MacDonald MH, Tesch AM, et al.: In vitro evaluation of the effect of dimethyl sulfoxide on equine articular cartilage matrix metabolism, *Vet Surg* 29:347–357, 2000.

Smith MJ: Arthroscopic treatment of the septic knee, *Arthroscopy* 2:30–34, 1986.

Smith RL, Kajiyama G, Schurman DJ: Staphylococcal septic arthritis: Antibiotics and nonsteroidal anti-inflammatory drug treatment in a rabbit model, *J Orthop Res* 15:919–926, 1997.

Snyder JR, Pascoe JR, Hirsch DC: Antimicrobial susceptibility of microorganisms isolated from equine orthopaedic patients, *Vet Surg* 16:197–201, 1987.

Spiers S, May SA, Harrison LJ, et al.: Proteolytic enzymes in equine joints with infectious arthritis, *Equine Vet J* 26:48–50, 1994.

Steel CM, Hunt AR, Adams PLE, et al.: Factors associated with prognosis for survival and athletic use in foals with septic arthritis: 93 cases (1987–1994), *J Am Vet Med Assoc* 215:973–977, 1999.

Stengel D, Bauwens K, Sehouli J, Ekkernkamp A, Porzsolt F: Systematic review and meta-analysis of antibiotic therapy for bone and joint infections, *Lancet Infectious Diseases* 1:175–188, 2001.

Stutz G, Kuster MS, Kheinstück F, et al.: Arthroscopic management of septic arthritis: Stages of infection and results, *Knee Surg Sports Traumatol Arthrosc* 8:270–274, 2000.

Theoret CL, Barber SM, Moyana T, et al.: Repair and function of synovium after arthroscopic synovectomy of the dorsal compartment of the equine antebrachiocarpal joint, *Vet Surg* 25:142–153, 1996.

Thiery JA: Arthroscopic drainage in septic arthritides of the knee: A multi-centre study, *Arthroscopy* 5:65–69, 1989.

Trumble TN: Orthopedic disorders in neonatal foals, *Vet Clin N Am: Equine Pract* 21:357–385, 2005.

Videman T: Changes in compression and distances between tibial and femoral condyles during immobilization of rabbit knee, *Arch Orthop Trauma Surg* 98:289–291, 1981.

Vispo Seara JL, Barthel T, Smitz H, et al.: Arthroscopic treatment of septic joints: Prognostic factors, *Arch Orthop Traum Surg* 122:204–211, 2002.

Wereszka MM, White NA, Furr MO: Factors associated with outcome following treatment of horses with septic tenosynovitis: 51 cases (1986-2003), *J Am Vet Med Ass* 1195–1200, 2007.

Werner LA, Hardy J, Berton AL: Bone gentamicin concentration after intra-articular injection or regional intravenous perfusion in the horse, *Vet Surg* 32:559–565, 2003.

Whitehair KL, Bowerstock TL, Blevins WE, et al.: Regional limb perfusion for antibiotic treatment of experimentally induced septic arthritis, *Vet Surg* 21:367–373, 1992b.

Wilson DG, Cooley AJ, McWilliams PS, et al.: Effects of 0.05% chlorhexidine lavage on the tarsocrural joints of horses, *Vet Surg* 23:442–447, 1994.

Wirtz DC, Marth M, Miltner O, et al.: Septic arthritis of the knee in adults: Treatment by arthroscopy or arthrotomy, *Int Orthopaed* 25:239–241, 2001.

Wright IM, Phillips TJ, Walmsley JP: Endoscopy of the navicular bursa: A new technique for the treatment of contaminated and septic bursae, *Equine Vet J* 31:5–11, 1999.

Wright IM, Scott M: The management of synovial penetrations in the horse, *Equine Vet Educ* 1:15–22, 1989.

Wright IM, Smith MRW, Humphrey DJ, et al.: Endoscopic surgery in the treatment of contaminated and infected synovial cavities, *Equine Vet J* 35:613–619, 2003.

Yanmiş I, Özkan H, Koca K, Kilingçoğlu V, Bek D, Tunay S: The relation between the arthroscopic findings and functional outcomes in patients with septic arthritis of the knee joint, treated with arthroscopic debridement and irrigation, *Acta Orthop Traumatol Turc* 45:94–99, 2011.

CHAPTER 15

Problems and Complications of Diagnostic and Surgical Arthroscopy

Arthroscopy involves, in most circumstances, hospitalization of horses and general anesthesia, which can both result in complications to case management. In addition, there are a number of intraoperative and postoperative complications that are of particular importance with respect to arthroscopy. The nature and incidence of complications in human arthroscopy have been documented for the most commonly operated joints, but reports of complications in equine arthroscopy are limited (Goodrich & McIlwraith, 2009; McIlwraith, 1990). Overall complication rates in humans vary between joints. The most common joint for human arthroscopy is the knee, for which complication rates of 0.8% (DeLee, 1985), 0.56% (Small, 1986), and 1.68% (Small, 1988) have been documented. Complication rates of 9% for arthroscopy of the ankle and 9.8% for foot and ankle combined were published by Ferkel et al in 1996 and 2001, respectively. Complications occurred in only 1.6% of hip arthroscopies reported by Griffin & Villar (1999), most of which were attributed to use of traction techniques. Kelly et al (2001) reported serious complications in 0.8% and minor complications (that resolved) in 11% of arthroscopic procedures in the elbow, whereas Reddy et al (2000) documented an overall incidence of 1.6% at this site. The highest reported incidence of complications in humans appears to be associated with arthroscopy of the shoulder—Berjano et al (1998) reported a 10.6% incident. The specific complications encountered in humans vary within individual joints and also with the surgical techniques used. The most common complications associated with arthroscopy of the human knee are presented in Box 15-1. The commonest complication associated with foot, ankle (Ferkel et al, 2001), elbow (Kelly et al, 2001), and wrist (Deal & Poehling, 2010) arthroscopy is iatrogenic damage to adjacent neural trunks.

PREOPERATIVE PROBLEMS AND PLANNING

The principal preoperative predispositions to complications in human arthroscopy include incorrect diagnosis, lack of preoperative planning, failure to obtain appropriate preoperative studies (Ferkel et al, 2001), and lack of clinical correlation (Dandy, 2011). All of these are salient to equine arthroscopy.

Box • 15-1	

Commonest Reported Complications in Arthroscopy of the Human Knee

Hemarthrosis	Ligament injury
Infection	Neurologic injury
Thromboembolism	Iatrogenic chondral injury
Anesthetic complications	Fracture
Wrong site surgery	Adhesion formation
Instrument breakage and/or failure	Postoperative effusion
Articular pain	Wound-healing complications
Complex regional pain syndrome	Ecchymoses

Data from DeLee (1985), Sherman et al (1986), and Small (1986, 1988), reviewed by Allum (2002) and from Bert & Bert (2010).

Appropriate positioning of the patient and limb(s) is critical to safe and effective arthroscopy in all species. In humans neural injury can result from inappropriate patient positioning or manipulation (Kim et al, 2002) and in horses, postanaesthetic hindlimb neurapraxia and myopathy are well recognized (Mayhew, 2009). Importance of thorough, three-dimensional anatomic knowledge has been emphasized in humans (Boardman & Cofield, 1999; Ferkel et al, 2001) and is equally appropriate in the horse.

Allum (2002) made four specific recommendations to minimize complications associated with arthroscopy of the human knee:

1. Use of a sharp trocar should be avoided.
2. Instruments should be used only if they can be seen clearly.
3. Tissue should never be cut blindly but always under direct visualization.
4. Care should be taken with power instruments, particularly when suction is applied, because this can rapidly result in joint evacuation and compromise visibility.

INTRAOPERATIVE PROBLEMS

Hemarthrosis

Hemarthrosis is not usually a significant problem. Distal limb hemorrhage is invariably reduced when animals are in dorsal recumbency compared with those positioned laterally. Use of an Esmarch bandage and tourniquet may be of benefit when dealing with lesions in which hemorrhage may be anticipated. Examples include contaminated and infected synovial cavities and tenoscopy of the digital flexor tendon sheath. In most other situations, hemorrhage is controlled by the pressure generated by irrigating fluids. One author (A.J.N.) uses epinephrine in the fluid as an additional aid. However, if the joint is exited, left undistended, and then reentered, the surgeon will encounter hemorrhage, particularly from debrided tissues. In such instances, flushing with an open egress cannula, followed by closure of the cannula and redistention, is all that is necessary to eliminate the problem. The same procedure is performed if hemarthrosis is present at the time of initial entry.

The fact that hemorrhage is minimized with distention is important to note, particularly with reference to debridement of subchondral defects. During curettage of subchondral bone, hemorrhage (as seen during arthrotomy) is not evident while the joint is distended. The surgeon must therefore either use other criteria to evaluate an appropriate depth of debridement or release fluid pressure in order to assess bleeding from subchondral bone.

Obstruction of View by Synovial Villi

Within each synovial cavity there are regions of villous and avillous synovium. Synovial villi may obstruct arthroscopic visualization throughout a synovial cavity, or this may be a localized problem. When generalized, this problem is usually associated with either inadequate distention or excessive fluid movement. Distention may be limited by inadequate delivery of fluid, capsular fibrosis, or the development of extrasynovial extravasation of fluid. Excessive fluid movement can occur with an open outflow portal. This is seen most commonly with an open egress cannula or an excessively large and patent

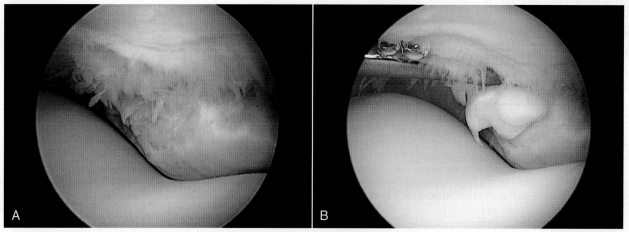

Figure 15-1 A, Joint capsule and proliferative synovium obscuring fragmentation of the dorsoproximal articular surface of the proximal phalanx. **B,** Visualization by raising the joint capsule with an arthroscopic probe.

instrument portal. The latter can occur as a technical error but more commonly follows removal of large intraarticular fragments. For these reasons, initial arthroscopic examination should be performed before surgical procedures, following initial lavage/clearance of the cavity and with a closed egress cannula. Whenever feasible, large fragments should be removed after small fragments. If necessary, the surgeon should also complete other procedures such as debridement before large fragments are moved. Many mechanical pumps will deliver fluids at rates up to 1 L/min. These will compensate for excessive fluid outflow in many situations, but at high flow rates bubbles are frequently produced, which also result in diminished visualization. Fluid exit through a large, patent instrument portal can also be controlled to some degree by retention of an instrument within the portal. However, the surgeon must try not to prevent fluid outflow by placing a finger over the instrument portal because this will result in rapid extrasynovial extravasation, which is counterproductive.

Proliferative synovial villi may obscure articular margins and lesions in these locations. Common examples include fragmentation of the dorsoproximal and plantaroproximal articular margins of the proximal phalanges and osteochondritis dissecans of the lateral trochlear ridge of the femur. Assessment of these sites can usually be made using a probe to displace the villi (Fig. 15-1), but frequently sufficient visualization to permit confident and accurate surgical interference will require local synovial resection (Fig. 15-2). This is performed most efficiently with motorized apparatus with suction attached. Resection should always be limited because, although the clinical implications are unknown, it has been demonstrated that regeneration of normal villous synovium does not occur (Doyle-Jones et al, 2002; Theoret et al, 1996). In addition, overzealous use of motorized apparatus may result in trauma to the fibrous capsule.

Many of the problems associated with obstructing synovial villi are reduced or eliminated by use of gas distention.

Extrasynovial Extravasation of Fluid

Extravasation of irrigating fluid into the subcutis and other fascial planes is a problem commonly encountered when learning arthroscopic techniques but occurs, to some degree, even with the most experienced surgeon. The principal predisposing factors are the shape of instrument portals, excessive perfusion pressure in the presence of obstructed outflow, and instrument manipulation.

Instrument portals in which the incision in the skin and extraarticular tissues is smaller than the opening into the joint will result in dissecting lines of fluid through fascial planes.

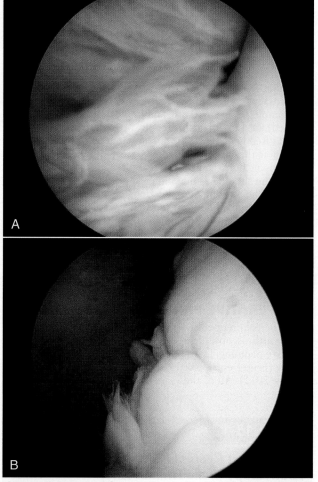

Figure 15-2 A, Proliferative synovial villi overlying the middle one third of the lateral trochlear ridge of the femur. **B,** The same field of view imaged in **A** following local synovial resection, revealing osteochondritis dissecans of the lateral trochlear ridge of the femur.

This can occur quickly and may be controlled effectively by minimizing perfusion pressure at the time of portal creation and also by completing the incision through the skin before the blade is advanced into the joint. The shape of a No. 11 blade assists also because this creates a triangular incision with the apex of the triangle at the point of the blade. An obstructed outflow with excessive perfusion pressure can occur while instruments (particularly large instruments) are being inserted or manipulated. It also results during removal of large fragments, while these are being pulled through the instrument portal. Selective reduction in perfusion pressure at this time will reduce the severity of the problem significantly. Similarly, repeated instrument entry or a large range of instrument movement through a portal, or both, will open up and weaken fascial planes with the same result. Noyes & Spievack (1982) demonstrated that excessive intraarticular fluid pressure potentiates subcutaneous extravasation of fluid.

The site at which surgeons experience most difficulties with extravasation of fluid is the scapulohumeral joint. Here, caudal instrument portals must traverse not only the skin and subcutis but also several centimeters of muscle and multiple fascial planes. The ability of the periarticular muscles and their fascial planes to imbibe fluid can result in restricted articular distention and thus loss of visibility and surgical access, particularly to lesions that are axial in the joint. Because this joint generally requires a high perfusion pressure to maintain arthroscopic access, particular care should be taken in the creation and use of instrument portals. Some degree of extraarticular extravasation is inevitable. The surgeon should be cognizant of its occurrence and plan surgical procedures such that more axially located lesions are treated first. Also, once extravasation has begun, surgical access time will be limited. Extrasynovial fluid accumulation can also hamper instrument entry to the stifle joints and both carpal and tarsal tendon sheaths. These areas can be reduced considerably by temporary cessation of ingress fluid and firm massage of fluid from skin portals. Surgery can then recommence. At the end of surgery large quantities of subcutaneously extravasated fluid may result in excessive tension in skin sutures. This can usually be ameliorated by simple hand massage of the site before closure.

In most circumstances extravasated fluid dissipates within 24 hours of surgery. Occasionally, when associated with large fascial planes such as those adjacent to the femoropatellar joint, this may take longer.

Iatrogenic Damage to Articular Cartilage

Full- and partial-thickness defects in articular cartilage can be created iatrogenically: This occurs most commonly when the joint is being entered and particularly when there is minimal distention. It can be limited by careful technique and use of a conical obturator (rather than a sharp trocar) in the arthroscopic sleeve.

Arthroscopic portals should be made using a blade directly into synovium, and the sleeve can then be passed along this pathway with minimal resistance. Use of two hands, one to advance the cannula and the second positioned adjacent to the skin portal to act as a bridge or brake, is recommended. In addition, the surgeon should angle entry of the arthroscopic sleeve and subsequent instruments away from the direct line of articular surfaces. When minor scuffing of the cartilage does occur, it does not appear to be of major significance (Dick et al, 1978; McIlwraith & Fessler, 1978).

In humans, iatrogenic damage to articular cartilage is considered the most frequent unreported complication of arthroscopy of any joint (Ferkel et al, 2001). As in horses, small joints are most susceptible; long-term sequelae are unknown (Ferkel et al, 2001).

Iatrogenic Damage to Other Tissues

Perisynovial structures may be damaged inadvertently during creation of arthroscope or instrument portals, or both. Obviously, the risk is dependent on proximity to portal sites. Elements of the palmar/plantar neurovascular bundle may be traumatized in surgery of the digital flexor tendon sheath.

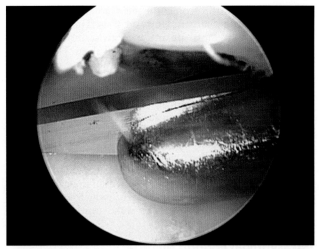

Figure 15-3 Removing a broken No. 11 scalpel blade from the palmar pouch of a metacarpophalangeal joint.

Use of an Esmarch bandage and tourniquet makes the bundle more difficult to identify, particularly in draught breeds and cobs, which have thick skin. However, with careful palpation and inspection of the skin incision before a deeper portal is created, the risk is limited. The surgeon may be unaware of damage during surgery. Laceration of the palmar/plantar artery may become apparent on release of the tourniquet or by the presence of postoperative hemorrhage during recovery from general anesthesia. This is usually controlled by the application of counterpressure. Damage to the palmar/plantar nerve may be clinically silent, but a painful neuroma may develop at the site.

The carpal sheaths of extensor carpi radialis and common digital extensor tendons can be penetrated by injudicious placement of arthroscope and instrument portals during both middle and antebrachiocarpal joint surgery. This is usually apparent to the surgeon as intraoperative and postoperative distention of the sheath. These sheaths can also be traumatized during removal of large fragments from the dorsodistal margin of the radius. The tendon sheath of the common digital extensor is most commonly affected when fragments are removed from the dorsolateral margin (intermediate facet) of the radius.

Intrasynovial Instrument Breakage

The most common cause of instrument breakage is the use of inappropriate force. It follows that the incidence of this problem usually decreases as a surgeon gains experience. If loose pieces are created within the synovial environment, then fluids should be stopped immediately or the perfusion rate reduced dramatically in order to maintain the fragment in the visible field. An appropriate grasping instrument should then be inserted and the fragment removed. If the piece disappears from view, a systematic search should follow, bearing in mind that most pieces will be metallic and therefore will gravitate to dependent areas (Fig. 15-3). If this fails to locate the debris, then intraoperative radiography should be employed. Magnetic retrievers have been employed (Jansson, 2009), but the limited frequency of their use makes the cost hard to justify.

Prevention is certainly better than cure. Instruments should be of an appropriate size (Ferkel et al, 2001) and only used in the purpose for which they are designed, and the surgeon should avoid excessive bending or lever movements. The use of fixed rather than disposable blade cutting instruments within joints is also recommended. Disposable No. 15 scalpel blades and the shafts of small angled spoon curettes are considered to be particularly vulnerable to intraarticular breakage.

Ferris-Smith arthroscopic rongeurs are a workhorse of equine arthroscopic surgery. However, if used inappropriately, particularly if attempts are made to twist firmly attached bone, then the pin linking the blades will shear. This disarms the instrument completely but does not produce debris. The pin can be replaced by manufacturers.

Minor trauma to the distal window of the arthroscope will result in cumulative image artifacts and loss of clarity, whereas major trauma can cause complete loss of image. There is generally no intrasynovial debris. Trauma to the glass is minimized principally by careful surgical techniques, and it is vital to maintain a direct view of instruments during surgical procedures. Protection of the distal window is aided also by a slightly recessed arthroscope position within the cannula.

Sudden movement during surgery, which occurs most commonly if an animal begins to wake, can bend or break instruments.

Intrasynovial Foreign Material

Tiny metallic fragments have been seen following impact of instruments on the arthroscopic sleeve or sometimes following other "metal-on-metal" contact. Such debris is usually flushed out with the irrigating fluid or may become embedded in the synovial membrane. No detrimental effects have been recognized.

Contamination of joints with hair and other debris has been demonstrated with needle centesis in horses (Adams et al, 2010; Wahl et al, 2012) and during arthroscopy in man (Glaser et al, 2001). This is also commonly observed in equine arthroscopy when needles are used either to inflate a synovial cavity or to determine sites for appropriate instrument portals. It is seen most frequently with stiletted needles; these may cut small pieces of skin, which are carried into the synovial space. If adhesive drapes are employed, then needles will also carry small pieces of plastic into the synovial space. Such debris is readily flushed from the synovial environment, and no adverse effects have been recognized. The risk of pushing larger pieces of plastic into the synovial cavity or adjacent tissues can be reduced by removing the adhesive material from the immediate vicinity of portals. Plastic fragments can result in swelling and discharge when lodged in the subcutis.

POSTOPERATIVE COMPLICATIONS

Infection

In a retrospective study of 682 horses that had undergone arthroscopic surgery on noninfected/contaminated joints in a single hospital between 1994 and 2003, Olds et al (2006) reported 8 of 932 (0.9%) joints in 7 of 682 (1%) horses to have a postoperative intraarticular infection. Draught breeds and tarsocrural joints represented significant risk factors. Interestingly, the ankle also appears to have the highest incidence in man (Kirchhoff et al, 2009). Intraarticular infection developed in 1 of 269 (0.4%) horses that received preoperative antimicrobials and in 6 of 413 (1.5%) that did not ($P = 0.21$). It was thus concluded that preoperative antimicrobial administration did not significantly affect the development of postarthroscopy infective arthritis. Gram-positive cocci, particularly staphylococci, were the commonest cultured organism (Olds et al, 2006).

A retrospective case review of 353 elective arthroscopic procedures in 305 small animals (294 dogs and 11 cats) revealed 3 cases (0.85%) of postoperative articular infection (Ridge, 2011). Postoperative infection is the commonest complication of human arthroscopy. A review of the literature produced rates of between 0.01% and 0.48% for procedures involving the knee (Babcock et al, 2002). When culture results were available, staphylococcus species dominated (Babcock et al, 2002; Babcock et al, 2003). These authors concluded that the most important control methods for infection are strict adherence

to aseptic technique and instrument sterilization. Other risk factors identified included the complexity of the procedure(s), perioperative intraarticular corticosteroid administration, and razor shaving of surgical sites. The latter was ascribed to iatrogenic skin damage; instigation of clipping as an alternative was reported to reduce the incidence in one hospital.

The potential for contaminated instruments to be responsible for postarthroscopic infections is considered to be low but has been identified in "outbreaks" of such in humans (Babcock et al, 2003).

The use of perioperative antimicrobial agents in clean orthopedic procedures (such as arthroscopy without the use of implants) remains contentious in all species including man (Alerany et al, 2005; American Society of Health-System Pharmacists, 1999; Bert et al 2007; Bratzler and Houck, 2005; Kurzweil, 2006). A single randomized, placebo-controlled, blinded clinical trial of 437 cases in man did not identify a difference in the incidence of postarthroscopy infections with or without perioperative antimicrobial prophylaxis and concluded that these were not justified (Wieck et al, 1997). A similar conclusion was reached in a retrospective comparative study of 3231 human knee arthroscopies in which infection rates of 0.15% and 0.16% were found in patients that received and did not receive perioperative antimicrobials, respectively (Bert et al, 2007).

However, in addition to prophylactic use with regard to the surgery site(s) there is a potential role in horses for reducing the risks associated with atelectasis and pulmonary congestion, which is an inevitable consequence of recumbent general anesthesia (Nyman et al, 1990). Use is commonplace and, when practiced, the authors recommend intravenous preoperative administration (within 1 hour of surgery) and less than 24 hours "therapy." Prolonged administration has been shown in humans to be of no benefit (Mini et al, 2001) while it may be associated with emergence of resistant bacteria (Harbarth et al, 2000; Hecker et al, 2003). The potential benefits should always be weighed against risks of antimicrobial use both to the individual in terms of gastrointestinal disturbances, principally colitis, and to the hospital populous (Cohen & Woods, 1999; House et al, 1999; Weese & Cruz, 2009) by increasing resistance in hospital microbial populations.

Infected cellulitis or fasciitis, or both, have been documented as uncommon sequelae to arthroscopic surgery most commonly involving the stifle. Difficulty in maintaining sterile covers to portals and accumulation of extravasated fluid in fascial planes are potential predisposing factors. All cases appear to have resolved following systemic administration of antimicrobial drugs. Drainage from skin portals or surgically created sites may or may not occur.

Occasionally, small skin abscesses or suture sinuses are encountered. These almost invariably require no treatment and resolve when sutures are removed, although in some cases a small fibrous lump may persist at the site. Infection can also follow suture removal if this is not performed appropriately.

Postoperative Distention/Synovitis

Postoperative hemarthrosis is reported to have an incidence of 1% in human arthroscopy (Allum, 2002). It is undocumented but appears uncommon in horses. In humans postoperative effusion is considered a sign of unresolved lesions (Dandy, 1987). Distention usually signifies persistent synovitis, which, in turn, requires a "drive." However, there is variability according to site (e.g., in the femoropatellar joint, persistent distention is frequently a sign of continued intraarticular lesions, but this may not be so in the tarsocrural joint). Mild synovial distention may persist without clinical significance (e.g., when preoperative distention has been long-standing. In the absence of additional clinical signs, such as lameness and reduced or resented flexion, mild distention usually does not justify further investigation or treatment. Marked synovial distention is more likely to result when active intrasynovial lesions persist and reevaluation is indicated. If causative lesions are not identified, then treatment of the synovitis may be beneficial.

Synovial Herniae

Synovial herniae are an uncommon sequel to arthroscopic portals. There is a single case report associated with the middle carpal joint (Wilson, 1989). The authors have also seen clinically inconsequential synovial herniae at other sites.

Failure to Remove Fragments

In surgery for removal of traumatic or developmental fragments it is possible, particularly in cases with multiple fragmentation, that all pieces are not removed. A number of possible explanations fall into two broad categories: those fragments that may be identified immediately after surgery and those that are identified later. The former category includes the simple surgical error of failing to identify lesions. Predisposing factors include inadequate preoperative examination (e.g., failure to identify fragments that may be medial and lateral in a joint and incomplete arthroscopic evaluation of the joint). At some sites (e.g., the dorsoproximal margin of the proximal phalanx), fragmentation can be covered by proliferative synovium and may not be apparent until this is lifted with a probe. In some animals there is a distinct dorsal recess of the joint capsule at this site, which can also obscure fragments. At other sites (e.g., in animals with multiple, loose osteochondral fragments in the femoropatellar joint), it may be difficult to determine accurately from preoperative radiographs the exact number of fragments that need to be accounted for (Fig. 15-4). It should also be appreciated that some fragments identified radiographically may be embedded within the joint capsule. Current opinion suggests that the dissection necessary to identify and remove these is not justified. Failure to remove fragments is limited by a thorough preoperative evaluation and the surgeon should ensure that all identified fragments are accounted for at surgery. Within individual joints, loose fragments move frequently to consistent locations [e.g., into the suprapatellar pouch of the femoropatellar joint, (Fig. 15-5) or the intercondylar fossa of the medial femorotibial joint (Fig. 15-6)]. These

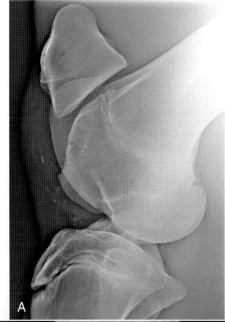
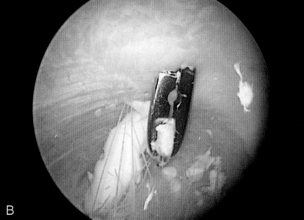

Figure 15-5 Osteochondral fragments that have migrated into the suprapatellar pouch in an animal with osteochondritis dissecans of the lateral trochlear ridge of the femur. **A,** Lateromedial radiograph. **B,** Detached fragments removed with arthroscopic rongeurs through a suprapatellar portal.

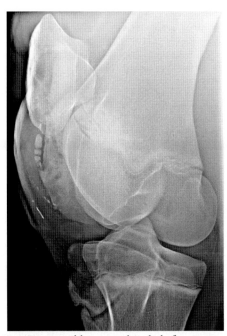

Figure 15-4 Innumerable osteochondral fragments displaced from the lateral trochlear ridge of the femur and scattered throughout the femoropatellar joint.

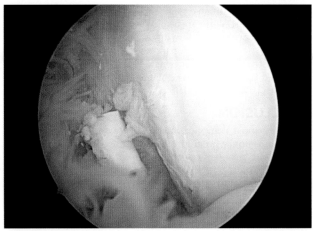

Figure 15-6 Osteochondral debris in the cranial medial femorotibial joint that has migrated into the cul-de-sac of the intercondylar fossa during evacuation and debridement of a femoral subchondral bone cyst.

sites should always be assessed at the end of each surgery and debris removed. Use of intraoperative and postoperative radiography has been recommended (and can help avoid litigation) but is not necessarily an assurance.

Lesions that may be identified after surgery and misinterpreted as failure to remove fragments include new bone deposits at the site of previous lesions, fragmentation of the same, additional new fragments, and dystrophic mineralization in adjacent soft tissues.

Postoperative Capsulitis, Entheseous New Bone, and Soft Tissue Mineralization

In many instances capsulitis may be present preoperatively, such as when there is tearing of the fibrous joint capsule, or can be anticipated when articular damage is severe. Problems can also develop with surgical trauma to the joint capsule. Attempts at removing intracapsular fragments, trauma to the capsule during debridement, particularly with motorized apparatus, and undue trauma to the sensitive transition zone of the joint can all cause problems.

Problems Associated with Positioning

Transient failure to extend hindlimb joints on recovery from general anesthesia has been noted following long surgical procedures in which (usually both) hindlimbs are fixed in an extended position. Some cases are thought to be associated with a femoral neuropathy or neuromyopathy involving the quadriceps muscle. Others, which may be peroneal neurapraxia, appear able to fix the proximal joints but fail to extend the metatarsophalangeal and interphalangeal joints. In both instances, symptoms generally subside quickly with symptomatic care. The problem is readily controlled by minimizing intraoperative traction, supporting extended limbs during surgery, and flexing the contralateral limb while not undergoing surgery.

Pain

Anesthetists frequently report that distention of the digital flexor tendon sheath is more painful than joint distention. Postoperatively, the degree of pain exhibited by horses appears proportional to soft tissue (particularly tendon and ligament) involvement. However, this is usually transient and requires little more than analgesia provided by nonsteroidal antiinflammatory drugs for 24 hours after surgery. It has been reported that horses with extensive articular or tendon sheath derangements can be maintained on lower levels of inhaled anesthetic agents and have improved recovery by using bupivacaine or mepivacaine for initial synovial inflation. One author (A.J.N.) now uses such a protocol routinely.

Similarly in humans, pain is considered uncommon after diagnostic arthroscopy or simple surgical procedures, although it may be a problem following extensive soft tissue interference such as meniscal repair, synovectomy, or intraarticular reconstruction of ligaments (Allum, 2002). This may be controlled by intraarticular opiates (Joshi et al, 1992) or local analgesics (Chirwa et al, 1989).

CONCLUSION

Generally, most complications can be avoided by good technique and none preclude the advantages of arthroscopic surgery. The problems with equine arthroscopic surgery are mainly technical and anatomic. Good technique comes with training and experience, and the benefits of practice on cadaver limbs cannot be overemphasized.

REFERENCES

Adams SB, Moore GE, Elrashidy Mohammed, et al.: Effect of needle size and type, reuse of needles, insertion speed, and removal of hair on contamination of joints with tissue debris and hair after arthrocentesis, *Vet Surg* 39:667–673, 2010.

Alerany C, Campany D, Monterde J, Semeraro C: Impact of local guidelines and an integrated dispensing system on antibiotic prophylaxis quality in a surgery centre, *J Hosp Infect* 60:111–117, 2005.

Allum R: Complications of arthroscopy of the knee, *J Bone Joint Surg (Br)* 84B:937–945, 2002.

American Society of Health-System Pharmacists: ASHP therapeutic guidelines on antimicrobial prophylaxis in surgery, *AM J Health-Syst Pharm* 56:1839–1888, 1999.

Babcock HM, Matavia MJ, Fraser V: Postarthroscopy surgical site infections: Review of the literature, *Clin Infect Dis* 34:65–71, 2002.

Babcock HM, Carroll C, Matavia M, L'Ecuyer P, Fraser V: Surgical site infections after arthroscopy: Outbreak investigations and case control study, *Arthroscopy* 19:172–181, 2003.

Berjano P, González BG, Olmedo JF, Perez-Espana LA, Munilla MG: Complications in arthroscopic shoulder surgery, *Arthroscopy* 14:785–788, 1998.

Bert JM, Giannini D, Nace L: Antibiotic prophylaxis for arthroscopy of the knee: Is it necessary? arthroscopy, *J Arthroscopic Rel Surg* 23:4–6, 2007.

Bert JM, Bert TM: Complications of knee arthroscopy. In Hunter RE, Sgaglione NA, editors: *The Knee; AANA Advanced Arthroscopy*, Philadelphia, 2010, Saunders, Elsevier, pp 37–44.

Boardman ND, Cofield RH: Neurologic complications of shoulder surgery, *Clin Orthop Del Res* 368:44–53, 1999.

Bratzler DW, Houck PM: Antimicrobial prophylaxis for surgery; an advisory statement from the National Surgical Infection Prevention Project, *Am J Surg* 189:395–404, 2005.

Chirwa SS, MacLeod BA, Day B: Intra-articular bupivacaine (Marcaine) after arthroscopic meniscectomy: A randomised double-blind controlled study, *Arthroscopy* 5:33–35, 1989.

Cohen ND, Woods AM: Characteristics and risk factors for failure of horses with acute diarrhea to survive: 122 cases (1990-1996), *J Am Vet Med Assoc* 214:382–390, 1999.

Dandy DJ: Complications and technical problems. In Dandy DJ, editor: *Arthroscopic management of the knee*, ed 2, Edinburgh, 1987, Churchill Livingstone, pp 64–71.

Dandy D: Imaging and clinical judgement, *Equine Vet J* 42(4):287, 2010.

Deal D Nicole, Poeling GG: Complications of wrist arthroscopy. In Savoie III FE, Field LD, editors: *The Elbow and Wrist; AANA Advanced Arthroscopy*, Philadelphia, 2010, Saunders, Elsevier, pp 300–306.

DeLee JC: Complications of arthroscopy and arthroscopic surgery: Results of a national survey, *J Arthroscopic Rel Surg* 1:214–220, 1985.

Dick W, Glinz W, Henche HR, et al.: Komplikationen in Arthroskopie, *Arch Orthop Trauma Surg* 92:69–73, 1978.

Doyle-Jones PS, Sullins KE, Saunders GK: Synovial regeneration in the equine carpus after arthroscopic, mechanical or carbondioxide laser synovectomy, *Vet Surg* 31:331–343, 2002.

Ferkel RD, Heath DD, Guhl JF: Neurological complications of ankle arthroscopy, *Arthroscopy* 12:200–208, 1996.

Ferkel RD, Small HN, Gittins JE: Complications in foot and ankle arthroscopy, *Clin Orthop Rel Res* 391:89–104, 2001.

Glaser DL, Schildhorn JC, Bartolozzi AR, et al.: The inadvertent introduction of skin into the joint during intra-articular knee injections: Do you really know what is on the tip of your needle? *Proc Am Acad Orth Surgery* 68:130–131, 2001.

Goodrich LR, McIlwraith CW: Complications associated with equine arthroscopy, *Vet Clin Equine* 24:573–589, 2009.

Griffin DR, Villar RN: Complications of arthroscopy of the hip, *J Bone Joint Surg (Br)* 81B:604–606, 1999.

Harbarth S, Samore MH, Lichtenberg D, Carmeli Y: Prolonged antibiotic prophylaxis after cardiovascular surgery and its effect on surgical site infections and antimicrobial resistance, *Circulation* 101:2916–2921, 2000.

Hecker MT, Aron DC, Patel NP, Lehmann MK, Donskey CJ: Unnecessary use of antimicrobials in hospitalized patients: Current activity, *Arch Inter Med* 163:928–972, 2003.

House JK, Mainar-Jaime RC, Smith BP, et al.: Risk factors for nosocomial salmonella infection among hospitalized horses, *J Am Vet Med Assoc* 214:1511–1516, 1999.

Jansson N: Arthroscopic removal of metallic foreign body from the talocrural joint using a magnetic retriever in a horse, *Veterinary Surgery* 38:620–622, 2009.

Joshi GP, McCarroll SM, Cooney CM, et al.: Intra-articular morphine for pain relief after knee arthroscopy, *J Bone Joint Surg (Br)* 74B:749–751, 1992.

Kelly EW, Morney BF, O'Driscoll SW: Complications of elbow arthroscopy, *J Bone Joint Surg (Am)* 83A:25–34, 2001.

Kim TK, Sarino RM, McFarland EG, Cosgarea AJ: Neurovascular complications of knee arthroscopy, *Am J Sports Med* 30:619–629, 2002.

Kirchhoff C, Braunstein V, Paul J, Imhoff AB, Hinterwimmer S: Septic arthritis as a severe complication of elective arthroscopy: Clinical management strategies, *Patient Safety in Surgery* 3:1–6, 2009.

Kurzweil P: Antibiotic prophylaxis for arthroscopic surgery, *Arthroscopy* 22:452–454, 2006.

Mayhew IG: Multifactional and idiopathic disorders. In: *Large Animal Neurology* 2nd, Chichester, 2009, IG Joe Mayhew, Wiley – Blackwell, pp 392–429.

McIlwraith CW, Fessler JF: Arthroscopy in the diagnosis of equine joint disease, *J Am Vet Med Assoc* 172:263–268, 1978.

McIlwraith CW In: *Diagnostic and surgical arthroscopy in the horse*, ed 2, Philadelphia, 1990, Lea and Febiger.

Mini E, Grassi F, Cherubino P, Nobili S, Periti P: Preliminary results of a survey of the use of antimicrobial agents as prophylaxis in orthopedic surgery, *J Chemother* 13:73–79, 2001.

Noyes FR, Spievack ES: Extra-articular fluid dissection in tissues during arthroscopy: A report of clinical cases and a study of intra-articular and thigh pressures in cadavers, *Am J Sports Med* 10:346–351, 1982.

Nyman G, Funkquist B, Kvart C, et al.: Atelectasis causes gas exchange impairment in the anaesthesized horse, *Equine Vet J* 22:317–324, 1990.

Olds AM, Stewart AA, Freeman DE, Schaeffer DJ: Evaluation of the rate of development of septic arthritis after elective arthroscopy in horses: 7 cases (1994-2003), *J Am Vet Med Assoc* 229:1949–1954, 2006.

Reddy AS, Kritre RS, Yocum LA, et al.: Arthroscopy of the elbow: A longterm clinical review, *Arthroscopy* 16:588–594, 2000.

Ridge PA: A retrospective study of the rate of postoperative septic arthritis following 353 elective arthroscopies, *Journal of Small Animal Practice* 52:200–202, 2011.

Scott Weese J: Cruz. A retrospective study of perioperative antimicrobial use practices in horses undergoing elective arthroscopic surgery at a veterinary teaching hospital, *Can Vet J* 50:185–188, 2009.

Sherman OH, Fox JM, Snyder SJ, et al.: Arthroscopy "No problem surgery", an analysis of complications in two thousand six hundred and forty cases, *J Bone Joint Surg (Am)* 68A:256–265, 1986.

Small NC: Complications in arthroscopy: The knee and other joints, 1986, *Arthroscopy* 2:253–258, 1986.

Small NC: Complications in arthroscopic surgery performed by experienced arthroscopists, *Arthroscopy* 4:215–221, 1988.

Theoret CL, Barber SM, Moyana T, Townsend HG, Archer JF: Repair and function of synovium after arthroscopic synovectomy of the dorsal compartment of the equine antebrachiocarpal joint, *Vet Surg* 25:142–153, 1996.

Wahl K, Adams SB, Moore GE: Contamination of joints with tissue debris and hair after arthrocentesis: The effect of needle insertion angle, spinal needle gauge, and insertion of spinal needles with and without a stylet, *Veterinary Surgery* 41:391–398, 2012.

Weese Scott J, Cruz A: Retrospective study of perioperative antimicrobial use practices in horses undergoing elective arthroscopic surgery at a veterinary teaching hospital, *Can Vet J* 50:185–188, 2009.

Wieck JA, Jackson JK, O'Brien TJ, Lurate RB, Russell JM, Dorchak JD: Efficacy of prophylactic antibiotics in arthroscopic surgery, *Orthopedics* 20:133–134, 1997.

Wilson DG: Synovial hernia as a possible complication of arthroscopic surgery in a horse, *J Am Vet Med Assoc* 194:1071–1072, 1989.

CHAPTER 16

Arthroscopic Methods for Cartilage Repair

CARTILAGE RESPONSE TO INJURY

Articular cartilage rarely reforms a functional hyaline surface after injury. Most simple cartilage lacerative injuries reach a benign nonhealing phase, which remains unchanged over time (Hunziker & Rosenberg, 1996; Mankin, 1982). Deeper cartilage lesions, violating the tidemark and extending into the subchondral bone plate, result in an improved healing response (Campbell, 1969). This is largely due to the proliferation of undifferentiated mesenchymal cells from the deeper tissues. In horses, spontaneous healing in cartilage defects progresses from granulation to fibrous tissue and finally fibrocartilage, at least in the deeper layers (Riddle, 1970). The fibrous tissue undergoes progressive chondrification to form a fibrocartilaginous mass, loosely attached to the original cartilage edges. The subchondral bone plate occasionally reforms to the same approximate level as the adjacent undamaged bone, but in cartilage lesions that do not involve substantial erosion of the underlying bone, the reformed subchondral bone plate may be higher than the surrounding normal bone plate (Frisbie et al, 1999). Immediately above the reformed subchondral plate, areas of cartilage proliferation predominate. The deeper cartilage layers and surface fibrous tissue generally follow a pattern of decreasing cellularity as the defect matures. At 12 months, type II collagen content approaches normal but proteoglycan levels are only about half that of normal (Howard et al, 1994). The phenomenon of matrix flow, an intrinsic repair mechanism, may also contribute to healing of articular cartilage defects by centripetal collapse of the perimeter of the lesion (Ghadially & Ghadially, 1975). In small defects, this can result in significant reduction in lesion size, but in defects over 9 mm in diameter, matrix flow is proportionally insignificant (Convery et al, 1972).

Depth of injury (full or partial thickness), the area of the defect, location in relation to weight-bearing or non-weight-bearing areas, and the age of the animal influence the repair rate and resiliency of new cartilage surfaces. The healing of chondral and osteochondral defects is more complete in young animals due to the increased mitotic capacity of chondrocytes, more active matrix synthesis, and closer proximity to the vascular supply in the depths of the articular-epiphyseal complex cartilage (Madsen et al, 1983). Examples of improved repair capacity are easily seen in the resurfacing potential following osteochondritis dissecans (OCD) flap removal in weanlings compared with debridement of articular erosions in adults. The area of the lesion is critical. Convery et al (1972) showed that lesions in the equine femorotibial joint less than 3 mm in diameter healed with little residual deformity (Convery et al, 1972). More recently, Hurtig et al (1988) determined that lesions larger than 15 mm^2 in surface area (3 × 5 mm rectangle) tended to show reasonably good repair at 5 months but degenerated with increasing time (Hurtig et al, 1988). These studies indicate that most clinically relevant defects in adults cannot be expected to heal well. The metaplasia of fibrous tissue to fibrocartilage is not always evident, and depending on the time of examination, degeneration to fibrous tissue and later mechanical erosion of the repair tissue can occur. Repair tissue is biomechanically inferior to normal articular cartilage, even though the histologic appearance is often fibrocartilage or even hyaline-like tissue (Ahsan & Sah, 1999). Repair tissue generally has significantly less proteoglycan and to some extent type II collagen

than normal cartilage. Additionally, the development of subchondral architecture and reestablishment of a tidemark is often irregular and inconsistent. This creates stress risers and susceptibility to cartilage deterioration with normal joint activity. Poor-quality, relatively short-lived repair cartilage has led to the development of pharmacologic and surgical methods to improve the repair process.

REPAIR METHODS

Techniques that enhance the quantity and hyaline characteristics of cartilage repair tissue would allow the surgeon to improve the long-term outcome when debriding cartilage lesions, particularly in challenging conditions of the stifle, carpus, and shoulder. These techniques should meet several important criteria:

1. Achievable arthroscopically
2. Result from local manipulations or use of simple transplant tissues
3. Available to surgical specialists with minimal delay between the diagnosis, decision for surgery, and the institution of the surgical repair
4. Reasonably economical
5. Tested in a research setting and able to offer advantages in durability and hyaline quality in the repair tissue
6. Amenable to the variety of shapes and locations of acute, subacute, and in some instances chronic, cartilage lesions that occur in clinical disease

No one arthroscopic system routinely provides all of these advantages. Those with inherent simplicity such as cartilage debridement, forage, and microfracture meet many of the criteria for simplicity, economy, and minimal delay between diagnosis and repair but provide less assured hyaline cartilage and cartilage durability than many of the more complex transplant methods. Techniques for cartilage repair that are clinically used or have been studied in a research setting can be subdivided into two categories: local manipulative procedures or cell and tissue transplantation techniques.

Local Manipulative Procedures

Surgical techniques that rely on simple manipulative procedures include the following:

- Cartilage debridement
- Chondroplasty to remove partial-thickness fibrillation
- Cartilage reattachment
- Forage or drilling of the subchondral bone to provide a uniform diameter perforation through the subchondral plate
- Microfracture or micropick, which uses a tapered surgical awl to perforate the subchondral bone and open marrow spaces
- Abrasion arthroplasty, using a motorized burr to remove a uniform layer of eburnated cartilage and bone
- Spongialization (saucerization) of the subchondral plate to open up larger marrow spaces by removal of greater thicknesses of the subchondral bone

Cartilage Debridement

Some form of cartilage debridement is common during arthroscopic surgery. As a simple rule, fibrous interpositional tissue or exposed loose bone should be removed from full-thickness defects. Debridement should continue down to firm, normal-appearing, subchondral bone plate. Maintaining

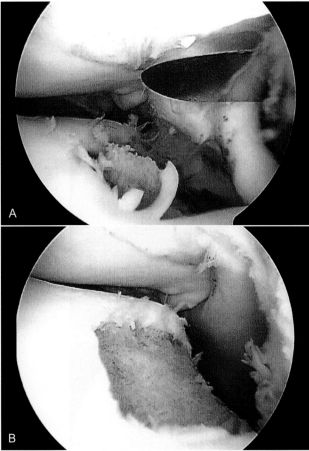

Figure 16-1 Cartilage and bone debridement of a stifle osteo-chondritis dissecans. **A,** The cartilage flap has been elevated using a periosteal elevator, revealing fibrous tissue and degenerate bone. **B,** The flap and underlying tissue, including degenerate loose bone, are removed, leaving perpendicular cartilage walls and normal subchondral bone. *(From Nixon AJ: Arthroscopic Techniques for Cartilage Repair, Clinical techniques in equine practice 1(4): 257-269, 2002.)*

damaged cartilage leaching degraded cartilage matrix fragments, including collagen, proteoglycan, and cellular components to the synovial fluid, where they increase synovitis and concurrent lameness (Thompson, 1975).

Full-thickness cartilage lesions are debrided to remove residual portions of the calcified cartilage layer, which tends to retard the development of well-attached cartilage repair tissue from the subchondral bone and surrounding cartilage (Frisbie et al, 2006). The most appropriate tools for cartilage debridement include a series of spoon and ring curettes that allow adequate removal of residual fibrous areas attached to the subchondral bone while leaving perpendicular cartilage defect walls (Fig. 16-2). A controlled study in dogs indicated the benefit of perpendicular cartilage walls following debridement, compared with beveled edges, which tended to increase the overall dimension of the healing defect (Rudd et al, 1987).

Exposed subchondral surfaces can be smoothed with either hand tools, which include curettes, rasps, and rongeurs, or motorized burrs. Several types of burr heads are available, varying from spherical to oval acromioplasty or notchplasty blades, which have an elongated profile for maximum bone removal effect (see Chapter 2). Hand tools are generally preferred to avoid excessive bone loss; however, for large areas of irregular hard bone, a burr may expedite the procedure and provide a better end result. Because the need for substantial bone removal in horses is low, an inventory of a single burr type is recommended.

Chondroplasty

Resection of the protruding surface strands of partial-thickness cartilage fibrillation has been promoted as a mechanism to reduce cartilage-derived detritus entering the synovial environment (Altman et al, 1992; Childers & Ellwood 1979; Kim et al, 1991; Thompson 1975). Motorized synovial abraders are used to smooth the surface of the more seriously damaged cartilage. The residual cartilage then presents a more uniform nonclefted surface, which may be more durable and incites less synovitis than the large surface area presented by multiple strands of fibrillated cartilage. The concept seems simple, but there is a paucity of evidence documenting any discrete benefit, either in reducing synovial levels of fragmented proteoglycan and collagen or in abrogating the symptoms of synovitis. Despite this, the technique has empirical benefits and has been used in equine arthroscopy for trimming extensive areas of partial-thickness fibrillated cartilage. The most frequent site for application in the horse is the stifle (Fig. 16-3). Trochlear ridge OCD in mature horses (>3 years) can be accompanied by fibrillation of the surrounding cartilage and the patella. Chondroplasty has been used to trim these areas to smooth articular cartilage and seems to reduce the incidence of persistent effusion when these horses reenter competition. No controlled clinical or experimental data support chondroplasty in the horse, so its use remains controversial. It may be preferable to doing nothing, but the resection depth should only involve the fibrillated surface and not be aggressively pursued down to the subchondral bone because the ensuing repair tissue rarely has the hyaline characteristics of the original deep cartilage layers that were resected.

Chondroplasty cannot be efficiently performed without sharp motorized abraders. Disposable cutting heads are recommended. Attached suction is also helpful in drawing and holding the cartilage fronds into the shaver blades. A "whisker" technique is used to avoid penetration of the intact deeper layers of cartilage. Benefits in man have been described for months to years after chondroplasty; however, as much as 6 months symptomatic relief has also been attributed to synovial washout using a saline lavage (Hubbard, 1996).

as much subchondral bone as possible keeps the bone and overlying cartilage repair tissue contoured to the normal congruency of the opposing joint surface, thereby enhancing the chance of healing cartilage tissue persistence. However, the remaining bone must be viable; crumbly, brownish bone should always be removed by debridement, using either hand instruments or motorized equipment (Fig. 16-1). At least for the carpus, the amount of residual bone after debridement is an important parameter in determining the prognosis for return to athletic activity (McIlwraith, 1990; McIlwraith et al, 1987). Several studies indicate the advantage of removal of full-thickness fibrillated cartilage. However, more debate surrounds the potential advantages of debriding partial-thickness cartilage defects down to subchondral bone, in efforts to encourage new cartilage formation from subchondral bone cellular and growth factor elements (Baumgaertner et al, 1990; Hubbard, 1996). Consensus appears to favor *not* debriding partial-thickness fibrillated cartilage, but rather leaving it attached to the calcified cartilage and underlying bone (McIlwraith, 1990). Partial-thickness defects have been shown to remain physically unchanged for at least 2 years (Mankin, 1982). Conversely, some symptomatic benefit for several months can be derived from chondroplasty of the obviously fibrillated portion of partial-thickness defects, which is described in more detail later (Kim et al, 1991; Thompson, 1975). In summary, chondroplasty reduces the possibility of

Cartilage Reattachment

Some cartilage flaps in the stifle, hock, and fetlock can be potentially salvaged and reattached (Nixon et al, 2004). Although not common, an OCD cartilage flap that is relatively smooth and has not detached on its entire perimeter can be secured with polydioxanone (PDS) pins (OrthoSorb, Depuy, Johnson & Johnson, New Brunswick, NJ). The technique has been detailed and illustrated in Chapter 6, and long-term results for stifle OCD have been recently presented (Sparks et al, 2011). Reattachment of partly mineralized flaps that have a smooth surface contour has been achieved more recently and can salvage the joint contour and avoid patellar

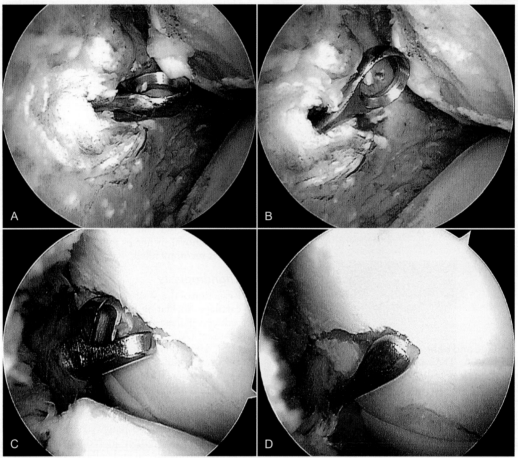

Figure 16-2 A, Debridement of cartilage using a ring curette. The aperture allows better visual control of the cutting edge, and the ring can also be used to provide a rasping effect. **B,** The curette cutting surface should be angled to provide a perpendicular cartilage edge. **C,** Biopsy punch rongeurs with a central vacuum channel can be effective for cleaning up debris along the cartilage edge. **D,** Spoon curettes are indicated for fine-edge debridement.

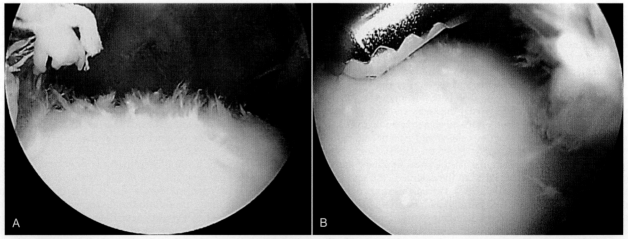

Figure 16-3 Chondroplasty. A, Extensive partial-thickness fibrillation of the lateral trochlear ridge of a 5-year-old horse with chronic gonitis from an untreated osteochondritis dissecans. **B,** Debridement with a motorized synovial resector has smoothed the fibrillated cartilage down to intact cartilage.

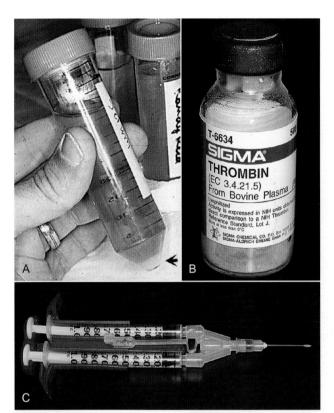

Figure 16-7 A, Autogenous fibrinogen derived by centrifugation of thawing plasma (cryoprecipitate) is ready to use after discarding the supernatant and saving the fibrinogen pellet *(arrowhead).* **B,** Bovine thrombin from commercial sources (250 or 500 units). Polymerization requires mixing calcium activated thrombin 1:1 with fibrinogen. **C,** A dual syringe holder (Baxter Healthcare, Arnold, MO) and Y-connector allows simultaneous mixing and injection of the fibrinogen-chondrocyte component and the thrombin–IGF-1 component.

congenital deformities. Cartilage slices are harvested aseptically from the stifle, shoulder, or elbow, and the cells isolated from their matrix by overnight collagenase digestion (Nixon et al, 1992). The cells are then counted, and dimethyl sulfoxide (DMSO) is added to the culture medium prior to freezing and storage in liquid nitrogen. When the cells are required, 48 hours' lead time is necessary to thaw the cells and then briefly culture to allow removal of any dead cells, before collection for use in surgery.

MSC Isolation and Banking. Harvest of autologous bone marrow–derived MSCs has become routine in university and practice laboratories, and several commercial laboratories offer harvest and frozen storage solutions for MSC use in cartilage repair. Several groups also utilize other sources of stem cells, including adipose tissue, synovial membrane, tendon, muscle, umbilical cord, and more recently fetal and induced pluripotent stem cell (iPS) sources. Although MSC immunophenotyping allows selection of potentially more appropriate predifferentiated cell types for cartilage repair, the use of stem cells has other broad effects, including antiinflammatory, immune suppressant, trophic anabolic, and anti-apoptotic effects, that suggest chondrogenesis of MSCs is not the primary target in MSC therapy in joint disease (Caplan, 2009). This provides rationale for surgical implantation of MSCs to cartilage, meniscus, and subchondral bone voids, as well as primary and follow-up injection of MSCs after the index surgery. Banked MSCs can be thawed and propagated in chondrogenic media containing dexamethasone and TGF-β3 before implantation.

Clinical Application. At the time of surgery the chondrocytes or MSCs are mixed with fibrinogen or PRP and stored at 4° C prior to injection. IGF-1 (50 μg) is added to 250 or 500 units of activated thrombin, to provide a two-component system for immediate injection. Thrombin is obtained from Sigma-Aldrich Corporation or MP Biomedicals (Fig. 16-7B), and the lyophilized powder reconstituted with calcium chloride (40 mmol) and sterilized by filtration through a 0.2-μm millipore syringe filter. At surgery, the polymerization process develops immediately upon injection of the two components into the articular defect (Fig. 16-7C). Arthroscopic lesion debridement is followed by helium or CO_2 gas insufflation for the few minutes required for fibrin or PRP injection. This allows drying of the defect using Q-tips® or surgical sponges applied to the end of a hemostat. Drying of the subchondral bed and surrounding intact cartilage allows better application of the naturally adhesive properties of fibrin and PRP. The polymerizing liquid nature of fibrin allows contouring of the cell transplant to the irregularities of many joint surfaces (Fig. 16-8).

Clinical application of chondrocyte grafting in horses has included traumatic cartilage lesions of the third carpal bone, metacarpal condylar fractures, and osteochondritis dissecans (OCD) or subchondral cystic lesions of the fetlock (14 horses) and stifle (49 horses) (Ortved et al, 2012). Chondrocyte augmentation following third carpal bone slab fracture repair and shoulder OCD debridement has resulted in few improvements in the number of horses capable of returning to athletic work. However, results for stifle OCD and subchondral cyst grafting of the stifle and fetlock have been generally good (Ortved et al, 2012). Complete radiographic filling has occurred in more than half of the stifle subchondral cysts radiographed at or beyond 12 months postoperatively (Fig. 16-9), and 73% of stifle subchondral cysts, including failures of previous simple debridement alone, have also been in athletic work for a minimum of 2 years. Similarly, fetlock subchondral cysts have been treated using arthroscopic extirpation and grafting (Fig. 16-10). Radiographic filling of the fetlock cysts can be slow, and residual deeper lytic regions can remain despite athletic performance (Fig. 16-11). All but two horses more than 12 months postoperative have entered athletic work. Both of these cases had evidence of remodeling due to osteoarthritis at the time of grafting.

Autologous MSCs have now largely replaced allograft chondrocytes for equine cartilage repair. Targeted implantation to cartilage and meniscus lesions has improved the outcome compared with ungrafted defects (Fig. 16-12), but retrospective data comparing MSC grafting to chondrocyte implantation have yet to be published. Predifferentiation of MSCs to the chondrocyte lineage with TGF-β3 and hypoxic conditions for articular repair is routine in one of the authors' laboratories (A.J.N.).

Future Directions

Numerous tissue-engineered cartilage composites have been developed for cartilage repair using the concept of artificial implantable hyaline-like cartilage, but none have entered clinical practice. The predominant reason for failure with preformed cartilage analogues is the lack of integration of the cartilage-like material to the subchondral bone and, most particularly, the surrounding cartilage. Most composites that begin to take on the biomechanical characteristics of cartilage before integration will fail. For this reason, soft, self-polymerizing and self-contouring grafts that are placed as liquids or soft composites and attach to the surrounding tissues are more likely to succeed. These grafts accumulate intrinsic mechanical competency as the cells synthesize their own matrix, which allows a better stress transition to adjacent cartilage. Although allograft chondrocytes from foals can potentially offer younger, more metabolically active cells (Kopesky et al, 2010), there has been a move to the use of autologous MSCs

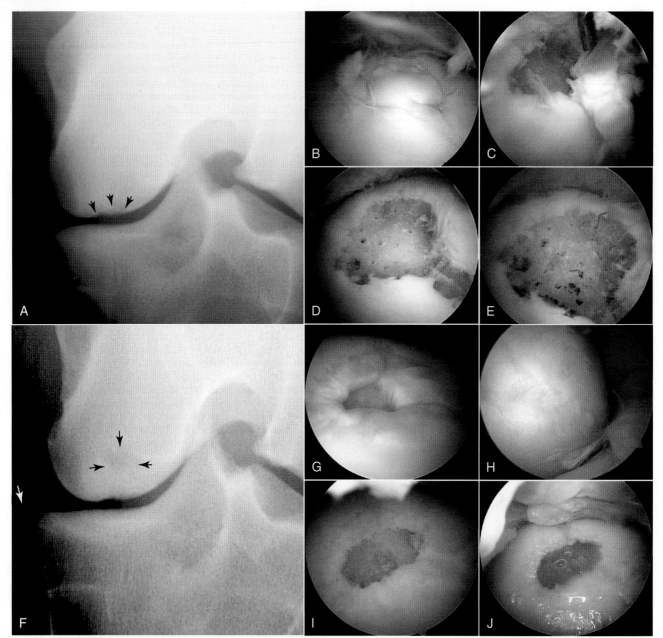

Figure 16-8 Mesenchymal stem cell (MSC) graft of failed medial femoral condyle debridement in a 5-year-old warmblood. **A,** Radiographs at original presentation show a shallow subchondral cyst *(arrows)*. **B-E,** Surgical debridement of necrotic cartilage and bone, followed by microfracture of the bone bed, shown with fluid distension **(D)** and fluid line closed **(E),** with active bleeding. Two years later the horse remained lame. **F,** New radiographs show residual crater, formation of a cyst deeper in the condyle *(black arrows)*, and osteoarthritis with osteophyte formation *(white arrow)*. At second surgery, the crater had partially filled **(G),** leaving a residual central cyst. **H,** Generalized cartilage fibrillation has developed on the medial condyle, and the medial meniscus has a minor tear. **I** and **J,** Debridement of the central defect revealed entry to deeper portion of the cyst. **J,** Graft of MSCs in platelet-rich plasma to the debrided cyst under gas distension. Other cartilage and meniscal defects were also debrided and selectively grafted. The horse returned to jumping and is still competing 6 years later.

to induce chondrogenesis (McIlwraith et al, 2011). The future will include more efficient culture methods, typing of the best primordial stromal cells for cartilage repair, and use of an autogenous bone marrow origin that has been extensively programmed using a combination of growth factor, peptide, and gene modulations to provide a better chondrocyte (Nixon et al, 2000). Moreover, the addition of anabolic growth factors to the cell mixture, including IGF-1 and several from the transforming growth factor superfamily, particularly BMP7 or BMP2, or both, will promote long-term matrix synthesis and

chondrocyte persistence (Nixon et al, 2000). Studies of IGF-I and BMP 7 gene–enhanced chondrocyte function in equine models suggest both stimulate extraordinary early healing, beyond that seen in unstimulated chondrocyte implanted cartilage defects (Goodrich et al, 2002; Hidaka et al, 2003). Long-term provision of an anabolic growth factor (IGF-I) and an anticatabolic factor (IL-1 receptor antagonist) using gene therapy has shown encouraging results in vitro (Haupt et al, 2005 ; Nixon et al, 2005) and more recently a postitive effect on cartilage repair in vivo (Morisset et al, 2007).

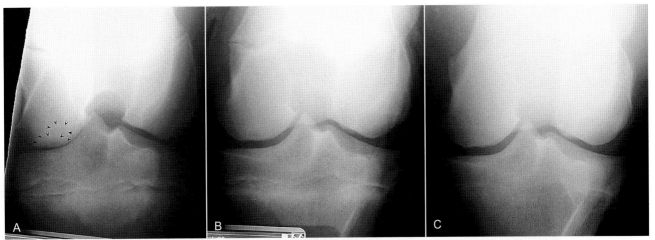

Figure 16-9 Chondrocyte-IGF-1 grafting of subchondral bone cysts of the medial femoral condyle. **A,** Radiographs of a yearling Quarter Horse showing a recently formed series of subchondral cysts of the medial condyle of the femur prior to surgery. **B,** Nine months after chondrocyte/IGF-1 grafting, some residual bone remodeling and lysis are evident. **C,** Radiographic filling and remodeling progressing 2 years after surgery.

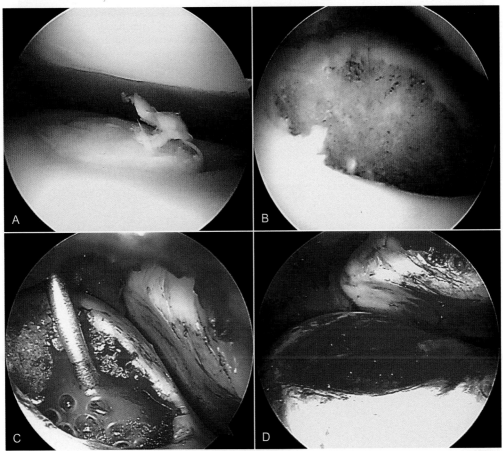

Figure 16-10 Chondrocyte-IGF-1 grafting of a subchondral bone cyst in the metacarpophalangeal joint. **A,** Arthroscopic appearance of a subchondral cyst in the medial condyle of the third metacarpal bone of a yearling Thoroughbred. **B,** Appearance of the cyst after debridement. **C,** The fibrin vehicle containing chondrocytes and IGF-1 is being injected. **D,** After polymerization, the grafted surface is congruous with surrounding cartilage.

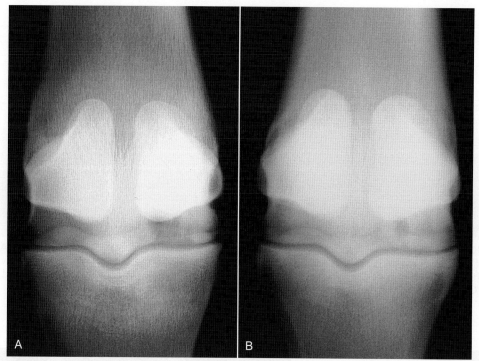

Figure 16-11 A, Preoperative radiographs of horse in Figure 16-10, showing a subchondral cyst with a wide opening (cloaca) to the articular surface of the third metacarpal bone. **B,** Radiographic appearance 2 years after grafting, showing return of subchondral bone density and residual small cyst. The filly was racing and had won at least one race despite this residual lesion.

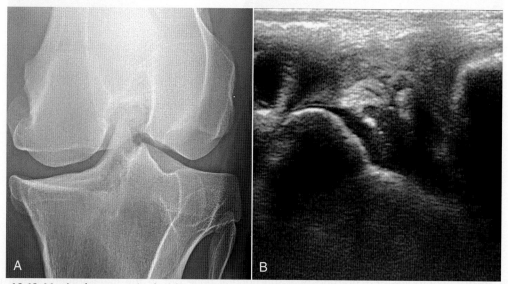

Figure 16-12 Meniscal tear repaired with mesenchymal stem cell (MSC) graft. **A** and **B,** Preoperative radiographs and ultrasound examination show osteoarthritis and void in the cranial horn of the medial meniscus.

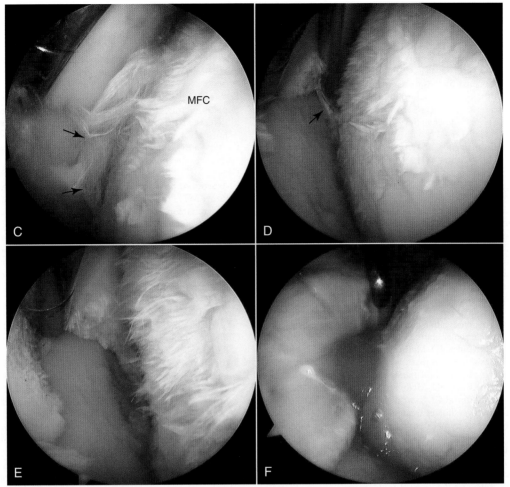

Figure 16-12, cont'd C, Arthroscopic examination shows extensive fibrillation of the medial femoral condyle *(MFC)* and shredded edge of meniscus *(arrows)*. **D,** Retraction of the cranial horn allows more exposure and motorized resection of the grade 3 tear *(arrow)*. **E,** Completed tear debridement. **F,** Implantation of MSCs in platelet-rich plasma vehicle to the meniscus void and debrided articular cartilage.

REFERENCES

Ahsan T, Sah RL: Biomechanics of integrative cartilage repair, *Osteoarthritis. Cartilage* 7:29–40, 1999.

Altman RD, Kates J, Chun LE, et al.: Preliminary observations of chondral abrasion in a canine model, *Ann Rheum Dis* 51:1056–1062, 1992.

Aubin PP, Cheah HK, Davis AM, Gross AE: Long-term followup of fresh femoral osteochondral allografts for posttraumatic knee defects, *Clin. Orthop* 391(Suppl):S318–S327, 2001.

Baumgaertner MB, Cannon WD, Vittori JM, Schmidt ES, Maurer RC: Arthroscopic debridement of the arthritic knee, *Clin Orthop* 253:197–202, 1990.

Blevins FT, Steadman JR, Rodrigo JJ, Silliman J: Treatment of articular cartilage defects in athletes: an analysis of functional outcome and lesion appearance, *Orthopedics* 21:761–767, 1998.

Bodo G, Hangody L, Szabo Z, et al.: Arthroscopic autologous osteochondral mosaicplasty for the treatment of subchondral cystic lesion in the medial femoral condyle in a horse, *Acta Vet Hung* 48:343–354, 2000.

Bodo G, Kaposi AD, Hangody L, et al.: The surgical technique and the age of the horse both influence the outcome of mosaicplasty in a cadaver equine stifle model, *Acta Vet Hung* 49:111–116, 2001.

Bodo G, Hangudy L, Modish, Hurtig M: Autologous osteochondral grafting (mosaic arthroplasty) for treatment of subchondral cystic lesions in the equine stifle and fetlock joints, *Vet Surg* 33:588–596, 2004.

Bouwmeester PS, Kuijer R, Homminga GN, Bulstra SK, Geesink RG: A retrospective analysis of two independent prospective cartilage repair studies: autogenous perichondral grafting versus subchondral drilling 10 years post-surgery, *J Orthop Res* 20:267–273, 2002.

Breinan HA, Martin SD, Hsu HP, Spector M: Healing of canine articular cartilage defects treated with microfracture, a type-II collagen matrix, or cultured autologous chondrocytes, *J Orthop Res* 18:781–789, 2000.

Breinan HA, Minas T, Hsu HP, et al.: Effect of cultured autologous chondrocytes on repair of chondral defects in a canine model, *J Bone Joint Surg* 79A:1439–1451, 1997.

Brittberg M, Lindahl A, Nilsson A, et al.: Treatment of deep cartilage defects in the knee with autologous chondrocyte transplantation, *N Engl J Med* 331:889–941, 1994.

Brittberg M, Tallheden T, Sjogren-Jansson B, Lindahl A, Peterson L: Autologous chondrocytes used for articular cartilage repair: an update, *Clin Orthop* 391(Suppl):S337–S348, 2001.

Bruns J, Kersten P, Lierse W, Silbermann M: Autologous rib perichondrial grafts in experimentally induced osteochondral lesions in the sheep-knee joint: morphological results, *Virchows Archiv A Pathol Anat* 421:1–8, 1992.

Butnariu-Ephrat M, Robinson D, Mendes DG, Halperin N, Nevo Z: Resurfacing of goat articular cartilage by chondrocytes derived from bone marrow, *Clin Orthop* 330:234–243, 1996.

Campbell CJ: The healing of cartilage defects, *Clin Orthop* 64:45–63, 1969.

Caplan AI: Why are MSCs therapeutic? New data: new insight, *J Pathol* 217:318–324, 2009.

Chen H, Hoemann DC, Sun J, Chebrier A, McKee MD, Shive MS, Hurtig M, Buschmann MD: Depth of subchondral perforation influences the outcome of bone marrow stimulation cartilage repair, *J Orthop Res* 29:1178–1184, 2011.

Chen H, Sun J, Hoemann CD, Lascau-Coman V, Ouyang W, McKee MD, Shive MS, Buschmann MD: Drilling and microfracture lead to different bone structure and necrosis during bone-marrow stimulation for cartilage repair, *J Orthop Res* 27:1432–1438, 2009.

Childers JC, Ellwood SC: Partial chondrectomy and subchondral bone drilling for chondromalacia, *Clin Orthop* 144:114–120, 1979.

Chu CR, Convery FR, Akeson WH, Meyers M, Amiel D: Articular cartilage transplantation. Clinical results in the knee, *Clin Orthop* 360:159–168, 1999.

Cole BJ, Farr J, Winalski CS, Hosea T, Richmond J, Mandelbaum B, De Deyne PG: Outcomes after a single-stage procedure for cell-based cartilage repair, *Am J Sports Med* 39:1170–1179, 2011.

Convery FR, Akeson WH, Keown GH: The repair of large osteochondral defects, *Clin Orthop* 82:253–262, 1972.

Coutts RD, Woo SLY, Amiel D, von Schroeder HP, Kwan MK: Rib periochondrial autografts in full thickness articular cartilage defects in rabbits, *Clin Orthop* 275:263–273, 1992.

Elves MW: A study of the transplantation antigens on chondrocytes from articular cartilage, *J Bone Joint Surg* 56-B:178–185, 1974.

Elves MW, Zervas J: An investigation into the immunogenicity of various components of osteoarticular grafts, *Br J Ex Path* 55:344–351, 1974.

Ferris DJ, Frisbie DD, Kisiday JD, McIlwraith CW: In vivo healing of meniscal lacerations using bone marrow derived mesenchymal stem cells and fibrin glue, *Stem Cell International* 2012:691605, 2012.

Ferris DJ, Frisbie DD, Kisiday JD, McIlwraith CW, Hague BA, Major MD, Schneider RK, Zubrod CJ, Kawcak CE, Goodrich LR: Clinical follow-up of thirty three horses treated for stifle injury with bone marrow derived mesenchymal stem cells intra-articularly, *Vet Surg*, 2013. In Press.

Ficat RP, Ficat C, Gedeon P, Toussaint JB: Spongialization: a new treatment for diseased patellae, *Clin Orthop* 144:74–83, 1979.

Foley RL, Nixon AJ: Insulin-like growth factor-1 peptide elution profiles from fibrin polymers determined by high performance liquid chromatography, *Am J Vet Res* 58:1431–1435, 1997.

Fortier LA, Cole BJ, McIlwraith CW: Science and animal models of marrow stimulation for cartilage repair, *J Knee Surg* 25:3–8, 2012.

Fortier LA, Lust G, Mohammed HO, Nixon AJ: Coordinate upregulation of cartilage matrix synthesis in fibrin cultures supplemented with exogenous insulin-like growth factor-I, *J Orthop Res* 17:467–474, 1999.

Fortier LA, Lust G, Mohammed HO, Nixon AJ: Insulin-like growth factor-I enhances cell-based articular cartilage repair, *J Bone Joint Surg* 84-B:276–288, 2002a.

Fortier LA, Nixon AJ, Lust G: Phenotypic expression of equine articular chondrocytes grown in three-dimensional cultures supplemented with supraphysiologic concentrations of insulinlike growth factor-1, *Am J Vet Res* 63:301–305, 2002b.

Fortier LA, Nixon AJ, Mohammed HO, Lust G: Altered biological activity of equine chondrocytes cultured in a three-dimensional fibrin matrix and supplemented with transforming growth factor B1, *Am J Vet Res* 58:66–70, 1997.

Fortier LA, Nixon AJ, Williams J, Cable CS: Isolation and chondrocytic differentiation of equine bone marrow-derived mesenchymal stem cells, *Am J Vet Res* 59:1182–1187, 1998.

Frisbie DD, Bowman SM, Calhoun HA, DiCarlo EF, Kawcak CE, McIlwraith CW: Evaluation of autologous chondrocyte concentration via a collagen membrane in equine articular defects – results at 12 and 18 months, *Osteoarthritis Cartilage* 16:667–679, 2008.

Frisbie DD, Lu Y, Kawcak CE, DiCarlo EF, Binette F, McIlwraith CW: In vivo evaluation of autologous cartilage fragment-loaded scaffold implanted into equine articular defects and compared with autologous chondrocyte implantation, *Am J Sports Med* 37:71S–80S, 2009.

Frisbie DD, Morisset S, Ho CP, Rodkey WG, Steadman JR, McIlwraith CW: Effects of calcified cartilage on healing of chondral defects treated with microfracture in horses, *Am J Sports Med* 34:1824–1831, 2006.

Frisbie DD, Nixon AJ: Insulin-like growth factor 1 and corticosteroid modulation of chondrocyte metabolic and mitogenic activities in interleukin 1-conditioned equine cartilage, *Am J Vet Res* 58:524–530, 1997.

Frisbie DD, Oxford JT, Southwood L, et al.: Early events in cartilage repair after subchondral bone microfracture, *Clin Orthop* 215–227, 2003.

Frisbie DD, Trotter GW, Powers BE: Arthroscopic subchondral bone plate microfracture technique augments healing of large chondral defects in the radial carpal bone and medial femoral condyle of horses, *Vet Surg* 28:242–255, 1999.

Gertzbein SD, Tait JH, Devlin SR, Argue S: The antigenicity of chondrocytes, *Immunology* 33:141–145, 1977.

Ghadially JA, Ghadially FN: Evidence of cartilage flow in deep defects in articular cartilage, *Arch B Cell Path* 18:193–204, 1975.

Ghazavi MT, Pritzker KP, Davis AM, Gross AE: Fresh osteochondral allografts for post-traumatic osteochondral defects of the knee, *J Bone Joint Surg* 79-B:1008–1013, 1997.

Goodrich LR, Nixon AJ, Hidaka C, Robbins PD, Evans CH: Enhanced early healing of articular cartilage with genetically modified chondrocytes expressing insulin-like growth factor-I, *Vet Surg* 31:482, 2002.

Grande DA, Southerland SS, Manji R, et al.: Repair of articular cartilage defects using mesenchymal stem cells, *Tissue Eng* 1:345–353, 1995.

Gross AE, Aubin P, Cheah HK, Davis AM, Ghazavi MT: A fresh osteochondral allograft alternative, *J Arthroplasty* 17:50–53, 2002.

Gudas R, Stankebicius E, Monastyrsekiene E, Branys D, Kalesinskas RJ: Osteochondral autologous transplantation vs. microfracture in the treatment of articular cartilage defects in the knee joint in athletes, *Knee Surg Sports Traumatol Arthros* 14:834–842, 2006.

Hale BW, Goodrich LR, Frisbie DD, McIlwraith CW, Kisiday JD: Effect of scaffold dilution on migration of mesenchymal stem cells from fibrin hydrogels, *Am J Vet Res* 73:313–318, 2012.

Hangody L, Feczko P, Bartha L, Bodo G, Kish G: Mosaicplasty for the treatment of articular defects of the knee and ankle, *Clin Orthop* 391(Suppl):S328–S336, 2001a.

Hangody L, Kish G, Karpati Z, Szerb I, Udvarhelyi I: Arthroscopic autogenous osteochondral mosaicplasty for the treatment of femoral condylar articular defects, *Knee Surg Sports Traumatol Arthrosc* 5:262–267, 1997.

Hangody L, Kish G, Karpati Z, et al.: Mosaicplasty for the treatment of articular cartilage defects: application in clinical practice, *Orthopedics* 21:751–756, 1998.

Hangody L, Kish G, Modis L, et al.: Mosaicplasty for the treatment of osteochondritis dissecans of the talus: two to seven year results in 36 patients, *Foot Ankle Int* 22:552–558, 2001b.

Harris JD, Siston RA, Pan X, Flanigan DC: Autologous chondrocyte implantation: a systematic review, *J Bone Joint Surg Am* 92:2220–2230, 2010.

Haupt JL, Frisbie DD, McIlwraith CW, Robbins PD, Ghivizzani S, Evans CH, Nixon AJ: Dual transduction of insulin-like growth factor-1 and interleukin-1 receptor antagonist protein controls cartilage degradation in an osteoarthritic culture model, *J Orthop Res* 23:118–126, 2005.

Hendrickson DA, Nixon AJ, Grande DA, et al.: Chondrocyte-fibrin matrix transplants for resurfacing extensive articular cartilage defects, *J Orthop Res* 12:485–497, 1994.

Heyner S: The significance of the intercellular matrix in the survival of cartilage allografts, *Transplantation* 8:666–677, 1969.

Hidaka C, Goodrich LR, Chen C-T, et al.: Acceleration of cartilage repair by genetically modified chondrocytes over-expressing bone morphogenetic protein-7, *J Orthop Res* 21:573–583, 2003.

Howard RD, McIlwraith CW, Trotter GW: Arthroscopic surgery for subchondral cystic lesions of the medial femoral condyle in horses: 41 cases (1988–1991), *J Am Vet Med Assoc* 206:842–850, 1995.

Howard RD, McIlwraith CW, Trotter GW, et al.: Long-term fate and effects of exercise on sternal cartilage autografts used for repair of large osteochondral defects in horses, *Am J Vet Res* 55:1158–1168, 1994.

Hubbard MJS: Articular debridement versus washout for degeneration of the medial femoral condyle, *J Bone Joint Surg* 78:217–219, 1996.

Hulse DA, Miller D, Roberts D, et al.: Resurfacing canine femoral trochleoplasties with free autogenous periosteal grafts, *Vet Surg* 15:284–288, 1986.

Hunziker EB, Rosenberg LC: Repair of partial-thickness defects in articular cartilage: cell recruitment from the synovial membrane, *J Bone Joint Surg* 78-A:721–733, 1996.

Hurtig M, Pearce S, Warren S, Kalra M, Miniaci A: Arthroscopic mosaic arthroplasty in the equine third carpal bone, *Vet Surg* 30:228–239, 2001.

Hurtig MB: Experimental use of small osteochondral grafts for resurfacing the equine third carpal bone, *Equine Vet J*(Suppl 6)23–27, 1988.

Hurtig MB, Fretz PB, Doige CE, Schnurr DL: Effects of lesion size and location on equine articular cartilage repair, *Can J Vet Res* 52:137–146, 1988.

Im GI, Kim DY, Shin JH, Hyun CW, Cho WH: Repair of cartilage defect in the rabbit with cultured mesenchymal stem cells from bone marrow, *J Bone Joint Surg (Br)* 83:289–294, 2001.

Insall J: The Pridie debridement operation for osteoarthritis of the knee, *Clin Orthop* 101:61–67, 1974.

Jackson DW, Simon TM: Donor cell survival and repopulation after intraarticular transplantation of tendon and ligament allografts, *Microsc Res Tec* 58:25–33, 2002.

Jakob RP, Franz T, Gautier E, Mainil-Varlet P: Autologous osteochondral grafting in the knee: indication, results, and reflections, *Clin Orthop* 401:170–184, 2002.

Johnson LL: Arthroscopic abrasion arthroplasty historical and pathologic perspective: present status, *Arthroscopy* 2:54–69, 1986.

Johnson LL: Characteristics of the immediate postarthroscopic blood clot formation in the knee joint, *Arthroscopy* 7:14–23, 1991.

Johnson LL: Arthroscopic abrasion arthroplasty: a review, *Clin Orthop* 391(Suppl):S306–S317, 2001.

Johnstone B, Yoo JU: Autologous mesenchymal progenitor cells in articular cartilage repair, *Clin Orthop* 367(Suppl):S156–S162, 1999.

Kawabe N, Yoshinao M: The repair of full-thickness articular cartilage defects. Immune responses to reparative tissue formed by allogeneic growth plate chondrocyte implants, *Clin Orthop* 268:279–293, 1991.

Kim HKW, Moran ME, Salter RB: The potential for regeneration of articular cartilage in defects created by chondral shaving and subchondral abrasion, *J Bone Joint Surg* 73A(9):1301–1315, 1991.

King PJ, Bryant T, Minas T: Autologous chondrocyte implantation for chondral defects of the knee: indications and technique, *J Knee Surg* 15:177–184, 2002.

Knutsen G, Drogset JO, Engebretsen L, et al.: A randomized trial comparing autologous chondrocyte implantation with microfracture: findings at five years, *J Bone Joint Surg Am* 89:2105–2112, 2007.

Kopesky PW, Lee HY, Vanderploeg EJ, Kisiday JD, Frisbie DD, Plaas AH, Ortiz C, Grodzinsky AJ: Adult equine bone marrow stromal cells produce a cartilage-like ECM mechanically superior to animal-matched adult chondrocytes, *Matrix Bio* 29:427–438, 2010.

Kreuz PC, Erggelet C, Steinwachs MR, Krause SJ, Lahm A, Niemeyer P, Ghane MN, Uhl M, Südkamp N: Is microfracture of chondral defects in the knee associated with different results of patients aged 40 years or younger? *Arthroscopy* 22:1180–1186, 2006b.

Kreuz PC, Steinwachs MR, Erggelet C, Krause SJ, Konrad G, Uhl M, Südkamp N: Results after microfracture of full-thickness chondral defects in different compartments in the knee, *Osteoarthritis Cartilage* 14:1119–1125, 2006a.

Krych AJ, Robertson CM, Williams RJ: Return to athletic activity after osteochondral allograft transplantation in the knee, *Am J Sports Med* 40:1053–1059, 2012.

Kwan MK, Coutts RD, Woo SLY, Field FP: Morphological and biomechanical evaluations of neocartilage from the repair of full-thickness articular cartilage defects using rib perichondrium autografts: a long term study, *J Biomech* 22:921–930, 1989.

Lance EM, Kimura LH, Manibog CN: The expression of major histocompatibility antigens on human articular chondrocytes, *Clin Orthop* 291:266–282, 1993.

Lee CR, Grodzinsky AJ, Hsu HP, Martin SD, Spector M: Effects of harvest and selected cartilage repair procedures on the physical and biochemical properties of articular cartilage in the canine knee, *J Orthop Res* 18:790–799, 2000.

Lindahl A, Brittberg M, Peterson L: Health economics benefits following autologous chondrocyte transplantation for patients with focal chondral lesions of the knee, *Knee Surg Sports Traumatol Arthrosc* 9:358–363, 2001.

Luyten FP, Hascall VC, Nissley SP, Morales SP, Reddi AH: Insulin-like growth factors maintain steady state metabolism of proteoglycans in bovine articular cartilage explants, *Arch Biochem Biophys* 276:416–425, 1988.

Madsen K, Moskalewski S, von der Mark K, Friberg U: Synthesis of proteoglycans, collagen, and elastin by cultures of rabbit auricular chondrocytes-relation to age of the donor, *Dev Biol* 96:63–73, 1983.

Mankin HJ: The response of articular cartilage to mechanical injury, *J Bone Joint Surg* 64A:460–466, 1982.

Mankin HJ, Jennings LC, Treadwell BV, Trippel SB: Growth factors and articular cartilage, *J Rheumatol* 18(Suppl 27):66–67, 1991.

McIlwraith CW: Surgery of the hock, stifle, and shoulder, *Vet Clin North Am* 5:350–354, 1983.

McIlwraith CW: *Diagnostic and surgical arthroscopy in the horse*, ed 2, Philadelphia, 1990, Lea and Febiger.

McIlwraith CW, Frisbie DD, Rodkey WG, Kisiday JD, Werpy NM, Kawcak CE, Steadman JR: Evaluation of intra-articular mesenchymal stem cells to augment healing of microfractured chondral defects, *Arthroscopy* 27:1552–1561, 2011.

McIlwraith CW, Yovich JV, Martin GS: Arthroscopic surgery for the treatment of osteochondral chip fractures in the equine carpus, *J Am Vet Med Assoc* 191:531–540, 1987.

Menche DS, Frenkel SR, Blair B, et al.: A comparison of abrasion burr arthroplasty and subchondral drilling in the treatment of full-thickness cartilage lesions in the rabbit, *Arthroscopy* 12:280–286, 1996.

Mendicino RW, Catanzariti AR, Hallivis R: Mosaicplasty for the treatment of osteochondral defects of the ankle joint, *Clin Podiatr Med Surg* 18:495–513, 2001.

Meyers MH, Akeson W, Convery FR: 1989 Resurfacing of the knee with fresh osteochondral allograft, *J Bone Joint Surg* 71A:704–713, 2001.

Minas T: Chondrocyte implantation in the repair of chondral lesions of the knee: economics and quality of life, *Am J Orthop* 27:739–744, 1998.

Minas T: Autologous chondrocyte implantation for focal chondral defects of the knee, *Clin Orthop* 391(Suppl):S349–S361, 2001.

Minas T, Chiu R: Autologous chondrocyte implantation, *Am J Knee Surg* 13:41–50, 2000.

Minas T, Peterson L: Advanced techniques in autologous chondrocyte transplantation, *Clin Sports Med* 18, 1999. 13-vi.

Moran ME, Kim HKW, Salter RB: Biological resurfacing of full-thickness defects in patellar articular cartilage of the rabbit, *J Bone Joint Surg* 74B:659–667, 1992.

Morisset S, Frisbie DD, Robbins PD, Nixon AJ, McIlwraith CW: IL-1Ra/IGF-1 gene therapy modulates repair of microfractured chondral defects, *Clin Orthop Related Res* 462:221–228, 2007.

Moskalewski S, Kawiak J, Rymaszewska T: Local cellular response evoked by cartilage formed after auto-and allogeneic transplantation of isolated chondrocytes, *Transplantation* 4:572–581, 1966.

Niedermann B, Boe S, Lauritzen J, Rubak JM: Glued periosteal grafts in the knee, *Acta Ortho Scand* 56:457–460, 1985.

Nixon AJ, Begum L, Mohammed HO, Huibregtse B, O'Callaghan MM, Matthews GL: Autologous chondrocyte implantation drives early chondrogenesis and organized repair in extensive full- and partial-thickness cartilage defects in an equine model, *J Orthop Res* 29:1121–1130, 2011.

Nixon AJ, Rickey EJ, Butler TJ, Scimeca MS, Moran N, Matthews GL: A chondrocyte infiltrated collagen type I/III membrane (MACI® implant) improves cartilage healing in the equine patellofemoral joint model, *Osteoarthritis Cartilage*, 2014. In press.

Nixon AJ, Brower-Toland BD, Bent SJ, et al.: Insulin-like growth factor-I gene therapy applications in cartilage repair and degenerative joint diseases, *Clin Orthop* 379S:S201–S213, 2000.

Nixon AJ, Fortier LA, Goodrich LR, Ducharme NG: Arthroscopic reattachment of select OCD lesions using resorbable polydioxanone pins, *Equine Vet J* 36:376–383, 2004a.

Nixon AJ, Haupt JL, Frisbie DD, et al.: Gene mediated restoration of cartilage matrix by combination insulin-like growth factor-I/interleukin-1 receptor antagonist therapy, *Gene Therapy* 12:177–186, 2005.

Nixon AJ, Fortier LA, Williams J, Mohammed HO: Enhanced repair of extensive articular defects by insulin-like growth factor-I laden fibrin composites, J Orthop Res 17:475–487, 1999.

Nixon AJ, Lillich JT, Burton-Wurster N, Lust G, Mohammed HO: Differentiated cellular function in fetal chondrocytes cultured with insulin-like growth factor-I and transforming growth factor-B, J Orthop Res 16:531–541, 1998.

Nixon AJ, Lust G, Vernier-Singer M: Isolation, propagation and cryopreservation of equine articular chondrocytes, Am J Vet Res 53:2364–2370, 1992.

O'Connor WJ, Botti T, Khan SN, Lane JM: The use of growth factors in cartilage repair, Orthop Clin North Am 31:399–410, 2000.

O'Driscoll SW: Healing and regeneration of articular cartilage, J Bone Joint Surg 80A:1795–1812, 1998.

O'Driscoll SW: Articular cartilage regeneration using periosteum, Clin Orthop 367(Suppl):S186–S203, 1999.

O'Driscoll SW, Keeley FW, Salter RB: The chondrogenic potential of free autogenous periosteal grafts for biological resurfacing of major full-thickness defects in joint surfaces under the influence of continuous passive motion, J Bone Joint Surg 68A:1017–1035, 1986.

O'Driscoll SW, Salter RB: The induction of neochondrogenesis in free intra-articular periosteal autografts under the influence of continuous passive motion, J Bone Joint Surg 66A:1248–1257, 1984.

O'Driscoll SW, Salter RB: The repair of major osteochondral defects in joint surfaces by neochondrogenesis with autogenous osteoperiosteal grafts stimulated by continuous passive motion, Clin Orthop 208:131–140, 1986.

Ohlsen L, Widenfalk B: The early development of articular cartilage after perichondrial grafting, Scand J Plast Reconstr Surg 17:163–177, 1983.

Orth P, Goebel L, Wolfram J, Ong FF, Graber S, Kohn D, Cucchiarini M, Ignatius A, Pape D, Madr Y: Effect of subchondral drilling on the microarchitecture of subchondral bone: analysis in a large animal model of six month, Am J Sports Med 40:828–836, 2012.

Ortved KO, Nixon AJ, Mohammed HO, Fortier LA: Treatment of subchondral cystic lesions of the medial femoral condyle of mature horses with growth factor enhanced chondrocyte grafts: A retrospective study of 49 cases, Equine Vet J 44:606–613, 2012.

Ostrander RV, Goomer RS, Tontz WL, et al.: Donor cell fate in tissue engineering for articular cartilage repair, Clin Orthop 389:228–237, 2001.

Pearce SG, Hurtig MB, Clarnette R, et al.: An investigation of 2 techniques for optimizing joint surface congruency using multiple cylindrical osteochondral autografts, Arthroscopy 17:50–55, 2001.

Peterson L, Brittberg M, Kiviranta I, Akerlund EL, Lindahl A: Autologous chondrocyte transplantation. Biomechanics and long-term durability, Am J Sports Med 30:2–12, 2002.

Peterson L, Minas T, Brittberg M, Nilsson A, Sjogren-Jansson E, Lindahl A: Two-to 9-year outcome after autologous chondrocyte transplantation of the knee, Clin Orthop 374:212–234, 2000.

Pridie KH: A method of resurfacing osteoarthritic knee joints, J Bone Joint Surg 41B:618, 1959.

Richardson JB, Caterson B, Evans EH, Ashton BA, Roberts S: Repair of human articular cartilage after implantation of autologous chondrocytes, J Bone Joint Surg Br 81:1064–1068, 1999.

Riddle WE: Healing of articular cartilage in the horse, J Am Vet Med Assoc 157:1471–1479, 1970.

Ritsila VA, Santavirta S, Alhopuro S, et al.: Periosteal and perichondral grafting in reconstructive surgery, Clin Orthop 302:259–265, 1994.

Robert H, Bahuaud J: Autologous chondrocyte implantation. A review of techniques and preliminary results, Rev Rhum Engl Ed 66:724–727, 1999.

Rodrigo JJ, Steadman JR, Silliman JF, Fulstone HA: Improvement of full-thickness chondral defect healing in the human knee after debridement and microfracture using continuous passive motion, Am J Knee Surg 7:109–116, 1994.

Rogachefsky RA, Dean DD, Howell DS, Altman RD: Treatment of canine osteoarthritis with insulin-like growth factor-1 (IGF-1) and sodium pentosan polysulfate, Osteoarthritis Cart 1:105–114, 1993.

Rubak JM: Reconstruction of articular cartilage defects with free periosteal grafts. An experimental study, Acta Orthop Scand 53:175–180, 1982.

Rudd RG, Visco DM, Kincaid SA, Cantwell HD: The effects of beveling the margins of articular cartilage defects in immature dogs, Vet Surg 16:378–383, 1987.

Sams AE, Minor RR, Wootton JAM, Mohammed H, Nixon AJ: Local and regional matrix responses to chondrocyte laden collagen scaffold implantation in extensive articular cartilage defects, Osteoarthritis Cart 3:61–70, 1995.

Sams AE, Nixon AJ: Chondrocyte-laden collagen scaffolds for resurfacing extensive articular cartilage defects, Osteoarthritis Cart 3:47–59, 1995.

Saris DBF, Vanlauwe J, Victor J, Almqist KF, Verdonk R, Bellemans J, Luyten FP: Treatment of symptomatic cartilage defects of the knee: Characterized chondrocyte implantation results in better clinical outcome at 36 months in a randomized trial compared to microfracture, Am J Sports Med 37:10S–19S, 2009.

Shamis LD, Bramlage LR, Gabel AA, Weisbrode S: Effect of subchondral drilling on repair of partial-thickness cartilage defects of third carpal bones in horses, Am J Vet Res 50:290–295, 1989.

Sparks HD, Nixon AJ, Fortier LA, Mohammed HO: Arthroscopic reattachment of osteochondritis dessicans cartilage flaps of the femoropatellar joint: long-term results, Equine Vet J 43:650–659, 2011.

Steadman JR, Rodkey WG, Briggs KK: Microfracture to treat full-thickness chondral defects: surgical technique, rehabilitation, and outcomes, J Knee Surg 15:170–176, 2002.

Steadman JR, Rodkey WG, Rodrigo JJ: Microfracture: surgical technique and rehabilitation to treat chondral defects, Clin Orthop 391(Suppl):S362–S369, 2001.

Strong DM, Friedlaender GE, Tomford WW, et al.: Immunologic responses in human recipients of osseous and osteochondral allografts, Clin Orthop 326:107–114, 1996.

Thompson RC: An experimental study of surface injury to articular cartilage and enzyme responses within the joint, Clin Orthop 107:239–248, 1975.

Trippel SB, Coutts RD, Einhorn TA, Mundy GR, Rosenfeld RG: Growth factors as therapeutic agents, J Bone Joint Surg 78A:1272–1286, 1996.

Tyler JA, Bird JLE, Giller T, Benton HP: Cytokines, growth factors and cartilage repair. In Russel RGG, Dieppe PA, editors: Osteoarthritis. Current research and prospects for pharmacological intervention, Sheffield, 1989, IBC Technical Services, pp 144–153.

Vachon A, Bramlage LR, Gabel AA, Weisbrode S: Evaluation of the repair process of cartilage defects of the equine third carpal bone with and without subchondral bone perforation, Am J Vet Res 47:2637–2645, 1986.

Vachon A, McIlwraith CW, Trotter GW, Norrdin RW, Powers BE: Neochondrogenesis in free intraarticular, periosteal, and perichondrial autografts in horses, Am J Vet Res 50:1787–1794, 1989.

Vachon AM, McIlwraith CW, Keeley FW: Biochemical study of repair of induced osteochondral defects of the distal portion of the radial carpal bone in horses by use of periosteal autografts, Am J Vet Res 52:328–332, 1991a.

Vachon AM, McIlwraith CW, Trotter GW, et al.: Morphologic study of induced osteochondral defects of the distal portion of the radial carpal bone in horses by use of glued periosteal autografts, Am J Vet Res 52:317–327, 1991b.

van Beuningen HM, van der Kraan PM, Arntz OJ, van den Berg WB: Transforming growth factor-β1 stimulates articular chondrocyte proteoglycan synthesis and induces osteophyte formation in the murine knee joint, Lab Inves 71:279–290, 1994.

van den Berg WB: Growth factors in experimental osteoarthritis: transforming growth factor ß pathogenic? J Rheumatol 22:143–145, 1995.

van den Berg WB, van Osch GJ, van der Kraan PM, van Beuningen HM: Cartilage destruction and osteophytes in instability-induced murine osteoarthritis: role of TGF beta in osteophyte formation? Agents Actions 40:215–219, 1993.

Wakitani S, Goto T, Pineda SJ: Mesenchymal cell-based repair of large, full-thickness defects of articular cartilage, J Bone Joint Surg 76A:579–592, 1994.

White NA, McIlwraith CW, Allen D: Curettage of subchondral bone cysts in medial femoral condyles of the horse, Equine Vet J 6(Suppl):120–124, 1988.

Wilke M, Nixon AJ, Adams TA: Enhanced early chondrogenesis in equine cartilage defects using implanted autologous mesenchymal stem cells, Vet Surg 30:508–509, 2001.

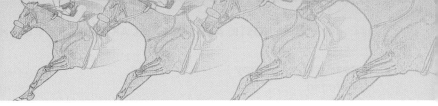

CHAPTER 17

Postoperative Management, Adjunctive Therapies, and Rehabilitation Procedures

IMMEDIATE POSTOPERATIVE MANAGEMENT

Bandaging

The maintenance of sterile bandages is critical in the immediate postoperative period. Ideally sterile bandages should be maintained for all joints from carpus and tarsus distally for 2 weeks. Typically a recommendation is to remove sutures at 10 to 12 days and then maintain the sterile bandage for at least 2 days beyond this. As illustrated in Chapter 6 the use of postoperative covers after stifle arthroscopy is also recommended. The two main risk factors for postoperative infection, other than asepsis during arthroscopic surgery itself, are loss of bandage cover and lack of a sterile preparation when removing sutures.

Nonsteroidal Antiinflammatory Drugs

The use of nonsteroidal antiinflammatory drugs (NSAIDs) to control postoperative inflammation and pain is appropriate. Administration times vary between 3 and 7 days and the usual drug is phenylbutazone. A drug blocking cyclooxygenase (COX) affects prostaglandins alone and therefore represents a focused antiinflammatory therapy. It is currently considered standard care for first-line treatment of traumatically induced inflammation, and the authors use it both preoperatively and postoperatively. It is recognized that phenylbutazone inhibits both COX-1 and COX-2, but side effects are rare. Newer COX-2 preferential inhibitors are now available, and topical application has been shown to be beneficial in an equine osteoarthritis (OA) model (Frisbie et al, 2009). Phenylbutazone is relatively nontoxic at repeated doses of 2.2 mg/kg, and 4.4 mg/kg daily (Collins and Tyler, 1984). A single dose of 4.4 g/kg phenylbutazone markedly reduced PGE2 levels and production in exudate for up to 24 hours (Higgins & Lees, 1983). This is due to an accumulation of phenylbutazone in inflammatory exudate (probably explained by a high degree of protein binding of phenylbutazone and the proteinaceous nature of inflammatory fluid) leading to an elimination T½ in exudate of 24 hours (Lees et al, 1986). The use of this dose of phenylbutazone has been shown to have a significant effect on lameness in horses with experimentally induced synovitis, including joint temperature, synovial fluid volume, and synovial fluid PGE_2 levels. Furthermore, in a comparative study the effects produced by phenylbutazone were significantly greater compared with ketoprofen (Owens et al, 1996). In the authors' experience, phenylbutazone is a clinically effective analgesic for orthopedic pain in horses.

LONGER-TERM POSTOPERATIVE MANAGEMENT

This section includes the period from postsurgery until training is commenced in the equine athletic patient. Therapies and rehabilitative techniques that are discussed include parenteral medications, intraarticular medications, oral medications, and physical therapies including exercise that the authors use.

Systemic Medications

Polysulfated Glycosaminoglycan

Polysulfated glycosaminoglycan (PSGAG) administered intramuscularly (IM) is still popular, but evidence is limited to anecdotal opinion. Intramuscular injections of 500 mg were commonly recommended by the first author postoperatively until a controlled study in experimentally induced equine OA showed no significant difference in the administration of PSGAG IM every 4 days for 28 days as a positive control treatment in an evaluation of extracorporeal shock wave treatment on experimentally induced OA in the middle carpal joints of horses (Frisbie et al, 2009). Consequently this recommendation is no longer made.

Pentosan Polysulfate

Intramuscularly administered sodium pentosan polysulfate (NaPPS) has been commonly used outside the United States both postoperatively and for the treatment of OA. Recently, NaPPS at a dose of 3 mg/kg IM at 15, 22, 29, and 36 days after induction of experimental carpal OA caused a significant reduction in articular cartilage fibrillation and an increase in chondroitin sulfate 846 epitope (a synthetic biomarker) in the synovial fluid of both osteoarthritic and nonosteoarthritic joints. This indicated that NaPPS has some beneficial disease-modifying effects (McIlwraith et al, 2012). The product is available as Pentosan Equine Injectionr® (250 mg/mL; Ceva, Australia) and as Pentosan Gold® and PentAussie® (125 mg/mL in combination with N-Acetyl Glucosamine 200 mg/mL; International Veterinary Supplies, Australia). The reader should be aware that at the time of writing, licensing for these products is restricted.

Intravenous Hyaluronan

The administration of intravenous hyaluronan (HA) (40 mg IV) postoperatively is used by some clinicians, and scientific evidence supports its use. With a study in the equine osteochondral fragment–OA model three treatments of 40 mg were given intravenously 13, 20, and 27 days after osteochondral fragment creation. There was a significant decrease in lameness, synovial fluid protein and PGE_2 levels, synovial membrane vascularity, and synovial membrane cellular infiltration at day 72 compared with the control group given 4 mL of saline intravenously at those same times (Kawcak et al, 1997).

Oral Hyaluronan

A number of nutraceuticals are used following arthroscopic surgery. All of these products are unlicensed and, with the exception of oral HA (Conquer®), there is no scientific evidence to support their use. Oral HA (Conquer®) has been shown to reduce postoperative effusion after arthroscopic surgery for tarsocrural OCD (Bergin et al, 2006). In 24 yearlings (with 27 joints operated) 100 mg of oral HA were given daily for 30 days postoperatively, and another 24 yearlings (30 joints operated) were treated with placebo daily for 30 days. An examiner blinded to the treatment groups scored the effusion 30 days post surgery on a scale of 0 to 5. The mean 30-day effusion score in the treated group was 0.67 compared with 2.05 in the placebo group ($P < 0.0001$).

Intraarticular Therapy

Hyaluronan

Although the authors do not routinely recommend the use of intraarticular HA after surgery, it is commonly practiced and can be defended scientifically. In an experimental study of equine OA induced by osteochondral fragmentation in the middle carpal joint, eight horses received 20 mg of HA (Hyvisc®, Anika Therapeutics Inc., Woburn, MA) intraarticularly 14, 21, and 28 days after fragment creation (Frisbie et al, 2009). No adverse treatment-related events were detected. No changes in clinical signs were seen with HA compared with control horses, but histologically at day 70 there was significantly less fibrillation with HA treatment compared with controls. The potential is certainly there for reduction of early postoperative OA following arthroscopic surgery with such a treatment.

Polysulfated Glycosaminoglycan

The first author has routinely recommended the use of intraarticular polysulfated glycosaminoglycan (PSGAG) (Adequan IA®, Luitpold Pharmaceuticals Inc., Animal Health Division, Shirley, NY) following arthroscopic surgery when there is any degree of subchondral bone debridement. The latter tends to cause persistent postoperative effusion and hemarthrosis, and a clinical observation had been made that this could be corrected quickly with the use of one to two injections of 250 mg of PSGAG (typically these were middle carpal joints). Again, studying the potential value in a controlled study using the equine osteochondral fragment–OA model, eight horses received PSGAG (250 mg) and amikacin sulfate (125 mg) intraarticularly at 14, 21, and 28 days after induction of OA and eight control horses received 2 mL of saline (0.9% NaCl) solution and amikacin sulfate (125 mg) intraarticularly on study days 14, 21, and 28. No adverse treatment-related effects were seen. Although there were no significant changes in clinical signs seen with PSGAG compared with control horses, the degree of synovial membrane vascularity and subintimal fibrosis was significantly reduced with PSGAG treatment and there was a trend for reduced fibrillation at day 70. This implied beneficial disease-modifying effects and usefulness postoperatively (Frisbie et al, 2009).

Corticosteroids

Intraarticular corticosteroids were the original intraarticular therapy for equine OA and are still used frequently for traumatic arthritis (including posttraumatic OA). Historically, the untoward effects of corticosteroids have been generalized and are often unsubstantiated. More recently, effects of the commonly used corticosteroids have been carefully evaluated. A study with betamethasone esters (Betavet Soluspan®; Celestone® Soluspan®, Schering-Plough Animal Health Corp, Union, NJ) administered in a 2.5-mL (3.9 mg betamethasone sodium phosphate and 12 mg betamethasone acetate per milliliter) dose 14 and 35 days after experimental osteochondral fragmentation showed that there were no deleterious side effects on the articular cartilage and that preservation of glycosaminoglycan staining with safranin O was better in the group treated with betamethasone and exercise compared with control groups that were injected with saline or betamethasone but were not exercised (Foland et al, 1994). It is to be noted that Betavet Soluspan® is no longer available and Celestone® Soluspan® is now used. Each milliliter of Celestone® injectable suspension contains 3 mg of betamethasone as betamethasone sodium phosphate and 3 mg of betamethasone acetate. On the other hand, evaluation of methylprednisolone acetate (MPA, Depo Medrol®) (at a dose of 100 mg given 14 and 28 days) postoperatively in the osteochondral fragment OA model showed that, although there was decrease in inflammatory indices, MPA caused articular degeneration in middle carpal joints even when it was injected in the opposite joint (Frisbie et al,

1998). A third study with triamcinolone acetonide (Vetalog®) tested with the same experimental design as MPA showed significant reduction in lameness after intraarticular injection of 12 mg at 14 and 28 days, as well as disease-modifying effects on articular cartilage with a reduction in the modified Mankin score compared with saline-injected controls (Frisbie et al, 1997). The suggestion from these studies is that if evidence of continued inflammation is present a number of weeks after arthroscopic surgery, the use of betamethasone esters or triamcinolone acetonide could be an appropriate treatment.

Autologous Conditioned Serum (IRAP® or IRAP II®)

Autologous conditioned serum (ACS) was initially developed for the treatment of human OA as a product called Orthokine® and was initially tested in horses in Europe and shown to be particularly beneficial in OA (of the distal interphalangeal joint) not responding to triamcinolone and HA (Weinberger personal communication, 2003). Orthokine® was subsequently distributed in the United States as IRAP® (initially marketed by Arthrex, and now marketed by another company Dechra), and an experimental study demonstrated benefit in osteochondral fragment–induced equine OA (Frisbie et al, 2007). Horses received 6 mL of ACS at 14, 21, 28, and 38 days after treatment (control horses received 6 mL of saline intraarticularly at the same time). Horses treated with ACS were observed to have significantly reduced lameness in the OA limbs even 5 weeks after the last treatment compared with placebo-treated horses. There was also a significant reduction in synovial membrane hyperplasia in treated compared with placebo joints at day 70. A trend for improvement ($P < 0.10$) in cartilage gross score and cartilage histochemistry was also noted in ACS compared with placebo-treated OA joints. The hypothesis that the main effect of this therapy was due to significant increases in interleukin 1 receptor antagonist protein (IL-1ra) was confirmed with increases seen at days 35 and 71.

A newer product, IRAP II® (developed and now marketed by Arthrex Vet Systems), has since been produced with a modified technique, including a newly designed device with dual ports, and a comparative study done on the cytokine profiles of IRAP® and IRAP II® using equine blood (Hraha et al, 2011). The level of IL-1ra and the ratio of IL-1ra to IL-1β in IRAP II® were significantly increased compared with IRAP®. On the other hand, there was a significantly increased level of TNF-α in IRAP® compared with IRAP II® but no significant difference in IL-1β levels. There was no significant difference in production of IGF-1 and TGF-β between the two products, but both were significantly increased over serum alone. On the basis of the extrapolation of doses used in this study, the recommendation for IRAP following arthroscopic surgery is 6 mL in knees, fetlocks, distal interphalangeal joints, and tendon sheaths 10 to 12 mL in femoropatellar or femorotibial joints. Treatment in the latter joints would therefore require two preparations (two preparations of IRAP® or IRAP II®) to provide three intraarticular injections at this dose rate.

Platelet-Rich Plasma

Platelet-rich plasma (PRP) has been advocated as a way to introduce increased concentrations of growth factors and other bioactive molecules to injured tissues in an attempt to optimize the local environment. There are various definitions of PRP, but the consensus now is simply that the product should have an increase in platelet content over the level in blood. The initial enthusiasm for PRP was based on growth factors within the α-granules, including TGF-β, PDGF, IGF-1 and IGF-2, FGF epidermal growth factor, and FEGF, as well as interthelial growth factor. A number of other bioactive factors are contained in the dense granules of platelets (Foster et al, 2009), and there is an emerging paradigm that more than just platelets are playing a role in PRP (Boswell et al, 2012).

The use of PRP to treat joint disease is currently increasing in the horse. Good clinical results have been reported with OA in humans (Kon et al, 2011), and recent in vitro work showed beneficial effects on cartilage metabolism (Kisiday et al, 2012). More recently, a comparison between HA and PRP intraarticularly in the treatment of knee OA showed that local injection of a low platelet count PRP product called ACP® (Arthrex) had a significant effect shortly after the final infiltration. There was also a sustained effect up to 24 weeks (WOMAC score 65.1 and 36.5 in the HA and ACP groups, respectively, $P <$ 0.001) where the clinical outcomes were better compared with the results with HA (Cerza et al, 2012). Also in the HA group the worst results were obtained for grade III gonarthrosis, whereas the clinical results obtained in the ACP group did not show any statistically significant difference in terms of the grade of gonarthrosis. The mean WOMAC scores for grade III gonarthrosis were 74.85 in the HA group and 41.20 in the ACP group ($P < 0.001$).

Recent work has suggested that although a higher number of platelets are seen in some PRP products, this also brings with it higher white cell count levels and higher catabolic cytokine levels (Sundman et al, 2011). In another study looking at the anabolic and catabolic activities of cartilage and meniscal explants in vitro and the effect of a single-spin PRP (Arthrex ACP® system) compared with a double-spin product (Harvest Technologies Smart Prep II), $ADAMTS-4$ (aggrecanase-1) gene expression was lowest for single-spin PRP (Kisiday et al, 2012). Aggrecanase is considered a major factor in articular cartilage degeneration. Also, radiolabel incorporation with 35-sulfate (an index of glycosaminoglycan synthesis) and 3H-proline incorporation (as an indication of collagen synthesis) were significantly enhanced with the single-spin system. Therefore, there is growing scientific support for the potential use of PRP (at least the ACP® product) postoperatively, but good clinical evidence in the horse is needed.

Mesenchymal Stem Cells

The use of mesenchymal stem cells (MSCs) or mesenchymal stromal cells has become popular as an adjunctive therapy in equine orthopedics. Most work has concentrated on the undifferentiated multipotent cells present in adult bone marrow stem cells (BMSCs) that have the potential to differentiate along mesenchymal lineages, including bone, cartilage, muscle, ligament, tendon, adipose, and stroma (Pittenger et al, 1999). Multiple different pathways of multipotent MSCs and the proteins involved in their transcriptional control have been described in a review of MSC therapy in equine musculoskeletal disease (Taylor et al, 2007). The clinical use of MSCs in horses, justification for their use, and issues surrounding their use have been reviewed by Frisbie and Smith (2010). Early work with labeled MSCs has shown that they have an affinity for damaged joint tissue, and more recent work in humans has confirmed their ability to localize and participate in the repair of damaged joint structures, including cruciate ligaments, menisci, and cartilage lesions (Agung et al, 2006).

Most in vivo studies done in animals other than horses have focused on meniscal repair. A particularly significant study involved intraarticular injection with beneficial effects to meniscus and secondary OA (Murphy et al, 2003). This led to the initiation of a clinical study at CSU with intraarticular BMSCs plus HA therapy in clinical cases of femorotibial joint trauma where meniscal injury (and other soft tissue injury) with secondary OA is a common problem (Ferris et al, 2013). It has been demonstrated that experimental equine meniscal lacerations can heal when treated with equine BMSCs in fibrin glue and show increased vascularization, decreased thickness in repair and increased total bonding (Ferris et al, 2012). The authors also examined the use of BMSCs in the equine osteochondral fragment model (Frisbie et al, 2009).

In a comparative study it was shown that there was significant improvement in synovial fluid PGE$_2$ levels using BMSCs with nominal improvement in symptoms and disease-modifying effects. On the other hand, there was an interesting negative response with adipose-derived stromal vascular fraction cells in that there was an increase in synovial fluid TNF-α levels and no significant change in PGE$_2$ levels. This antiinflammatory effect with BMSCs was another good example of trophic effects with MSCs, which in addition to cellular differentiation also secrete a variety of cytokines and growth factors that have both paracrine and autocrine activities (Caplan & Dennis, 2006). These secreted bioactive factors suppress the local immune response, inhibit fibrosis (scar formation) and apoptosis, enhance angiogenesis, and stimulate mitosis and differentiation of tissue-intrinsic reparative or stem cells.

The trophic effects of BMSCs have been further demonstrated by a recent study in the horse in which an intraarticular injection of 20 million BMSCs in 20 mg of HA (Hyvisc®) was compared with HA alone administered at 4 weeks in the repair of full-thickness microfractured defects on the medial femoral condyle (McIlwraith et al, 2011). There was enhancement of the firmness of the repair tissue at 6 and 12 months, as well as a significant increase in aggrecan content in the repair tissue.

Rehabilitation with Aquatic Therapy

Aquatic therapy has become increasingly popular in its use for rehabilitation of equine musculoskeletal injuries. One of the authors (C.W.M.) routinely recommends underwater treadmilling as part of the postarthroscopic rehabilitation in racehorses. The mechanisms of actions of aquatic therapy and its potential use in the clinical management of equine OA has been recently reviewed (King et al, 2013).

Recent human research has increased our understanding of neuromuscular responses to joint pain (Templeton et al, 1996). Joint mechanoreceptors are characterized as sensory receptors within periarticular tissues that respond to changes in joint position and motion and are also important in regulating neuromuscular control associated with joint stability (Hurley, 1997). Pain, inflammation, and joint effusion alter the normal sensory input from articular mechanorecpetors, which may cause motor neuron excitability and reduced muscle activation (Johansson et al, 1991). Experimentally induced knee effusion produced significant quadriceps muscle inhibition (Hopkins et al, 2001; Iles et al, 1990; Palmieri et al, 2004). Joint instability alters the distribution of weight-bearing forces across articular surfaces and induces an increase in the recruitment of adjacent muscles to help aid in joint stability (Shultz et al, 2004). The resulting functional imbalance and paired agonist-antagonist muscle groups contributed to increased joint instability and altered limb biomechanics, which led to further progression of OA and chronic maladaptive compensatory mechanisms (Wu et al, 2008). Aquatic therapy is frequently prescribed in humans for rehabilitation following orthopedic injury to both improve the overall function of the affected limb and prevent further injuries (Giaquinto et al, 2007). There is an increasing perception among veterinarians that joint injuries may recur or be exacerbated due to muscle weakness, reduced joint range of motion, and poor proprioception as exemplified by immobilization of the equine metacarpophalangeal joint. In addition to treating the primary injury with arthroscopic surgery, the entire musculoskeletal system needs to be rehabilitated to return the horse to optimal performance (King et al, 2012). Aquatic therapy such as underwater treadmill exercise and swimming (Fig. 17-1) has been reported in humans to increase cardiovascular endurance, improve muscle strength and timing, decrease limb edema, improve joint range of motion, decrease pain, and reduce mechanical stresses applied to the limb (Kamioka et al, 2010). Previous work has shown that in horses, water at

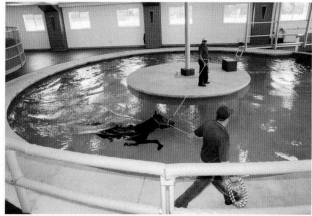

Figure 17-1 A horse undergoing swimming rehabilitation (Pegasus Training and Equine Rehabilitation Center, Seattle). *(Courtesy of Pegasus Training and Equine Rehabilitation Center, Seattle, WA, USA.)*

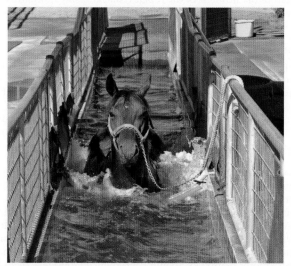

Figure 17-2 A horse undergoing underwater treadmilling rehabilitation. Note that the water is up to the point of the shoulder (Bonnie Acres Rehabilitation Center, Hemet, CA).

the level of the point of the shoulder produces a 50% to 60% reduction in body weight (Fig. 17-2) (McClintock et al, 1987). Increased buoyancy reduces the effects of weight-bearing stress placed on the joints and helps reduce pain and inflammation associated with impact loading exercises. Underwater kinematic analysis in man has also demonstrated that increased buoyancy improves joint range of motion. Recently the use of underwater treadmilling has been assessed in the equine OA model and both decrease in OA, as well as improved proprioception, was demonstrated (King, 2010 PhD Thesis) (Fig. 17-3). This was the first demonstration of benefit to posttraumatic OA, as well as proprioception reported before. Otherwise there is limited work comparing ascending loading exercise regimens with underwater treadmilling.

Clinical Use of Underwater Treadmills
Use of underwater treadmilling is increasing, and the first author has most of his racehorse patients go through underwater treadmilling postoperatively. At one rehabilitation facility that the author uses, both swimming and underwater treadmilling (Hydrohorse®) are used with swimming commencing at 14 days and going to 30 days and swimming plus Aqua Tred being commenced at 30 days and proceeding daily for 30 days.

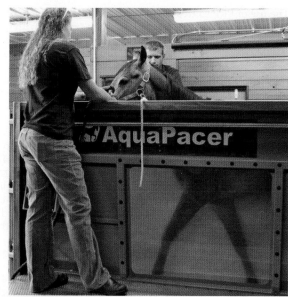

Figure 17-3 Use of portable underwater treadmill (AquaPacer®) at Orthopaedic Research Center, Colorado State University.

Swimming starts off at 2 laps and 1 or 2 laps a week are added depending on how the horse is handling the exercise. For underwater treadmilling at 30 days the protocol is 3 minutes a day and then increases to 5 minutes the second week, and 2 to 5 minutes a week are added each subsequent week up to a maximum of 20 minutes. Horses are treated with this protocol 6 days a week and just walk on the seventh day.

More commonly, underwater treadmilling is used as the sole aquatic therapy technique. Typically the first author starts horses in underwater treadmilling at 30 to 60 days, and they get a 30- to 45-day protocol. If the horse has experience with underwater treadmilling, it is started at 10 minutes daily and moved up to 20 minutes daily over a 10-day period. A horse can undergo treadmilling 7 days a week. If it is unaccustomed to the underwater treadmill, the horse is started at 5 minutes a day for 3 days followed by 8 minutes a day for 3 days and then 10 minutes a day for 3 days adding 2-minute increments up to 20 minutes.

REFERENCES

Agung M, Ochi M, Yanada S, Adachi N, Izuta Y, Yamasaki T, Toda K: Mobilization of bone marrow-derived mesenchymal stem cells into the injured tissues after intra-articular injection and their contribution to tissue regeneration, *Knee Surg Sports Traumatol Arthrosc* 14:1307–1314, 2006.

Bergin BJ, Pierce SW, Bramlage LR, Stromberg A: Oral hyaluronan gel reduces post operative tarsocrural effusion in the yearling Thoroughbred, *Equine Vet J* 38:375–378, 2006.

Boswell SG, Cole BJ, Sundman EA, Karas V, Fortier LA: Platelet-rich plasma: a milieu of bioactive factors, *Arthroscopy* 28:429–439, 2012.

Caplan AI, Dennis JE: Mesenchymal stem cells as trophic mediators, *J Cell Biochem* 98:1076–1084, 2006.

Cerza F, Carni S, Carcangiu A, Di Vavo I, Schiavilla V, Pecora A, De Biasi G, Ciuffreda M: Comparison between hyaluronic acid and platelet-rich plasma, intra-articular infiltration in the treatment of gonarthrosis, *Am J Sports Med* 40:2822–2827, 2012.

Collins LG, Tyler DE: Phenylbutazone toxicosis in the horse: a clinical study, *J Am Vet Med Assoc* 184:699–703, 1984.

Ferris DJ, Frisbie DD, Kisiday JD, McIlwraith CW: In vivo healing of meniscal lacerations using bone marrow derived mesenchymal stem cells and fibrin glue, *Stem Cell International* 2012:691605, 2012.

Ferris DJ, Frisbie DD, Kisiday JD, McIlwraith CW, Hague BA, Major MD, Schneider RK, Zubrod CJ, Kawcak CE, Goodrich LR: Clinical follow-up of thirty three horses treated for stifle injury with bone marrow derived mesenchymal stem cells intra-articularly, *Vet Surg*, 2013, In Press.

Ferris DJ, Frisbie DD, McIlwraith CW, Kawcak CE: Current joint therapy usage in equine practice a survey of veterinarians 2009, *Equine Vet J* 43:530–535, 2011.

Foland JW, McIlwraith CW, Trotter GW, Powers BE, Lamar CH: Effect of betamethasone and exercise on equine carpal joints with osteochondral fragments, *Vet Surg* 23:369–376, 1994.

Foster TE, Puskas BL, Mandelbaum BR, Gerhardt MB, Rodeo SA: Platelet-rich plasma: from basic science to clinical applications, *Am J Sports Med* 37:2259–2272, 2009.

Frisbie DD, Kawcak CE, Baxter GM, Trotter GW, Powers BE, Lassen ED, McIlwraith CW: Effects of 6alpha-methylprednisolone acetate on an equine osteochondral fragment exercise model, *Am J Vet Res* 59:1619–1628, 1998.

Frisbie DD, Kawcak CE, McIlwraith CW, Werpy NM: Evaluation of polysulfated glycosaminoglycan or sodium hyaluronan administered intra-articularly for treatment of horses with experimentally induced osteoarthritis, *Am J Vet Res* 70:203–209, 2009.

Frisbie DD, Kawcak CE, McIlwraith CW: Evaluation of the effect of extracorporeal shockwave treatment on experimentally induced osteoarthritis in middle carpal joints of horses, *Am J Vet Res* 70:449–454, 2009.

Frisbie DD, Kawcak CE, Trotter GW, Power BE, Walton RM, McIlwraith CW: Effects of triamcinolone acetonide on an *in vivo* equine osteochondral fragment exercise model, *Equine Vet J* 29:349–359, 1997.

Frisbie DD, Kawcak CE, Werpy NM, Park RD, McIlwraith CW: Clinical, biochemical and histologic effects of intra-articular administration of autologous conditioned serum in horses with experimentally induced osteoarthritis, *Am J Vet Res* 68:290–296, 2007.

Frisbie DD, McIlwraith CW, Kawcak CE, Werpy NM, Pearce GL: Evaluation of topically administered diclofenac liposomal cream for treatment of horses with experimentally induced osteoarthritis, *Am J Vet Res* 70:210–215, 2009.

Frisbie DD, Smith RKW: Clinical update on the use of mesenchymal stem cells in equine orthopaedics, *Equine Vet J* 42:86–89, 2010.

Giaquinto S, Ciotola E, Margutti F, Valentini F: Gait during hydrokinesitherapy following total hip arthroplasty, *Disabil Rehabil* 29:743–749, 2007.

Higgins AJ, Lees P: Phenylbutazone inhibition of prostaglandin E2 production in equine acute inflammatory exudate, *Vet Rec* 113:622–623, 1983.

Hopkins J, Ingersoll C, Drause B, Edwards J, Cordova M: Effect of knee joint effusion on quadriceps and soleus motoneuron pool excitability, *Med Sports Sci Sports Exerc* 33:123–126, 2001.

Hraha TH, Doremus KM, McIlwraith CW, Frisbie DD: Autologous conditioned serum: The comparative cytokine profiles of two commercial methods (IRAP and IRAP II) using equine blood, *Equine Vet J* 43:516–521, 2011.

Hurley MV: The effects of joint damage on muscle function, proprioception and rehabilitation, *Man Ther* 2:11–17, 1997.

Iles J, Stokes M, Young A: Reflex actions of knee joint afferents during contraction of the human quadriceps, *Clin Physiol* 10:489–500, 1990.

Johansson H, Sjolander P, Sojka P: A sensory role for the cruciate ligaments, *Clin Orthop* 268:161–178, 1991.

Kamioka H, Tsutanji K, Okuizumi H, Mutoh Y, Ohta M, Handa S, Okada S: Effectiveness of aquatic exercise and balneotherapy: a summary of systematic reviews based on randomized controlled trials of water immersion therapies, *J Epidemiol* 20:2–12, 2010.

Kawcak CE, Frisbie DD, Trotter GW, et al.: The effects of intravenous administration of sodium hyaluronate on carpal joints in exercising horses after arthroscopic surgery and osteochondral fragmentation, *Am J Vet Res* 58:1132–1140, 1997.

King MR, Haussler KK, Kawcak CE, McIlwraith CW, Reiser RF: Mechanisms of aquatic therapy and its potential use in managing equine osteoarthritis, *Equine Vet Edu 2012* 25(4):204–209, 2013.

Kisiday JD, McIlwraith CW, Rodkey WR, Frisbie DD, Steadman JR: Effects of platelet-rich plasma composition on anabolic and catabolic activities in equine cartilage and meniscal explants, *Cartilage* 2012, doi:10.1177/1947603511433181.

Kon E, Mandelbaum B, Buda R, Filardo G, Delcogliano M, Timoncini A, Fornasari PM, Giannini S, Marcacci M: Platlet-rich plasma intra-articular injection versus hyaluronic acid viscosupplementation as treatments for cartilage pathology: from early degeneration to osteoarthritis, *Arthroscopy* 27:1490–1501, 2011.

Lees P, Higgins AJ, Mawhinney IC, Reid DS: Absorption of phenylbutazone from a paste formulation administered orally to the horse, *Res Vet Sci* 41:200–206, 1986.

McClintock SA, Hutchins DR, Brownlow MA: Determination of weight reduction in horses in flotation tanks, *Equine Vet J* 19:70–71, 1987.

McIlwraith CW, Frisbie DD, Kawcak CE: Evaluation of intramuscularly administered sodium pentosan polysulfate for treatment of experimentally induced osteoarthritis in horses, *Am J Vet Res* 73:628–633, 2012.

McIlwraith CW, Frisbie DD, Rodkey WG, Kisiday JD, Werpy NM, Kawcak CE, Steadman JR: Evaluation of intra-articular mesenchymal stem cells to augment healing of microfractured chondral defects, *Arthroscopy* 27:1552–1561, 2011.

Murphy JM, Fink DJ, Hunziker EB, Barry FP: Stem cell therapy in a caprine model of osteoarthritis, *Arthritis Rheum* 48:3464–3474, 2003.

Owens JG, Kamerling SG, Stanton SR, Keowen ML, Prescott-Mathews JS: Effects of pretreatment with ketoprofen and phenylbutazone on experimentally induced synovitis in horses, *Am J Vet Res* 57:866–874, 1996.

Palmieri R, Tom J, Edwards J, Weltman A, Saliba E, Mistry D, Ingersoll C: Arthrogenic muscle response induced by an experimental knee joint effusion is mediated by pre- and post-synaptic spinal mechanism, *J Electromyogr Kinesiol* 14:631–640, 2004.

Pittenger MF, Mackay AM, Beck SC, Jaiswal RK, Douglas R, Mosca JD, Moorman MA, Simonetti DW, Craig S, Marshak DR: Multilineage potential of adult human mesenchymal stem cells, *Science* 284:143–147, 1999.

Shultz SJ, Carcia CR, Perrin DH: Knee joint laxity affects muscle activation patterns in the healthy knee, *J Electromyogr Kinesiol* 14:475–483, 2004.

Sundman EA, Cole BJ, Fortier LA: Growth factor and catabolic cytokine concentrations are influenced by the cellular composition of platelet-rich plasma, *Am J Sports Med* 39:2135–2140, 2011.

Taylor SE, Smith RKW, Clegg PD: Mesenchymal stem cell therapy in equine musculoskeletal disease: scientific fact or clinical fiction? *Equine Vet J* 39:172–180, 2007.

Templeton MS, Booth DL, O'Kelly WD: Effects of aquatic therapy on joint flexibility and functional ability in subjects with rheumatic disease, *J Orthop Sports Phys Ther* 23:376–381, 1996.

Wu S-H, Chu N-K, Liu Y-C, Chen C-K, Tang SFT, Cheng C-K: Relationship between the EMG ratio of muscle activation and bony structure in osteoarthritis knee patients with and without patellar malalignment, *J Rehabil Med* 40:381–386, 2008.

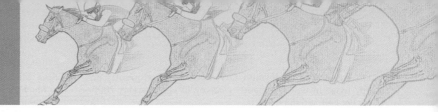

INDEX

Page numbers followed by *b*, *t*, and *f* indicate boxes, tables, and figures, respectively.